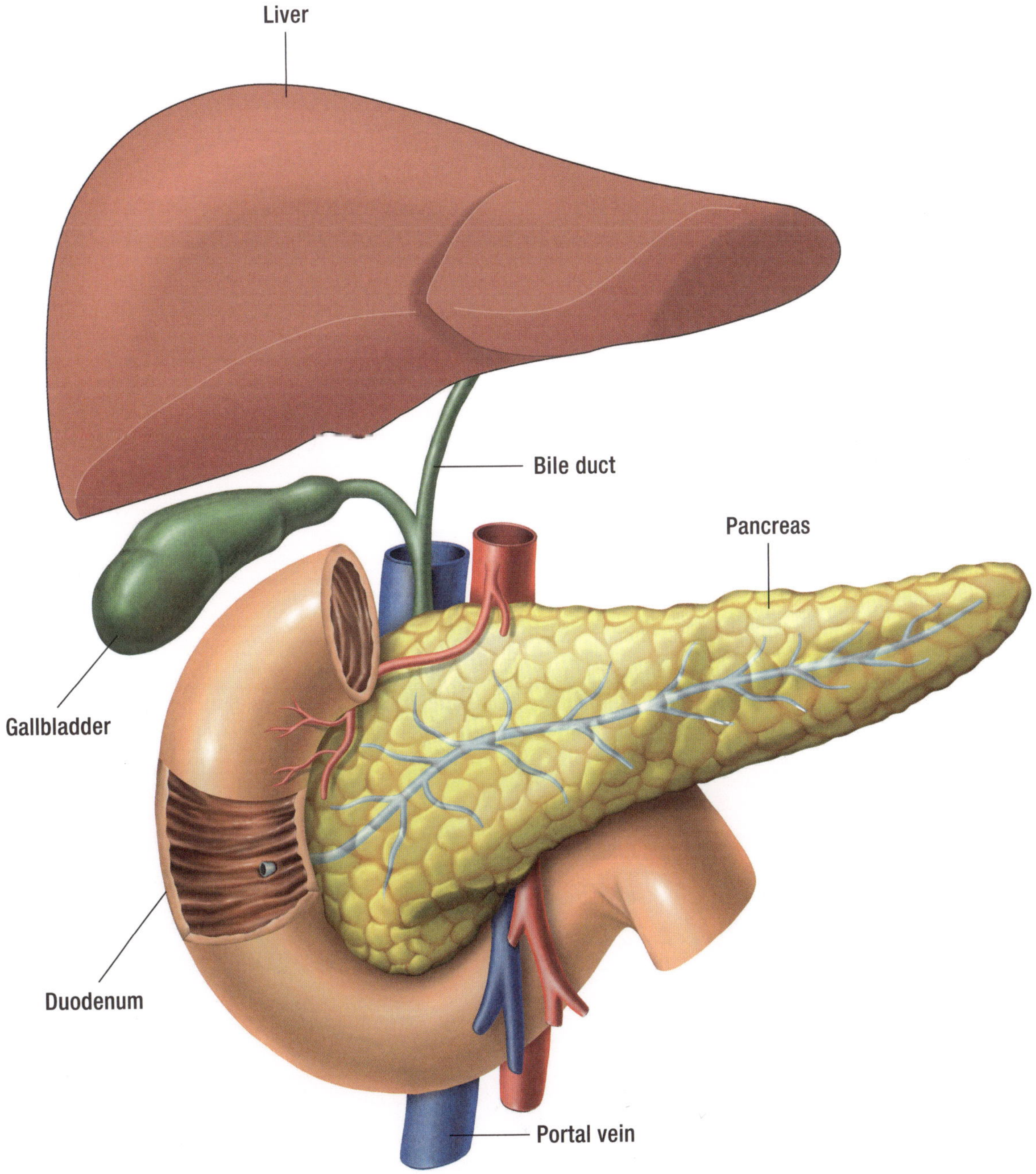
Liver
Bile duct
Pancreas
Gallbladder
Duodenum
Portal vein

VETERINARY INTERNAL MEDICINE

EDITORS-IN-CHIEF
EDWARD FELDMAN
FEDERICO FRACASSI

CANINE HEPATOBILIARY AND EXOCRINE PANCREATIC DISEASES

EDITOR
Penny Watson

edra
PUBLISHING

VETERINARY INTERNAL MEDICINE SERIES - Edward Feldman, Federico Fracassi. Editors-in-chief.
Penny Watson – Canine Hepatobiliary and Exocrine Pancreatic Diseases

ISBN: 978-1-957260-74-7
eISBN: 978-1-957260-79-2

Book Publishing Manager: Costanza Smeraldi

Paper, printing and Binding Manager: Paolo Ficicchia

Cover: Laura Barzacca

Layout: T&T studio s.a.s, Milano

Copyediting: Mercedes González Fernández de Castro – Science & Health Publications

edra
PUBLISHING

Edra Publishing US LLC
3309 Northlake Boulevard
Suite 203, Palm Beach Gardens
FL, 33403
EIN: 844113980
info@edrapublishing.com
www.edrapublishing.com

Printed in Italy by "Erregiemme printing" S.r.l., May 2024

Series editors

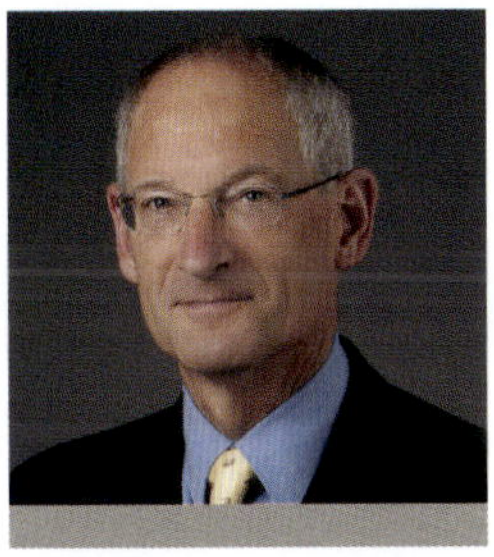

Edward C. Feldman
DVM, ACVIM Diplomate (SAIM), Emeritus Professor of Small Animal Internal Medicine,
University of California, Davis, USA

Dr. Feldman earned his DVM from the University of California in 1973. He joined the Davis faculty in 1979 after an internship at the Animal Medical Center in New York City, a Residency with Dr. Stephen Ettinger in the world's first referral only private veterinary practice in Berkeley California, a year in general practice and another on faculty at the University of Saskatchewan, in Canada. He has authored more than 160 peer-reviewed scientific publications, 110 scientific abstracts, and 75 book chapters.

Dr. Feldman has coedited the last six editions of The Textbook of Veterinary Internal Medicine with Dr. Stephen Ettinger and the last two also with Dr. Etienne Côté. He coauthored the four editions of Canine and Feline Endocrinology with Dr. Richard Nelson and the 4th edition also with Drs. Claudia Reusch, Catharine Scott-Moncrieff, and Ellen Behrend. He coedited Feline Endocrinology with Dr. Fracassi and Dr. Peterson.

Dr. Feldman has lectured in more than 45 of the 50 United States and 43 countries.

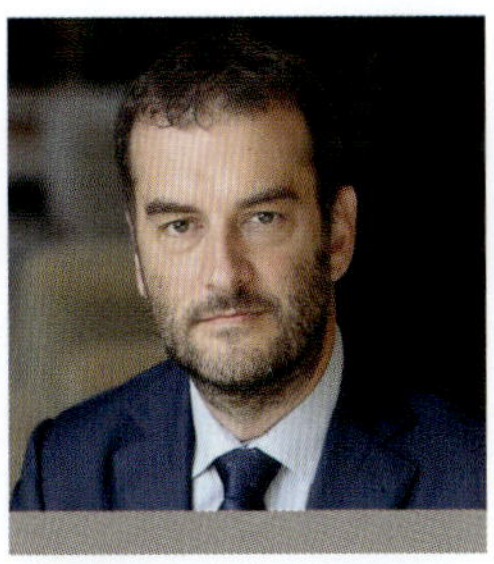

Federico Fracassi
DVM, ECVIM Diplomate (SAIM)
Professor of Small Animal Internal Medicine
University of Bologna, Italy

Dr. Fracassi graduated in Veterinary Medicine (DVM) at the University of Bologna, Italy. In 2005 he defended his PhD thesis and then completed a Residency in Internal Medicine at the University of Zurich, Switzerland, with Prof Claudia Reusch.

He is now an Associate Professor of Veterinary Internal Medicine at the University of Bologna.

He has been president of the European Society of Veterinary Endocrinology, and he is director of the international Master "Canine and Feline Endocrinology".

He has authored more than 100 peer-reviewed scientific publications and 10 book chapters. He is the editor of Veterinaria and associate editor of the Journal of Small Animal Practice. He coedited Feline Endocrinology with Dr. Feldman and Dr. Peterson. He has edited the book "Diagnostic and therapeutic algorithms in internal medicine for dogs and cats".

Dr. Fracassi has lectured in 22 countries.

Book editor

Penny Watson

MA, VetMD, CertVR, DSAM, ECVIM, FRCVS

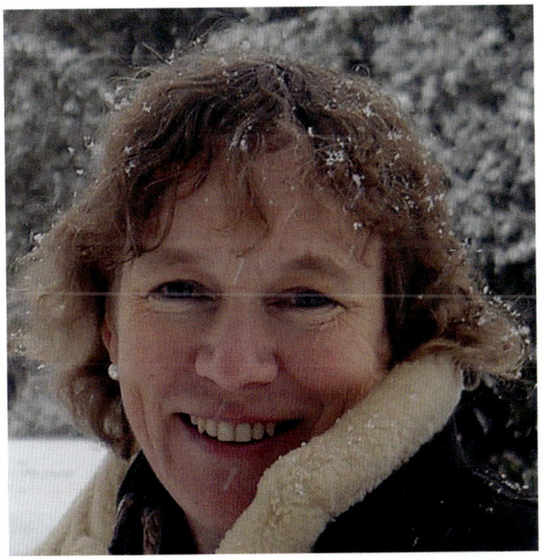

After graduating from Cambridge in 1989, Dr. Penny Watson spent 4 years in farm, equine and small animal practice before returning to Cambridge to undertake a small animal medicine residency. She spent 29 years at the Queen's Veterinary School Hospital, becoming an RCVS and ECVIM Diplomate and recognized specialist in small animal medicine. She became a Fellow of the RCVS in 2016. She recently retired from clinical practice but continues with research and lecturing. Penny is ECVIM Past President and a former chair of the ECVIM Internal Medicine Diploma examination committee and former Honorary Secretary of BSAVA. Penny's research focuses on liver and pancreas disease in dogs and cats, particularly chronic disease and fibrosis and she has published widely in these areas. Recent research has focused on copper storage disease in a variety of breeds and feline chronic cholangitis. She was a member of the group which produced the ACVIM Consensus Statement on Canine Chronic hepatitis. This group is now working to increase awareness of copper storage disease in dogs and to improve regulation of the amount of copper in dog foods.

Contributors

Frederik Allan, BVMedSci (Hons), BVM BVS (Hons), MRCVS
Department of Clinical Science and Services
Royal Veterinary College
University of London – Hertfordshire, UK

Daniel Batchelor, BVSc, PhD, DSAM, DECVIM-CA (Internal Medicine), SFHEA, MRCVS
Institute of Veterinary and Ecological Sciences
University of Liverpool – Neston, UK

Asaf Berkowitz, DVM, DACVP
Department of Clinical Sciences and Pathobiology
School of Veterinary Medicine
University of Pennsylvania – Philadelphia, PA, USA

Karyn Bischoff, DVM, DABVT
College of Veterinary Medicine
Cornell University – Ithaca, NY, USA

Abby Caine, MA, VetMB, CertVDI, DECVDI, FRCVS
Dick White Referrals
Cambridgeshire, UK

Giulia Cattaneo, MA VetMB MRCVS,
Senior Clinical Training, Scholar in Small Animal, Internal Medicine, (ECVIM-CA Resident)
The Queen's Veterinary School Hospital
Department of Veterinary Medicine
University of Cambridge – Cambridge, UK

Daniel L. Chan, DVM, DACVECC, DECVECC, DACVIM (Nutrition), FHEA, MRCVS
Department for Clinical Science and Services
Royal Veterinary College
University of London – Hertfordshire, UK

Harry Cridge, MVB, MS, PGCert Vet Ed, DACVIM (SAIM), DECVIM-CA (Internal Medicine), FHEA, MRCVS
Department of Small Animal Clinical Sciences
College of Veterinary Medicine
Michigan State University – East Lansing, MI, USA

Jane Dobson, MA BVetMed, DVetMed, DECVIM-CA (IntMed, Oncol, RadOnc), FRCVS
The Queen's Veterinary School Hospital
Department of Veterinary Medicine
University of Cambridge – Cambridge, UK

Floris Dröes, DVM (Hon), MRCVS, PGCert VMS
School of Veterinary Medicine & Biomedical Sciences
Texas A&M University – College Station, TX, USA

Antonio Giuliano, VM, MS, PgCert(CT), GpCert(SAM), DECVIM-CA (Oncology), DACVIM (Oncology), MRCVS
CityU Department of Veterinary Clinical Sciences (VCS)
Sham Shui Po, Kowloon, Hong Kong

Adam G. Gow, BVM&S, PhD, DSAM, DECVIM-CA (Internal Medicine), FHEA, FRCVS
Zoetis UK
Leatherhead, UK

Cassia Hare, MA, VetMB, AFHEA, DACVP (Clin Path), DECVCP, MRCVS
The Queen's Veterinary School Hospital
Department of Veterinary Medicine
University of Cambridge – Cambridge, UK

Ben Harris, MA, VetMB, CertSAM, FLS, DECVIM-CA (Internal Medicine), MRCVS
Wear Referrals
County Durham, UK

Andre Kortum, BVSc, MANZCVS(SAM), SFHEA, DECVIM-CA (Internal Medicine), MRCVS
The Queen's Veterinary School Hospital
Department of Veterinary Medicine
University of Cambridge – Cambridge, UK

Sharon Kuzi, DVM, DECVIM-CA (Internal Medicine)
Hebrew University Veterinary Teaching Hospital
Koret School of Veterinary Medicine
Hebrew University of Jerusalem – Rehovot, Israel

Rommaneeya Leela-arporn, DVM, PhD
Department of Clinical Sciences
College of Veterinary Medicine and Biomedical Sciences
Colorado State University – Fort Collins, CO, USA

Becca Leung, BVSc, PhD, DACVIM (Nutrition)
Veterinary Nutrition Group
Sydney, Australia

Francesco Lotti, DVM, MSc, DECVIM-CA (Internal Medicine)
Clinica Veterinaria Valdinievole
Monsummano Terme (PT), Italy

Angela Marolf, DVM, DACVR
Department of Clinical Sciences,
College of Veterinary Medicine
The Ohio State University-Columbus, OH, USA

Marina Martín-Ambrosio Francés, DVM, DECVIM-CA (Internal Medicine), MRCVS
Veterinary Hospital
CEU Cardenal Herrera University, Valencia, Spain

Carlo Masserdotti, DVM, DECVCP
IDEXX Laboratories

Katie McCallum, BVM&S, PGCertSAM, FHEA, DECVIM-CA (Internal Medicine), MRCVS
The Queen's Veterinary School Hospital
Department of Veterinary Medicine
University of Cambridge – Cambridge, UK

Sean McDonough, DVM, PhD, DACVP
Department of Population Medicine and Diagnostic Sciences
College of Veterinary Medicine
Cornell University – Ithaca, NY, USA

Yvonne McGrotty, BVMS, CertSAM, DECVIM-CA (Internal Medicine), MRCVS
Clinique VetRef AniCura
Beaucouzé, France

Susana Monforte Monteiro, DVM, MSc, CertAVP PGCertVPS AFHEA, DECVN, PhD candidate University of Cambridge
The Queen's Veterinary School Hospital
Department of Veterinary Medicine
University of Cambridge – Cambridge, UK

Ran Nivy, DVM, DECVIM-CA (Internal Medicine)
Koret School of Veterinary Medicine
Hebrew University of Jerusalem – Rehovot, Israel

Laura J. Owen, BVSc, AFHEA, DECVS, MRCVS
The Queen's Veterinary School Hospital
Department of Veterinary Medicine
University of Cambridge – Cambridge, UK

Fabio Procoli, DMV, MVetMed, DACVIM, DECVIM-CA (Internal Medicine), MRCVS
Veterinary Hospital AniCura I Portoni Rossi
Bologna, Italy

Sofia Rapastella, DVM, MRCVS, DECVIM-CA (Internal Medicine)
Davies Veterinary Specialist
Hertfordshire, UK

Beatrice Ruggerone, DVM, PhD, DECVIM-CA (Internal Medicine)
Veterinary Hospital AniCura I Portoni Rossi
Bologna, Italy

Luca Schiavo, DVM, MRCVS, DECVIM-CA (Oncology)
Davies Veterinary Specialist
Hertfordshire, UK

Ian Self, BSc. BVSc, CertVA, DECVAA, PGCertVetEd, PGCert, MAPP, MAcadMedEd FHEA, FRCVS
Harper & Keele Veterinary School
Keele University, Keele, UK

Mellora Sharman, BVSc, MVM, PGradCert, PhD, FANZCVSt, DECVIM-CA (Internal Medicine), FHEA, MRCVS RCVS
VetCT Teleconsulting Hospital

Jörg M. Steiner, MedVet, DrMedVet, PhD, DACVIM, DECVIM-CA (Internal Medicine), AGAF
School of Veterinary Medicine & Biomedical Sciences
Texas A&M University, College Station, TX, USA

Alice Tamborini, DVM, MRCVS, DECVIM-CA (Internal Medicine),
IDEXX Laboratories Italia
Milano, Italy

Mickey S. Tivers, BVSc, PhD, CertSAS, DECVS, MRCVS
Paragon Veterinary Referrals
Wakefield, UK

Cynthia RL Webster, DVM, DACVIM (SAIM)
Department of Clinical Sciences
Cummings School of Veterinary Medicine
Tufts University – North Grafton, MA, USA

Melanie Werner, DVM, DECVIM-CA (Internal Medicine)
Marigin Clinic for Small Animals
Feusisberg, Switzerland

Panagiotis G. Xenoulis, DVM, DrMedVet, PhD
Faculty of Veterinary Science
University of Thessaly, Karditsa, Greece
School of Veterinary Medicine & Biomedical Sciences
Texas A&M University, College Station, TX, USA

Sue Yee Lim, DVM, PhD
School of Veterinary Medicine & Biomedical Sciences
Texas A&M University, College Station, TX, USA

Series preface

"Oh! You are a veterinarian? I (or my brother, my sister, my son, my daughter...) always wanted to be a veterinarian." All of us, as veterinary students and later as veterinarians, have often heard comments like this. Becoming a veterinarian seems to be such a wonderful career to nonveterinarians: helping helpless dogs and cats. Veterinarians should be happy and satisfied in their *chosen* profession because they are able to earn a living by caring for loved pets. The journey to satisfaction and happiness for veterinarians, however, never seems to follow an obvious, straight, or level path.

The 1950s witnessed a dramatic growth in the popularity of pet dogs and in the number of veterinarians who cared exclusively for pets. The popularity of cats soon followed. Today, more dogs and cats are considered "members of the family" than ever before in human history, and their owners want to protect their family members from illness or to resolve any illness. There are more veterinarians who care for dogs and cats currently than ever before in human history. Veterinary medicine has evolved remarkably to meet the ever-growing medical care expectations and demands of dog and cat owners.

When learning of a diagnosis, prognosis, treatment, and/or the cost of care for their ill pet, some owners become distressed. These emotions are often directed at the "messenger" of the bad news: the veterinarian. The veterinarian, in turn, may not respect their own knowledge and feel inadequate. One reason that a veterinarian may feel inadequate is the realization that it is impossible for anyone in general practice to be expert and current on all the canine and feline conditions encountered in a day, week, or month: everything from orthopedics to oncology, from vaccinology to dermatology, from ophthalmology to cardiology. Nor is it possible for an internal medicine specialist to be expert and current in each condition they encounter, from endocrinology to gastroenterology or from respiratory conditions to chronic kidney disease. Further, it is clear that cats are not small dogs. Perceived "knowledge deficiencies" can cause veterinarians to feel they are failing to meet their clients' expectations.

The internal medicine textbooks in this new series offer one approach for enjoying veterinary practice. We encourage colleagues to embrace developing expertise in one area. By focusing on and studying one organ system in either the dog or cat, one can achieve greater knowledge and skills and, in turn, greater confidence. Each book in this series offers a clear path to learning current opinions on pathophysiology, diagnosis, treatment, prognosis, and costs associated with illnesses involving one system in one species. Confidence gained in a focused area can be sensed by devoted owners. Further, confidence in one area of internal medicine also creates confidence in sharing limitations: "I am extremely confident in diagnosing and managing some conditions but I lack that level of expertise in all other conditions".

The books in this series have been constructed to help build expertise in one organ system in either the dog or the cat. Each book is edited by one or two specialists with outstanding international credentials. Each editor was tasked with building a text that contains all the information found in general internal medicine textbooks, but with much more in-depth discussions on each condition. Each book has early chapters focusing on differential diagnoses of owner concerns, physical examination findings, and laboratory and/or imaging results. These are excellent for students as they begin to apply their basic knowledge to clinical cases. These chapters also provide a quick review for experienced general practitioners and specialists. Each chapter provides at least one algorithm designed to take the reader from a vague owner concern, physical examination finding, or laboratory abnormality to a specific diagnosis with step-by-step instructions. The "techniques section" in each text teaches currently employed procedures, most with videos. In-depth chapters on known illnesses comprise 70 to 80% of each book's content. The editors have provided a larger number of chapters, a larger number of expert contributors, and greater depth on each organ system than any general textbook can supply. The material has a level of credibility that no internet site can claim. Each book can guide the reader through a more complete journey of understanding than is available in any other veterinary resource.

Edward Feldman
Federico Fracassi

Preface

Once in a while, if you are lucky, you are asked to contribute to a really worthwhile project. This textbook on canine hepatobiliary and pancreatic diseases has been such a project. There has long been a need for a book dedicated solely to these diseases and aimed at the interested small animal veterinarian in both first and second opinion practice. I am honored to have been asked to edit a textbook addressing diseases in these two organs, which have dominated my clinical and research work for nearly three decades.

The layout of this book is, I believe, unique –inspired by the series editors Edward Feldman and Frederico Fracassi, whose vision was integral to the book's design. I thank them most sincerely for their patience and wise help during the planning of this book.

There are very few, if any, clinical signs that are pathognomonic for liver or pancreas disease, and the clinician must consider differential diagnoses for presenting signs. The first section allows this with problem-orientated algorithms addressing the owner's presenting concerns and physical examination findings, guiding the clinician into the appropriate workup, and ensuring that other potential causes of these signs are not forgotten. The book is then divided into a section on pancreatic diseases and a section on liver diseases. The organ sections start with a detailed consideration of clinical pathology, imaging, and biopsy acquisition, with additional chapters on the interpretation of cytology and histology in the liver section, all written by experts in their fields. This is followed by chapters on specific diseases of the pancreas and liver. There are many helpful algorithms, tables, figures, and videos, both in the printed book and ebook, aimed to make this a practical resource for the busy veterinary practitioner.

Not only internal medicine specialists and residents but also specialist soft tissue surgeons, nutritionists, clinical pathologists, veterinary pathologists, oncologists, diagnostic imagers, an anesthetist, a toxicologist, and a neurologist have contributed to this work –so there is a sense that having this book on your bookshelf is like having all these specialists in your clinic to consult on those difficult cases.

The result is an up-to-date, and we hope complete, resource of pancreatic and liver diseases in dogs. Diseases of the liver and pancreas can cause a degree of despair in veterinary practitioners –so much about the causes and treatments of these diseases is poorly understood, and too many cases remain idiopathic. Nonetheless, over recent years, clinical research has started to improve our understanding, as detailed in this book, and it is clear that logical workup and treatment of our cases really can make a difference to both the quality and quantity of life. If this book results in increased enthusiasm amongst veterinarians in both first opinion and specialist practice to learn more about liver and pancreas disease in dogs, to treat their cases more carefully and positively, and to undertake more vital clinical research in this area, it will have achieved its goals.

Enormous thanks are due to the really talented group of authors who have been kind enough to contribute to this book. You have all been wonderful to work with. I hope you have enjoyed our interactions as much as I have. You have given this book so much time and effort, and I have learned a lot from reading your work. I thank you all most sincerely. In addition, this would not have been possible if it were not for the extraordinary work and passion of the team from Edra and, in particular, Costanza Smeraldi, whose enthusiasm, wise and patient guidance, and hard work have made this the smoothest, most efficient, and high-quality process imaginable. Thank you all!

Penny Watson

Abbreviations

AAA aromatic amino acids
AAFCO Association of American Feed Control Officials
ACHES aminoaciduric canine hypoaminoacidemic hepatopathy syndrome
ACT activated clotting time
ACTH adrenocorticotropic hormone
ADH antidiuretic hormone
ADPKD autosomal dominant polycystic kidney disease
AKI acute kidney injury
ALD acute liver disease
ALF acute liver failure
ALI acute liver injury
ALP alkaline phosphatase
ALT alanine aminotransferase
AP acute pancreatitis
APSS acquired portosystemic shunting
aPTT activated partial thromboplastin time
ARDS acute respiratory distress syndrome
ARPKD autosomal recessive polycystic kidney disease
AST aspartate aminotransferase
BAs bile acids
BAST bile acid stimulation test
BCAA branched-chain amino acids
BCS body condition score
BMBT buccal mucosal bleeding time
CA cholic acid
CAV canine adenovirus
CBC complete blood count
CBPI Canine Brief Pain Inventory
CC choledochal cysts
CCK cholecystokinin
CDCA chenodeoxycholic acid
CDI central diabetes insipidus
CE chronic enteropathy
CEUS contrast-enhanced ultrasound
CDV canine distemper virus
CH chronic hepatitis
CHF congenital hepatic fibrosis
CK creatine kinase
CKCS Cavalier King Charles Spaniel
CNS central nervous system
CP chronic pancreatitis
CPDA citrate phosphate dextrose adenine
cPL canine pancreas-specific lipase
cPLI canine pancreatic lipase immunoreactivity
CPSS congenital portosystemic shunts
CPV canine parvovirus
CRI constant rate infusion
CRP C-reactive protein
CRTZ chemoreceptor trigger zone
CSOM Client-Specific Outcome Measures
CT computerized tomography
CTA computed tomography angiography
CuCH copper-associated chronic hepatitis
DAMS dyserythropoietic anemia and myopathy syndrome
DCA deoxycholic acid
DDAVP water deprivation test and desmopressin
DDx differential diagnoses
DGGR lipase 1,2-o-dilauryl-rac-glycero glutaric acid-(6'-methylresorufin) ester lipase
DHA docosahexaenoic acid
DIC disseminated intravascular coagulation
DM diabetes mellitus
DM dry matter
DPM ductal plate malformations
DW dry weight
EHCPSS extrahepatic congenital portosystemic shunt
EHBDO extrahepatic biliary duct obstruction
ELISA enzyme-linked immunosorbent assay
EMG electromyography
EMH extramedullary hematopoiesis
EPA eicosapentaenoic acid
EPI exocrine pancreatic insufficiency
ERCP endoscopic retrograde cholangiopancreatography
FDPs fibrin degradation products
FEDIAF European Pet Food Industry Federation
FeLV feline leukemia virus
FFP fresh frozen plasma
FHTG familial hypertriglyceridemia
FIP feline infectious peritonitis
FISH fluorescence *in situ* hybridization
FIV feline immunodeficiency virus
FMF familial Mediterranean fever
FNA fine-needle aspiration
FNCS fine-needle capillary sampling
FRE food-responsive enteropathy
fT_4 free thyroxine
GABA γ-aminobutyric acid
GBM gallbladder mucocele
GBS gallbladder sludge
GFR glomerular filtration rate
GGT gamma-glutamyl transferase
GI gastrointestinal
GLDH glutamate dehydrogenase
GSD German Shepherd dog
GUE gastrointestinal ulceration/erosion
HA hyaluronic acid
HAC hyperadrenocorticism
HAVM hepatic arteriovenous malformation

HCC hepatocellular carcinoma
HCPI Helsinki Chronic Pain Index
HCT hematocrit
HE hepatic encephalopathy
HGE hemorrhagic gastroenteritis
HPC hepatic progenitor cell
HS harmonic scalpel
IASP International Association of Pain
IBD inflammatory bowel disease
IGF-2 insulin-like growth factor 2
ICH infectious canine hepatitis
ICH intracranial hypertension
IHCPSS intrahepatic congenital portosystemic shunt
ICP intracranial pressure
IHC immunohistochemistry
IMHA immune-mediated hemolytic anemia
IMTP immune-mediated thrombocytopenia
IOMP intraoperative mesenteric portovenogram
IRIS International Renal Interest Society
IVFT intravenous fluid therapy
LBM lean body mass
LCA lithocholic acid
LDH lactate dehydrogenase
LDH lobular dissecting hepatitis
LDDST low-dose dexamethasone suppression test
LL lower limit
LPL lipoprotein lipase
MAS multiple acquired shunts
MAT microscopic agglutination testing
MCHC mean cell hemoglobin concentration
MCS muscle condition score
MCV mean corpuscular volume
MDA maternally-derived antibody
ME metabolizable energy
MER maintenance energy requirements
MGG May-Grünwald Giemsa
MMM masticatory muscle myositis
MODS multiorgan dysfunction
MRCP magnetic resonance cholangiopancreatography
MRI magnetic resonance imaging
MVD microvascular dysplasia
N/A not applicable
NAPQI N-acetyl-p-benzoquinone imine
NCC nucleated cell count
NDI nephrogenic diabetes insipidus
NEFA nonesterified fatty acids
NDI nephrogenic diabetes insipidus
NMDA N-methyl-D-aspartate
NPY neuropeptide Y
NRC National Research Council
NSAID nonsteroidal anti-inflammatory drugs
OSPT one-stage prothrombin time
PAA pancreatic acinar atrophy
PAMP pathogen-associated molecular pattern
PANS postattenuation neurological signs
PARR PCR for antigen receptor rearrangements
PCR polymerase chain reaction
PCV packed cell volume
PD polydipsia
PDV patent ductus venosus
PERT pancreatic enzyme replacement therapy
PH portal hypertension
PKHD1 polycystic kidney and hepatic disease 1
PLD polycystic liver disease
PLE protein-losing enteropathy
PLI pancreatic lipase immunoreactivity
PLL pretied ligature loop
PLN protein-losing nephropathy
ppm parts per million
PPVH primary portal vein hypoplasia
PSS portosystemic shunt
PSTI pancreatic secretory trypsin inhibitor
PT prothrombin time
PTE pulmonary thromboembolism
PU polyuria
PU/PD polydipsia/polyuria
PVH portal vein hypoperfusion
RAAS renin-angiotensin-aldosterone system
RBC red blood cell
RDW red blood cell distribution width
RER resting energy requirements
RI reference interval
RIA radioimmunoassay
ROM range of motion
SAA serum amyloid A
SAMe S-adenosyl methionine
SDMA symmetric dimethyl arginine
SH steroid hepatopathy
SIRS systemic inflammatory response syndrome
SLE systemic lupus erythematosus
SPAID Shar Pei autoinflammatory disease
SPINK1 serine peptidase inhibitor Kazal type 1
TAP trypsin activation peptide
TBCT total body computed tomography
TEG thromboelastography
TENS toxic epidermal necrolysis
TFB thin film band
TGFβ transforming growth factor-beta
TIBC total iron binding capacity
TLI trypsin-like immunoreactivity
TMJ temporomandibular joint
TNCC total nucleated cell count
TP total protein
TPR temperature, pulse, respiration
TSH thyroid stimulating hormone
tT_4 total thyroxine
UA urinalysis
UDCA ursodeoxycholic acid
UL upper limit
UOsm urine osmolality
UPCR urine protein to creatinine ratio
US ultrasound
USG urine specific gravity
VCE video capsule endoscopy
VH vacuolar hepatopathy
VMC Von Meyenburg complex
vWD von Willebrand disease
vWF von Willebrand factor
vWF:Ag von Willebrand factor antigen testing
vWF:CBA von Willebrand factor collagen binding assay
WHO World Health Organization
WSAVA World Small Animal Veterinary Association

Table of contents

SECTION I Differential diagnoses for owner chief concerns and physical examination findings

SECTION II Diagnosis of exocrine pancreatic disease

SECTION IV Diagnosis of hepatobiliary disease

SECTION V Diseases of the liver, gallbladder, and biliary tract

Vomiting

Melanie Werner
Dr. med. vet.,
DECVIM-CA
(Internal Medicine)

Pathophysiology

Vomiting, or emesis, is a common clinical presentation in veterinary practice and can be a distressing experience for both dogs and their owners. It is an intricate physiological process involving a combination of neurological, gastrointestinal, and metabolic pathways. Understanding the pathophysiology and clinical signs of vomiting is essential for a small animal veterinarian to perform a precise diagnosis and plan effective management.

The pathophysiology of vomiting is a complex reflex action initiated in the emetic center of the brain, comprising several nuclei situated in the medulla oblongata. These nuclei house various receptors, including serotonergic (5HT1), adrenergic (alpha-2), and neurokinergic (NK1). Activation of these receptors triggers the complex reflex action of vomiting, serving as a protective mechanism against the ingestion of potentially harmful substances. The emetic center receives input from various sources, including indirect activation through humoral pathways via the chemoreceptor trigger zone (CRTZ) or direct stimulation via neural pathways originating from the gastrointestinal tract, cerebral cortex, vestibular system, or other parts of the body. The CRTZ, located in the postrema area on the floor of the fourth ventricle, lacks a blood-brain barrier, making it sensitive to detecting chemical stimuli in the bloodstream. Both endogenous (e.g., uremic or hepatoencephalic toxins resulting from renal failure or hepatic encephalopathy) and exogenous substances (e.g., drugs, environmental toxins, or endotoxins) can reach the CRTZ. The detection of these substances by the CRTZ signals the need for emesis as a protective response.

The vomiting reflex can also be triggered by neural stimulation of the emetic center through various pathways, including afferent vagal, sympathetic, vestibular, and cerebrocortical paths. Disorders affecting the gastrointestinal tract can stimulate vomiting by triggering the release of serotonin from enterochromaffin cells located in the gut mucosa. The released serotonin binds to 5HT3 receptors on afferent vagus nerves, leading to the stimulation of emesis.[1] Therefore, conditions causing gastrointestinal (GI) inflammation or obstruction may result in vomiting due to an increase in serotonin release. Furthermore, the coordination of various muscles during vomiting involves the pharynx, diaphragm, and abdominal muscles. The diaphragm contracts to increase intra-abdominal pressure, while the abdominal muscles contract to expel the gastric or duodenal contents. Simultaneously, the lower esophageal sphincter relaxes to allow the contents to move upward, and the larynx closes to prevent aspiration of vomitus, showing the importance of the reflex.[2]

In addition to the central and peripheral mechanisms described, vomiting may also occur due to increased intracranial pressure or following stimulation of the vestibular apparatus, commonly seen in conditions like vestibular syndrome.

Clinical signs

Vomiting refers to the forceful expulsion of gastric or duodenal contents through the oral cavity. The nature of vomitus can offer clues to the pathophysiology. For instance, the presence of undigested food observed several hours or even a day after ingestion suggests delayed gastric emptying due to gastric outflow obstruction or hypomotility. Conversely, bile-laden vomit indicates a patent gastric outflow tract with an open pylorus, signifying intact small intestinal motility. Blood-tinged vomit, whether fresh blood or coffee-ground appearance, raises suspicion of small gastrointestinal or esophageal erosions, ulcers, or potential bleeding neoplasia.[3] A thorough physical examination during a vomiting episode may reveal abdominal pain and distension. Abdominal pain can be indicative of inflammatory processes such as pancreatitis or obstructive lesions. Frequent or prolonged vomiting can lead to dehydration and electrolyte imbalances, manifested by dry mucous membranes, sunken eyes, and reduced skin turgor. Consequent weakness and lethargy may further complicate the clinical presentation. Chronic vomiting may result in weight loss, as the dog experiences nutrient and caloric deficits over time. If an intracranial process is the cause of vomiting, neurological signs may accompany vomiting, such as circling, head pressing, or seizures. The presence of fever is rare in the vomiting dog but may signal systemic infections or inflammatory conditions such as pancreatitis or hepatitis, warranting vigilant monitoring and further workup. Moreover, it is critical to distinguish between regurgitation and emesis. Regurgitation is characterized by effortless expulsion of undigested food from the esophagus, which points towards esophageal dysfunction or obstruction, while emesis involves active retching and abdominal contractions, indicating underlying gastric or intestinal disturbances. For aspects helping to differentiate vomiting and regurgitation, see Table 1.1.

TABLE 1.1 Differentiation of regurgitation and vomiting.

Aspect	Regurgitation	Vomiting
Definition	Effortless expulsion of undigested food from the esophagus, passive	Forceful expulsion of gastric or duodenal contents, coordinated reflex
Clinical significance	Points towards esophageal issues	Suggests underlying gastric, intestinal, metabolic, visceral, or neurological causes for the clinical sign
Associated actions	No retching or abdominal contractions	Active retching and abdominal contractions
Nausea and salivation	No	Common
Presence of bile	No	Possible
Presence of fresh blood	Possible	Possible
Presence of coffee-ground-like digested blood	No	Possible
Amount of material	Variable	Variable
Timing after eating	Variable	Variable
Risk of aspiration	High	Low

Diagnostic approach

Establishing whether the dog is vomiting or regurgitating is crucial. This is a critical first step, as the causes and subsequent diagnostic pathways for vomiting and regurgitation are significantly different. Remember, vomiting is a reflex, whereas regurgitation is passive, so with vomiting, there is usually evidence of nausea, and abdominal contractions precede the expulsion of gastric or duodenal contents. Regurgitation typically occurs without warning and involves the expulsion of food or fluid from the esophagus without abdominal effort.[4] Owners sometimes confuse coughing with vomiting, but the history should make this clear.

The diagnostic workup of a dog presenting with vomiting requires a meticulous and systematic strategy and is summarized in Algorithm 1.1.

Algorithm 1.1 Note 1 Begin with a thorough history taking and comprehensive physical examination. The veterinary practitioner should pay attention to the character of the vomitus, frequency and duration of vomiting, and any relationships to eating or drinking. Differentiating chronic and acute vomiting (persisting for over 7 days) is crucial, as it can provide valuable insights into the underlying etiology. Other relevant history might include previous episodes of vomiting, concurrent diarrhea, changes in appetite or drinking habits, weight loss, or behavioral changes.

Algorithm 1.1 Note 2 The dietary history is equally important, encompassing any recent changes, brand and type of food used, or the opening of a new food bag or can. The history should also include any potential exposure to toxins, foreign body ingestion, access to garbage, or feeding of table scraps.

Algorithm 1.1 Note 3 The physical examination includes general observations about the dog's body condition and hydration status, followed by a systematic examination. Abnormalities such as abdominal pain or the presence of a mass could provide clues to the underlying cause of vomiting.

Algorithm 1.1 Note 4 Laboratory tests are invaluable in the initial evaluation, including a complete blood count (CBC), serum biochemistry profile, specific pancreatic lipase (cPLi or DGGR-lipase) and urinalysis. These tests provide a general health assessment and may identify underlying systemic or metabolic diseases, such as kidney disease or liver function abnormalities, diabetic ketoacidosis, electrolyte imbalances or pancreatitis, which might be causing the vomiting. Moreover, especially if additional diarrhea is present, fecal examination for parasites or specific tests for infectious diseases (e.g., parvovirosis or leptospirosis) should be undertaken.[9,10]

Algorithm 1.1 Note 5 Blood gas analysis, although not essential in all cases, can help to identify metabolic hypochloremic alkalosis as an indicator for a potential gastric outflow obstruction.

Algorithm 1.1 Note 6 Imaging studies, including radiographs and abdomen ultrasound, are often the next step in the diagnostic process. Specific markers can be utilized in these imaging modalities when pyloric or intestinal obstruction is suspected. These findings may prompt further investigation with contrast studies or ultrasound. On ultrasound examination, the pylorus can be assessed for dilation, wall thickness, and the presence of intraluminal contents. Intestinal obstruction can also be visualized through ultrasound, with the identification of distended loops of the intestine, fluid-filled or gas-filled segments. Changes may also be seen in the liver, pancreas or other abdominal organs.[6,7]

Algorithm 1.1 Note 7 Depending on the initial findings, more specific diagnostic tests might be required. These could include workup in the direction of other uncommon diseases causing vomiting (e.g., hypoadrenocorticism).[8]

Algorithm 1.1 Note 8 Endoscopy may be indicated in chronic cases when extraintestinal diseases have been ruled out to visualize the GI tract directly (more in the chronic cases) and biopsy to diagnose conditions like chronic gastritis, chronic enteropathy, or neoplasia. Measuring cobalamin and folate and evaluating the dysbiosis index can give hints on any intestinal involvement in the disease in chronic cases.[11–13]

In conclusion, understanding the pathophysiology, recognizing the clinical signs, and adopting a systematic diagnostic approach is fundamental for effectively managing dogs with vomiting. Although vomiting is a common clinical sign, it can often be a challenge to determine its cause due to the wide variety of underlying conditions. Therefore, a meticulous, organized, and patient-centered approach is critical to reaching an accurate diagnosis and formulating an effective treatment plan, ultimately improving the quality of life for the affected canine patients.

ALGORITHM 1.1

Diagnostic workup of the vomiting dog.

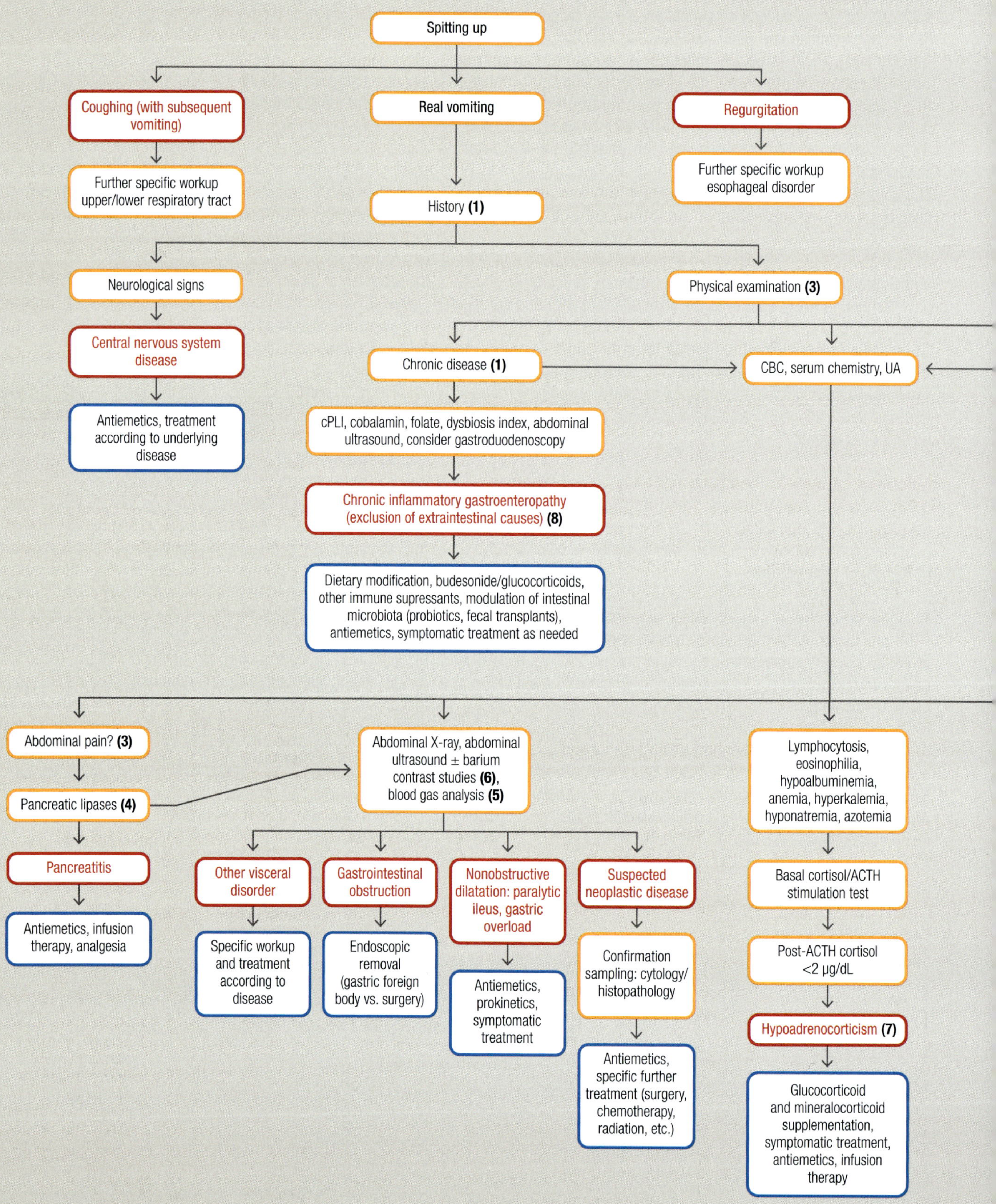

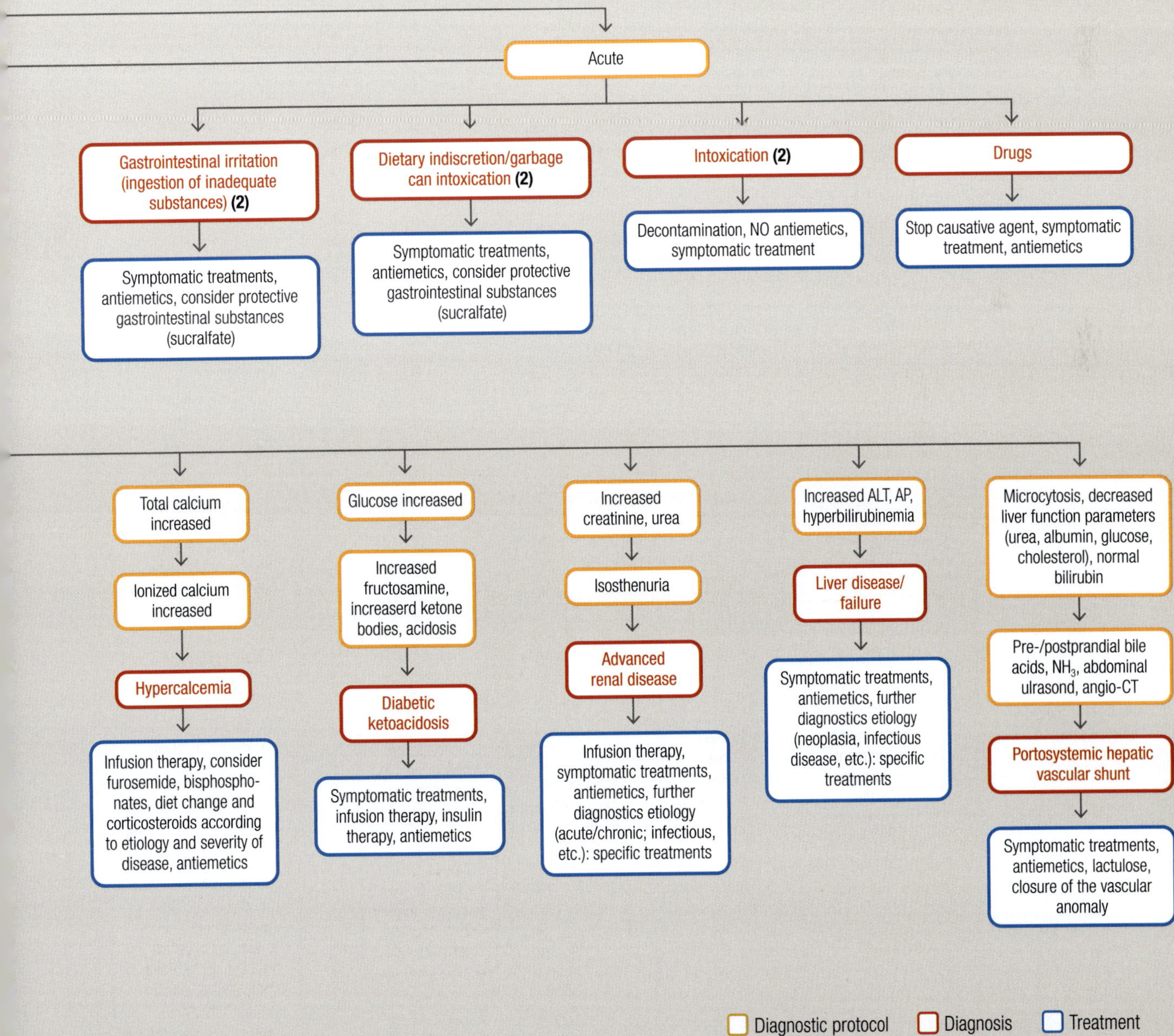
Acute
Gastrointestinal irritation (ingestion of inadequate substances) (2)
Symptomatic treatments, antiemetics, consider protective gastrointestinal substances (sucralfate)
Dietary indiscretion/garbage can intoxication (2)
Symptomatic treatments, antiemetics, consider protective gastrointestinal substances (sucralfate)
Intoxication (2)
Decontamination, NO antiemetics, symptomatic treatment
Drugs
Stop causative agent, symptomatic treatment, antiemetics
Total calcium increased
Ionized calcium increased
Hypercalcemia
Infusion therapy, consider furosemide, bisphospho-nates, diet change and corticosteroids according to etiology and severity of disease, antiemetics
Glucose increased
Increased fructosamine, increaserd ketone bodies, acidosis
Diabetic ketoacidosis
Symptomatic treatments, infusion therapy, insulin theraphy, antiemetics
Increased creatinine, urea
Isosthenuria
Advanced renal disease
Infusion therapy, symptomatic treatments, antiemetics, further diagnostics etiology (acute/chronic; infectious, etc.): specific treatments
Increased ALT, AP, hyperbilirubinemia
Liver disease/ failure
Symptomatic treatments, antiemetics, further diagnostics etiology (neoplasia, infectious disease, etc.): specific treatments
Microcytosis, decreased liver function parameters (urea, albumin, glucose, cholesterol), normal bilirubin
Pre-/postprandial bile acids, NH_3, abdominal ulrasond, angio-CT
Portosystemic hepatic vascular shunt
Symptomatic treatments, antiemetics, lactulose, closure of the vascular anomaly
Diagnostic protocol
Diagnosis
Treatment

References

1. Fukui H, Yamamoto M, Sato S. Vagal afferent fibers and peripheral 5-HT3 receptors mediate cisplatin-induced emesis in dogs. *Jpn J Pharmacol* 59(2):221-226, 1992.
2. Washabau RJ. Vomiting. In Washabau RJ, Day MJ (editors). Canine and Feline Gastroenterology [E-book]. Saint Louis, W.B. Saunders, 2013, pp. 167-173.
3. Ettinger SJ, Feldman EC, Côté E. Textbook of Veterinary Internal Medicine-Inkling E-Book. Elsevier Health Sciences, 2016.
4. Kook PH. Esophagitis in cats and dogs. *Vet Clin North Am Small Anim Pract* 51(1):1-15, 2021.
5. Boag AK, Coe RJ, Martinez TA, Hughes D. Acid-base and electrolyte abnormalities in dogs with gastrointestinal foreign bodies. *J Vet Intern Med* 19(6):816-821, 2005.
6. Hayes G. Gastrointestinal foreign bodies in dogs and cats: A retrospective study of 208 cases. *J Small Anim Pract* 50(11):576-583, 2009.
7. Aronson LR, Brockman DJ, Brown DC. Gastrointestinal emergencies. *Vet Clin North Am Small Anim Pract* 30(3):555-579, 2000.
8. Hauck C, Schmitz SS, Burgener IA, Wehner A, Neiger R, Kohn B, et al. Prevalence and characterization of hypoadrenocorticism in dogs with signs of chronic gastrointestinal disease: A multicenter study. *J Vet Intern Med* 34(4):1399-1405, 2020.
9. Mylonakis ME, Kalli I, Rallis TS. Canine parvoviral enteritis: an update on the clinical diagnosis, treatment, and prevention. *Vet Med Auckl NZ* 7:91-100, 2016.
10. Mazzaferro EM. Update on canine parvoviral enteritis. *Vet Clin North Am Small Anim Pract* 50(6):1307-1325, 2020.
11. Kather S, Grützner N, Kook PH, Dengler F, Heilmann RM. Review of cobalamin status and disorders of cobalamin metabolism in dogs. *J Vet Intern Med* 34(1):13-28, 2020.
12. Heilmann RM, Steiner JM. Clinical utility of currently available biomarkers in inflammatory enteropathies of dogs. *J Vet Intern Med* 32(5):1495-1508, 2018.
13. AlShawaqfeh MK, Wajid B, Minamoto Y, Markel M, Lidbury JA, Steiner JM, et al. A dysbiosis index to assess microbial changes in fecal samples of dogs with chronic inflammatory enteropathy. *FEMS Microbiol Ecol* 93(11), 2017.

CHAPTER 2

Diarrhea

Melanie Werner
Dr. med. vet., DECVIM-CA (Internal Medicine)

Pathophysiology

Understanding the pathophysiology of canine diarrhea necessitates a clear grasp of normal physiological processes within a dog's gastrointestinal (GI) tract. The small intestine primarily handles food digestion and nutrient absorption. Conversely, the large intestine focuses more on water absorption, fermentation, and stool formation. Disruptions in these activities can result in diarrhea.

There are four key mechanisms by which diarrhea can occur: osmotic, secretory, motility-related, and increased permeability. Osmotic diarrhea arises from the inability to absorb dietary components and their breakdown products, as seen in lactose intolerance, where undigested lactose draws water into the gut or is secondary to any problem causing small intestinal maldigestion and malabsorption. Secretory diarrhea results from excessive secretion of electrolytes and water into the intestinal lumen, often stimulated by bacterial toxins and exemplified by acute hemorrhagic diarrhea syndrome caused by *C. perfringens* and its pore-forming net-F toxins.[1-3] Motility-related diarrhea happens when food moves too quickly through the intestines, commonly occurring in intestinal parasitism or concurrently with other conditions such as inflammatory bowel disease. Permeability diarrhea occurs when there is increased permeability of the gut wall. If this is mild, fluid and proteins are lost into the small intestine, whereas if it is severe, red blood cells can also cross the leaky gut wall. Gut wall edema secondary to portal hypertension in liver disease can cause mild permeability diarrhea, whereas acute hemorrhagic diarrhea syndrome is a good example where there is a severe increase in small intestinal permeability in addition to secretory diarrhea. In reality, many diseases cause diarrhea by several mechanisms concurrently. For example, in exocrine pancreatic insufficiency, there is an element of osmotic diarrhea because of unabsorbed nutrients in the small intestine and secretory diarrhea in the colon stimulated by the irritant bacterial breakdown products of undigested fat.

The two types of diarrhea—small intestinal and large intestinal—manifest differently due to the distinct roles of these GI sections. Small intestinal diarrhea results in large volume but less frequent defecations due to increased fluid content and rapid transit time. In contrast, large intestinal diarrhea presents with more frequent but smaller volume defecations, as the large intestine's water reabsorption function is compromised (Table 2.1). Cases of small intestinal maldigestion/malabsorption can present with features of both small and large intestinal disease because unabsorbed nutrients passing to the large intestine (particularly fat and protein) are fermented by bacteria in the colon to irritant metabolites.

Clinical signs

Diarrhea, whether acute or chronic, is characterized by changes in the frequency, volume, and consistency of stool. The clinical signs can be either generalized or specific, depending on the underlying cause.

Acute diarrhea, typically lasting less than one week, may cause dogs to defecate more frequently, produce watery or loose stools, and possibly show an increased urgency to defecate. Some dogs might also display systemic signs like lethargy, loss of appetite, and vomiting. Most cases of acute diarrhea are self-limiting and may resolve with minimal or supportive treatment. Severe cases may require fluid and electrolyte therapy, particularly in puppies.

Chronic diarrhea persists for over three weeks and is often linked to more serious underlying conditions like chronic inflammatory enteropathies, food intolerance, or neoplasia.[4] Affected dogs with small intestinal diarrhea may also show signs such as weight loss, poor body condition, a deteriorating hair coat, and changes in appetite. Moreover, chronic small intestinal diarrhea may lead to malabsorption, manifesting as larger volumes of stool, while chronic colonic diarrhea might present with increased frequency and urgency of defecation, sometimes accompanied by fresh blood or mucus (Table 2.1).

Diagnostic approach

The diagnostic approach for canine diarrhea should be tailored to each patient based on the severity, duration, and accompanying clinical signs, as well as the age, breed, and overall health status of the patient. In uncomplicated patients with acute diarrhea, only history and clinical examination might be enough for the first steps of tailoring in symptomatic management of the clinical signs.
The diagnostic approach to the dog with diarrhea is shown in Algorithm 2.1.

Algorithm 8.1 Note 1 Diagnosing canine diarrhea starts with a comprehensive history and thorough physical examination. Understanding factors like duration, frequency, and consistency of the stool, as well as any concurrent systemic signs, helps differentiate between acute and chronic and large and small intestinal diarrhea (Table 2.1). Information about the dog's diet, exposure to foreign materials, recent medication use, vaccination status, and interaction with other animals is also crucial. Physical examination can yield significant insights, extending beyond the GI tract. Abdominal palpation may reveal pain, masses, or organ enlargement. Other systems should be evaluated, as diarrhea could be a secondary clinical sign of systemic diseases like pancreatitis, liver disease, or renal disease.

Algorithm 8.1 Note 2 Baseline diagnostics in chronic or acute diarrhea that does not resolve with symptomatic treatment should include a complete blood count (CBC), serum biochemical profile, and urinalysis. These tests are crucial for identifying systemic or extraintestinal diseases that might present with diarrhea and electrolyte abnormalities, which need treatment if the diarrhea is severe. Anemia may indicate chronic GI bleeding, while elevated white blood cell counts could suggest inflammation or infection.

Algorithm 8.1 Notes 3 and 4 Biochemical tests can reveal liver or kidney disease, as indicated by elevated liver enzymes combined with hyperbilirubinemia or azotemia, respectively. In cases of elevated kidney parameters, prerenal azotemia (due to dehydration) must be ruled out using urine specific gravity.

Algorithm 8.1 Note 5 Chronic conditions may show hypoalbuminemia, potentially indicating a protein-losing enteropathy, especially when accompanied by normo- or mild hyperglobulinemia .[5]

Algorithm 8.1 Note 6 In cases of hemorrhagic diarrhea, increased packed cell volume (PCV) symbolizing severe dehydration is a hallmark of acute hemorrhagic diarrhea syndrome.

Algorithm 8.1 Note 7 In juvenile dogs, inadequately vaccinated individuals, and dogs with severe neutropenia, suspicion of parvovirus infection must arise, leading to adequate testing.[6]

Algorithm 8.1 Note 8 In acute or chronic diarrhea, measurement of pancreatic lipases together with abdominal ultrasound could diagnose pancreatitis.

TABLE 2.1 Clinical differences between small and large intestinal diarrhea. Note dogs may have signs of both small and large intestinal disease (see text), in which case the workup should initially focus on the small intestine.

	Small intestine	Large intestine
Tenesmus	Absent	Present
Frequency	Increased or normal	Severely increased
Urgency	None	Present
Stool volume	Normal or increased	Decreased predefecation
Hematochezia	Absent	May be present
Melena	Maybe present	Absent
Mucus	Absent	Present
Appetite changes (polyphagia or anorexia)	Common	Very uncommon*
Weight loss	Common	Very uncommon*

* Weight loss and appetite changes are hallmarks of small intestinal disease and not seen in colitis. The exception is histiocytic colitis in Boxer dogs, which is such a severe inflammatory disease that it can lead to systemic clinical signs, e.g., weight loss.

Algorithm 8.1 Note 9 Fecal analysis is one of the most direct methods for evaluating the cause of diarrhea. Basic tests include fecal flotation and direct smears to identify common parasites. When parasites or ova are found, targeted deworming can swiftly resolve the diarrhea. Cultures and sensitivity tests on fecal samples might be carried out in cases of suspected bacterial enteritis. However, routine fecal cultures are generally not recommended due to the commensal nature of many intestinal bacteria and the risk of culture contamination. Quantitative cultures or PCR testing for particular pathogens (like *Salmonella* spp. or *Campylobacter* spp.) could be beneficial in specific situations. Parvovirus point-of-care (POC) antigen testing is specific but not highly sensitive for diagnosing parvovirus. If a negative POC test occurs, more sensitive PCR testing is recommended.[7]

Algorithm 8.1 Note 10 Cobalamin (vitamin B_{12}), folate levels, and serum TLI are particularly useful in cases of chronic diarrhea. Low serum cobalamin levels, irrespective of the cause, have been associated with poorer disease outcomes, underscoring its importance in the workup of chronic diarrhea.

Algorithm 8.1 Note 11 In chronic diarrhea, finding these typical clinicopathological changes should raise suspicion of hypoadrenocorticism, and measurement of basal cortisol or an ACTH stimulation test would be indicated.

Algorithm 8.1 Note 12 The dysbiosis index, a recent addition to the diagnostic toolkit, measures the abundance of various bacterial groups in the feces. This test helps diagnose dysbiosis, a condition marked by an imbalance of gut bacteria, which may underlie chronic diarrhea.[8]

Algorithm 8.1 Note 13 Imaging techniques become especially useful when physical examination and laboratory findings are inconclusive. Abdominal radiographs can help identify foreign objects, intestinal obstructions, or significant changes in organ size or position. In certain instances, contrast radiography may be required to better visualize the intestinal tract.

Abdominal ultrasound offers more detailed insights into the structure of the intestinal wall, the presence of masses, or changes in nearby organs like the liver or pancreas. It is now the preferred imaging modality for dogs with diarrhea. The technique is particularly useful for identifying conditions like protein-losing enteropathy (evidenced by mucosal striations) or neoplasia.[5]

Algorithm 8.1 Note 14 Endoscopy allows for direct visualization of the mucosal surface of the GI tract and enables biopsy sample collection. It is particularly valuable for diagnosing conditions like inflammatory bowel disease, intestinal lymphangiectasia, or neoplasia. Although less invasive than full surgical biopsies, endoscopy does require specialized equipment and an experienced operator to take diagnostic intestinal biopsies, making it better suited for chronic or severe cases where other diagnostic measures have failed. Histopathological examination of biopsy samples often provides a definitive diagnosis for chronic diarrhea cases. The observations made during this examination can guide the treatment plan. Special staining techniques can be employed to identify specific pathogens or to better characterize cellular changes in certain diseases (e.g., PAS reaction in histiocytic-ulcerative colitis).[9,10]

ALGORITHM 2.1

Diagnostic approach to the patient with diarrhea.

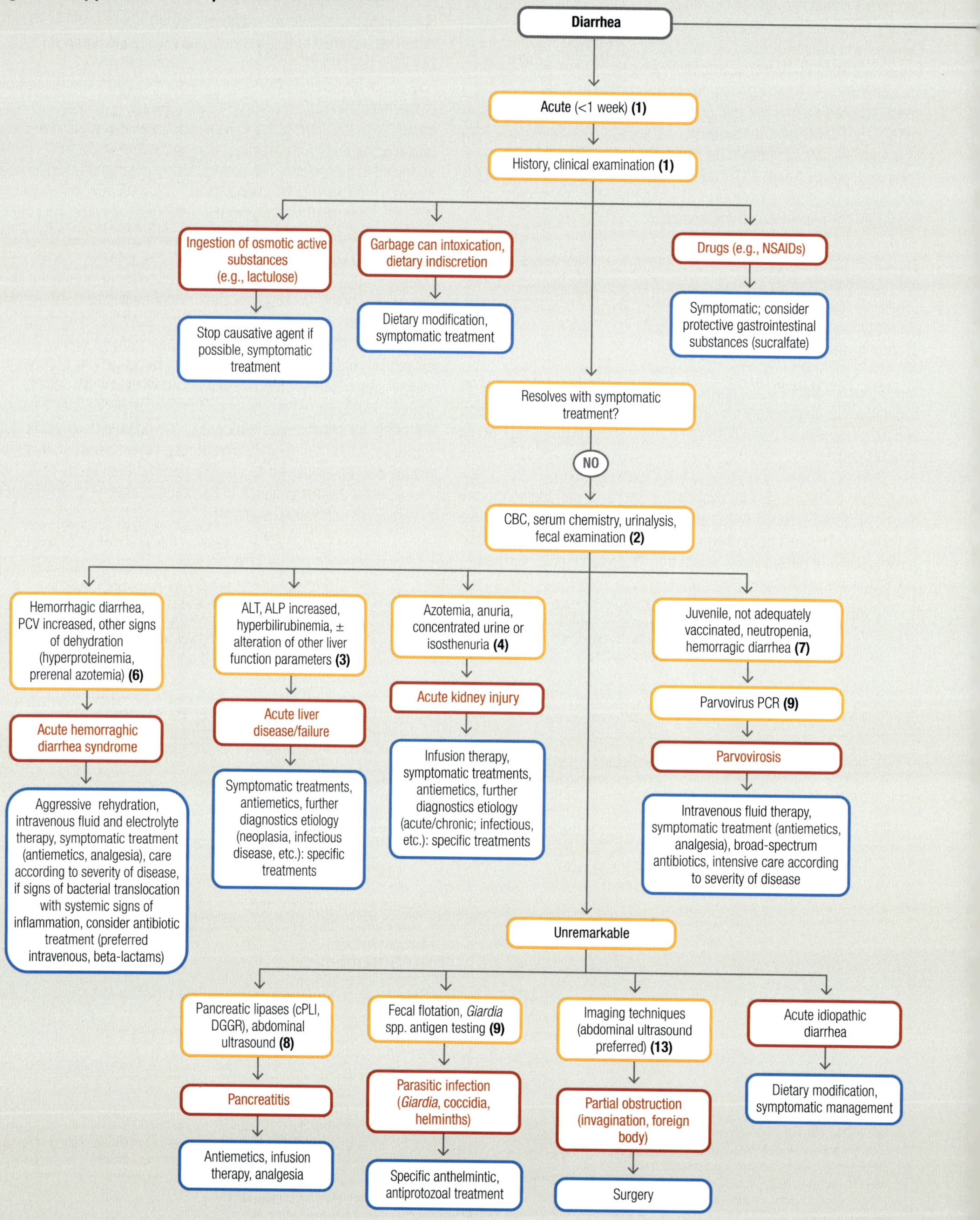

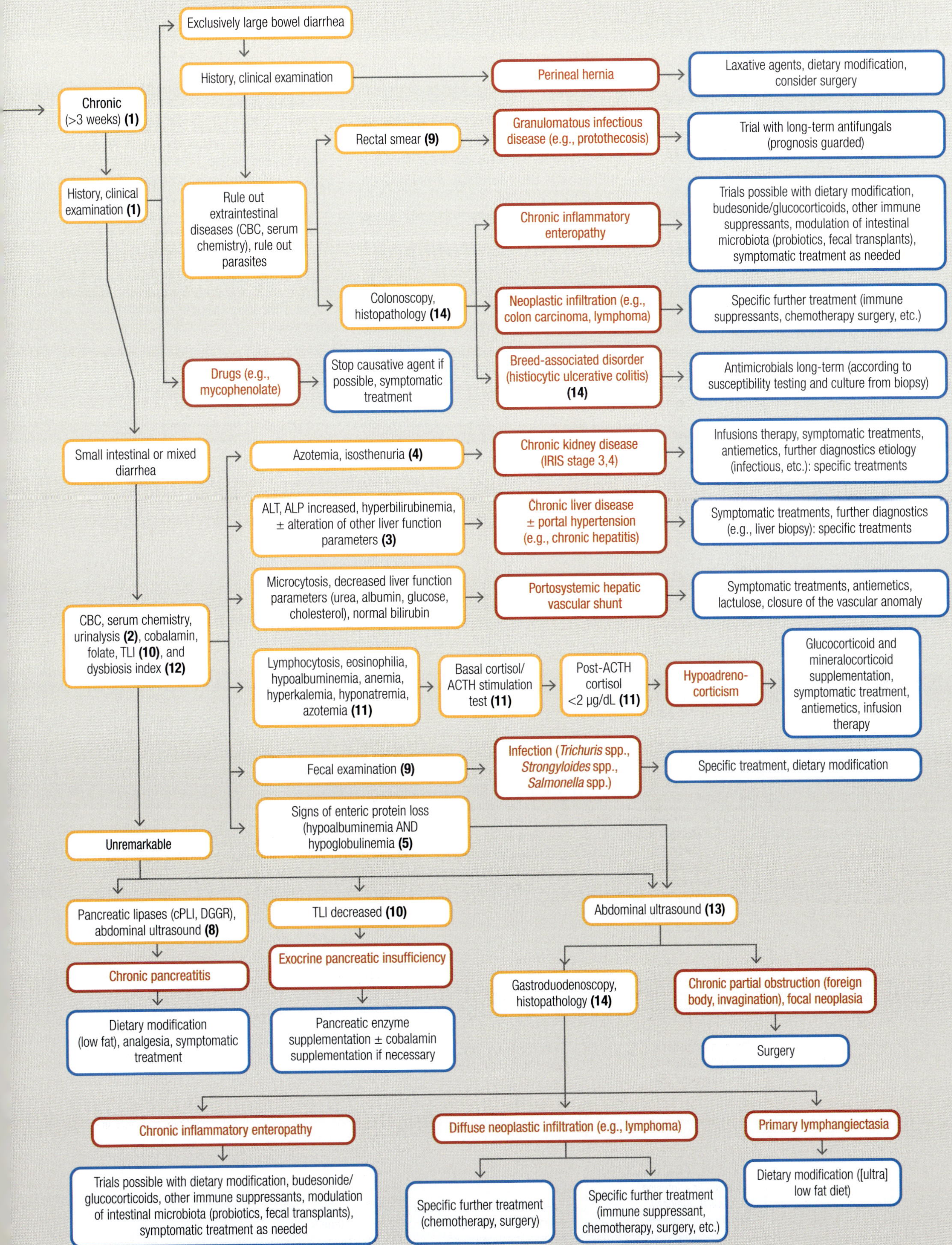
Chronic (>3 weeks) (1)
History, clinical examination (1)
Exclusively large bowel diarrhea
History, clinical examination
Perineal hernia
Laxative agents, dietary modification, consider surgery
Rule out extraintestinal diseases (CBC, serum chemistry), rule out parasites
Rectal smear (9)
Granulomatous infectious disease (e.g., protothecosis)
Trial with long-term antifungals (prognosis guarded)
Colonoscopy, histopathology (14)
Chronic inflammatory enteropathy
Trials possible with dietary modification, budesonide/glucocorticoids, other immune suppressants, modulation of intestinal microbiota (probiotics, fecal transplants), symptomatic treatment as needed
Neoplastic infiltration (e.g., colon carcinoma, lymphoma)
Specific further treatment (immune suppressants, chemotherapy surgery, etc.)
Breed-associated disorder (histiocytic ulcerative colitis) (14)
Antimicrobials long-term (according to susceptibility testing and culture from biopsy)
Drugs (e.g., mycophenolate)
Stop causative agent if possible, symptomatic treatment
Small intestinal or mixed diarrhea
CBC, serum chemistry, urinalysis (2), cobalamin, folate, TLI (10), and dysbiosis index (12)
Azotemia, isosthenuria (4)
Chronic kidney disease (IRIS stage 3,4)
Infusions therapy, symptomatic treatments, antiemetics, further diagnostics etiology (infectious, etc.): specific treatments
ALT, ALP increased, hyperbilirubinemia, ± alteration of other liver function parameters (3)
Chronic liver disease ± portal hypertension (e.g., chronic hepatitis)
Symptomatic treatments, further diagnostics (e.g., liver biopsy): specific treatments
Microcytosis, decreased liver function parameters (urea, albumin, glucose, cholesterol), normal bilirubin
Portosystemic hepatic vascular shunt
Symptomatic treatments, antiemetics, lactulose, closure of the vascular anomaly
Lymphocytosis, eosinophilia, hypoalbuminemia, anemia, hyperkalemia, hyponatremia, azotemia (11)
Basal cortisol/ ACTH stimulation test (11)
Post-ACTH cortisol <2 µg/dL (11)
Hypoadreno-corticism
Glucocorticoid and mineralocorticoid supplementation, symptomatic treatment, antiemetics, infusion therapy
Fecal examination (9)
Infection (Trichuris spp., Strongyloides spp., Salmonella spp.)
Specific treatment, dietary modification
Signs of enteric protein loss (hypoalbuminemia AND hypoglobulinemia (5)
Unremarkable
Pancreatic lipases (cPLI, DGGR), abdominal ultrasound (8)
Chronic pancreatitis
Dietary modification (low fat), analgesia, symptomatic treatment
TLI decreased (10)
Exocrine pancreatic insufficiency
Pancreatic enzyme supplementation ± cobalamin supplementation if necessary
Abdominal ultrasound (13)
Gastroduodenoscopy, histopathology (14)
Chronic partial obstruction (foreign body, invagination), focal neoplasia
Surgery
Chronic inflammatory enteropathy
Trials possible with dietary modification, budesonide/glucocorticoids, other immune suppressants, modulation of intestinal microbiota (probiotics, fecal transplants), symptomatic treatment as needed
Diffuse neoplastic infiltration (e.g., lymphoma)
Specific further treatment (chemotherapy, surgery)
Specific further treatment (immune suppressant, chemotherapy, surgery, etc.)
Primary lymphangiectasia
Dietary modification ([ultra] low fat diet)

References

1. Unterer S, Busch K. Acute hemorrhagic diarrhea syndrome in fogs. *Vet Clin North Am Small Anim Pract* 51(1):79-92, 2021.
2. Unterer S, Busch K, Leipig M, Hermanns W, Wolf G, Straubinger RK, et al. Endoscopically visualized lesions, histologic findings, and bacterial invasion in the gastrointestinal mucosa of dogs with acute hemorrhagic diarrhea syndrome. *J Vet Intern Med* 28(1):52-58, 2014.
3. Leipig-Rudolph M, Busch K, Prescott JF, Mehdizadeh Gohari I, Leutenegger CM, Hermanns W, et al. Intestinal lesions in dogs with acute hemorrhagic diarrhea syndrome associated with netF-positive *Clostridium perfringens* type A. *J Vet Diagn Investig Off Publ Am Assoc Vet Lab Diagn Inc* 30(4):495-503, 2018.
4. Marks SL. Diarrhea. In Washabau RJ, Day MJ (editors). Canine and Feline Gastroenterology. Saint Louis, W.B. Saunders, 2013, pp. 99-108.
5. Jablonski SA. Pathophysiology, diagnosis, and management of canine intestinal lymphangiectasia: A comparative review. *Anim Open Access J MDPI* 12(20):2791, 2022.
6. Mazzaferro EM. Update on canine parvoviral enteritis. *Vet Clin North Am Small Anim Pract* 50(6):1307-1325, 2020.
7. Mylonakis ME, Kalli I, Rallis TS. Canine parvoviral enteritis: an update on the clinical diagnosis, treatment, and prevention. *Vet Med Auckl NZ* 7:91-100, 2016.
8. Pilla R, Suchodolski JS. The role of the canine gut microbiome and metabolome in health and gastrointestinal disease. *Front Vet Sci* 6:498, 2019.
9. Craven M, Mansfield CS, Simpson KW. Granulomatous colitis of Boxer dogs. *Vet Clin North Am Small Anim Pract* 41(2):433-445, 2011.
10. Mansfield CS, James FE, Craven M, Davies DR, O'Hara AJ, Nicholls PK, et al. Remission of histiocytic ulcerative colitis in Boxer dogs correlates with eradication of invasive intramucosal *Escherichia coli*. *J Vet Intern Med* 23(5):964-969, 2009.

CHAPTER 3

Weight loss

Mellora Sharman
BVSc, MVM, PGradCert, PhD, FANZCVSt, DECVIM-CA (Internal Medicine), FHEA, MRCVS, RCVS

Marina Martín-Ambrosio
DVM, DECVIM-CA (Internal Medicine), MRCVS

Pathophysiology

Unintentional weight loss is frequently reported in clinical practice and reflects disorders that hinder food intake, impede nutrient absorption or metabolism, accelerate metabolic demand, or are associated with nutrient loss (Table 3.1). Regular monitoring of body weight should be regarded as an integral component of routine health assessments of dogs and cats. Loss of more than 5% of body weight should be considered significant enough to warrant further investigation.[1]

Maintenance of the body's overall mass and composition requires a balance between energy intake and energy expenditure. Both short-term and long-term control mechanisms regulate this equilibrium. Short-term mechanisms involve feelings of hunger and satiety, affected by environmental and psychogenic factors that influence specific centers of the brain, especially the hypothalamus. Long-term regulation involves feedback mechanisms controlled by the level of nutrients and amount of adipose tissue of the individual and their effect on food intake. Ambient temperature can also affect food intake. Thus, an increase or decrease in intake can occur when an animal is exposed to either cold or heat.[2] The physiologic regulation of food intake, including the influence of sensory, metabolic/hormonal, and environmental signals, is outlined in more detail in chapter 4.

Changes in body weight or condition can reflect starvation and/or cachexia, which are distinct physiologic processes. In starvation, healthy animals that are not receiving enough calories to meet their needs are able to make metabolic adjustments to enable the utilization of body fat as a primary fuel source, allowing relative preservation of lean body mass (LBM). Byproducts of this process are converted into ketone bodies, particularly β-hydroxybutyrate, which can traverse the blood-brain barrier and provide energy to brain cells. In comparison, in animals with chronic/inflammatory disease, amino acids from the muscle remain the primary energy source, leading to rapid breakdown of LBM and resulting in cachexia.[3]

In veterinary patients, cachexia has been particularly associated with cancer, renal, cardiac, and chronic respiratory disease, where the production of humoral factors (e.g., inflammatory cytokines, catecholamines, cortisol, insulin, glucagon) suppresses food intake but can also

TABLE 3.1 Pathophysiological classification of causes of weight loss in small animals.*

Factors related to food provided	Decreased caloric intake due to a reduced ability to eat or desire for food	Inability to utilize ingested calories	Increased metabolic demand	Accelerated energy loss

■ Insufficient quantity
■ Poor quality
	■ Fear/stress or food competition
	■ Reduced sense of smell:
	  ■ Aging
	  ■ Nasal disease
	  ■ Disease of the olfactory lobe
	■ Anatomic/neuromuscular disease that disrupts chewing/swallowing
	  ■ Dental disease
	  ■ Oropharyngeal neoplasia
	  ■ Neuromuscular disorders: cricopharyngeal achalasia or esophageal dysmotility
		■ Malabsorption: primary gastrointestinal disease
		■ Maldigestion: pancreatic disease
		■ Reduced capacity for synthesis: hepatic disease
		■ Diabetes mellitus
			■ Pregnancy, lactation
			■ Exercise
			■ Cardiac disease
			■ Respiratory disorders
			■ Chronic kidney disease
			■ Chronic inflammation/infection
			■ Hyperthyroidism (rare in dogs)
			■ Neoplasia
				■ Diabetes mellitus (due to glucosuria)
				■ Renal glucosuria/Fanconi syndrome
				■ Protein-losing enteropathy
				■ Protein-losing nephropathy

* Please note that weight loss in chronic kidney disease is multifactorial, including cachexia, a component of renal protein loss, and/or poor appetite due to uremia (nausea/vomiting, gastric ulceration, and lesions of the oral cavity).

impair metabolism, and/or lead to the disruption of nutrient processing.[3] Their contributions to nausea and vomiting can also affect nutrient intake and further contribute to weight loss.

In some illnesses, weight loss may be multifactorial. For example, hyporexia or anorexia may be concurrent with increased energy expenditure (i.e., cachexia), resulting in serious weight loss (i.e., wasting syndrome). It is also possible to see weight loss as a result of sarcopenia as defined by a loss of lean body mass (LBM) related to age. This can occur independently of disease or coexist with cachexia in older individuals.[3]

Clinical signs

Monitoring of body weight and body condition score (BCS), together with taking a dietary history, is integral to a physical examination. The goal for most pets is a BCS of 4 to 5/9, where the ribs are palpable without excessive covering fat and where the waist and abdominal tuck are easily visible.[4] Body condition assessment should also include a separate evaluation of muscle mass (i.e., a muscle condition score [MCS]) as a subjective means of assessing lean tissue status. This includes visual examination and palpation over the temporal bones, scapulae, lumbar vertebrae, and pelvic bones. The World Small Animal Veterinary Association (WSAVA) offers excellent body and muscle condition score tools for dogs and cats to aid in accurate patient assessment.[4]

A low BCS indicates a suboptimal body weight, with loss of subcutaneous fat, prominent skeletal structures, and an emaciated appearance (Fig. 3.1). In cachectic patients, this will often be characterized by disproportionate muscle loss compared to fat. Recognition of cachexia is important because muscle loss is greater in patients with most acute and chronic diseases (i.e., stressed starvation) compared to healthy animals deprived of food where primarily fat is lost (i.e., simple starvation), and as animals with cachexia may not respond as expected to therapeutic interventions and nutritional support.[3]

As unintentional weight loss is nonspecific and rather an indicator of either inadequate nutrition or underlying illness, it is always important to assess for accompanying clinical signs that might provide clues to reflect a more specific underlying pathological process.

Diagnostic approach

Algorithm 3.1 shows the approach to patients presenting with weight loss.

Algorithm 3.1 Note 1 Diagnosing the reason behind unintended weight loss in dogs and cats can pose a challenge in the absence of specific clinical signs or examination findings. As an initial step, a careful review of the patient's dietary history, appetite, and ability to eat should be collected. This should include details regarding the dietary quality and calorie content, caloric intake relative to maintenance energy requirements (MER) provided, the amount of daily exercise, and the patient's environment (food competition or other psychological factors that might impede intake).

Algorithm 3.1 Note 2 Comparing estimated MER with daily caloric intake is useful to estimate whether the animal is consuming enough calories. The RER should be calculated using the following equation: RER $= 70 \times (\text{body weight [kg]})^{0.75}$. The RER is then multiplied by different factors (Table 3.2) to calculate the maintenance energy requirements (MER), which are mainly influenced by age, neuter status, life stage, and activity levels.[4,5] It should be remembered that this is only an estimate, and individual animals usually have requirements that are less or more than this.

Algorithm 3.1 Note 3 Clarifying interest and ability to eat can require direct observation of food consumption to evaluate for conditions that impede prehension, chewing, and swallowing of food. When appetite is normal, or if polyphagia is reported, the index of suspicion for excessive nutrient loss or overutilization of nutrients due to physiological or pathologic causes will be increased. If hyporexia or anorexia are reported, a broad range of underlying conditions may need to be considered.

Algorithm 3.1 Note 4 Physical examination might also identify abnormalities that offer insights into the underlying cause of weight loss. Particular attention should be paid to the oral cavity, cardiopulmonary auscultation, palpation of the cervical/thyroid area, and the abdominal

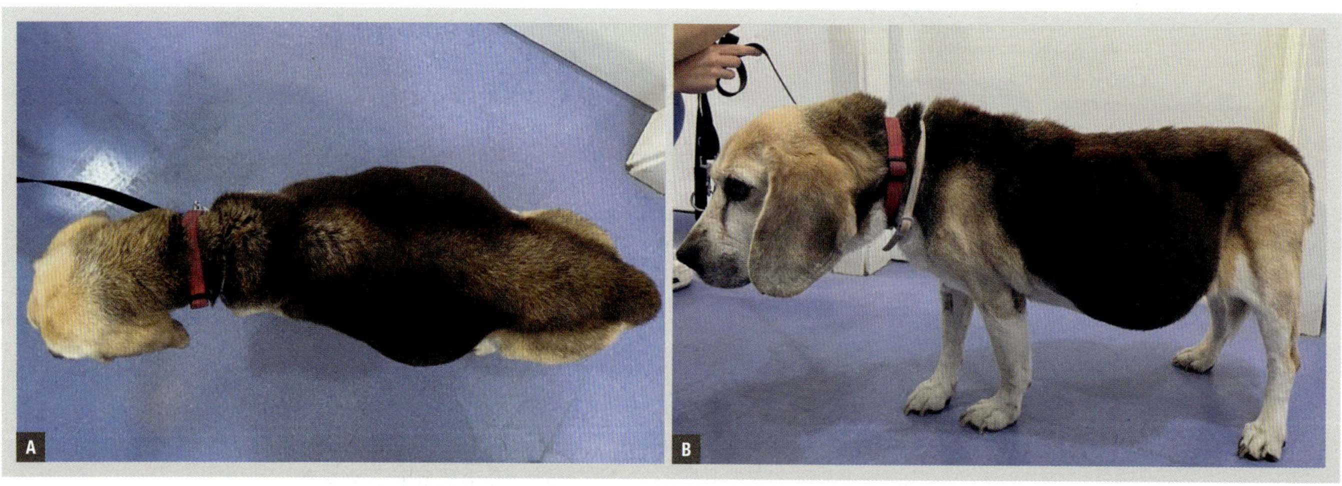

FIG. 3.1 A 16-year-old, spayed female Beagle dog presenting with marked cachexia despite a pendulous abdomen and an estimated body condition score of 2/9. The underlying cause was an adrenocortical carcinoma with metastatic disease involving the liver.

ALGORITHM 3.1

Diagnostic approach to unintentional weight loss.

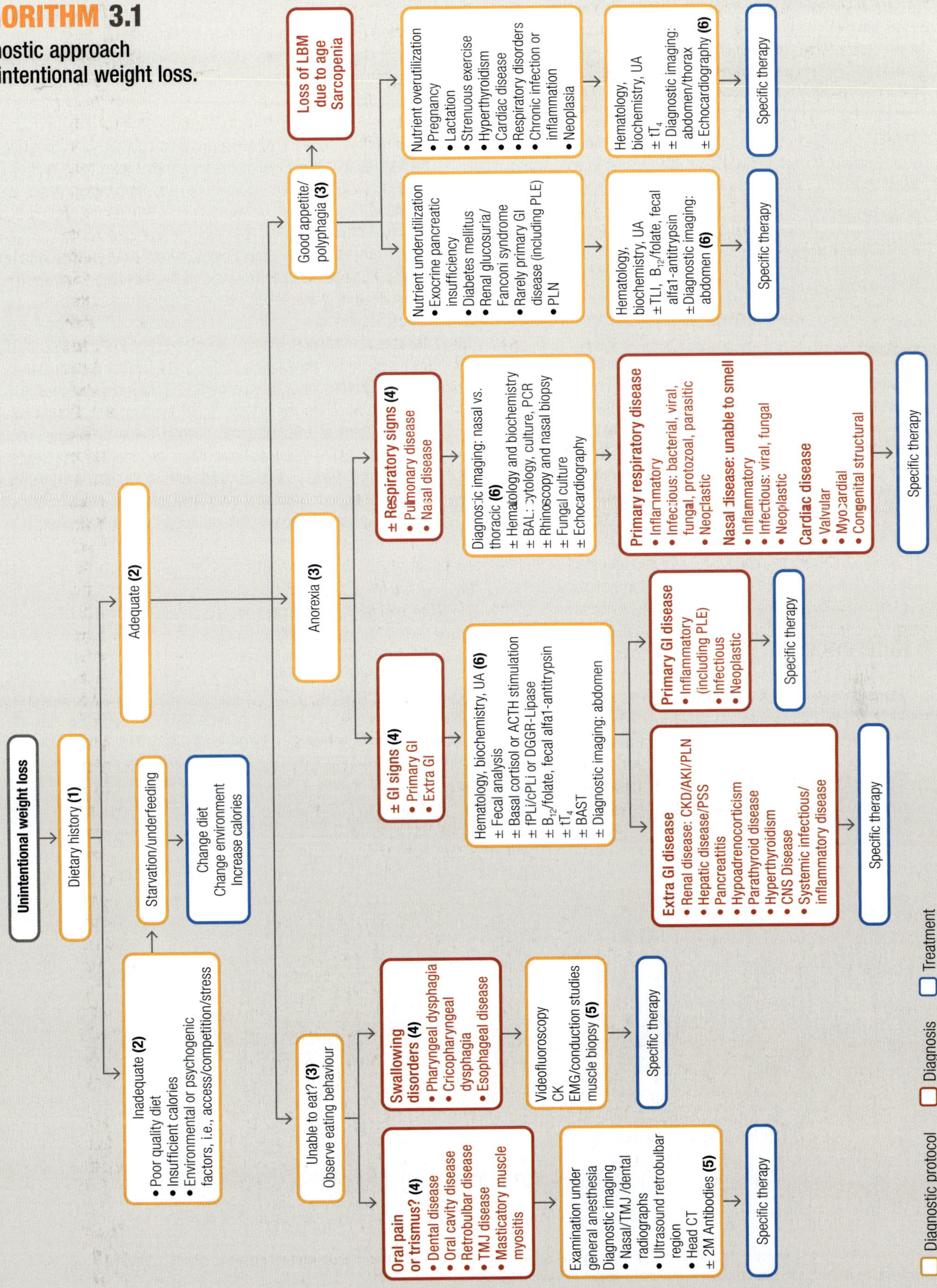

TABLE 3.2 Coefficients to calculate the estimated daily energy requirements in dogs and cats*.

Nutritional assessment factors	Dogs	Cats
	(to be multiplied by RER)	
Growth	0-4 months: ×3 4 months-adult: ×2	×2.5
Intact adult	×1.6-1.8	×1.4-1.6
Neutered adult	×1.4-1.6	×1.2-1.4
Inactive/obese-prone	×0.8	×1
Working adult	Light: ×1.6-2 Moderate: ×2-5 Heavy: ×5-11	
Gestation	×3 (last 3 weeks)	×1.6-2
Lactation (based on number of offspring and weeks of lactation)	×3-≥6	×2-6

* Please note that these are estimated energy requirements based on the patient's life stage and activity levels; adjustments may be needed based on regular monitoring of the patient's body weight and BCS.

cavity. Depending on the constellation of presenting findings, a more targeted physical examination (e.g., neurological or orthopedic examination) may be necessary. Other clinical findings, such as the presence of gastrointestinal or respiratory signs, might help pinpoint an organ system of interest.

Algorithm 3.1 Note 5 If an oral cavity or swallowing disorder is suspected, further investigation under general anesthetic and/or imaging studies, including videofluoroscopy and electrodiagnostic, might be indicated.

Algorithm 3.1 Note 6 Hematology, serum biochemistry, and urinalysis findings may be nonspecific, but equally, they might uncover the underlying cause of presentation. However, additional diagnostics can be required depending on preliminary clinicopathologic findings. For example, markers of malabsorption (i.e., cobalamin and folate levels), maldigestion (i.e., trypsin-like immunoreactivity), and intestinal protein loss (i.e., fecal alfa-1-antitrypsin) may be considered if a chronic gastrointestinal disease is suspected. Detection of persistent hyperglycemia might lead to the measurement of fructosamine. Beyond these preliminary steps, and where no specific cause is yet evident, or to further evaluate identified underlying disease as a cause, radiographic or ultrasonographic studies might be needed. Additional diagnostic steps to explore potential diagnoses in greater detail will depend upon these initial results.[1]

References

1. Schermerhorn T. Weight loss as a chief complaint. In Ettinger SJ, Feldman EC, Côté E (editors). Textbook of Veterinary Internal Medicine 8th edition. St. Louis, Elsevier, 2017, pp. 85-88.
2. Hall JE. Dietary balances; regulation of feeding; obesity and starvation; vitamins and minerals. In Hall JE (editor). Guyton and Hall Textbook of Medical Physiology 13th edition. Philadelphia, Elsevier, 2015, pp. 887-902.
3. Freeman LM. Cachexia and sarcopenia: emerging syndromes of importance in dogs and cats. *J Vet Intern Med* 26(1):3-17, 2011.
4. WSAVA Nutritional Assessment Guidelines Task Force Members; Freeman L, Becvarova I, Cave N, et al. WSAVA Nutritional Assessment Guidelines. *J Small Anim Pract* 52(7):385-396, 2011.
5. Cline MG, Burns KM, Coe JB, Downing R, Durzi T, Murphy M, Parker V. 2021 AAHA nutrition and weight management guidelines for dogs and cats. *J Am Anim Hosp Assoc* 57(4):153-178, 2021.

CHAPTER 4

Poor appetite/no appetite

Sofia Rapastella
DVM, MRCVS,
DECVIM-CA
(Internal Medicine)

Mellora Sharman
BVSc, MVM, PGradCert,
PhD, FANZCVS,
DECVIM-CA
(Internal Medicine),
FHEA, MRCVS

Anorexia is a term used to describe lack of appetite or inability to eat, while hyporexia defines a reduction of appetite. Both anorexia and hyporexia are common, nonspecific findings in dogs and can be seen in either acute or chronic presentations. When prolonged anorexia or hyporexia occurs, inadequate nutritional intake can contribute to serious sequelae, such as immune suppression and secondary organ dysfunction.

Pathophysiology

Regulation of food intake is a complex process involving the integration of endogenous and exogenous factors that affect the central nervous system (CNS), particularly the hypothalamus and brainstem, resulting in hunger or satiety. The lateral hypothalamic nuclei represent the "feeding center", while the ventromedial hypothalamic nuclei are considered the "satiety center". In general, the feeding center is constantly active unless inhibited by the satiety center. The brainstem nucleus of the solitary tract and area postrema have secondary coordinating roles.

Signals affecting CNS centers for hunger and satiety can be grouped into three major categories, including sensory, metabolic, and environmental inputs.[1] Sensory signals include orosensory factors, such as flavor, smell, and physical attributes of the food, such as its temperature, water content, texture, and consistency. These factors also contribute to the palatability of a meal, which is considered specific to each patient. Preferences towards specific food characteristics develop over time, with avoidance of others.

Metabolic signals are driven by hormones, mostly produced by neurons, as well as those produced by gastrointestinal and pancreatic cells, which in turn have effects on the hypothalamus. Among the orexigenic (that is, appetite-stimulating) factors, neuropeptide Y (NPY) has a central role in regulating hunger. Other hormones affect hunger indirectly by either stimulating or suppressing NPY production. For example, secretion of NPY is induced by low insulin concentration (e.g., during starvation or in pathologic processes such as diabetes), as well as endogenous and exogenous glucocorticoids. Leptin, produced mainly by adipocytes, is conversely the main factor that induces a reduction of NPY secretion, thereby contributing to satiety.

Additional gastrointestinal hormones that affect the hypothalamus include cholecystokinin (CCK), which is produced in response to fat and protein content in a meal and suppresses food intake, most likely to allow digestion of these substances. Ghrelin, produced primarily by the stomach when empty, has orexigenic properties that are thought to be secondary to stimulation of the orexigenic agouti-related protein (AGRP) neurons and concurrent inhibition of the anorexigenic pro-opiomelanocortin (POMC) neurons. Other gastrointestinal hormones can act either locally or have central actions within the CNS to reduce CNS-derived hunger signals. This includes insulin, glucagon, PYY, and pancreatic peptide.[2]

Environmental factors can affect appetite and sometimes override both sensory and metabolic signals. These can include the timing and location of meals and psychological factors such as ambient noise, type of bowls, and the presence of people or other pets during feeding. Equally, learned behaviors and past experiences can affect food intake. Thus, a variety of psychological components can ultimately interfere with food consumption and lead to so-called "learned food aversion".

Clinical signs

It is important to differentiate anorexia from pseudoanorexia. Pseudoanorexia occurs when there is still interest in food, but the type of food or environmental conditions are changed such that they impact consumption. True anorexia occurs when there is a refusal of food despite encouragement and modifications of environmental factors. Sometimes, concurrent hypersalivation or lip smacking is reported when offering food, which can reflect one of the main contributors to lack of appetite and/or nausea. Nausea is a complex mechanism finely regulated by several regions within the CNS that are also involved in the regulation of appetite. This includes the cerebral cortex, the chemoreceptor trigger zone, the oculovestibular system, the nucleus tractus solitarius and the emetic center in the medulla oblongata.[3] These areas can be stimulated directly or indirectly via gastrointestinal stimuli (more details can be found in chapter 1). Nausea secondary to a variety of systemic diseases can significantly reduce appetite.

Duration of hyporexia and anorexia can mirror chronicity associated with the underlying disease. Duration of appetite change should be correlated with changes in body weight and the body condition score, as these factors can be indicative of disease severity.

In most cases, a lack of appetite is not the only presenting complaint, and additional signs are described that help to point towards an underlying disease process. For example, hyporexia or anorexia are commonly reported in dogs with primary gastrointestinal disease or pancreatic diseases, organ failure, neoplasia or conditions causing inflammatory states or pyrexia. Often, the underlying mechanism is linked with the production of cytokines (e.g., TNF-α, IL-1) or accumulation of substances normally metabolized by the diseased organ (e.g., uremic toxins accumulating secondary to renal dysfunction or bilirubin/neurotoxins accumulating secondary to hepatic dysfunction) that then affect the hypothalamic feeding center either directly or indirectly.[3]

Chronic or acute pain, particularly abdominal, e.g., associated with pancreatitis or due to obstructive choledocolithiasis, or pain localized in the mouth, e.g., dental disease or stomatitis, can also negatively impact food consumption.

Hyporexia and anorexia can also be sequelae to various medications prescribed to manage a variety of diseases that, for example, cause gastric irritation, ulceration, or functional ileus. Therefore, a careful audit of currently administered therapeutics is important to determine if this is likely.

Diagnostic approach

The approach to the patient with hyporexia or anorexia is shown in Algorithm 4.1.

Algorithm 4.1 Note 1 Differential diagnoses for alterations in appetite can be broad and include any acute or chronic disease. In patients presenting with anorexia or hyporexia, a more directed diagnostic approach can be facilitated by careful collection of historical information and a thorough physical examination. In doing so, a more specific problem may be identifiable to direct diagnostics towards, or it may be possible to determine if a patient has pseudoanorexia/hyporexia due to either situational or iatrogenic factors (environmental, anorexigenic drugs).

Dietary history should, ideally, include diet type, how much of what is offered is consumed, whether the animal is eating its calculated resting energy requirements (RER) (see chapter 3 for more details), and feeding management/environment, as this can help pinpoint specific dietary or environmental factors such as fear or food competition. Physical examination should always include an assessment of the patient's body condition and muscle score.

Algorithm 4.1 Note 2 Environmental triggers resulting in pseudoanorexia can include changes in the person in charge of feeding, introduction of new people or pets, or changes in the food bowl or feeding schedule. Food competition or interactions with other household pets may also have significant impacts.

Algorithm 4.1 Note 3 Dietary factors causing pseudoanorexia vary from type of diet offered, palatability, and physical characteristics (e.g., warmth, water content, wet/dry form). Mixing medications into meals can also make food less palatable and negatively impact the perceived palatability of the diet.

TABLE 4.1 Medications commonly causing anorexia and hyporexia in dogs.

- Antibiotics: amoxicillin, ampicillin, cephalexin, chloramphenicol, erythromycin, tetracycline, trimethoprim/sulfadiazine
- Omeprazole
- Nonsteroidal anti-inflammatories
- Chemotherapeutic agents: cisplatin, doxorubicin, vincristine and others
- Narcotic analgesic agents (opioids)
- Diuretics
- Cardiac glycosides
- Chelating agents: penicillamine
- Supplements such as zinc and iron

Algorithm 4.1 Note 4 Various medications can negatively affect appetite. Table 4.1 summarizes anorexigenic drugs or drugs that can result in gastrointestinal side effects and lack of appetite. Discontinuation of medications with a potential to negatively impact appetite is recommended, i.e., where nausea or anorexia are observed immediately after initiation and/or administration. Where this is not possible, treatments aimed at reducing nausea and improving gastrointestinal motility can be considered.

Algorithm 4.1 Note 5 Careful clinical questioning and/or observation of eating behaviors can also be of benefit to assess prehension, mastication, bolus formation, and swallowing. Direct evaluation of eating can be useful in addition to an owner's description to determine if oral pain, dysphagia, or regurgitation are present, and this can then lead to oral cavity examination, assessment of cranial nerve function, or swallowing studies.

Algorithm 4.1 Note 6 Oral pain could be secondary to dental disease, stomatogingivitis (primary or secondary to systemic diseases), oral ulcers, abscesses, or masses that cause discomfort during prehension, chewing, or swallowing. The presence of oral foreign bodies can result in similar signs. Pain when opening the mouth or trismus can also contribute to anorexia and be secondary to a plethora of diseases, including masticatory muscle myositis (MMM), temporomandibular joint (TMJ) disease, fractures, or retrobulbar disease, amongst others.

Algorithm 4.1 Note 7 Dysphagia, especially affecting the oropharyngeal phase of eating, can result in anorexia, although these patients may demonstrate a keenness but inability to eat or have pseudoanorexia. Underlying causes can include polyneuropathies, trigeminal or facial nerve diseases, as well as trauma. Regurgitation or esophagitis associated with esophageal dysphagia can also result in anorexia, often associated with nausea.

Algorithm 4.1 Note 8 A neurologic examination with particular attention to cranial nerve deficits could be useful to determine the origin of dysphagia. Other tests, e.g., electromyographies (EMGs) or AchR autoantibodies or infectious diseases tests (e.g., *Toxoplasma* spp., *Neospora* spp.) could also be considered based on presentation/neurologic findings to investigate neuropathies further. Fluoroscopy is sometimes useful to

ALGORITHM 4.1

Diagnostic approach to lack of appetite or poor appetite.

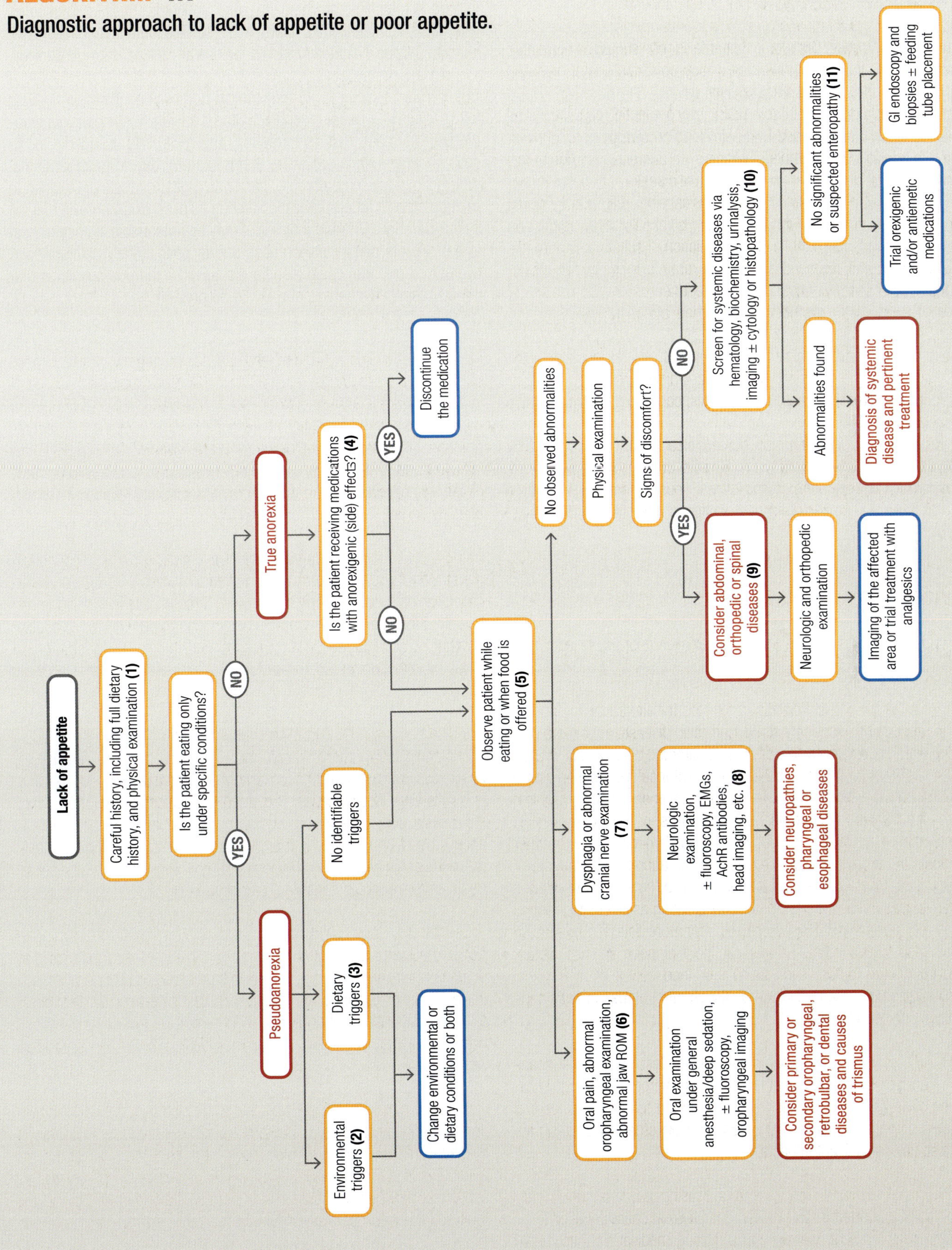

understand the cause of dysphagia, possibly in association with head and esophageal/thoracic imaging.

Algorithm 4.1 Note 9 Pain is a common cause of reduced appetite. A thorough physical examination helps to locate a source of pain and may direct the clinician toward a specific disease. For example, cranial abdominal discomfort can be seen with pancreatitis or gastrointestinal diseases, whilst retroperitoneal discomfort is more frequently demonstrated in conditions affecting the kidneys (e.g., pyelonephritis). Generalized abdominal discomfort is more difficult to interpret and can reflect primary GI disease or peritonitis, although referred pain due to spinal disease should not be dismissed (see chapter 11 for more details on cranial abdominal pain).

Some painful conditions, such as orthopedic or neurological diseases, can impact the ability to reach food physically.

Algorithm 4.1 Note 10 The minimum diagnostic workup should ideally include hematology, biochemistry, and urinalysis. Further diagnostics (e.g., cPLI, TLI, cobalamin, folate, ACTH stimulation test) and diagnostic imaging may be indicated based on the overall clinicopathologic findings.

Algorithm 4.1 Note 11 Where clinical and clinicopathologic findings fail to identify a cause definitively, the clinician might consider supportive treatment trials (antiemetics, analgesia, and orexigenic medications) where signs are acute and potentially due to gastroenteritis. Where signs are more chronic, performing gastrointestinal biopsies to exclude chronic enteropathy manifesting as hyporexia/anorexia may be a consideration. Offering a new diet may be reasonable in case refusal to eat reflects dietary preferences and/or poor dietary palatability. A hydrolyzed diet trial could also be discussed if there is suspicion that a food-responsive enteropathy could be present.

References

1. Washabau RJ, Day MJ (editors). Canine and Feline Gastroenterology. Elsevier Saunders, 2013.
2. Hall JE (editor). Guyton and Hall Textbook of Medical Physiology (Guyton and Hall) 13th edition. Elsevier, 2016.
3. Ettinger SJ, Feldman EC, Côté E (editors). Textbook of Veterinary Internal Medicine 8th edition. Elsevier, 2017.

CHAPTER 5

Polyphagia

Beatrice Ruggerone
DVM, PhD, DECVIM-CA

Fabio Procoli
DMV, MVetMed, DACVIM, DECVIM-CA, MRCVS

Pathophysiology

Polyphagia is defined by an increased food intake and can be further classified according to the etiology into three groups: (1) physiologic, which satisfies the need for a normal increase in metabolic rate (e.g., intense exercise, pregnancy, cold temperatures); (2) pathologic, when associated with diseases and, generally, with weight loss or gain; or (3) iatrogenic, secondary to drug administration (e.g., phenobarbital, corticosteroids, mirtazapine, antihistamines, progestins). In addition, breed-related differences in appetite exist: e.g., Labrador Retrievers and Flat-Coated Retrievers can suffer from a deletion in the pro-opiomelanocortin (POMC) gene, and this seems to be associated with adiposity and a greater food motivation;[1] on the other hand, smaller dogs often show more selective appetite.

Several neuronal centers in the hypothalamus participate in the control of food intake: polyphagia can be induced when the lateral nucleus is stimulated, whereas a total lack of interest in food can be seen following its destruction.[2] The ventromedial nucleus is the major satiety center and can transmit a nutritional satisfaction impulse inhibiting the feeding center. Moreover, hypothalamic nuclei can control the secretion of hormones involved with the regulation of metabolism and appetite, such as thyroidal, adrenal, and pancreatic hormones.

Neural signs from the gastrointestinal tract, chemical signs from nutrients in the blood, hormones produced by the gastrointestinal tract and adipose tissue, and signals from the cerebral cortex reach the hypothalamic nuclei, controlling food intake. Orexigenic (i.e., appetite-stimulating) hormones such as endorphins, cortisol, and ghrelin or anorexigenic (i.e., appetite suppressing) hormones such as leptin, serotonin, insulin, cholecystokinin influence the satiety center by altering appetite and feeding behavior.

A short-term system to regulate food intake exists: for example, cholecystokinin, released when lipids and proteins reach the duodenum, stimulates gallbladder contractions and gastric acid secretion and sends signals to the brain through the vagus nerve, ultimately contributing to satiety. Conversely, ghrelin is released by gastric oxyntic cells mainly during fasting and induces an increase in food intake in animals. An intermediate/long-term regulation of food intake is also present: glucose, amino acids, and lipids in the bloodstream can interfere with satiety and hunger; cold environmental temperatures can increase food intake, whereas leptin released by adipose tissue can decrease food intake, although this action is less effective in overweight animals.[3]

Nutritional deficiency can cause polyphagia; for example, dogs fed poorly balanced home-made diets or insufficient quantities of manufactured diet for their caloric needs. In addition, some dog breeds, such as Labrador Retrievers, are less able to regulate their appetites than other breeds. When physiologic, environmental, breed-related, and iatrogenic causes of polyphagia are excluded, some diseases typically associated with polyphagia in dogs and cats should be considered.

For example, dogs affected by hyperadrenocorticism, unlike humans and cats, show polyphagia because of an increased level of serum cortisol. Polyphagia in humans with diabetes mellitus is explained by the incapacity of glucose to enter the satiety center neurons in the absence of insulin and, as a consequence, the absence of intracellular glucose to reduce the feeling of hunger, in addition to weight loss due to glycosuria.[4] It is likely that the same mechanisms exist in dogs to justify polyphagia as one of the typical symptoms of diabetes mellitus. Insulin excess (e.g., insulinoma) can lead to polyphagia commonly associated with weight gain, whereas hypoglycemia (e.g., hepatic dysfunction arising from congenital or acquired liver diseases) can cause polyphagia associated with poor body condition. In cases of hyperthyroidism (rarely reported in dogs and typically caused by thyroid carcinoma), an increased metabolic rate is responsible for polyphagia associated with weight loss and behavioral and gastrointestinal alterations. Polyphagia may also occur due to an increase in metabolic rate caused by other neoplastic processes using energy inefficiently.

Polyphagia may occur due to maldigestion/malabsorption of food. Appetite changes are common in small intestinal inflammatory bowel disease, and affected dogs may show either a reduced or increased appetite. Exocrine pancreatic insufficiency (EPI) is another relevant cause of polyphagia, either caused by pancreatic acinar atrophy

or tissue destruction in chronic pancreatitis, with other rare causes including pancreatic duct obstruction, juvenile pancreatic hypoplasia and selective enzyme deficiency (see chapter 20 for more details).[5,6,7,8] In end-stage chronic pancreatitis, both EPI and diabetes mellitus may be present and responsible for polyphagia.[9] Another example of polyphagia secondary to malnutrition and reduced food assimilation is megaesophagus (congenital or acquired), especially if appropriate assisted feeding measures are not implemented (e.g., vertical feeding, selection of better-tolerated food consistency).
Finally, increased loss of nutrients may be associated with polyphagia, for example, in protein-losing enteropathy or nephropathy, in addition to the glycosuria of diabetes mellitus.

Clinical signs

When presented with a dog with presumed polyphagia, it is important to consider the patient's age, sex, reproductive status, and exercise levels, together with diet and caloric intake. Some dogs can be particularly food-driven, showing an excellent appetite since early life, and this is more common in certain breeds, e.g., Labrador Retriever. Pregnant or lactating bitches and racing dogs may show increased appetite in response to increased caloric expenditure, while neutered dogs might develop increased appetite following neutering surgery. A full dietary history should be taken. Any dietary change and introduction of more palatable, highly caloric foods (in the case of weight gain) or feeding of insufficient calories (in the case of weight loss) will need to be ruled out. The duration of the perceived polyphagia and the presence or absence of accompanying clinical signs (e.g., polyuria and polydipsia, weight loss, or diarrhea) will need to be ascertained.
Clinical signs of EPI related to pancreatic acinar atrophy are usually seen in young adults (1-4 years) and certain breeds.[6] Moreover, an aged dog with a history of chronic pancreatitis or gastrointestinal signs should be tested for EPI in the presence of polyphagia and weight loss. The presence of gastrointestinal signs associated with polyphagia might give clues as to which is the underlying pathology: in the case of regurgitation, megaesophagus will need to be ruled out, whereas vomiting and diarrhea can indicate a chronic intestinal or pancreatic disease with malabsorption (parasitism, chronic inflammatory enteropathy, neoplasia, chronic pancreatitis).
If concurrent polyuria and polydipsia are reported, diabetes mellitus and hyperadrenocorticism should be considered; in cases of polyphagia associated with severe weight loss in an old dog, a neoplastic condition should be suspected, and full investigations for occult neoplasia are indicated, including neck palpation to rule out the presence of a cervical mass (functional thyroid carcinoma with subsequent hyperthyroidism).

TABLE 5.1 **Main causes of polyphagia in dogs according to their pathophysiological classification.**

Insufficient caloric intake	Increased metabolism/use	Increased loss	Iatrogenic
Inadequate quantity of food	Lactation	Exocrine pancreatic insufficiency (EPI)	Phenobarbital
Inadequate quality of food	Cold temperatures	Chronic enteropathy (FRE, dysbiosis, IBD, PLE)	Corticosteroids
Megaesophagus or diseases causing dysphagia	Intense exercise	Parasitic disease	Mirtazapine
	Growth	PLN	Antihistamines
	Hyperadrenocorticism	Diabetes mellitus	Progestins
	Neoplasia	Hepatic dysfunction	
	Hyperthyroidism		
	Insulinoma		

FRE, food-responsive enteropathy; IBD, inflammatory bowel disease; PLE, protein-losing enteropathy; PLN, protein-losing nephropathy.

Diagnostic approach

The diagnostic approach to polyphagia is shown in Algorithm 5.1 (and summarized also in Table 5.1).

Algorithm 5.1 Note 1 To best define the initial diagnostic approach, it is advisable first to determine whether polyphagia is occurring in the face of weight loss or weight gain, as this will affect the list of differential diagnoses and the choice of diagnostic tests and their relative order.

Algorithm 5.1 Note 2 Moreover, the signalment could help to understand if the quality and quantity of food are adequate for the patient; in a young dog, it is important to evaluate its growing curve and definitive weight because polyphagia can mask an inappropriate energy intake. Not only the quantity but also the quality of food should be considered in a growing puppy, considering the different food composition for adults. Calculating the dog's energy requirement is possible using the formulae detailed in chapter 3 and Table 3.2, although any formula is only an average value and not an exact figure for every dog. Owners should be encouraged to use this as a starting point and then feed to maintain adult body weight. Therefore, the metabolizable energy of the administered food can be used to evaluate if the dog is assuming a correct intake after calculating its daily energy requirement.

Algorithm 5.1 Note 3 If the history shows vomiting, diarrhea, or regurgitation and/or if the dog shows a poor coat suggestive of fat maldigestion, the investigation will focus on ruling our maldigestion/malabsorption.

Algorithm 5.1 Note 4 A TLI value less than the cutoff for EPI defined by the laboratory indicates EPI, whereas if the TLI value is in the gray zone, it should be reassessed within one month or after trial therapy with pancreatic enzymes in animals with consistent clinical signs (for more details see chapter 20). Moreover, if EPI is strongly suspected, but TLI is within normal reference intervals, it is suggested that potential chronic pancreatitis be considered and an appropriate workup pursued (see chapters 19 and 20). A trial course of pancreatic enzymes might be indicated in suspected chronic pancreatitis.

Algorithm 5.1 Note 5 Cobalamin or vitamin B_{12} should be supplemented whenever serum cobalamin concentration is suboptimal (less than 400 ng/L). Acquired hypocobalaminemia in dogs is generally due to a decreased absorption from the ileum (chronic inflammation,

ALGORITHM 5.1

Diagnostic approach to polyphagia.

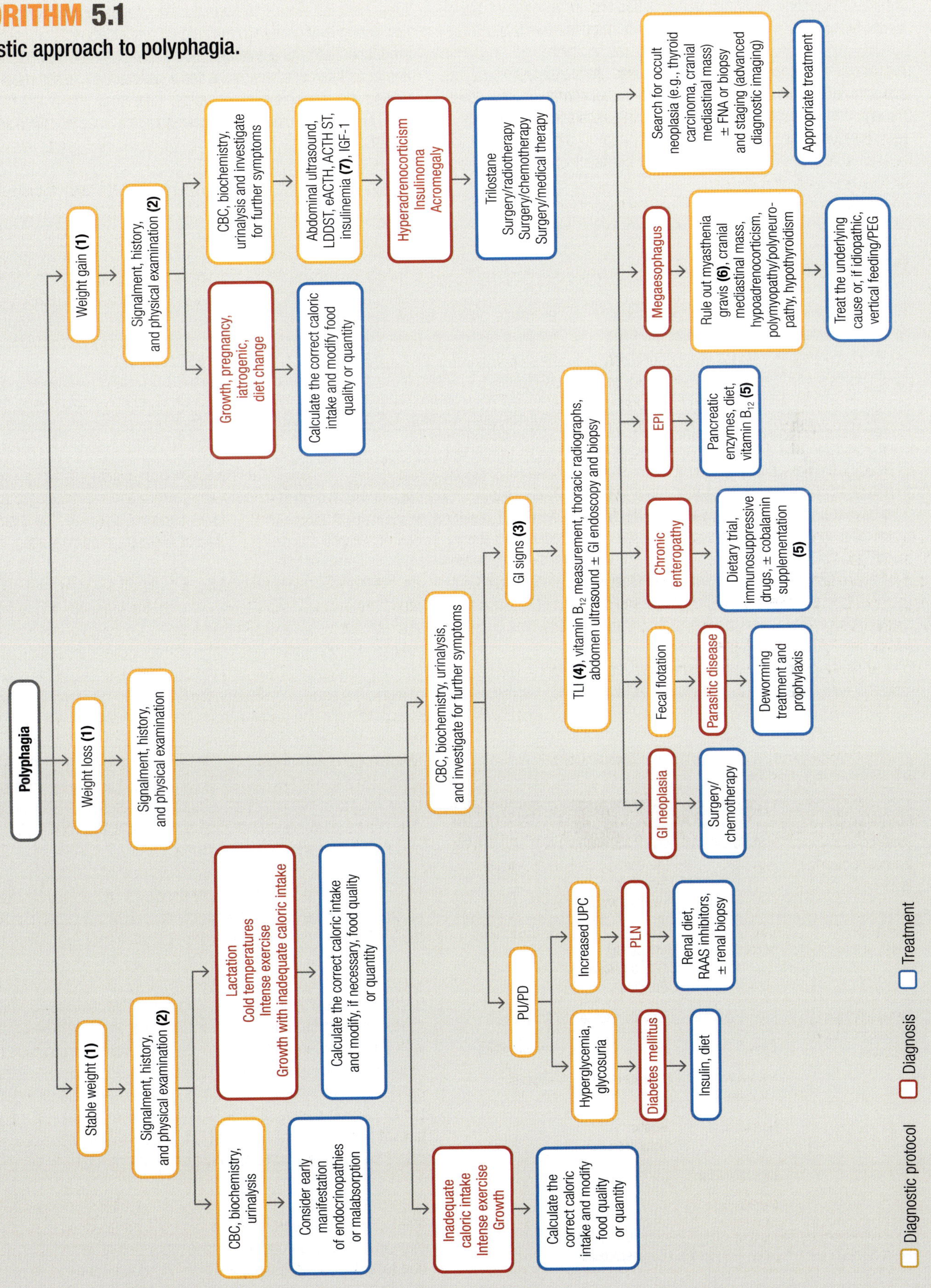

surgical resection), microbial consumption, or an absence of the intrinsic factor, which is mainly produced by the pancreas (e.g., EPI).[10]

Algorithm 5.1 Note 6 Among the causes of megaesophagus, myasthenia gravis should be considered. Its confirmation is possible through the measurement of acetylcholine receptor autoantibody by radioimmunoassay.[11]

Algorithm 5.1 Note 7 A normal or increased serum insulin concentration during hypoglycemia (<40 mg/dL) can confirm an abnormal insulin production and, as a consequence, strengthen the suspicion of insulinoma. In this case, searching for a pancreatic mass through imaging (abdominal ultrasound examination, total body computed tomography [TBCT], or abdominal magnetic resonance imaging, MRI) is strongly suggested.

References

1. Raffan E, Dennis RJ, O'Donovan CJ, et al. A deletion in the canine POMC gene is associated with weight and appetite in obesity-prone Labrador retriever dogs. *Cell Metabolism* 23:893-900, 2016.
2. Hall JE. Dietary balances; regulation of feeding; obesity and starvation; vitamins and minerals. In Hall JE (editor). Guyton and Hall. Textbook of Medical Physiology 14th edition. Philadelphia, Elsevier Saunders, 2021, pp. 879-880.
3. Cortese L, Terrazzano G, Pelagalli A. Leptin and immunological profile in obesity and its associated diseases in dogs. *Int J Molecular Sci* 20:2392, 2019.
4. Nelson RW. Canine diabetes mellitus. In Feldman EC, Nelson RW, Reusch C, Scott-Moncrieff JC, Behrend E (editors). Canine and Feline Endocrinology 4th edition. St. Louis, Elsevier Saunders, 2015, p. 217.
5. Westermarck E, Wiberg M. Exocrine pancreatic insufficiency in the dog: historical background, diagnosis, and treatment. *Top Companion Anim Med* 27:96-103, 2012.
6. Westermarck E, Saari SA, Wiberg ME. Heritability of exocrine pancreatic insufficiency in German Shepherd dogs. *J Vet Int Med* 24:450-452, 2010.
7. Wiberg ME, Saari SA, Westermarck E. Exocrine pancreatic atrophy in German Shepherd dogs and Rough-coated Collies: an end-result of lymphocytic pancreatitis. *Vet Pathol* 36:530-541, 1999.
8. Viviano KR, Ziglioli V. Suspected isolated pancreatic enzyme deficiency in dogs. *J Vet Intern Med* 27:588-592, 2013.
9. Davison LJ. Diabetes mellitus and pancreatitis – cause of effect? *J Small Anim Pract* 56(1): 50-59, 2015.
10. Kather S, Grützner, Kook P, et al. Review of cobalamin status and disorders of cobalamin metabolism in dogs. *J Vet Intern Med* 34:13-38, 2020.
11. Shelton GD. Myasthenia gravis and disorders of neuromuscular transmission. *Vet Clin North Am Small Anim Pract* 32:189-206, 2002.

CHAPTER 6

Polyuria/polydipsia

Beatrice Ruggerone
DVM, PhD, DECVIM-CA

Fabio Procoli
DVM, DACVIM, DECVIM-CA

Pathophysiology

Water is essential for life, and several mechanisms exist in humans and animals to maintain its homeostasis. It is introduced in the organism by ingesting liquids and in food but is also synthesized by carbohydrate oxidation. It is lost normally through breath, urine, and feces. Several conditions (e.g., environmental temperature, physical activity, drugs, or diseases) can affect water intake or loss.[1]

Water homeostasis is controlled by complex interactions involving plasma osmolarity, the hypothalamus, the neurohypophysis, and the kidneys. The two main players in the maintenance of water balance are thirst and the antidiuretic hormone (ADH), also known as arginine-vasopressin. ADH is produced by the hypothalamic supraoptic and paraventricular nuclei and transported to the neurohypophysis in neurons, from which it is released after stimulation of osmoreceptors in the hypothalamus. Osmoceptors perceive subtle changes in body fluid concentration and induce ADH release to maintain stable blood osmolarity. ADH exerts its antidiuretic effect on the kidneys by stimulating the insertion of both water channels (aquaporins) and urea transporters into the luminal membrane of the renal collecting ducts, thus increasing the ability of the collecting ducts to reabsorb water and retain it within the body. The result is decreased plasma osmolarity and more concentrated urine. Conversely, in the absence of ADH, the renal collecting ducts become impermeable to water, which is thus lost in more diluted urine, reducing overall body fluid content.[2] Two other main stimuli can concur to induce ADH release: a drop in blood pressure and a loss of blood volume. In the normal dog, arterial baroreceptors and atrial and venous stretch receptors stimulate the hypothalamus and inhibit ADH release. In the case of systemic hypotension or a large drop in blood volume, the firing of these receptors is reduced, which will induce ADH release. In these circumstances, ADH acts as a vasoconstrictor in addition to increasing water retention, both of which increase or maintain blood pressure in the case of sudden loss of blood volume, such as acute hemorrhage.

Thirst is an important part of water balance as it is the only way to increase water intake rather than just preserve what is already present in the body. It is controlled by the thirst center in the hypothalamus and, like ADH, is stimulated by a change in osmolarity or a large drop in blood volume.

In dogs, polydipsia (PD) is defined by a water intake greater than 100 mL/kg/day. Normal water intake is 50 mL/kg/day, so there is a gray area in between. Polyuria (PU) is defined by a urine output exceeding 50 mL/kg/day. Both polyuria and polydipsia can be primary or secondary.

Causes of primary polyuria in dogs can be classified according to the underlying physiopathology (Table 6.1) and include primary central (pituitary) diabetes insipidus (CDI), primary nephrogenic diabetes insipidus (NDI), secondary NDI, interference with the hypothalamic release of ADH, and osmotic diuresis-induced.[3] Primary CDI is uncommon and derives from a partial or complete lack of ADH production. Trauma, neoplasia, cysts, inflammation, aberrant parasite migration, or congenital defects involving supraoptic and paraventricular nuclei and/or axons carrying ADH to the neurohypophysis can all be responsible for CDI. An idiopathic form of CDI affecting dogs of any breed, age, and sex is also recognized. An impaired response of nephrons to ADH causes NDI. A congenital form is very rarely reported in dogs, whereas acquired NDI is by far more frequent, caused by various pathophysiological mechanisms: (1) bacterial endotoxins during infections (e.g., pyometra, pyelonephritis, prostatitis) can compete with ADH for its receptors leading to absent or reduced downstream response which may be reversible after the resolution of the infection; (2) excess of endogenous or exogenous glucocorticoids inhibits ADH release and decreases renal response; (3) significant and persistent hyponatremia (e.g., associated with hypoadrenocorticism and subsequent mineralocorticoid deficiency) or low plasma urea nitrogen concentration (e.g., during hepatic dysfunction) will disrupt the renal medullary osmotic gradient resulting in decreased ability to concentrate urine; (4) hypercalcemia can compete with ADH for its renal receptors and downregulates water channel numbers in collecting ducts; (5) in patients with hepatic dysfunction, the mechanisms for polyuria are poorly understood but altered cortisol metabolism can contribute. Polyuria can be a consequence of osmotic diuresis caused by (1) severe glycosuria, as seen during diabetes mellitus (DM) or primary renal glycosuria; (2) chronic kidney disease (CKD), where the remaining functioning nephrons will increase the glomerular filtration rate to compensate for the progressive loss of renal function, but causing loss of urea and sodium responsible for maintaining the renal medullary osmotic gradient; (3) hypoadrenocorticism as a result of reduced reabsorption of sodium in the kidneys and postobstructive diuresis, as a consequence of severe azotemia and electrolyte disturbances. Polyuria (with secondary polydipsia) can also be induced by drugs, such as glucocorticoids, mineralocorticoids, diuretics, and phenobarbital.

Polydipsia can be "primary" (Table 6.1) or "psychogenic" when related to behavioral disorders (e.g., environmental stress, mainly in young animals), or hepatic encephalopathy, "secondary" when caused by fever, nausea[4] or gastrointestinal diseases,[5,6,7,8] or compensating for polyuria. It is important to rule out physiological polydipsia, e.g., due to a high salt diet, dried food, or heat. In dogs with or at risk of pancreatitis, polydipsia is reported, although the mechanisms are poorly understood. It could be induced by nausea or be a consequence of comorbidities or drugs (e.g., endocrinopathies, phenobarbital administration), and chronic pancreatitis appears to resolve with a change of diet.[8] Polydipsia has also been reported in gastrointestinal diseases in excess of that expected with diarrhea. The mechanism is not clear, but the control of gastrointestinal symptoms seems to be associated with the resolution of polydipsia.[5]

Clinical signs

The owner should ideally be asked to measure water intake to confirm the presence of PU/PD and confirm if PU is associated with PD. Owners may report the development of urinary incontinence as a consequence of a larger amount of urine production or the tendency to drink any liquid. The concurrent presence of other clinical signs can be helpful in localizing the primary disease responsible for polyuria/polydipsia (e.g., weight loss and hyporexia in CKD, polyphagia in hyperadrenocorticism (HAC) or DM, abdominal pain and/or diarrhea in pancreatitis or gastrointestinal diseases). Neurological signs (e.g., disorientation, blindness, circling) can be due to the presence of a pituitary mass or head trauma, whereas a change in the coat (trunk symmetrical alopecia) and other dermatological alterations are generally present in dogs with HAC.

In the case of idiopathic or congenital DI, dogs are bright and alert, and if water access is not restricted, their hydration status is normal. On the other hand, a dog with CKD or severe gastrointestinal signs can appear dehydrated and in poor body condition.

Diagnostic approach

The diagnostic approach to the patient with polydipsia/polyuria is shown in Algorithm 6.1.

Algorithm 6.1 Note 1 Polyuria and polydipsia are commonly reported by owners and usually present concurrently. The first step is to check USG to confirm the suspicion and then to establish which is the primary problem; when primary polydipsia is suspected, it is suggested to investigate a behavioral, physiological, or psychogenic stimulus but also to consider the presence of chronic or acute gastroenteric/pancreatic signs. Conversely, if the main symptom is polyuria, different systems should be evaluated.

Algorithm 6.1 Note 2 It is important to quantify water intake to confirm PU/PD.

Algorithm 6.1 Note 3 Remember to determine neutering status, dietary and drug history, recent trauma, and the presence of other clinical signs such as weight loss, loss of appetite, and GI signs. The signalment can be helpful: older dogs are more likely to develop CKD, HAC, and DM, whereas younger dogs are more predisposed to congenital hypothalamic/pituitary malformations, portosystemic shunts, and hypoadrenocorticism. Breeds more predisposed to chronic pancreatitis (e.g., Cavalier King Charles Spaniels, Collies, Cocker Spaniel, and Boxer)[9] could have a higher risk of developing diabetes mellitus[10] as a cause of polyuria/polydipsia. Females with vulval discharge or with signs of sepsis could have developed a pyometra or, in the case of hematuria, pyelonephritis. In adult entire males with acute abdomen and fever the presence of prostatitis should be promptly investigated.

Algorithm 6.1 Note 4 Concurrent blood and urine samples should be analyzed to check electrolytes, including calcium, and to identify azotemia. Urinalysis, including culture to rule out infection, is advised.

Algorithm 6.1 Note 5 Depending on clinical signs and laboratory results, a definitive diagnosis can be achieved through:

TABLE 6.1 Differential diagnoses for polyuria/polydipsia in dogs divided according to pathophysiology.

Acquired nephrogenic diabetes insipidus	Primary diabetes insipidus	Osmotic diuresis	Primary/secondary polydipsia	Drug-induced
■ Bacterial endotoxins, mainly produced by *Escherichia coli* ■ Hypercalcemia ■ Hyperadrenocorticism ■ Hyperthyroidism (rare) ■ Hepatic dysfunction ■ Hyperaldosteronism ■ Pheochromocytoma (rare) ■ Acromegaly ■ Polycythemia	■ Nephrogenic: rare congenital disorder of aquaporin insertion in renal collecting ducts ■ Central: hypothalamic or pituitary lesion (see text) or idiopathic ■ Hypophysectomy	■ Diabetes mellitus ■ Fanconi syndrome ■ Primary renal glycosuria ■ Postobstructive diuresis ■ Chronic kidney disease ■ Hypoadrenocorticism	■ Psychogenic ■ Physiological (high salt diet, dried food, heat) ■ Fever ■ Gastrointestinal disease or pancreatitis ■ Hepatic encephalopathy	■ Glucocorticoids ■ Diuretics ■ Phenobarbital ■ Mannitol ■ Levothyroxine ■ Desoxycortone pivalate

ALGORITHM 6.1

Diagnostic approach to the patient with polydipsia/polyuria.*

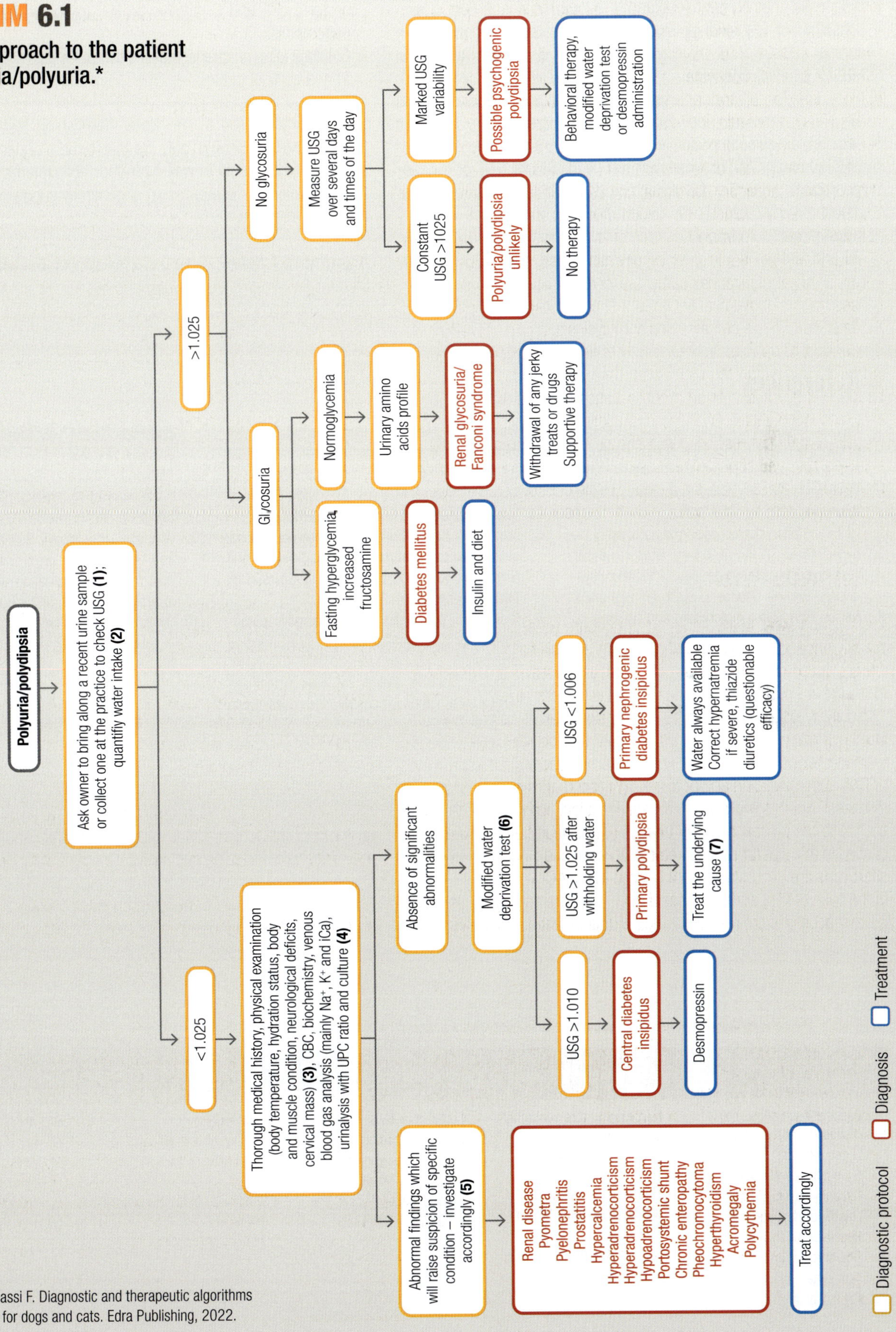

*Adapted from Fracassi F. Diagnostic and therapeutic algorithms in internal medicine for dogs and cats. Edra Publishing, 2022.

- Diagnostic imaging (ultrasonography to look for uterine fluid distention, signs of acute kidney injury, prostatic disease, adrenomegaly or adrenal masses, PSS; CT imaging for cervical or adrenal mass, PSS; MRI for pituitary adenoma).
- More specific laboratory examinations (bile acid stimulation test (BAST) or ammonia test for PSS/hepatic dysfunction; low-dose dexamethasone suppression test (LDDST) for HAC, endogenous ACTH (eACTH) and/or ACTH stimulation test (ACTHST) for HAC or hypoadrenorticism; urinary or plasmatic normetanephrine measurement for pheochromocytoma; tT_4 for hyperthyroidism; aldosterone or IGF-1 measurement for hyperaldosteronism and acromegaly, respectively; TLI and vitamin B_{12} in case of gastrointestinal signs; DGGR lipase or Spec cPL and C-reactive protein to search for acute or chronic pancreatitis).
- Cytology (e.g., of adrenal masses to differentiate a pheochromocytoma from a cortical tumor).

Algorithm 6.1 Note 6 The water deprivation test is laborious and not risk-free; it should only be performed under strict veterinary surveillance and only in well-hydrated, nonazotemic dogs. The direct administration of desmopressin is generally suggested as a safer and simpler alternative.

Algorithm 6.1 Note 7 Consider a behaviorist evaluation.

References

1. Hall JE. Regulation of body fluid compartments: extracellular and intracellular fluids; edema. In Hall JE (editor). Guyton and Hall. Textbook of Medical Physiology 14th edition. Philadelphia, Elsevier Saunders, 2021, pp. 305-320.
2. Hall JE. Pituitary hormones and their control by the hypothalamus. In Hall JE (editor). Guyton and Hall. Textbook of Medical Physiology 14th edition. Philadelphia, Elsevier Saunders, 2021, pp. 929-940.
3. Nelson RW. Water metabolism and diabetes insipidus. In Feldman EC, Nelson RW, Reusch C, Scott-Moncrieff JC, Behrend E (editors). Canine and Feline Endocrinology 4th edition. St. Louis, Elsevier Saunders, 2015, pp. 1-37.
4. Rothuizen J, Meyer HP. History, physical examination, and signs of liver disease. In Ettinger SJ, Feldman EC, Côté E (editors). Textbook of Veterinary Internal Medicine 5th edition. St. Louis, Elsevier Saunders, 2000, pp. 1272-1277.
5. Henderson SM, Elwood CM. A potential causal association between gastrointestinal disease and primary polydipsia in three dogs. *J Small Anim Pract* 44(6):280-284, 2003.
6. Craven M, Washabau RJ. Comparative pathophysiology and management of protein-losing enteropathy. *J Vet Intern Med* 33:383-402, 2019.
7. Cridge H, Scott N, Steiner JM. Risk factors and clinical presentation in dogs with increased serum pancreatic lipase concentration – A descriptive analysis. *Animals* 12:1581, 2022.
8. Watson PJ, Archer J, Roulois AJ, et al. Observational study of 14 cases of chronic pancreatitis in dogs. *Vet Rec* 167:968-976, 2010.
9. Watson PJ, Roulois AJ, Scase T, et al. Prevalence and breed distribution of chronic pancreatitis at post-mortem examination in first-opinion dog. *J Small Anim Pract* 48(11):609-618, 2007.
10. Davison LJ. Diabetes mellitus and pancreatitis – cause of effect? *J Small Anim Pract* 56(1): 50-59, 2015.

CHAPTER 7

Lethargy/stupor/pacing

Susana Monforte
DVM, MSc, CertAVP
PGCertVPS AFHEA,
DECVN, PhD candidate

Pathophysiology

Hepatic dysfunction due to liver disease or urea cycle disorders or, most commonly in dogs, portosystemic shunt (PSS) can lead to an abnormal neurological presentation referred to as hepatic encephalopathy (HE). The pathophysiology of HE encompasses both endogenous and exogenous factors, with abnormal mental status and/or behavior arising from changes in neurotransmission, cell energy metabolism, and, in severe cases, raised intracranial pressure (ICP). The most widely accepted cause of HE is hyperammonemia-induced astrocytic failure.[1,2,3]

TABLE 7.1 Precipitating factors for hepatic encephalopathy.

Gastrointestinal hemorrhage/ excessive protein intake	■ Increase in ammonia, GABA, aromatic amino acids (AAA)
Constipation	■ Increase in formation of bacterial breakdown products – ammonia, short-chain fatty acids, mercaptans
Infection/sepsis	■ Increase in protein metabolism –increase in ammonia and AAA ■ Potential increase in urease-producing bacteria –increase in ammonia ■ SIRS –increase in cytokines, increase in ammonia CNS diffusion, and expression of benzodiazepine binding sites
Renal dysfunction	■ Impaired clearance of ammonia and urea ■ Predisposition to acid-base disturbance, electrolyte imbalance, and reduced intravascular volume –contribution to altered mental status
Metabolic abnormalities Metabolic alkalosis Hypokalemia Hyponatremia Hypoglycemia	■ Increase in ammonia and CNS diffusion ■ Increase in ammonia ■ Renal ammoniogenesis ■ Reduction of myoinositol in CNS –cerebral edema ■ Neuroglycopenia –increased vulnerability to hyperammonemia
Dehydration	■ Activation of RAAS –hypokalemia
Anorexia	■ Increase in catabolism –loss of skeletal muscle mass, loss of hyperammonemia buffer ■ Hypokalemia, hypoglycemia, dehydration ■ Decrease in zinc –impairment of urea cycle
Medications with hepatic metabolism (opioids, benzodiazepines)	■ Accumulation of the drug and exacerbation of altered mental status
Furosemide	■ Depletion of intravascular volume, hypokalemia, alkalosis

Ammonia is largely produced in the gastrointestinal tract. This is mainly by the deamination of glutamine via glutaminase by the small intestinal enterocytes to provide energy, but it is also via bacterial metabolism of both urea and large proteins and nitrogenous dietary products.[2,3] Ammonia reaches the liver via the portal circulation, where detoxification occurs via two main mechanisms: 1) periportal hepatocytes have a high affinity for ammonia and convert it into urea via the urea cycle. Urea is then excreted renally or through enterohepatic circulation and bacterial metabolism, and 2) more centrilobular hepatocytes have a lower affinity for ammonia and use it to convert glutamate to glutamine.[2,3] Only with 65-70% loss of functional hepatic mass is the ammonia detoxification ability of the liver impaired. Alternatively, PSS allows blood to bypass the liver, avoiding these metabolic processes. The kidneys can also synthesize and break down glutamine from and to ammonia, respectively, and have an important role in eliminating both ammonia and urea via urine excretion.[1,2] Maintenance of acid-base balance is also closely related to the generation of ammonium and bicarbonate from glutamine metabolism in the kidneys coupled with changes in glutamine production in the liver. Finally, the skeletal muscle is able to use ammonia as a substrate for the production of glutamine, reducing blood ammonia.[2,3]

There are several mechanisms that can precipitate or exacerbate HE, most of them via their action on ammonia metabolism. These include causes of increased protein metabolism, acid-base changes, or electrolyte imbalances. More details on these can be found in Table 7.1.

Clinical signs

Dogs with HE can present with a vast spectrum of neurological abnormalities. The most common neurological signs are obtundation and altered behavior (Video 7.1), but ataxia, head pressing, seizures, lethargy, and visual deficits are also common findings.[4,5] HE, as a neurological presentation, is mainly believed to be due to the action of ammonia as a neurotoxin. An elevated ammonia concentration in the central nervous system (CNS) causes astrocytic dysfunction and, consequently,

Video 7.1

A 2-year-old Bichon with a PSS and neurological signs. Notice the marked change in the mental status (obtundation) and mild head bobbing. This dog had severe behavioral changes and focal seizures.

neuronal impairment. Other hypotheses have been proposed for the development of HE in dogs (Table 7.2), and the different mechanisms might work in synergy.

Astrocytes are the most numerous glial cells, responsible for supporting neurons via several different mechanisms, and are the only CNS cells able to detoxify ammonia.[2,3] Glutamine produced from ammonia is released from the astrocyte and utilized by the neuron in the intracellular production of glutamate used at the synapse. Released glutamate is reused, together with ammonia, by the astrocyte in the formation of more glutamine. With hyperammonemia, the production of glutamine by the astrocyte increases. The additional extracellular glutamine causes an inhibition of its release by the astrocyte, and consequent accumulation within the cell leads to mitochondrial oxidative damage (ROS production) and dysfunction. Furthermore, intracellular accumulation of ammonia in the astrocytes causes impairment of the tricarboxylic acid cycle with consequent lactate production. These processes ultimately lead to neuroastrocytic glutamate trafficking disruption, cellular metabolic failure, and accumulation of glutamine within the astrocyte causes an increase in the intracellular osmotic pressure and cell swelling –this gliopathy is referred to as "Alzheimer type II astrocytosis".[2,3]

Depending on how quickly this process takes place, the autoregulatory mechanisms of the brain might not be able to control and adapt to the volume expansion caused by the astrocyte dysfunction-associated cytotoxic cerebral edema.[1] In severe, acute cases, the sudden change of volume leading to an increase in ICP could cause brain herniation and consequent death. This extreme presentation can be associated with acute liver failure and is rarely seen in dogs. With the much more common chronic form, which is usually seen with PSS, signs can be subtle and episodic, but persistent and more marked neurological changes can also be found.[2]

TABLE 7.2 Other proposed pathophysiological causes for hepatic encephalopathy.

Manganese CNS accumulation	Alzheimer type II astrocytosis –dysfunction of the glutamatergic system and brain energy metabolism
Aromatic amino acids increased concentration	Synthesis of false neurotransmitters – catecholaminergic neurotransmission dysfunction
Altered serotonin metabolism	Reduced serotonergic neurotransmission
Neuroinflammation, increased levels of TNF-α	Increased ammonia diffusion, GABA (γ-aminobutyric acid), and glutamate receptor-mediated neurotoxicity
Increase in GABAergic tone	Increased activation of GABA receptors by neurosteroids. Controversial role of endogenous benzodiazepines

Diagnostic approach

Algorithm 7.1 provides the approach to the patient with altered mental status/behavior, which is the most common presentation for HE.

The diagnosis of HE is based mainly on two factors: 1) a neurological presentation compatible with a metabolic encephalopathy and 2) laboratory findings consistent with hepatic dysfunction or PSS. Diagnostic imaging findings and a positive response to treatment further support the diagnosis.

Algorithm 7.1 Note 1 Most cases of canine HE are seen in young dogs with congenital extrahepatic PSS. Some breeds are predisposed, such as Havanese, Yorkshire Terriers, and Miniature Schnauzers.[4,5] Other causes of HE include intrahepatic PSS, which is more common in large breeds, and acquired extrahepatic shunts. The latter are secondary to chronic portal hypertension, which may be due to end-stage chronic hepatitis/cirrhosis or a variety of congenital diseases, such as portal vein hypoplasia, ductal plate disease, and arteriovenous fistula. A typical history of HE can include episodic or persistent clinical signs, failure to gain weight, gastrointestinal signs, or exacerbation of neurological abnormalities with eating.[4,5]

Algorithm 7.1 Note 2 An altered mental status can be found in several debilitating conditions, including severe circulatory compromise/hypovolemia, endotoxemia, and cardiac or respiratory disease. A complete physical examination should uncover signs supportive of these disorders and guide the diagnostic plan.

Algorithm 7.1 Note 3 Reflex bradycardia secondary to systemic hypertension can be found in dogs with severe alteration of the mental status and indicate an increase in ICP. This presentation is called "Cushing's reflex" and is considered a medical emergency.

Algorithm 7.1 Note 4 If increased ICP is suspected, emergency treatment to target cerebral edema should start. Mannitol and hypertonic saline act as osmotic agents to reduce ICP, and IVFT aims to maintain normotension. Mild hypothermia can help avoid an increase in metabolic rate and cerebral blood flow. Hypercapnia must be avoided, as it increases cerebral blood flow and ICP. However, care should be taken not to hyperventilate and cause marked hypocapnia, as this could decrease cerebral perfusion. End-tidal CO_2 of 35 mmHg is typically the target of capnographic monitoring. Acid-base balance and blood glucose should be checked and corrected to avoid further neurological deterioration.[1]

If the dog is seizuring, levetiracetam, which is not extensively metabolized by the liver, is the preferred long-acting medication. Benzodiazepines such as midazolam can be used for a quicker effect, but with care.[9] Benzodiazepines undergo hepatic metabolism and have been shown to precipitate HE in people with severe hepatic disease. Should the dog continue seizuring, propofol should be started.

Algorithm 7.1 Note 5 The neurological examination will allow the classification of the suspected cause as focal/lateralized or nonfocal. HE typically has a diffuse distribution in the brain, although lateralized signs can be seen.[6]

Algorithm 7.1 Note 6 Several laboratory abnormalities can be found in the blood or urine of dogs with HE. More specific tests include the measurement of pre- and postprandial bile acid concentrations and ammonia

ALGORITHM 7.1

Diagnostic approach to the patient with altered mental status/behavior.

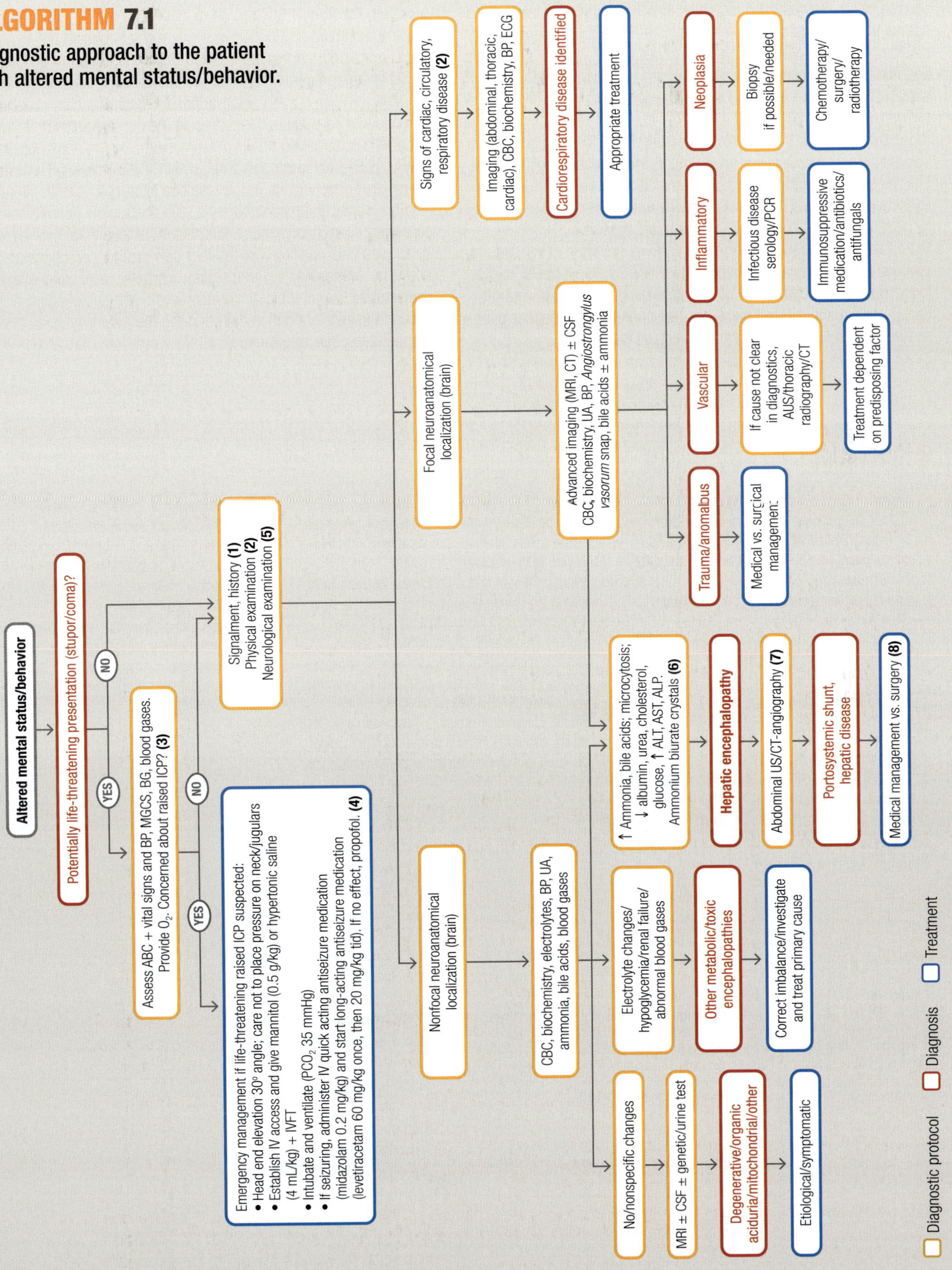

concentration. Both can be increased in HE, but not exclusively, and normal values do not exclude it. Fasting ammonia is considered a poor predictor of HE severity in dogs.[7] In a population of dogs with seizures and documented hepatopathy, preprandial bile acids were abnormal in about 60% of the cases, but postprandial were elevated in all cases.[8]

Algorithm 7.1 Note 7 Abdominal ultrasound and CT-angiography are common diagnostic imaging modalities in investigating dogs with HE. The use of portal scintigraphy and MRI angiography are also described.[4,5] Patients with acquired hepatic disease may require liver biopsies followed by histological characterization to achieve a diagnosis.
Brain imaging is rarely performed. On MRI of the brain, T1W bilateral symmetric hyperintensities at the level of the lentiform nuclei can be found due to the deposition of manganese, among other changes.[9] Certain patterns for HE can be recognized in magnetic resonance spectroscopy, as well as in electroencephalographic studies[10].

Algorithm 7.1 Note 8 HE can be managed medically, with treatment targeting ammonia production/absorption. Diets should not be highly protein-restricted, as this can lead to muscle catabolism and consequent hyperammonemia, but rather, they should incorporate highly digestible protein spread over multiple smaller meals. Lactulose, given orally or via enema, depending on the neurological presentation, promotes the formation of NH_4^+ (ammonium), which does not diffuse easily, creating an "ammonia trap" within the intestines. From its digestion result, fatty acids act as osmotic laxatives, remove ammonia and nitrogenous dietary components, and change the gut microbiome, decreasing ammoniagenesis. Care should be taken when administering lactulose, as possible consequent dehydration can aggravate HE. Neomycin, metronidazole, amoxicillin-clavulanic acid, and ampicillin are described to alter the gut microbiome and reduce ammoniagenesis, although typically are only required in the more severe cases that fail to respond to other treatment.[2,4]

References

1. Galvao J, Center S. Fluid, electrolyte, and acid-base disturbances in liver disease. In DiBartola SP (editor). Fluid, Electrolyte and Acid-base Disorders in Small Animal Practice 4th edition. St Louis, Elsevier Saunders, 2012, p. 15.
2. Gow A. Hepatic encephalopathy. *Vet Clin North Am Small Anim Pract* 47(3):585-599, 2017.
3. El Khiat A, El Hiba O, Aimrane A, Draoui A, Jayakumar AR, Norenberg MD, Gamrani H. Hepatic encephalopathy: an overview of basic concepts and mechanisms. *Front Med Case Rep* 3:1-19, 2022.
4. Lidbury JA, Cook AK, Steiner JM. Hepatic encephalopathy in dogs and cats. *J Vet Emerg Crit Care (San Antonio)* 26(4):471-487, 2016.
5. Dewey C. Encephalopathies: disorders of the brain. In Dewey C, da Costa R (editors). Practical Guide to Canine and Feline Neurology 3rd edition. Ames, Wiley-Blackwell, 2016, p. 7.
6. Windsor RC, Olby NJ. Congenital portosystemic shunts in five mature dogs with neurological signs. *J Am Anim Hosp Assoc* 43(6):322-331, 2007.
7. Lidbury JA, Ivanek R, Suchodolski JS, Steiner JM. Putative precipitating factors for hepatic encephalopathy in dogs: 118 cases (1991-2014). *J Am Vet Med Assoc* 247(2):176-183, 2015.
8. Fisher C, Harcourt-Brown T. Diagnostic utility of serum bile acids in dogs presenting with epileptic seizures consistent with a tier 1 confidence level diagnosis of idiopathic epilepsy. *Vet Rec* 10:e2585, 2023. Epub ahead of print.
9. Chandler S, Googs R. Metabolic encephalopathies. In Platt S, Garosi L (editors). Small Animal Neurological Emergencies 1st edition. Boca Raton, CRC Press, 2012, p. 27.
10. Wrzosek MA, Płonek MA, Nicpoń JÓ. Electroencephalographic features of metabolic encephalopathy in dogs. *Med Weter* 71:100-103, 2015.

CHAPTER 8

Jaundice

Frederik Allan
BVMedSci (Hons), BVM
BVS (Hons), MRCVS

Pathophysiology

Yellow discoloration of the skin and mucus membranes secondary to the deposition of bilirubin pigments is referred to as jaundice (or icterus). This is often most noticeable at the mucus membranes, sclera, inner aspect of the pinnae and the oropharyngeal mucosa, and can be detectable in other thin-skinned areas such as the inguinum, axillae, and ventral abdomen. Visible jaundice occurs once total bilirubin levels exceed 35-50 μmol/L (2.0-3.0 mg/dL; normal reference interval <4.2 μmol/L; <0.25 mg/dL).

A general understanding of the physiology of bilirubin metabolism is useful when considering the approach to the jaundiced patient. Bilirubin is the major endpoint of heme metabolism from red blood cell breakdown. Briefly, in the reticuloendothelial system in the spleen and liver, heme is cleaved to biliverdin which is then reduced to bilirubin. Unconjugated bilirubin is reversibly bound to albumin and transported to the liver where it is released from albumin and absorbed through the hepatocyte cell membrane. Bilirubin is then metabolized within hepatocytes to a conjugated form. Conjugated bilirubin is actively transported into bile canaliculi and stored in the gallbladder prior to excretion (via the common bile duct) into the duodenum. The intestinal microflora then converts bilirubin through a series of products until it reaches its terminal product, stercobilin, which is then eventually incorporated into feces and defecated.

Through consideration of the stages of bilirubin production and metabolism, the diagnostic approach to jaundice relies upon determining whether jaundice is prehepatic, hepatic, or posthepatic in origin (Table 8.1).

Prehepatic jaundice refers to hemolysis. Extravascular hemolysis is often the major contributor to this, as intravascular hemolysis produces only small amounts of bilirubin. In extravascular hemolysis, increased bilirubin production often overwhelms the excretory capacity of the liver and results in bilirubin deposition in the tissues. Hepatic jaundice results from hepatocellular dysfunction causing abnormal uptake, conjugation, or excretion of bilirubin. As the liver has an impressive

TABLE 8.1 Differential diagnoses of prehepatic, hepatic, and posthepatic jaundice.

Prehepatic	Hepatic	Posthepatic

■ Immune-mediated hemolytic anemia
  ▪ Nonassociative
  ▪ Associative: drug administration (carprofen, penicillins, methimazole, sulfonamides), infectious disease (viral, protozoal or bacterial), neoplasia, inflammatory disease
■ Infectious
  ▪ *Babesia* spp.
■ Heinz body
  ▪ Toxin (onion, garlic, paracetamol, zinc)
■ Hereditary
  ▪ Pyruvate kinase deficiency
  ▪ Phosphofructokinase deficiency
  ▪ Hereditary/familial stomatocytosis
■ Envenomation
■ Microangiopathic erythrocyte fragmentation disorders (hemangiosarcoma, disseminated intravascular coagulation)
■ Hemophagocytic histiocytic sarcoma
	■ Infectious
	  ▪ Bacterial – *Leptospira spp.*, rickettsial disease
	  ▪ Viral – canine infectious hepatitis (canine adenovirus-1)
	  ▪ Protozoal – *Toxoplasma gondii, Neospora caninum*
	  ▪ Fungal – *Histoplasma capsulatum, Coccidiodes* spp.
	■ Idiopathic
	  ▪ Chronic hepatitis
	  ▪ Copper-associated hepatopathy
	■ Toxin
	  ▪ Xylitol, *Amanita* spp., aflatoxin, blue-green algae, Cycad (*Sago* palm)
	  ▪ Drugs: azathioprine, azoles, barbiturates, carprofen, CCNU (lomustine), paracetamol, sulfonamides, tetracyclines
	■ Neoplasia
		■ Cholecystitis/cholangitis
		  ▪ Bacterial – *Escherichia coli, Enterococcus* spp., *Clostridium* spp., etc.
		  ▪ Protozoal – *T. gondii, N. caninum, Hammondia heydomi*
		  ▪ Fungal – *Candida albicans*
		■ Intraluminal obstructive
		  ▪ Gallbladder mucocele, cholelithiasis, biliary stricture, intraluminal neoplasia
		■ Extraluminal obstructive
		  ▪ Pancreatitis, duodenal foreign body, complete obstruction of the duodenal papilla, extraluminal constrictive neoplasia, lymphadenopathy
		■ Cholestasis of sepsis

metabolic reserve capacity, the degree of hepatocellular pathology must be marked, with a large proportion of hepatocytes affected to result in jaundice. Intrahepatic cholestasis due to canalicular obstruction by hepatocyte swelling with vacuolar hepatopathy or lymphoma can also result in hepatic jaundice. Finally, posthepatic jaundice is due to partial or complete biliary obstruction, or biliary rupture. This occurs due to pathology either within the biliary system or affecting organs in close proximity to the biliary tree. As an aside, sepsis can also result in jaundice due to cytokine-mediated inhibition of hepatocellular transporters involved in bilirubin transport. This is commonly termed "cholestasis of sepsis" and is particularly recognized in cats, for example, with pyothorax.

Clinical signs

Clinical signs associated with jaundice are reflective of the underlying pathology causing hyperbilirubinemia, rather than a result of jaundice itself. Despite this, there are rare reports of bilirubin encephalopathy in dogs with severe hyperbilirubinemia,[1-3] where bilirubin deposition in the central nervous system resulted in neurological symptoms including generalized ataxia, head bobbing, stupor, coma, seizures, and death. Bilirubin encephalopathy is the preferred term in the clinical patient, as kernicterus refers to the postmortem finding of bilirubin deposits in the gray matter of the brain.

Clinical signs in patients with prehepatic jaundice are attributable to hemolytic anemia, such as weakness, tachycardia, tachypnea, pale mucous membranes, and hyperkinetic pulses. Dogs with a hepatic cause of jaundice display clinical signs associated with liver dysfunction which relates to the severity of the primary pathology. This varies from mild and vague signs including lethargy and hyporexia to severe and life-threatening signs associated with hepatic encephalopathy, hypoglycemia, or coagulopathy. Abdominal pain, pyrexia, vomiting, and dehydration are suggestive of posthepatic causes such as pancreatitis, biliary obstruction, or biliary tract rupture.

Diagnostic approach

The approach to the jaundiced patient is outlined in Algorithm 8.1.

Algorithm 8.1 Note 1 Signalment, history, and thorough physical examination are essential building blocks upon which the diagnostic approach to jaundice can be focussed. For example, a jaundiced, unvaccinated, young Labrador Retriever with signs of hypovolemic shock and a history of contact with stagnant water raises suspicion for leptospirosis, whereas a jaundiced, middle-aged Cocker Spaniel with weakness, pallor, and hyperdynamic pulses raises suspicion for immune-mediated hemolytic anemia. History should include diet, vaccination status, travel history, exposure to drugs or toxins, current medications, and antiparasitic control. Onset, duration, and progression of clinical signs assist in narrowing differential diagnoses. A minimum database consisting of hematology, biochemistry, and urinalysis is essential for every jaundiced patient. Minimum database results alongside signalment, history, and physical examination findings then allow a refined approach to further investigations. Bile acid stimulation testing is of no diagnostic value in the jaundiced patient and should not be performed because bile acids are also excreted in bile.

Algorithm 8.1 Note 2 A moderate to marked regenerative anemia with other hematological evidence of hemolysis such as spherocytosis, ghost cells, evidence of erythrocyte agglutination or increased numbers of Heinz bodies guides investigations towards prehepatic causes of jaundice. It is important to be cognizant that mild to moderate elevations in hepatobiliary enzyme activities may be present in anemic patients.

Algorithm 8.1 Note 3 Alongside a minimum database and thorough history to rule out obvious inciting causes of hemolysis, it is recommended to perform bicavitary imaging and infectious disease testing to assess for both direct causes of hemolysis and for triggers of associative immune-mediated hemolysis.[4] Specific diagnostics for rarer causes of hemolysis, such as hereditary erythrocyte defects, should be performed where appropriate after more commonly encountered conditions have been ruled out.

Algorithm 8.1 Note 4 In patients without evidence of hemolysis where elevations in enzyme activities indicative of hepatocellular damage (ALT, AST) are similar in degree to, or more prominent than, elevations in cholestatic enzyme activities (ALP, GGT), then a hepatic cause of jaundice is suspected. Some dogs with advanced chronic liver disease can present with hepatobiliary enzyme activities within normal limits and dogs with vacuolar hepatopathies may have more marked elevations in ALP. Dogs with markedly reduced liver function frequently have other biochemical abnormalities indicative of primary hepatic diseases, such as reductions in urea, albumin, cholesterol, and glucose levels, and/or abnormal coagulation profiles.

In dogs with acute markedly elevated hepatocellular enzyme activities, it is essential to rule out toxic or infectious liver injury with a thorough history detailing any possibility of access to medications or environmental toxins, as discussed in chapters 31 and 32. Being aware of vaccine status is essential, but a history of being vaccinated does not rule out infectious causes, particularly in cases of leptospirosis. When confronted with a jaundiced patient with comorbidities such as acute kidney injury, acute lung injury, or bleeding disorders (such as thrombocytopenia or other coagulopathic disease), then testing for leptospirosis should be performed.

Algorithm 8.1 Note 5 Abdominal ultrasonography and liver histology are cornerstones in the workup of cases with hepatic jaundice. Fine-needle aspirate cytology may be helpful for diffuse diseases such as lymphoma or large masses but is not useful for diagnosis of chronic hepatitis or copper hepatopathy and may miss focal pathology or focal inflammatory infiltrates (see chapters 27 and 28).

Algorithm 8.1 Note 6 In cases where an obvious infectious, inflammatory, toxic, or neoplastic cause is not identified on initial investigations, liver biopsy represents the next diagnostic step. It is recommended that a coagulation assessment is performed prior to biopsy.[5] Laparoscopy is the favored method of acquiring liver biopsies, but surgical exploratory laparotomy and ultrasound-guided percutaneous biopsy are alternatives when laparoscopy is not feasible. More details on biopsy techniques are found in chapter 27.

Algorithm 8.1 Note 7 Dogs with posthepatic jaundice commonly have cholestatic enzyme activities (ALP, GGT) elevated to a greater degree than hepatocellular enzyme activities (ALT, AST) although this is not always the case. Routine blood biochemistry may reveal

ALGORITHM 8.1
The approach to the jaundiced patient.

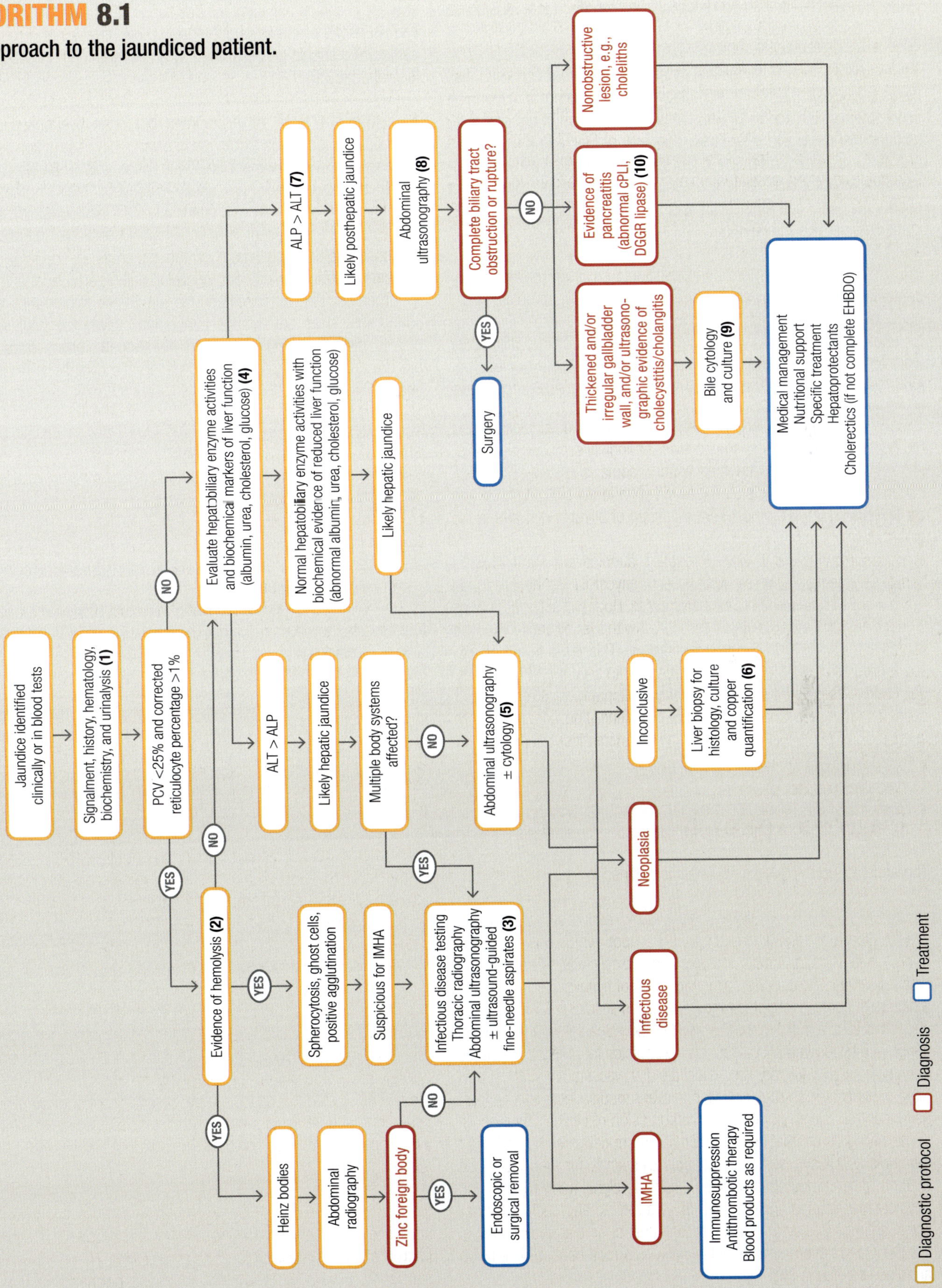

hypercholesterolemia without reductions in albumin, urea, or glucose unless other comorbidities exist.

Algorithm 8.1 Note 8 Abdominal ultrasonography is essential in these cases to elucidate the primary pathology resulting in jaundice. A thorough assessment of the abdomen with careful interrogation of the liver, gallbladder, bile ducts and biliary tree, duodenal papilla, and the pancreas and its surrounding mesentery is required, with sampling as necessary. Identification of biliary rupture or complete extrahepatic biliary duct obstruction, e.g., due to cholelithiasis, mucocele, or stricture, warrants immediate surgical intervention.

Algorithm 8.1 Note 9 Consideration should be given to cholecystocentesis for bile cytology and culture in cases without complete biliary duct obstruction and with ultrasonographic abnormalities suspicious for cholecystitis or cholangitis, such as thickening of the gallbladder wall, an irregular gallbladder wall lining or common bile duct distension.[6] In rare instances, cytological identification of fungal or protozoal species in canine bile samples has been reported.[7,8] Whilst the risk of complications of cholecystocentesis is low, this is not a routine procedure and should be performed by an experienced ultrasonographer (see chapter 26).

Algorithm 8.1 Note 10 A common but often overlooked cause of posthepatic jaundice is extrahepatic biliary duct obstruction secondary to pancreatitis. Assessment of DGGR lipase and/or canine pancreatic lipase immunoreactivity are useful diagnostic tools in these dogs, with favorable sensitivity and specificity.[9] Ultrasonographic pancreatic abnormalities are present in approximately two-thirds of cases,[9,10] but ultrasonographic assessment of the pancreas is impacted by both machine technical quality and operator skill. Therefore, it is important to remember that an unremarkable pancreatic appearance on ultrasonography does not exclude pancreatitis, given the poor sensitivity of this modality. Gallbladder and extrahepatic biliary tract disease are discussed in chapter 35, and pancreatic disease is discussed in chapters 18 and 19.

References

1. Tovar T, Deitschel S, Guenther C. The use of therapeutic plasma exchange to reduce serum bilirubin in a dog with kernicterus. *J Vet Emerg Crit Care (San Antonio)* 27(4):458-464, 2017.
2. Heffner GG, Cavanagh A, Nolan B. Successful management of acute bilirubin encephalopathy in a dog with immune-mediated hemolytic anemia using therapeutic plasma exchange. *J Vet Emerg Crit Care (San Antonio)* 29(5):549-557, 2019.
3. Sangster CR, Stevenson CK, Kidney BA, Montgomery DL, Allen AL. Kernicterus in an adult dog. *Vet Pathol* 44(3):383-385, 2007.
4. Garden OA, Kidd L, Mexas AM, Chang YM, Jeffery U, Blois SL, et al. ACVIM consensus statement on the diagnosis of immune-mediated hemolytic anemia in dogs and cats. *J Vet Intern Med* 33(2):313-334, 2019.
5. Webster CRL, Center SA, Cullen JM, Penninck DG, Richter KP, Twedt DC, et al. ACVIM consensus statement on the diagnosis and treatment of chronic hepatitis in dogs. *J Vet Intern Med* 33(3):1173-200, 2019.
6. Tamborini A, Jahns H, McAllister H, Kent A, Harris B, Procoli F, et al. Bacterial cholangitis, cholecystitis, or both in dogs. *J Vet Intern Med* 30(4):1046-1055, 2016.
7. Allan F, Blake D, Miller Z, Church D. Biliary protozoa in a dog with acute cholangiohepatitis fed a raw food diet. *J Vet Intern Med* 36(6):2177-2180, 2022.
8. Verwey E, Weltan SM, Whitehead Z. Candida albicans cholecystitis in a dog with diabetes mellitus. *Vet Rec Case Rep* e630, 2023.
9. Xenoulis PG. Diagnosis of pancreatitis in dogs and cats. *J Small Anim Pract* 56(1):13-26, 2015.
10. Cridge H, Sullivant AM, Wills RW, Lee AM. Association between abdominal ultrasound findings, the specific canine pancreatic lipase assay, clinical severity indices, and clinical diagnosis in dogs with pancreatitis. *J Vet Intern Med* 34(2):636-643, 2020.

CHAPTER 9

Dark feces or melena

Floris Dröes
DVM (Hon), MRCVS,
PGCert VMS

Pathophysiology

Melena is defined as dark to black, tarry, distinctly smelling stool. It is caused by oxidized hemoglobin (i.e., hematin) in the feces, which is derived from a hemorrhage in the oronasopharyngeal cavity or respiratory or gastrointestinal tract from which blood is entering the gastrointestinal tract. In experimental human studies, a minimum of 50-100 mL of blood was needed for melena to be appreciated. This means that for hemorrhage to be clinically obvious as melena, it requires first a significant amount of blood loss in a relatively short period, and second for it to remain in the gastrointestinal tract long enough for partial digestion before passing aboral. Of importance, severe acute intestinal hemorrhage can act as a cathartic, significantly decreasing gastrointestinal transit time and thus making blood appear less like melena and more like fresh blood. Melena could also be appreciated with delayed gastrointestinal transit time and retention of blood in the colon from lower gastrointestinal lesions (e.g., an ileal or proximal colonic hemorrhage). Other causes resembling melena are ingesting activated charcoal, antidiarrheal bismuth-containing medications, iron supplements, raw meat-based diets, and large quantities of blueberries or beets. Based on a thorough history, many of these can be excluded.

The etiologies of hemorrhage-causing melena are best classified by anatomical location to help focus diagnostic workup. However, with gastrointestinal hemorrhage as the main etiology of melena, causes for this hemorrhage can also be classified into three categories: diseases causing ulcers, diseases causing coagulopathies, and diseases associated with vascular anomalies. Gastrointestinal ulceration is the most common cause of melena. Medications (e.g., nonsteroidal anti-inflammatory drugs [NSAIDs] and corticosteroids), particularly with another risk factor (e.g., concurrent administration of NSAIDs), hepatic disease, neoplasia and mechanical etiologies (e.g., foreign bodies) are the leading risk factors for gastrointestinal ulceration in dogs (Table 9.1). Coagulation disorders leading to gastrointestinal hemorrhage are diverse, from intoxications to coagulation factor deficiencies and thrombocytopenia (Table 9.2). In dogs, thrombocytopenia is the most common coagulation disorder leading to gastrointestinal hemorrhage. Vascular anomalies (e.g., varices) are a common cause of gastrointestinal hemorrhage in humans; however, in small animals, these appear far less frequent.

TABLE 9.1 Causes for gastrointestinal ulceration in dogs leading to dark feces and melena.

Infections	Inflammation	Ischemia/ altered perfusion	Iatrogenic	Neoplasia
■ Viral: parvovirus, circovirus, distemper ■ Bacterial: *Campylobacter* spp., *Clostridium* spp., *Mycobacterium* spp., *Neorickettsia* spp., *Salmonella* spp. ■ Fungal: *Cryptococcus* spp., *Histoplasma* spp., *Pythium* spp., *Prototheca* spp. ■ Parasitic: *Spirocerca* spp., *Physaloptera* spp., *Ancylostoma* spp.*, *Uncinaria* spp.	■ Eosinophilic gastritis ■ Chronic enteropathy (CE)	■ Thrombosis/infarction (e.g., DIC) ■ Hypovolemia/decreased perfusion (e.g., pancreatitis, hypoadrenocorticism, DIC) ■ Secondary to trauma ■ Portal hypertension secondary to liver disease ■ Gastrointestinal intussusception ■ Gastrointestinal volvulus	■ Foreign body ■ Postsurgery ■ Drug-induced (e.g., corticosteroids, NSAIDs, etc.) ■ Racing sled dogs (after intense exercise)	■ Within the GI tract: adenocarcinoma, gastrointestinal stromal tumor, leiomyoma/ leiomyosarcoma, lymphoma ■ Outside the GI tract (producing ulcerogenic substances): mast cell tumor, gastrinoma

*Hemorrhage caused by hookworms is often largely ingested by them, obscuring melena.

TABLE 9.2 Coagulation disorders causing dark feces and melena in dogs.

Thrombocytopenia	Coagulation protein disorders
(See differential diagnosis in chapter 12: Petechiae and ecchymoses)	**Congenital/inherited** ■ Von Willebrand disease ■ Hemophilia A ■ Hemophilia B ■ Factor II (thrombin) disorder ■ Factor VII deficiency ■ Hypo-/dysfibrinogenemia ■ Other factor deficiencies (e.g., X, XI, XII) **Acquired** ■ Decreased or altered production ■ Vitamin K deficiency – Intoxication with rodenticides – Nutritional – Cholestasis (mostly in cats, uncommon in dogs) – Intestinal malabsorption (e.g., with exocrine pancreas insufficiency) ■ Hepatic disease: severe acute or end-stage chronic ■ Increased consumption ■ Inflammation – DIC (e.g., with severe organ inflammation such as severe acute pancreatitis or acute hepatitis) – Heatstroke ■ Envenomation ■ Medication/intoxication – Heparins, oral anticoagulants, anti-Xa inhibitors – NSAIDs ■ Significant blood loss ■ Dilution of proteins due to rapid excessive fluid therapy ■ Thrombosis

Clinical signs

Gastrointestinal ulceration and hemorrhage are the main causes of melena in small animals; thus, other signs of gastrointestinal diseases can be apparent, such as anorexia, nausea, and vomiting. Therefore, on physical examination guarding the abdomen, tenderness on palpation, induced nausea, identification of masses or foreign objects, organomegaly (e.g., spleen and liver), and abdominal distention could be observed when gastrointestinal diseases cause melena.

When hemorrhage from another location (e.g., nasal or oral cavity or airways) causes melena, clinical signs associated with that organ system might be observed. For example, with nasal cavity disease epistaxis, pawing at the nose and sneezing might be seen; with the oral cavity, reluctance to eat, difficulty swallowing, and oral blood loss; and with airways, abnormal breathing patterns, coughing or abnormal thoracic auscultation can be observed.

As a consequence of hemorrhage, physical examination might also show signs of shock, including tachypnea, tachycardia, thready or diminished arterial pulses, pale mucous membranes, prolonged capillary refill time, and cool extremities. If anemia and shock become severe, ataxia and weakness can be apparent. Active steps should be taken once signs of shock are observed to reverse this by fluid resuscitation while simultaneously localizing the site of hemorrhage. If just anemia without shock is present (e.g., due to more chronic low-grade hemorrhage), bounding pulses might be appreciated. Although anemia is not as obvious in most gastrointestinal hemorrhages, shock might still be observed in these patients due to hypovolemia (from vomiting and diarrhea), ulcer perforation, endotoxemia, severe inflammatory response, and sepsis.

Diagnostic approach

Algorithm 9.1 shows the approach to the melena patient.

Algorithm 9.1 Note 1 A thorough history and physical examination are important in patients presenting with melena. During the physical examination, specific emphasis should be placed on the different locations where hemorrhage could arise from the oro-, naso-, or pharyngeal cavity, respiratory system, or gastrointestinal tract (Table 9.1). Thorough and gentle abdominal palpation should be performed. Fecal consistency and localization of the blood or melena in relation to the fecal bolus can contribute to lesion localization. If the patient allows it, a careful rectal examination should be performed on a patient presenting with melena to identify frank blood, changes in mucosa, masses, and foreign bodies.

Algorithm 9.1 Note 2 Most animals with gastrointestinal hemorrhage may not be anemic on complete blood count (CBC). Anemia can be regenerative or nonregenerative (depending on the chronicity of the underlying disease), with often concurrent hypoalbuminemia. If blood loss is severe or chronic, microcytic, hypochromic anemia due to iron deficiency can be observed. Increased red blood cell distribution width (RDW) might be more sensitive than microcytemia to identify iron deficiency.

Algorithm 9.1 Note 3 High serum urea-to-creatinine ratio has been suggested to indicate gastrointestinal hemorrhage; however, studies are conflicting regarding its discriminatory power to identify covert hemorrhage and hemorrhage location. Other diseases that could increase serum urea-to-creatinine ratios should be considered, like fever, burns, infection, starvation, and administration of glucocorticoids.

Algorithm 9.1 Note 4 Leukocytosis and neutrophilia might be observed with perforated ulcers, peritonitis, enteritis, pancreatitis, gastrointestinal foreign bodies, and neoplasia. Leukopenia and neutropenia are more common in young puppies with parvoviral enteritis. Eosinophilia can be observed in patients with intestinal parasitism, food allergy, mastocytosis, and hypoadrenocorticism.

Algorithm 9.1 Note 5 Gastrointestinal bleeding secondary to thrombocytopenia occurs most often from tick-born rickettsia infections in endemic areas, immune thrombocytopenia (ITP), and systemic lupus erythematosus (SLE).

Algorithm 9.1 Note 6 The diagnostic utility of abdominal ultrasound for gastroduodenal ulceration is limited, especially for nonperforated mucosal ulceration. However, it could be helpful to identify signs of other abdominal diseases and portal hypertension.

Algorithm 9.1 Note 7 To exclude a meat-based diet as a false-positive cause for a fecal occult blood test, a meat-free diet should be fed for at least 72 hours before testing. A negative fecal occult blood test does not rule out significant gastrointestinal hemorrhage.

ALGORITHM 9.1

The approach to the patient with melena.

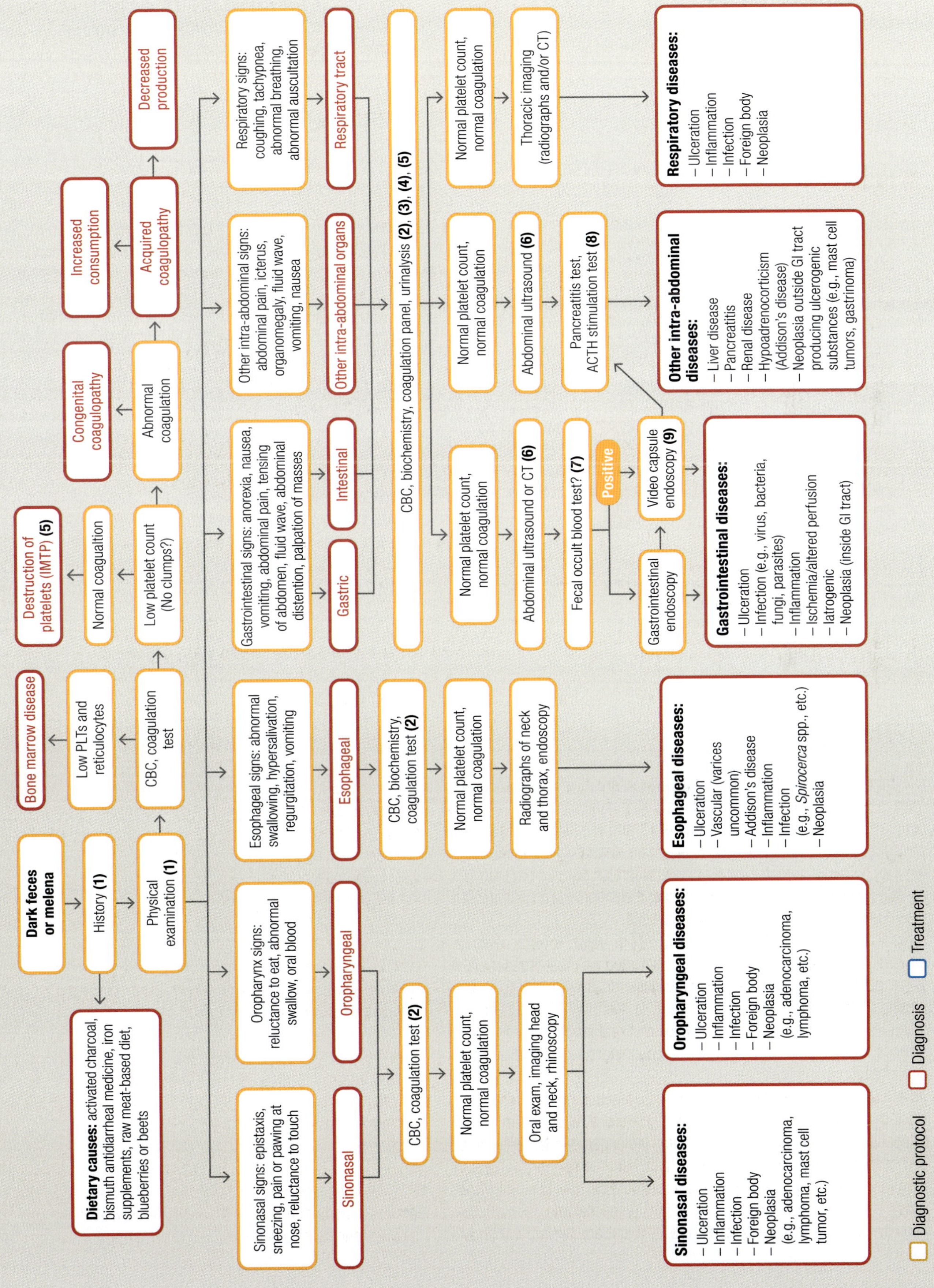

Algorithm 9.1 Note 8 If no cause of gastrointestinal hemorrhage can be found, an ACTH stimulation test should be performed to exclude hypoadrenocorticism.

Algorithm 9.1 Note 9 Video capsule endoscopy (VCE) is a minimally invasive method to evaluate for gastrointestinal hemorrhage usually performed after regular endoscopy. A 12-hour fast is recommended prior to VCE. The major challenge with VCE is incomplete studies due to gastric retention or altered gastrointestinal motility.

References

1. Tefft KM. Melena and hematochezia. In Ettinger SJ, Feldman EC, Côté E, editors. St. Louis, Elsevier, 2017:167-170.
2. Stiller J, Defarges AM, Brisson BA, et al. Feasibility, complications, and visualization quality using video capsule endoscopy in 40 dogs with overt or questionable gastrointestinal bleeding. *J Vet Intern Med* 35:1743-1753, 2021.
3. Stiller J, Defarges AM, Brisson BA, et al. Diagnostic evaluation of urea nitrogen/creatinine ratio in dogs with gastrointestinal bleeding. *J Vet Intern Med* 35:1427-1438, 2021.
4. Pavlova E, Gold RM, Tolbert MK, et al. Medical conditions associated with gastroduodenal ulceration or erosion in 168 dogs: 2008-2018. *J Vet Intern Med* 35:2697-2704, 2021.
5. O'Kell AL, Gallagher AE, Cooke KL. Gastroduodenal ulceration in dogs with liver disease. *J Vet Intern Med* 36:986-992, 2022.
6. Marks SL, Kook PH, Papich MG, et al. ACVIM consensus statement: Support for rational administration of gastrointestinal protectants to dogs and cats. *J Vet Intern Med* 32:1823-1840, 2018.
7. Mabry K, Hill T, Tolbert MK. Prevalence of gastrointestinal lesions in dogs chronically treated with nonsteroidal anti-inflammatory drugs. *J Vet Intern Med* 35:853-859, 2021.
8. Mabry K, Hill T, Marks SL, et al. Use of video capsule endoscopy to identify gastrointestinal lesions in dogs with microcytosis or gastrointestinal hemorrhage. *J Vet Intern Med* 33:1964-1969, 2019.
9. Fitzgerald E, Barfield D, Lee KCL, et al. Clinical findings and results of diagnostic imaging in 82 dogs with gastrointestinal ulceration. *J Small Anim Pract* 58:211-218, 2017.
10. Davignon DL, Lee ACY, Johnston AN, et al. Evaluation of capsule endoscopy to detect mucosal lesions associated with gastrointestinal bleeding in dogs. *J Small Anim Pract* 57:148-158, 2016.
11. Weston PJ, Maddox TW, Hõim S, et al. Diagnostic utility of abdominal ultrasound for detecting non-perforated gastroduodenal ulcers in dogs. *Vet Rec* 190:e199, 2022.

CHAPTER 10

Abdominal enlargement

Giulia Cattaneo
MA VetMB MRCVS, Senior Clinical Training Scholar in Small Animal Internal Medicine, (ECVIM-CA Resident)

Pathophysiology

Abdominal enlargement is a clinical finding or presenting complaint observed in several disease processes. Causes of abdominal enlargement can be subdivided into distinct categories including soft tissue, fluid, gastrointestinal contents, gas, and hypotonia of the abdominal musculature.[1] Soft tissue structures may include organomegaly (including liver, pancreas), fat deposition, neoplasia, pregnancy, granuloma, or other soft tissue inflammatory processes. Fluid may be observed in the form of an effusion (free fluid within the peritoneal and/or retroperitoneal spaces), within an encapsulated structure (cyst or abscess), or within a hollow viscus (pyometra or pregnancy, ileus, very large urinary bladder, or obstruction of the gastrointestinal tract). Increased quantities of solid gastrointestinal contents may result from constipation, obstipation, megacolon, ileus (functional or mechanical), increased dietary intake, or heavy parasitic burdens. Gas can accumulate freely within the abdomen (peritoneal and/or retroperitoneal space) secondary to gastrointestinal tract or body wall rupture (trauma, foreign body perforation), and surgical sequelae (laparoscopic inflation). Gas may also be contained within an organ structure, as is the case with emphysematous bacterial infections (liver, gallbladder, urinary bladder), or gastrointestinal obstruction (gastric dilation and volvulus, intestinal or mesenteric torsion). Hypotonia of the abdominal musculature is commonly observed in cases of hyperadrenocorticism.

For the purposes of this chapter, the focus will be on specific causes of hepatomegaly, cranial abdominal masses (hepatobiliary, pancreatic), and ascites (Table 10.1).

TABLE 10.1 Differential diagnoses for hepatomegaly, cranial abdominal mass (pancreatic and hepatobiliary), and ascites in the dog.

Hepatomegaly	Cranial abdominal mass: pancreatic	Cranial abdominal mass: hepatobiliary	Ascites
■ Drug-related: phenobarbital, glucocorticoids, general anesthetic agents ■ Neoplasia ■ Metabolic: lipid or glycogen deposition. ■ Hepatic venous congestion: right-sided congestive heart failure, caudal vena cava obstruction ■ Acute liver injury or failure: infectious, toxic, drug-related, copper storage disease, hypoxic damage ■ Biliary stasis/biliary tract obstruction (e.g., cholelithiasis, gallbladder mucocele, neoplasia) ■ Benign change: benign nodular hyperplasia, extramedullary hematopoiesis ■ Miscellaneous: cystic change, liver lobe torsion, hematoma, lysosomal storage disease, abscessation	■ Pancreatic adenocarcinoma ■ Pancreatic adenoma ■ Insulinoma ■ Metastatic neoplasia ■ Other non-neoplastic with mass effect (e.g., pancreatitis, pancreatolithiasis, pancreatic abscess) ■ Pancreatic edema/congestion secondary to portal hypertension? ■ Pancreatic cysts and pseudocysts (usually postinflammatory rather than congenital in dogs)	■ Hepatoma ■ Hepatocellular carcinoma ■ Malignant histiocytosis ■ Visceral mast cell tumor ■ Neuroendocrine tumor ■ Hepato-(splenic) lymphoma ■ Hemangioma ■ Hemangiosarcoma ■ Other mesenchymal ■ Biliary adenoma ■ Biliary adenocarcinoma ■ Metastatic: lymphoma, mast cell tumor, hemangiosarcoma, leukemia	■ Hemorrhage: trauma, coagulopathy, iatrogenic, neoplastic ■ Uroabdomen: trauma, urinary obstruction, iatrogenic, neoplasia ■ Bile peritonitis: trauma, biliary obstruction, iatrogenic, neoplasia ■ Neoplastic or paraneoplastic effusion ■ Septic peritonitis: trauma, gastrointestinal obstruction/perforation, foreign body migration, ruptured abscess ■ Chyloabdomen: primary (idiopathic), lymphatic obstruction (including neoplasia), right-sided congestive heart failure, trauma ■ Increased hydrostatic pressure: portal hypertension (prehepatic, intrahepatic or posthepatic causes) ■ Other inflammatory (septic or nonseptic): pancreatitis, steatitis, peritonitis ■ Reduced colloid osmotic pressure: hypoproteinemia (hypoalbuminemia)

Clinical signs

Clinical signs reported with abdominal enlargement are largely nonspecific including changes to body shape, weight gain, weakness, difficulty rising or ambulating. A thorough history and clinical examination will assist with further characterization of the disease process. When the abdominal enlargement is such that it impinges on the thoracic cavity and/or obstructs venous return, clinical signs such as alterations to the patient's breathing pattern, lethargy, collapse, and exercise intolerance can manifest. Clinical examination findings may therefore include tachypnea, dyspnea, hypotension, tachycardia, and impaired capillary refill time. Depending on the underlying cause, patients with abdominal enlargement may also exhibit abdominal pain or pyrexia (such as in traumatic, obstructive, or septic processes) (see chapter 11). Where fluid accumulation is present, a fluid thrill on ballottement of the abdomen may be palpable. Abdominal palpation may also raise concern over gas distension, increased solid gastrointestinal contents, or the presence of an abdominal mass.

Diagnostic approach

The basic diagnostic approach to abdominal enlargement requires a thorough history, clinical examination, and primary investigations to include complete blood count, serum biochemistry, urinalysis, and abdominal imaging. Further investigations (as described in Algorithm 10.1) can then be guided by the initial findings.

Algorithm 10.1 Note 1 Distinguishing between causes of abdominal enlargement may be difficult based on clinical examination alone; therefore, imaging may be performed in the first instance to confirm suspicion and to characterize or localize the pathology further. Abdominal ultrasonography is the initial modality of choice; radiography and/or CT can be considered at a later stage.

Algorithm 10.1 Note 2 Hepatomegaly, pancreatomegaly, splenomegaly, and lymphadenomegaly are some differential diagnoses for organomegaly. Further diagnostic testing or procedures may include specific blood tests and FNA cytology or ultrasound-guided needle biopsy, laparoscopic incisional biopsy, and surgical incisional or excisional biopsy for definitive diagnosis.

Algorithm 10.1 Note 3 Liver function testing includes bile acid stimulation, serum ammonia, and coagulation profiles (OSPT/APTT, thromboelastography; TEG). Other indirect measures of liver function include serum glucose, urea, albumin, and cholesterol. Prior to liver sampling (aspirates or biopsies), it is important to assess platelet count and coagulation profile (see chapters 24 and 25).

Algorithm 10.1 Note 4 Liver biopsies may be performed via laparoscopic incisional biopsy, surgical incisional or excisional biopsy, or ultrasound-guided needle biopsy (see chapters 26 and 27). FNA sampling may be most useful in the first instance when neoplasia is suspected, or a single mass is observed; however, it should not be relied upon for a definitive diagnosis. Further assessment of biopsy tissue may include fluorescence in-situ hybridization (FISH), immunohistochemistry (IHC), tissue culture, and copper quantification, depending on clinical suspicion of the underlying disease process. FISH and tissue culture may be considered in the case of an infectious process, whereas immunohistochemistry may aid in the identification of pathogens, a neoplastic or immune-mediated process. Copper quantification may be deemed useful in the case of a suspected acute toxic hepatopathy.

Algorithm 10.1 Note 5 Hepatic infectious disease testing may primarily include serology, PCR and/or culture of pathogens including bacteria (*Leptospira* spp., *Salmonella* spp., rickettsial diseases), viruses (canine adenovirus-1), protozoa (*Toxoplasma gondii*, *Neospora caninum*), fungi (*Histoplasma capsulatum*) or parasites (*Heterobilharzia americana*).

The diagnostic approach to ascites is outlined in Algorithm 10.2. More details on fluid analysis are available in chapters 13 and 24.

Algorithm 10.2 Note 1 Causes of portal hypertension are classified into prehepatic, intrahepatic, and posthepatic causes.[2] Prehepatic causes include congenital portal vein atresia or intraluminal/extraluminal obstruction including portal vein thrombus. Intrahepatic causes can be further subdivided into presinusoidal (portal vein hypoplasia, ductal plate anomalies, hepatic arteriovenous fistula), sinusoidal (cirrhosis, chronic hepatitis, chronic cholangiohepatitis), and postsinusoidal (veno-occlusive disease). Posthepatic causes include right-sided heart failure, caudal vena cava obstruction (intraluminal or extraluminal), or Budd-Chiari syndrome. Differential diagnoses for vasculitis may include various inflammatory, immune-mediated, infectious, drug/toxin-related, or neoplastic causes.

ALGORITHM 10.1

Diagnostic approach to abdominal enlargement, with a particular focus on hepatomegaly.

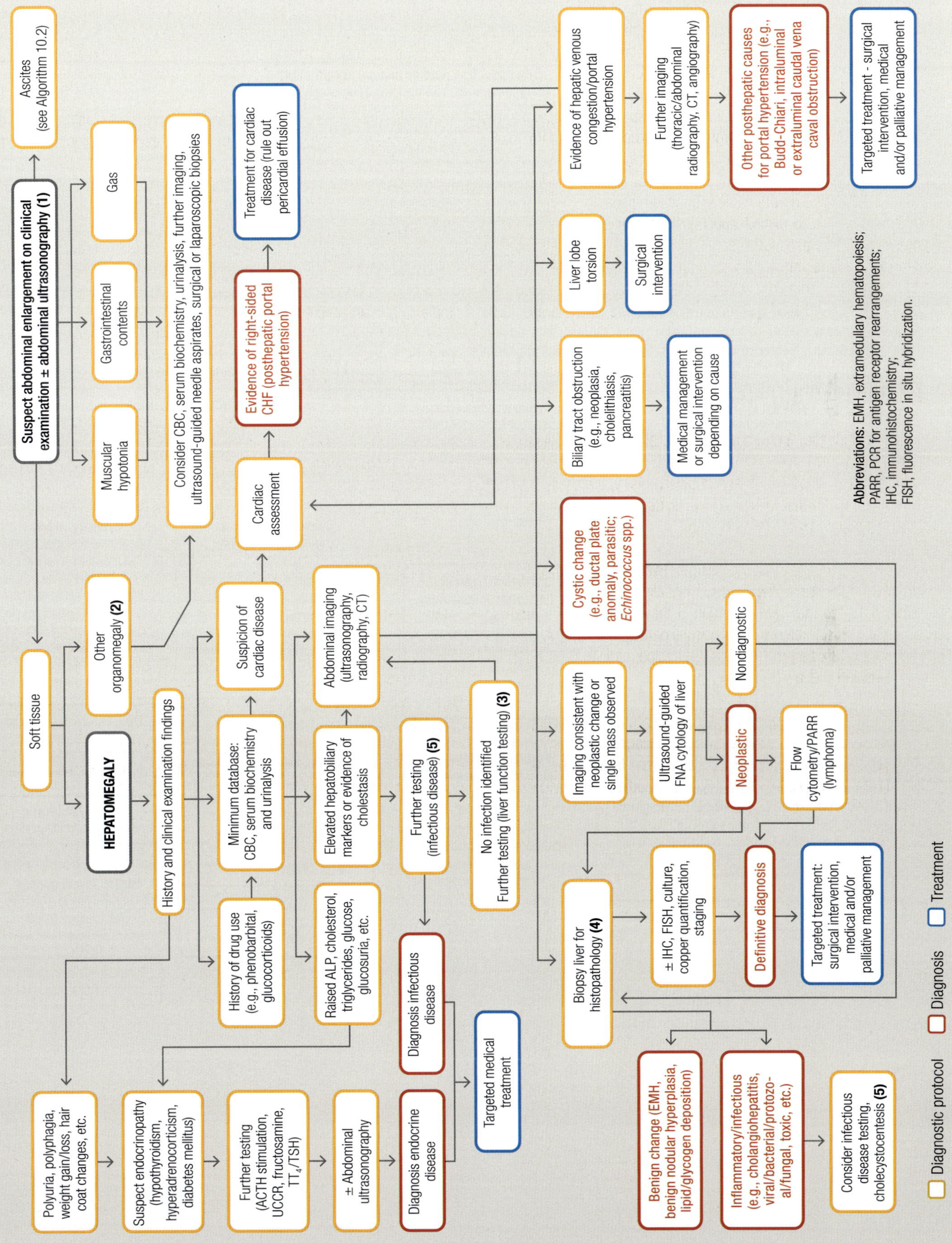

Abbreviations: EMH, extramedullary hematopoiesis; PARR, PCR for antigen receptor rearrangements; IHC, immunohistochemistry; FISH, fluorescence in situ hybridization.

ALGORITHM 10.2

Diagnostic approach to ascites.

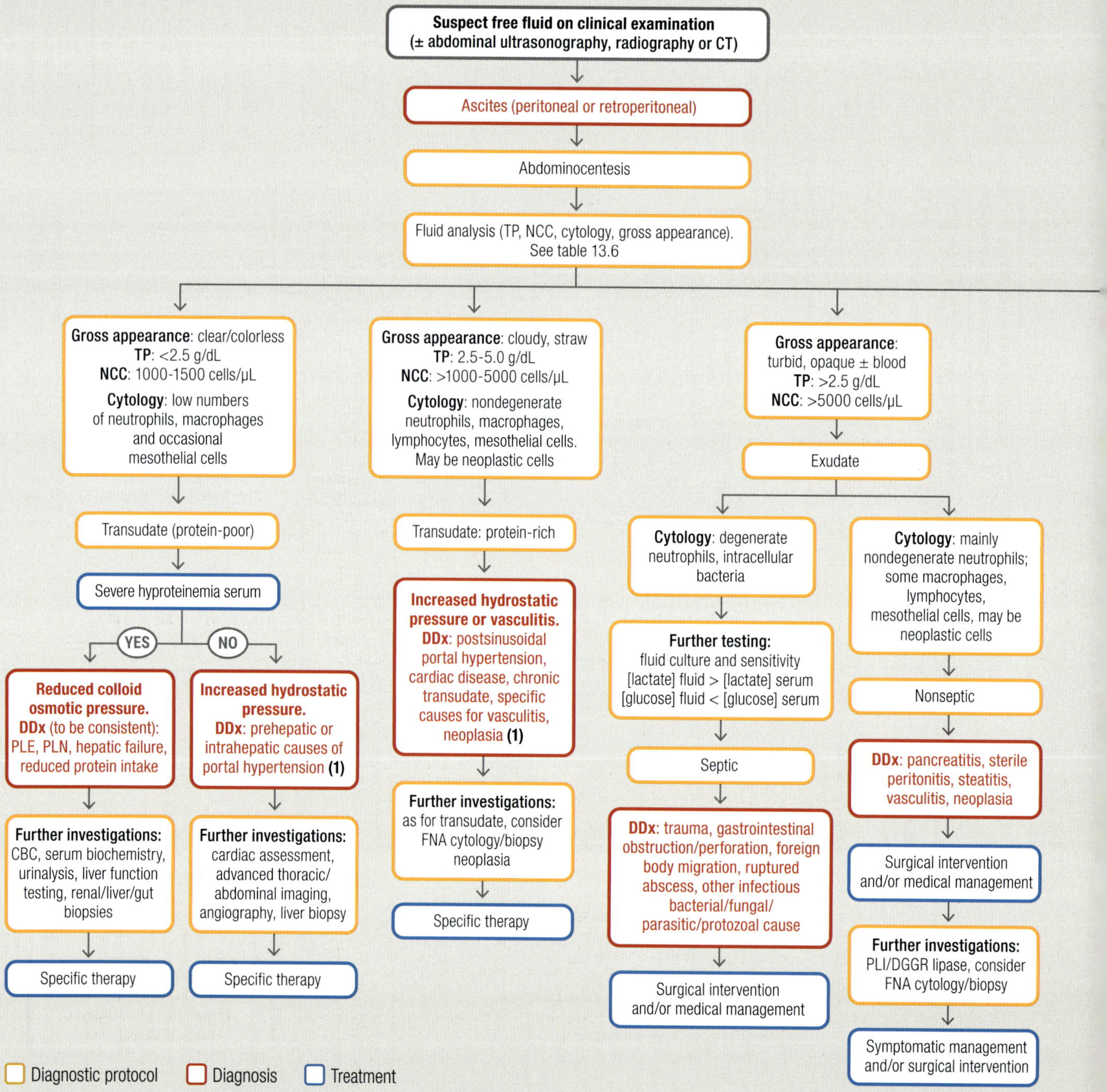

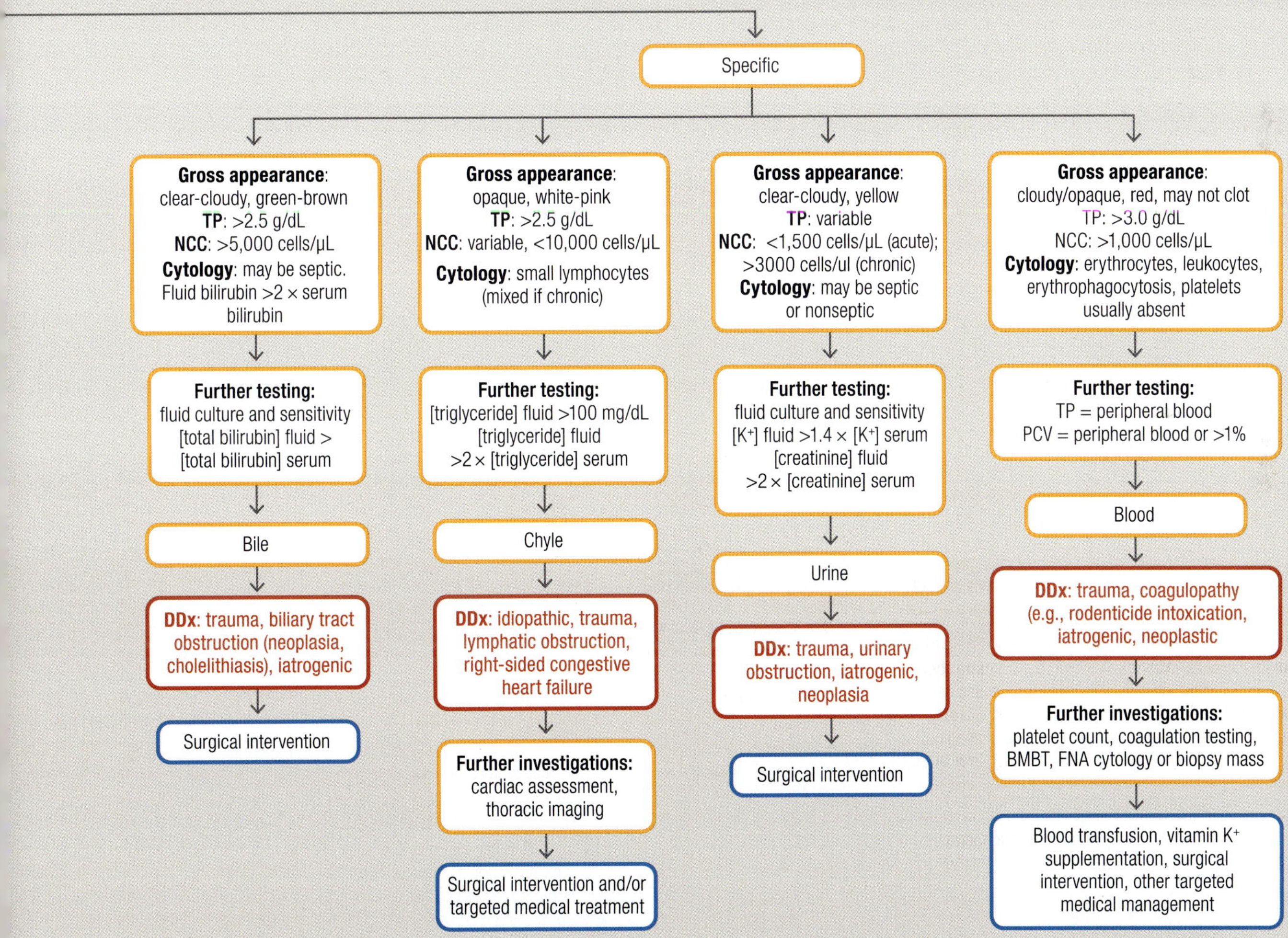
Specific
Gross appearance: clear-cloudy, green-brown
TP: >2.5 g/dL
NCC: >5,000 cells/μL
Cytology: may be septic.
Fluid bilirubin >2 × serum bilirubin
Further testing: fluid culture and sensitivity
[total bilirubin] fluid > [total bilirubin] serum
Bile
DDx: trauma, biliary tract obstruction (neoplasia, cholelithiasis), iatrogenic
Surgical intervention
Gross appearance: opaque, white-pink
TP: >2.5 g/dL
NCC: variable, <10,000 cells/μL
Cytology: small lymphocytes (mixed if chronic)
Further testing: [triglyceride] fluid >100 mg/dL
[triglyceride] fluid >2 × [triglyceride] serum
Chyle
DDx: idiopathic, trauma, lymphatic obstruction, right-sided congestive heart failure
Further investigations: cardiac assessment, thoracic imaging
Surgical intervention and/or targeted medical treatment
Gross appearance: clear-cloudy, yellow
TP: variable
NCC: <1,500 cells/μL (acute); >3000 cells/ul (chronic)
Cytology: may be septic or nonseptic
Further testing: fluid culture and sensitivity
[K+] fluid >1.4 × [K+] serum
[creatinine] fluid >2 × [creatinine] serum
Urine
DDx: trauma, urinary obstruction, iatrogenic, neoplasia
Surgical intervention
Gross appearance: cloudy/opaque, red, may not clot
TP: >3.0 g/dL
NCC: >1,000 cells/μL
Cytology: erythrocytes, leukocytes, erythrophagocytosis, platelets usually absent
Further testing: TP = peripheral blood
PCV = peripheral blood or >1%
Blood
DDx: trauma, coagulopathy (e.g., rodenticide intoxication, iatrogenic, neoplastic
Further investigations: platelet count, coagulation testing, BMBT, FNA cytology or biopsy mass
Blood transfusion, vitamin K+ supplementation, surgical intervention, other targeted medical management

References

1. Walter J. Abdominal enlargement. In Ettinger SJ, Feldman EC, Côté E, editors. Textbook of Veterinary Internal Medicine: Diseases of the Dog and Cat, Volume 1, 8th edition. St. Louis, Elsevier, 2017, pp 450-455.
2. Buob S, Johnston AN, Webster CR. Portal hypertension: pathophysiology, diagnosis, and treatment. *J Vet Intern Med* 25(2):171, 2011.

CHAPTER 11

Cranial abdominal pain

Giulia Cattaneo
MA, VetMB, MRCVS,
Senior Clinical Training Scholar in Small Animal Internal Medicine,
(ECVIM-CA Resident)

Pathophysiology

Visceral abdominal pain is mediated by sensory visceral afferent neurons of the autonomic nervous system. This response is elicited by various stimuli including strong contraction or dilation of an organ, inflammation, stretching of mesenteric attachments, and the presence of noxious substances within the gut lumen.[1,2] The afferents are located on serosal surfaces, within the mesentery and the muscular and mucosal layers of the gut to ultimately elicit a conscious perception of pain.[2] For example, acute liver or renal injury results in organ enlargement, subsequent capsular stretch, and associated abdominal pain. It is important to note that whilst the liver capsule and biliary tract are well-supplied with pain receptors, the parenchyma is not. On the other hand, musculoskeletal pain is mediated by sensory afferents of the somatic nervous system.

Cranial abdominal pain can be broadly divided into extra-abdominal and intra-abdominal causes. Extra-abdominal causes encompass the musculoskeletal system and integument, i.e., the skin, abdominal musculature, intercostal muscles, diaphragm, and ribs. Pain may also be referred from the thorax in intrathoracic disease (e.g., pleural space disease, pneumonia, and other causes of dyspnea). Given that spinal disease often presents with clinical signs that may be confused with abdominal pain, this should also be considered a differential diagnosis. Intra-abdominal causes of cranial abdominal pain are further subdivided into specific cranial abdominal organs based on whether they are intraperitoneal (liver, stomach, intestines, spleen, pancreas, peritoneum) or retroperitoneal (adrenals, kidneys, lymph nodes). Table 11.1 provides a summary of differentials for cranial abdominal pain.

Clinical signs

Clinical signs of cranial abdominal pain can be relatively nonspecific and include lethargy, reluctance to exercise or ambulate, hyporexia, anorexia, and other gastrointestinal signs (e.g., vomiting, diarrhea, nausea). More specifically, the patient may adopt a kyphotic posture, display tensing or guarding of the abdomen, or react behaviorally (e.g., vocalization, aggression, turning around) on palpation of the cranial abdomen. Dependent on the underlying pathological process, there may be evidence of abdominal enlargement, a distinct mass structure, organomegaly, or a fluid thrill within the abdomen on palpation or ballottement (see chapter 10). Other clinical examination findings such as tachypnea, tachycardia, arrhythmias, hypertension, and hyperthermia/pyrexia may also be observed in response to pain or inflammation and subsequent upregulation of the sympathetic nervous system. On the other hand, a patient presenting with bradycardia is not uncommon and can arise secondary to increased vagal tone in intra-abdominal disease states. Hypoadrenocorticism can present with apparent abdominal pain and is an important rule-out. Patients with a history of trauma may present with multi-organ involvement and subsequent cardiovascular, respiratory, neurological, or orthopedic signs. Patients with dermatological disease may have visible lesions on the skin with pain or discomfort elicited on examination. Spinal pain and abdominal pain can be difficult to differentiate. A thorough clinical history should always be undertaken to characterize the onset and duration of clinical signs, previous history of disease, trauma, known concurrent disease, dietary or scavenging history, drug administration or toxin ingestion, etc.

Pain elicited in a particular quadrant (right/left, ventral/dorsal) of the cranial abdomen may allow the clinician to narrow down the differential diagnoses: e.g., right-sided, ventral cranial abdominal pain, alongside a suggestive history or concurrent clinical signs, can increase suspicion for pancreatic disease. However, clinical examination alone is not deemed sufficient for a definitive diagnosis, and therefore subsequent investigations to support the suspicion should always be performed. It is also important to note that the phenomenon of "referred pain" can confound diagnosis, which further stresses the importance of careful interpretation of the initial clinical examination.

TABLE 11.1 Differential diagnoses for cranial abdominal pain subdivided into intra-abdominal (intraperitoneal vs. retroperitoneal), and extra-abdominal causes.

Intra-abdominal, intraperitoneal				
Liver (stretching of liver capsule or biliary pain)	**Stomach, proximal small intestine, transverse colon**	**Spleen**	**Pancreas**	**Peritoneum**
■ Acute liver injury or acute liver failure (e.g., toxic, infectious, hypoxic/ischemic/thrombosis) ■ Hepatobiliary neoplasia (e.g., hepatocellular carcinoma, biliary tract adenocarcinoma, hemangiosarcoma) ■ Trauma, diaphragmatic rupture with herniation ■ Liver lobe torsion ■ Hepatic congestion ■ Biliary tract obstruction/rupture (e.g., trauma, cholelithiasis, gallbladder mucocele) ■ Other causes of hepatomegaly ■ Hepatic abscessation	■ Hiatus hernia or diaphragmatic rupture with gastrointestinal herniation ■ Gastritis or enteritis (viral, bacterial, parasitic, protozoal, fungal, inflammatory/immune-mediated) ■ Gastrointestinal neoplasia (e.g., adenocarcinoma, leiomyoma, lymphoma) ■ Gastrointestinal obstruction, foreign body, intussusception (with or without perforation) ■ Trauma (blunt or penetrating) ■ Thrombosis/ischemic event ■ Mucosal ulceration or erosion	■ Splenic neoplasia (e.g., hemangiosarcoma, lymphoma, mast cell tumor) ■ Splenic torsion ■ Trauma (blunt or penetrating) ■ Other causes of splenomegaly (e.g., drug-related, hypersplenism) ■ Thrombosis/ischemic event	■ Pancreatitis (acute or chronic) ■ Pancreatolithiasis ■ Neoplasia (e.g., pancreatic carcinoma, metastatic) ■ Trauma ■ Pancreatic abscessation ■ Thrombosis/ischemic event	■ Septic peritonitis (e.g., gastrointestinal tract rupture, migrating foreign body, penetrating trauma) ■ Bile peritonitis ■ Uroperitoneum ■ Other sterile peritonitis (e.g., pancreatitis, steatitis) ■ Lymphadenopathy (reactive or neoplastic) ■ Portal hypertension (prehepatic, intrahepatic, posthepatic)

Intra-abdominal, retroperitoneal			Extra-abdominal
Adrenals	**Kidneys**	**Other**	**Musculoskeletal and skin (including referred from thorax)**
■ Neoplasia (e.g., pheochromocytoma) ■ Trauma ■ Thrombosis/ischemic event	■ Pyelonephritis ■ Trauma ■ Ureteral obstruction with or without hydronephrosis (e.g., ureterolithiasis, neoplasia) ■ Glomerulonephritis ■ Neoplasia (e.g., renal carcinoma, lymphoma) ■ Other causes of acute kidney injury (e.g., infectious, toxic, drug-related) ■ Thrombosis/ischemic event ■ Renal or pararenal cysts	■ Neoplasia (paraganglioma) ■ Lymphadenopathy (reactive or neoplastic) ■ Ectopic tissue	■ Trauma, including to the external body wall and diaphragm (e.g., diaphragmatic rupture) ■ Muscular overexertion (e.g., intercostals, ribs, cranial abdominal wall) ■ Dermatological disease, skin lesions or trauma ■ Spinal disease (e.g., intervertebral disc herniation, discospondylitis, neoplasia) ■ Referred pain from thorax (pleural fluid, pyothorax, pneumonia, or any other disease causing dyspnea)

Diagnostic approach

The basic diagnostic approach to cranial abdominal pain requires a thorough history, clinical examination, and primary investigations to include complete blood count, serum biochemistry, urinalysis, and abdominal imaging. Further investigations (as described in Algorithm 11.1) can then be guided by the initial findings.

Algorithm 11.1 Note 1 Careful clinical examination is vital. For example, spinal pain may manifest with clinical signs similar to abdominal pain such as a guarded abdomen, kyphotic posture, and painful response on abdominal palpation, therefore it is not uncommon for a clinician to confuse these two entities.

Algorithm 11.1 Note 2 Tissue biopsies may be performed via ultrasound-guided needle biopsy, endoscopic biopsies (in the case of the gut), laparoscopic incisional biopsy, and surgical incisional or excisional biopsy. Further assessment of tissue biopsies may include fluorescence in-situ hybridization (FISH), immunohistochemistry (IHC), and tissue culture, depending on clinical suspicion of the underlying disease process. FISH and tissue culture may be considered in the case of an infectious process, whereas immunohistochemistry may aid in the identification of pathogens or a neoplastic or immune-mediated process. For liver biopsies, staining for copper and quantification may also be undertaken. Where lymphoma may be suspected, flow cytometry or PARR may be run on FNA samples from tissues (e.g., liver, spleen, lymph nodes).

ALGORITHM 11.1

Diagnostic approach to cranial abdominal pain.

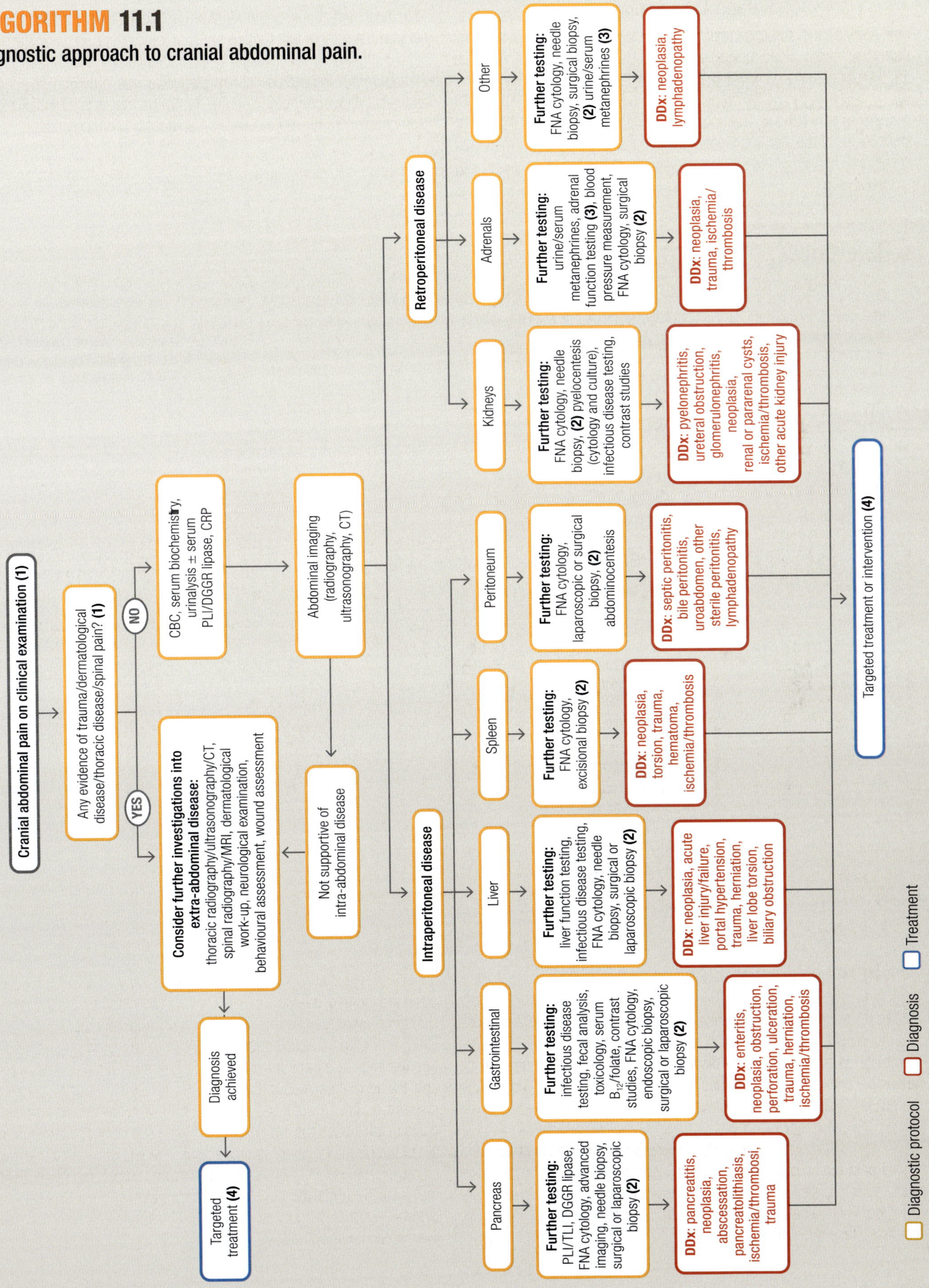

Algorithm 11.1 Note 3 Neuroendocrine tumors such as pheochromocytomas (and some paragangliomas) may secrete catecholamines; therefore, serial blood pressure measurements and serum or urine metanephrine testing should be considered.

Algorithm 11.1 Note 4 Treatment is very dependent on final diagnosis; whilst some of the aforementioned conditions can be medically managed (e.g., toxic, infectious, acute renal or hepatic injury, pancreatitis, diffuse neoplasias), others will require surgical intervention (e.g., solitary neoplasias, obstructive processes) or a combination of medical and surgical management. Regardless of the diagnosis, the provision of adequate analgesia with serial pain scoring forms the mainstay of initial therapy (see chapter 23 for more details on analgesia in pancreatitis).

References

1. Klein BG. The autonomic nervous system. In Klein BG, editor. Cunningham's Textbook of Veterinary Physiology 6th edition. St. Louis, Elsevier, 2020, pp 126-137.
2. Herdt TH. Regulation of gastrointestinal function. In Klein BG, editor. Cunningham's Textbook of Veterinary Physiology 6th edition. St. Louis, Elsevier, 2020, pp 284-291.
3. Burrows CF. The acute abdomen. In The Acute Abdomen: Proceedings from World Small Animal Veterinary Association World Congress, 24-27 October 2003, Bangkok, Thailand. College of Veterinary Medicine, Florida, USA.

CHAPTER 12

Petechiae and ecchymoses

Floris Dröes
DVM (Hon), MRCVS,
PGCert VMS

Pathophysiology

Petechiae (<3 mm), purpura (3-10 mm), and ecchymoses (>10 mm) are small to medium, round, red-brown to purple discolorations of the skin or mucous membranes. They occur where blood has extravasated the circulation either from capillaries (i.e., petechiae) or small arterioles and venules (i.e., purpura and ecchymoses). Hemostasis is tightly regulated in healthy animals, and signs of bleeding (such as petechiae and ecchymoses) should not be observed without an inciting event. If petechiae or ecchymoses are observed, it is suggestive of a defect in primary hemostasis, although secondary or generalized hemostatic disorders could have a similar clinical presentation.

Primary hemostasis involves a combination of vascular endothelial cells, von Willebrand factor (vWF) (an essential factor for platelet aggregation), and platelets. Blood vessels are lined with a single layer of vascular endothelial cells connected by tight junctions onto a basal membrane. Under physiologic conditions, these endothelial cells express anticoagulant properties; however, after an injury to the vessel, the subendothelial matrix is exposed, comprising collagen and different proteins. Circulating platelets adhere to the matrix and undergo shape and functional changes, attracting even more platelets to aggregate, forming a "platelet plug".

Functional or quantitative defects in any of the three parts of primary hemostasis (i.e., endothelial cells, vWF, and platelets) can cause petechiae or ecchymoses. For all parts, primary hereditary and secondary acquired causes have been identified (Table 12.1). However, a low platelet number (thrombocytopenia) is the most common cause of these clinical signs in small animals. Other causes, such as abnormal platelet function (thrombocytopathy), disorders with vWF (i.e., von Willebrand disease), and vascular disorders, should also be considered. Von Willebrand disease (vWD) is the most common hereditary hemostatic disorder in small animals.

Thrombocytopenia can be caused by four mechanisms: destruction, consumption, sequestration, or decreased production. Destruction of platelets, immune-mediated thrombocytopenia (IMTP), can be primary (i.e., idiopathic) or secondary to medication, infection, neoplasia, or inflammation (see memorizing tip). Idiopathic IMTP appears more common in middle-aged female dogs. Although some breed predispositions have been identified (e.g., Cocker Spaniels, Poodles, German Shepherd dogs, and Old English Sheepdogs), any dog breed could be affected.

Easy memorizing tip

When looking for secondary causes of petechiae and ecchymoses, ask yourself if there is a cause of the following acronym (MINI) present.

- Medication.
- Infection.
- Neoplasia.
- Inflammation.

Clinical signs

Petechiae are most commonly found on the inner pinnae, skin of the ventral abdomen, axillae, and inguinal regions, and mucous membranes of the oral cavity and genitalia. Ecchymoses, however, are most found on the skin of the ventral abdomen and inguinal region or at recent venipuncture sites.

Other signs of primary hemostatic disorders that can also be observed include gingival bleeding, gastrointestinal hemorrhage (e.g., hematemesis, melena, hematochezia), hematuria, epistaxis, ocular hemorrhage (e.g., scleral or fundic), and hematoma formation. Prolonged bleeding during or postsurgery or excessive blood loss during estrus could also be indicators of primary hemostatic disorders.

Dogs of any breed and age can develop petechiae and ecchymoses. In certain dog breeds, hereditary defects of primary hemostasis have been described (Table 12.1). The age at which these are observed could increase suspicion for congenital (i.e., young age) versus acquired causes. Congenital causes are more likely in pedigree dogs with affected relatives, presenting early in life, with (multiple) similar previous events and a fixed bleeding pattern each time. Acquired causes might be suspected in those patients with no (family) history of bleeding disorders and that may have signs of concurrent diseases.

TABLE 12.1 Causes of petechia and ecchymoses in dogs.

Thrombocytopenia	Thrombocytopathies	Von Willebrand disease (vWD –most common inherited hemostatic defect)	Vascular disorders	Secondary hemostasis disorders

Destruction of platelets
■ Immune-mediate thrombocytopenia (IMTP)
  ■ Primary (idiopathic)
  (Reported breeds: Cocker Spaniels, Poodles, Old English Sheepdogs, German Shepherd dogs)
  ■ Secondary
   – Medication: sulfonamide antibiotics, cephalosporins, penicillins, chloramphenicol, griseofulvin, methimazole, procainamide, quinidine, thiazide diuretics, phenobarbital, propylthiouracil, etc.
   – Infection: *Rickettsia* spp., *Anaplasma* spp., *Babesia* spp., *Bartonella* spp., *Cytauxzoon felis*, *Dirofilaria* spp., *Ehrlichia* spp., *Leishmania* spp., *Mycoplasma haemofelis*, *Histoplasma* spp., *Candida* spp., *Leptospira* spp., CDV, CPV, CAV, FIV, FeLV, FIP, diverse fungal and bacterial infections
   – Neoplasia: lymphoma, hemangiosarcoma, histiocytic sarcoma
   – Inflammation: chronic hepatitis, pancreatitis, SIRS
■ Disseminated intravascular coagulation (DIC)
Consumption of platelets
■ Thrombosis
■ Disseminated intravascular coagulation (DIC) caused by acute severe inflammation (e.g., severe acute pancreatitis, acute hepatitis)
■ Microangiopathic hemolytic anemia
Increased sequestration of platelets (secondary to)
■ Hepatomegaly
■ Splenomegaly (e.g., due to infectious agents, neoplasia, congestion due to portal hypertension or cardiac failure)
■ Hypotension
■ Endotoxemia
■ Hypothermia
Decreased platelet production
■ Structural
  ■ Bone marrow aplasia/hypoplasia
  ■ Bone marrow necrosis
  ■ Myelodysplasia
  ■ Bone marrow fibrosis/sclerosis
  ■ Hereditary macrothrombocytosis/-penia
  (Reported breeds: Cavalier King Charles Spaniel, Norfolk Terrier, Cairn Terrier)
■ Secondary to
  ■ Medication: chemotherapeutics, estrogen, chloramphenicol
  ■ Infection: FIV, FeLV, *Ehrlichia* spp.
  ■ Neoplasia: (e.g., myelophthisis, neoplastic bone marrow infiltration)
  ■ Inflammation
	Congenital/inherited
	■ Glanzmann's thrombasthenia *(Reported breeds: Great Pyrenees dogs and Otterhounds)*
	■ Thrombopathy *(Reported breeds: Basset hound, Spitz, Landseer)*
	■ Delta PLT granule storage pool deficiency *(Reported breed: American Cocker Spaniel)*
	Acquired
	■ Medication: carprofen, hydroxyethyl starch solutions, aspirin, clopidogrel, omega fatty acids, other NSAIDs (e.g., ibuprofen, phenylbutazone)
	■ Infection: *Rickettsia* spp., *Leishmania* spp., *Ehrlichia* spp., *Anaplasma* spp.
	■ Neoplasia
	■ Inflammation
	■ Other: hepatic dysfunction, uremia, anemia
		■ **Type 1** – partial quantitative vWF deficiency *(Reported breeds: Airedale Terrier, Akita, Bernese Mountain Dog, Dachshund, Doberman Pinscher, German Shepherd dog, Golden Retriever, Greyhound, Kerry Blue Terrier, Manchester Terrier, Mini Pinscher, Papillon, Pembroke Welsh Corgi, Poodle)*
		■ **Type 2** – qualitative vWF structure and function defect *(Reported breeds: German Short- and Wirehaired Pointers)*
		■ **Type 3** – absence or extremely low quantity of vWF *(Reported breeds: Dutch Kookier, Scottish Terrier, Shetland Sheepdog, Border Collie, Chesapeake Retriever, Cocker Spaniel, Labrador Retriever, Maltese, Pomeranian)*
			Congenital/inherited (primary)
			■ Ehlers-Danlos syndrome
			■ Familial vasculopathy *(Reported breeds: German Shepherd dog, Beagle, Scottish Terrier, Greyhound)*
			Acquired (secondary)
			■ Medication
			■ Infection
			■ Neoplasia
			■ Inflammation
				See Table 12.2

TABLE 12.2 Secondary hemostasis disorders causing ecchymoses.

Coagulation protein disorders	
Congenital/ inherited	■ Hemophilia A (factor VIII) ■ Hemophilia B (factor IX) ■ Factor II (thrombin) disorder ■ Factor VII deficiency ■ Hypo-/dysfibrinogenemia ■ Other factor deficiencies (e.g., X, XI, XII)
Acquired	■ Decreased (or altered) production ■ Hepatic disease: severe acute or end-stage chronic ■ Inadequate (or altered) function ■ Vitamin K deficiency – Intoxication with rodenticides – Nutritional – Cholestasis (mostly in cats, uncommon in dogs) – Intestinal malabsorption (e.g., with exocrine pancreas insufficiency) ■ Envenomation ■ Dilution of coagulation proteins – Rapid excessive fluid therapy or use of colloids ■ Medication/intoxication – Heparins, oral anticoagulants, anti-Xa inhibitors – NSAIDs ■ Increased consumption ■ Significant blood loss ■ Thrombosis ■ Inflammation – DIC (e.g., with severe organ inflammation such as severe acute pancreatitis) – Heatstroke

Diagnostic approach

The approach to the petechiae/ecchymoses is outlined in Algorithm 12.1.

Algorithm 12.1 Note 1 A thorough history including questions regarding historical bleeding tendencies (e.g., during teething, previous surgical procedures, and blood draws), recent trauma, medications, vaccinations, pedigree information, tick exposure, travel history, and other current or previous medical history is important. This information could help identify which kind of hemostatic disorder is more likely.
A detailed physical exam helps identify the distribution and extent of the hemorrhage as well as signs of any potential underlying or concurrent diseases. During this physical exam, there should be special attention on other common locations of petechiae or ecchymoses and other signs of primary hemostatic disorders (e.g., epistaxis, gingival or gastrointestinal bleeding). A fundoscopic examination and evaluation of the abdomen (for spleen and liver size) and lymph nodes should be included.

Algorithm 12.1 Note 2 The lower limit for a normal platelet count in dogs is around 150,000-200,000/μL. However, if thrombocytopenia is the sole cause, clinical bleeding often does not become apparent until the count is <30,000-35,000/μL.

Algorithm 12.1 Note 3 Most commercial hematology analyzers provide a platelet count. When platelet counts are abnormal, confirming these with microscopic blood smear evaluation is recommended to exclude platelet clumping.
A microscopic blood smear evaluation can obtain an estimated platelet count: multiply the average number of observed platelets in 10 high-power fields by 15,000/μL to obtain a platelet count estimate.

Algorithm 12.1 Note 4 Buccal mucosal bleeding time (BMBT) is a global insensitive test of platelet function, von Willebrand factor, and abnormalities in vascular integrity. It is subject to inter- and intraoperator variability, and standardization is highly recommended. BMBT should only be performed if platelet counts are normal because, in thrombocytopenic patients, BMBT is likely prolonged. Before performing a BMBT, it is recommended to evaluate hematocrit because BMBT might also be prolonged with concurrent anemia. Normal BMBT in dogs is <4 minutes.

Algorithm 12.1 Note 5 Von Willebrand factor (vWF) can be quantified by vWF antigen testing (vWF:Ag). This is a quantitative ELISA to identify patients with low concentrations of vWF (<50%). When there is a qualitative defect, vWF collagen binding assay (vWF:CBA) is the test of choice. Ratios of vWF:Ag to vWF:CBA help identify partial quantitative vWF deficiency.

Algorithm 12.1 Note 6 Platelet function testing requires fresh blood samples and specialized equipment and staff, which limits this test to specific centers. A bench-top version, PFA-100, makes this more readily available. Platelet aggregation testing is dependent on platelet number and function, as well as functional vWF. Therefore, normal platelet numbers and vWF defects should be evaluated before.

Algorithm 12.1 Note 7 If platelet number and function are normal, secondary hemostatic disorders should be explored by further coagulation testing.

ALGORITHM 12.1

Diagnostic approach to petechiae and ecchymoses.

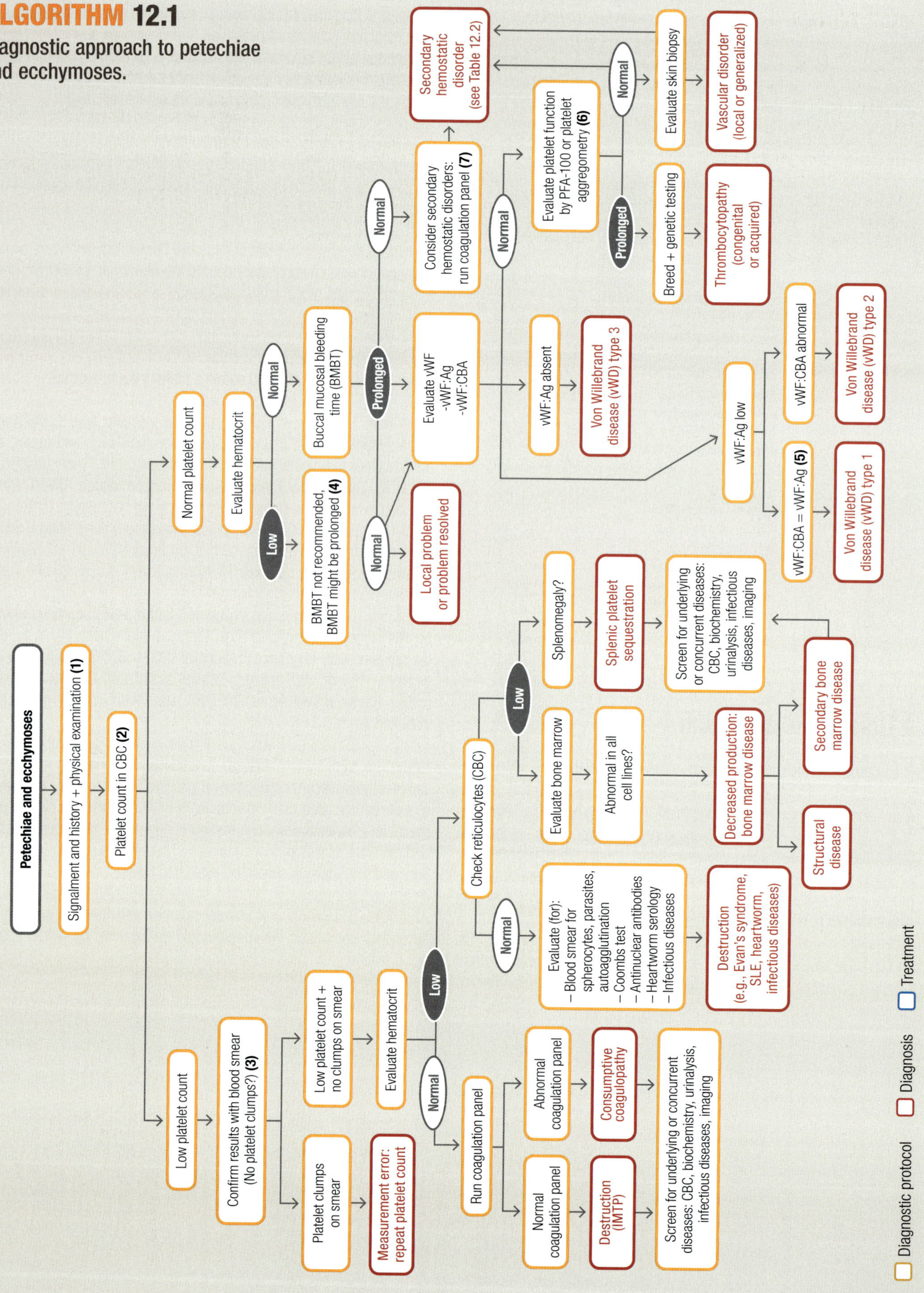

References

1. Blois S. Petechiae and ecchymoses. In Ettinger SJ, Feldman EC, Côté E, editors. Textbook of veterinary internal medicine. St. Louis, Elsevier, 2017, pp. 217-219.
2. Callan MB, Catalfamo JL. Immune-mediated thrombocytopenia, von Willebrand disease, and other platelet disorders. In Ettinger SJ, Feldman EC, Côté E, editors. Textbook of veterinary internal medicine. St. Louis, Elsevier, 2017, pp. 847-855.
3. Prater R, Tvedten H. Hemostatic abnormalities. In Willard MD, Tvedten H, editors. Small animal clinical diagnoses by laboratory methods. Missouri, Elsevier, 2004, pp. 92-112.
4. Brooks MB, Catalfamo JL. Current diagnostic trends in coagulation disorders among dogs and cats. *Vet Clin North Am Small Anim Pract* 43:1349-1372, 2013.
5. Burgess HJ, Woods JP, Abrams-Ogg ACG, et al. Evaluation of laboratory methods to improve characterization of dogs with von Willebrand disease. *Can J Vet Res* 73:252-259, 2009.
6. Herring J, McMichael M. Diagnostic approach to small animal bleeding disorders. *Top Companion Anim Med* 27:73-80, 2012.
7. Barr JW, McMichael M. Inherited disorders of hemostasis in dogs and cats. *Top Companion Anim Med* 27:53-58, 2012.

Nonspecific laboratory findings in pancreatic disease

Yvonne McGrotty
BVMS, CertSAM,
DECVIM-CA, MRCVS

The diagnosis and management of veterinary patients with pancreatitis have evolved significantly over the last two decades. Although specific markers for pancreatic inflammation exist (see chapter 14), it is also important to recognize nonspecific laboratory changes that can occur as a result of this complex inflammatory disease and will impact prognosis and treatment. Pancreatitis is associated with both local and systemic inflammatory responses, which can affect a wide range of body systems and lead to a variety of clinicopathological abnormalities (Table 13.1). Complete hematological analysis (with concurrent film examination), biochemical analysis, including lipid profiles, and contemporaneous urinalysis are strongly recommended in all cases of suspected or confirmed pancreatic inflammatory disease. Additional tests, including measurement of cobalamin, are also recommended in chronic exocrine pancreatic disease. If cavity effusions are identified, fluid analysis can prove instrumental in confirming a definitive diagnosis or excluding additional pathologies. In severe cases of pancreatitis, the release of proinflammatory cytokines can lead to coagulation abnormalities, and as such, coagulation tests are also recommended. Although these laboratory changes are also identified in many other diseases and are, therefore, not specific to pancreatic disease, assessment of these additional parameters is essential for a comprehensive evaluation of the patient with suspected or confirmed pancreatic disease.

TABLE 13.1 Nonspecific laboratory findings in pancreatic disease.

- Azotemia
- Increased liver enzymes
- Hyperbilirubinemia
- Hyperlipidemia
- Hypoalbuminemia
- Hypoglycemia
- Hyperglycemia
- Hypocalcemia
- Neutrophilia
- Thrombocytopenia
- Increased CRP
- Prolonged clotting times
- Hypocobalaminemia
- Proteinuria
- Glycosuria

Azotemia

Azotemia is defined as an excess of nonprotein nitrogenous compounds (such as urea and creatinine) in blood. These substances are usually filtered by the kidneys and subsequently excreted in the urine. Causes of azotemia can be divided into prerenal, renal, and postrenal causes. It is critical to differentiate between these three categories early on in investigations, as treatment and prognosis will vary considerably depending on the underlying cause (see Algorithm 13.1). Prerenal azotemia may be identified in dogs with pancreatitis due to fluid losses associated with vomiting, diarrhea, and decreased intake. Renal azotemia may also be recognized due to the systemic inflammatory response, concurrent unrelated kidney disease, or potentially as part of a syndrome of the immune-mediated disease recognized in English Cocker Spaniels.[1,2] Renal azotemia should be further subclassified as either acute or chronic. Both acute and chronic stable renal azotemia should be staged using the IRIS kidney classification.[3,4] Acute kidney injury is commonly identified in humans with pancreatitis and has also been suggested to be a comorbidity in canine acute pancreatitis, where it is associated with a poorer outcome.[5]

Algorithm 13.1 Note 1 A calibrated refractometer should be used to measure USG, as urine dipsticks are not accurate for veterinary use.

Algorithm 13.1 Note 2 If USG is higher than 1.030 (hypersthenuria) in an azotemic dog, then azotemia is confirmed as prerenal.

Algorithm 13.1 Note 3 Prerenal azotemia is commonly caused by dehydration and decreased renal perfusion. Contemporaneous measurement of urine specific gravity (USG) is imperative in the azotemic patient (before fluid therapy is initiated, where possible) to differentiate between renal and prerenal causes.

Algorithm 13.1 Note 4 An important exception to this rule includes dogs with hypoadrenocorticism; in such cases, azotemia is prerenal in origin, but due to sodium wasting and lack of medullary hypertonicity, urine is often poorly concentrated (typically USG around 1.018 to 1.020). Certain drug therapies, such as diuretics, and also underlying conditions, such as hypercalcemia, will interfere with the patient's ability to concentrate urine in the face of dehydration.

Algorithm 13.1 Note 5 A full medical history should be obtained before interpreting USG further. In cases where comorbidities or drugs may be interfering with the interpretation of USG, intravenous fluid therapy can be administered, followed by repeat biochemical analysis, which should demonstrate the resolution of prerenal azotemia.

Algorithm 13.1 Note 6 Contemporaneous measurement of USG is required to confirm renal azotemia. Dogs with renal azotemia will have isosthenuric urine (1.008-1.012), which is similar to the specific gravity of plasma. However, submaximally concentrated urine (USG 1.013-1.029) in an azotemic patient is also an indicator of subnormal renal function and should be investigated further (e.g., SDMA measurement, renal imaging, full urinalysis).

Algorithm 13.1 Note 7 Postrenal azotemia should initially be suspected based on a suggestive clinical history and physical examination. Dogs with postrenal azotemia may present with signs of dysuria, a distended bladder, or an abdominal effusion in cases of urinary tract rupture. In cases of suspected urinary tract rupture, the measurement of creatinine in the abdominal effusion can be compared to that of serum creatinine. Concurrent measurement of electrolytes is essential in animals with postrenal azotemia, as hyperkalemia is a common finding and can be life-threatening if left untreated.

Increased liver enzymes

There are four liver enzymes that are routinely measured in the dog – alanine aminotransferase (ALT), aspartate aminotransferase (AST), alkaline phosphatase (ALP) and gamma-glutamyl transferase (GGT). ALT and AST are considered to be hepatocellular leakage enzymes, while ALP and GGT are more associated with cholestasis. Please refer to chapter 25 for more detailed description of interpretation of raised liver enzymes.
ALT is released from the cytoplasm of hepatocytes after cell injury. Both primary hepatocellular damage (e.g., neoplasia, hepatitis, trauma) and secondary injury (e.g., pancreatitis, gastrointestinal inflammation, congestive heart failure, endocrine disease) can lead to increased levels of ALT.
AST is also located within hepatocytes but also in skeletal muscle, cardiac myocytes, and the kidneys and is therefore considered less "liver-specific" than ALT.
ALP is a membrane-associated enzyme that increases with liver, biliary, and bone disease. High levels are often found in dogs with cholestasis, pancreatitis, endocrine disease, bone disease, and due to steroid therapy. Immature dogs will also have increased ALP due to bone growth, and elderly dogs frequently have raised ALP due to nodular hyperplasia of the liver. Some dog breeds, such as the Scottish Terrier, have higher levels of ALP compared to others.[6] Increased ALP concentrations are very commonly identified in canine medicine but are nonspecific. A concurrent increase in GGT improves the specificity of increased ALP as a marker of hepatic disease in the dog.
GGT is also a membrane-associated enzyme found in high concentrations in the biliary tract. Concentrations are increased in dogs with cholestasis and biliary hyperplasia. In the dog, increased concentrations of GGT are more specific but less sensitive than increased ALP concentrations for liver disease.
In canine pancreatic disease, increased liver enzymes are often a secondary effect due to local inflammation, systemic inflammatory effects, and bile duct inflammation or obstruction.

Hyperbilirubinemia

Dogs with pancreatitis may present with jaundice due to hyperbilirubinemia. Pancreatitis is the most common cause of extrahepatic bile duct obstruction (EHBDO) in dogs.[7] Pancreatic inflammation leads to local swelling and blockage of the common bile duct, with resultant moderate-to-severe increases in bilirubin and concurrent elevation of ALP and GGT.[7] Treatment options include biliary decompression, such as ultrasound-guided cholecystocentesis, biliary stenting, and surgical decompression. Surgical interventions carry a significant risk of mortality in dogs with concurrent pancreatitis.[8] Recent studies suggest that many cases will respond favorably to medical management without the need for surgical intervention.[9] For more details on the investigation of the dog with increased bilirubin, see chapters 8 and 25.

Hyperlipidemia

Hyperlipidemia describes an increase in cholesterol and/or triglyceride concentrations in the blood and can be primary, secondary to disease (such as pancreatitis) or drugs, or associated with dietary fat content[10] (see Algorithm 13.2).
The association between pancreatitis and hyperlipidemia in dogs has not been fully elucidated. Hypertriglyceridemia is reported to be a trigger for pancreatitis in dogs, although published evidence to support this is lacking. It is not clear whether hypertriglyceridemia causes pancreatitis or if pancreatitis causes hypertriglyceridemia.[11] The exception is familial hypertriglyceridemia in Miniature Schnauzers, which appears to be a trigger for recurrent acute pancreatitis in affected dogs when triglycerides are moderate to markedly elevated, as in humans with familial hypertriglyceridemia.[12] In a prospective case study of 17 dogs with a clinical diagnosis of pancreatitis, most dogs were found to have both serum triglyceride and cholesterol levels within reference intervals.[11] When an increase in serum lipids was identified, these changes were generally mild. In another small study, hypercholesterolemia was noted to be elevated in 58% of dogs with chronic pancreatitis.[13]

Algorithm 13.2 Note 1 Elevated triglyceride and cholesterol levels can be identified in nonfasted samples.

Algorithm 13.2 Note 2 Postprandial hyperlipidemia can be confirmed or excluded by re-evaluating triglyceride and cholesterol levels after a minimum of 12 hours of fasting. Elevated lipids in animals that have been fasted for more than 12 hours are abnormal and should be investigated further.

ALGORITHM 13.1

Diagnostic approach to azotemia.

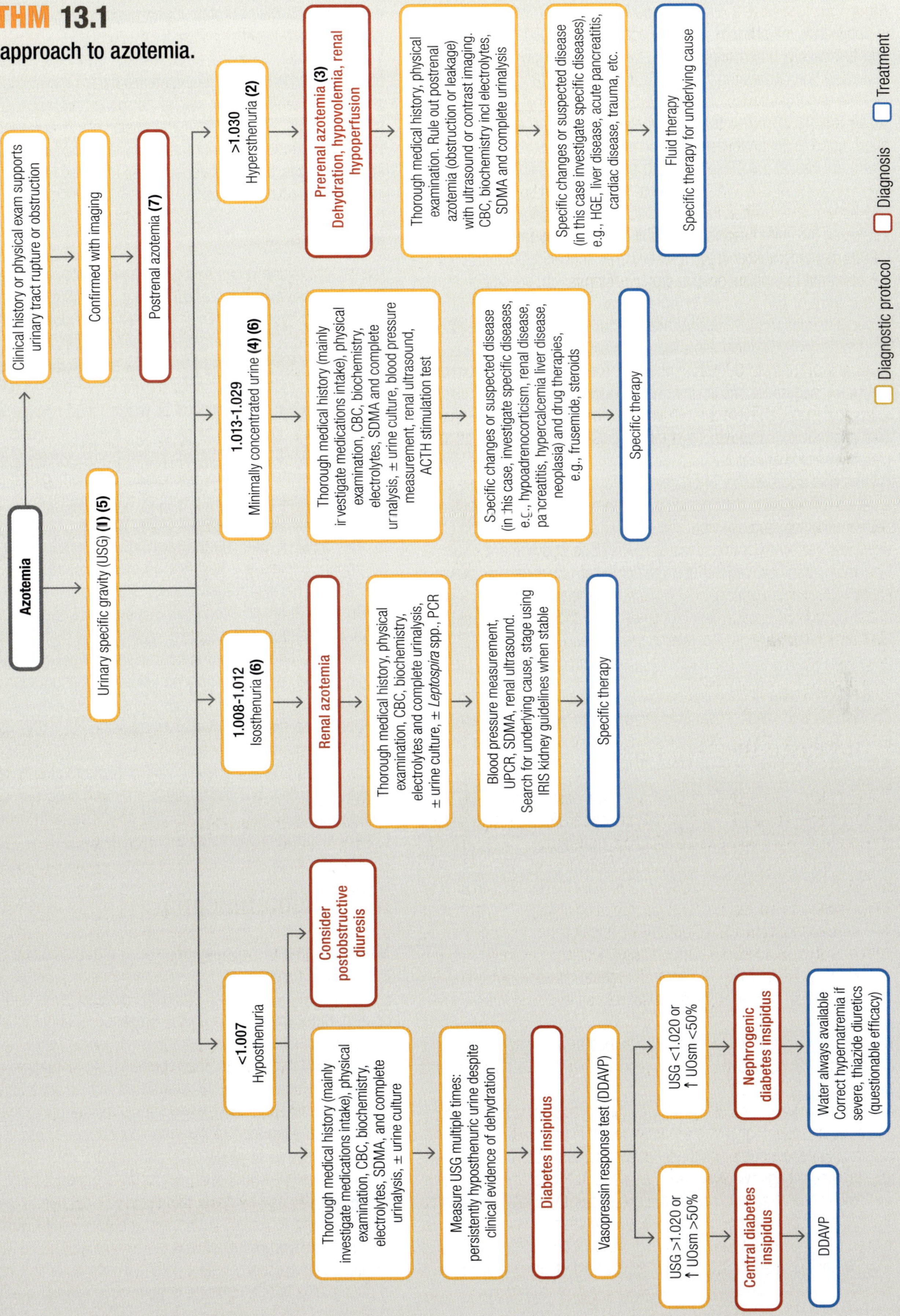

Algorithm 13.2 Note 3 Primary hyperlipidemias, due to an inborn error in lipoprotein metabolism, are less common than secondary disorders and are usually breed-related (e.g., familial hypertriglyceridemia in the Miniature Schnauzer).

Algorithm 13.2 Note 4 In cases where a secondary cause is not identified, specific lipoprotein panels and electrophoresis may help confirm a primary cause, but these are often not readily available.

Algorithm 13.2 Note 5 Treatment of hypertriglyceridemia consists of managing the underlying cause and introducing a low-fat diet (containing $<20\%$ metabolizable energy). If severe hypertriglyceridemia (triglyceride >5.65 mmol/L) persists despite dietary modification, specific treatment in the form of fish oils and/or fibrates can be considered.[14,15] Primary hyperlipidemias require lifelong therapy.

Algorithm 13.2 Note 6 Treatment of hypercholesterolemia should focus on the management of the underlying cause (e.g., endocrine disease) in combination with dietary modification (low-fat diet). If dietary therapy fails, then the use of statins has been proposed, but these can be associated with side effects such as lethargy, diarrhea, and hepatopathies.[15]
Canine lipid disorders are often detected fortuitously but can also cause a variety of clinical signs, including hepatomegaly, seizures, abdominal pain or vomiting, and diarrhea. Hyperlipidemias can also result in ocular signs such as lipid keratopathies or lipemic aqueous humor.[15]
The most common causes of hyperlipidemias in dogs are shown in Table 13.2.

Cholesterol

Hypercholesterolemia has been identified in canine pancreatitis and is associated with cholestasis secondary to pancreatic inflammation.[13] Cholestasis can result in variable increases in serum cholesterol levels.[14,15] Secondary hypercholesterolemia is more common than primary and is also identified in dogs consuming a high-fat diet (60% metabolizable energy fat), in obese dogs, and in those with endocrine disease or protein-losing nephropathy.[15,16] Primary hypercholesterolemia has been identified in Briards, Shetland Collies, Rough Collies, Dobermans, and Rottweilers.[15,16] The highest levels of cholesterol (>15 mmol/L) are generally found in dogs with hypothyroidism. Hypercholesterolemia is a common sequelae of protein-losing nephropathy, but the mechanism is not fully understood.[15]
The liver is the main site of cholesterol synthesis, but cholesterol can also be absorbed via the gastrointestinal tract from the diet. Cholesterol serves as a precursor for steroid hormone and bile acid synthesis and also is a component of cell membranes.
Hypercholesterolemia rarely causes any specific clinical signs other than ocular changes, and dogs appear to be relatively resistant to atherosclerosis compared to humans.[16]

TABLE 13.2 **Causes of hyperlipidemia in dogs.**

- Physiological, i.e., postprandial hyperlipidemia
- High-fat diets
- Primary hyperlipidemia
  - Breed-specific disorders, e.g., familial hypertriglyceridemia in Schnauzers
- Secondary hyperlipidemia
  - Pancreatitis
  - Diabetes mellitus
  - Hypothyroidism
  - Hyperadrenocorticism
  - Protein-losing nephropathy
  - Obesity
  - Cholestasis
  - Hepatic insufficiency
  - Lymphoma
  - Drugs, e.g., steroids, phenobarbital

Triglycerides

Hypertriglyceridemia can occur with pancreatitis, in nonfasted samples, in dogs consuming a high-fat diet (e.g., raw diet), and also in animals with primary hyperlipidemia or secondary to endocrine diseases or drug therapies (e.g., corticosteroids or phenobarbital).[16]
Triglycerides are synthesized from fatty acids in the liver, small intestine, mammary glands, and adipose tissue. Hypertriglyceridemia should be suspected when centrifugation of whole blood reveals lipemic plasma or serum. It is important to recognize lipemia in a blood sample, as it can interfere with certain hematological and biochemical assays, leading to falsely elevated calcium, phosphate, and hemoglobin concentrations and also increased measurement of total solids using a refractometer. Hypercholesterolemia does not cause lipemia.
In the case of persistent hypertriglyceridemia, both primary and secondary causes are possible. Primary idiopathic causes are more prevalent in certain breeds of dogs, such as the Miniature Schnauzer or Brittany Spaniel. Secondary hypertriglyceridemia is identified in dogs with various diseases (e.g., pancreatitis, hypothyroidism, diabetes mellitus, and hyperadrenocorticism) following exogenous steroid administration or may simply be linked to consumption of a diet with high-fat content. Where clinical signs are supportive, investigations for endocrine diseases should be considered in the investigation of persistent hypertriglyceridemia.
There may not be any specific clinical signs related to hypertriglyceridemia in the dog, but clinical signs are more likely associated with the underlying cause (e.g., polyuria and polydipsia with hyperadrenocorticism or alopecia and lethargy with hypothyroidism).

Hypoalbuminemia

Mild and transient hypoalbuminemia is often identified as part of the acute phase response in dogs with pancreatitis.[17] Serum albumin levels should always be assessed alongside globulin levels and interpreted in context with clinical signs. In the presence of acute inflammation, the production of albumin is temporarily switched off, while the production of globulins and major acute phase proteins, like C-reactive protein, is upregulated. Hypoalbuminemia, associated with an acute phase response, is generally mild and self-limiting but can contribute to the development of peripheral edema or ascites when concurrent illness is present.
Hypoalbuminemia in dogs with pancreatitis can also be associated with increased protein losses via the urinary tract if there is concurrent glomerular damage by or via the digestive tract due to local peritonitis. Globulins tend to remain within the reference range with renal protein losses, while hypoglobulinemia is more commonly found where intestinal protein loss is present. Another potential contributor to hypoalbuminemia in pancreatitis is third spacing in abdominal exudative effusions. Other

ALGORITHM 13.2

Diagnostic approach to hyperlipidemia.

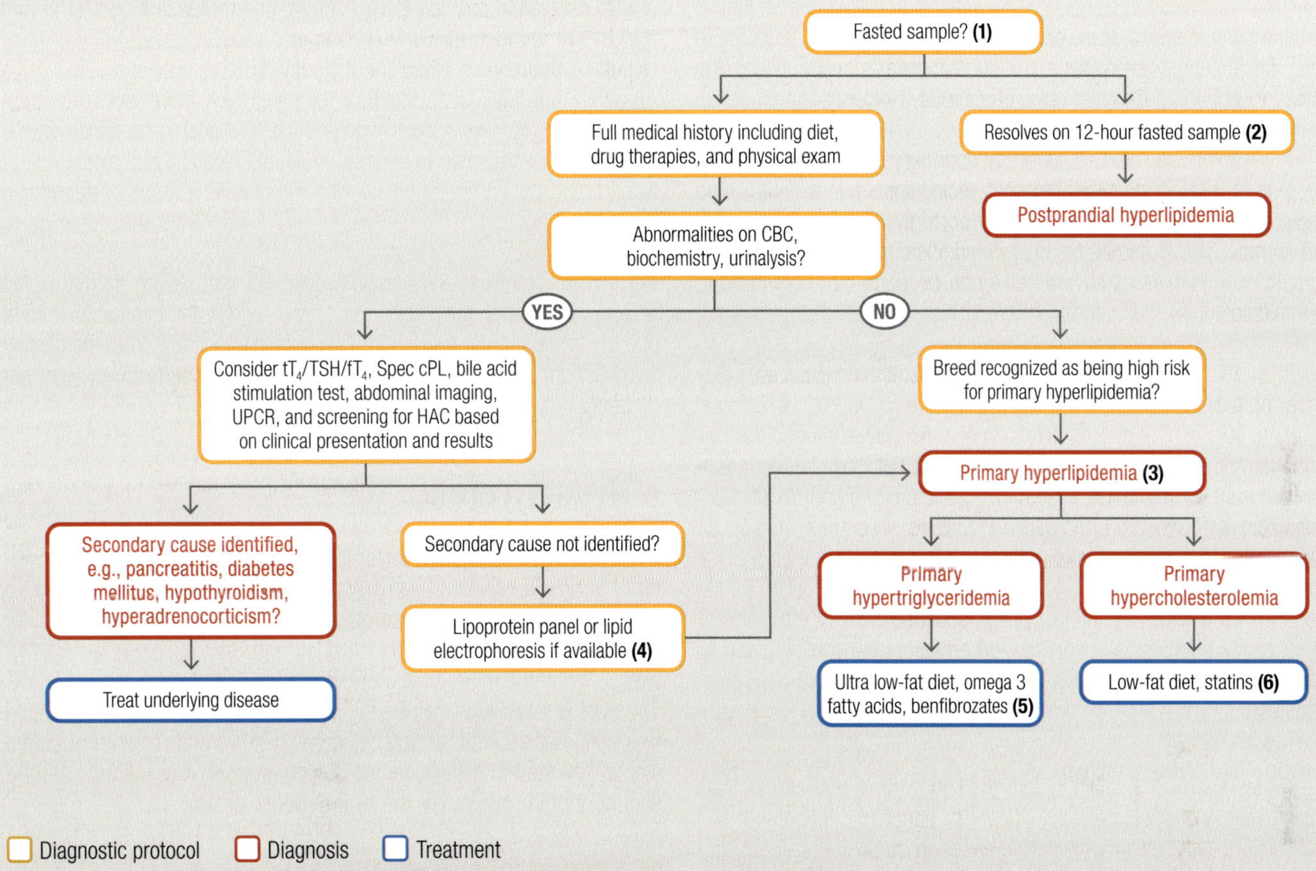

causes unrelated to pancreatitis include decreased production of albumin due to hepatic dysfunction or severe burns.
Approach to the hypoalbuminemic patient (see Algorithm 13.3):

Algorithm 13.3 Note 1 Confirm or exclude renal proteinuria. A logical approach to hypoalbuminemia commences by assessing urinary protein levels. An absence of protein on a urine dipstick usually allows the clinician to exclude significant renal proteinuria. However, the presence of proteinuria on a dipstick should lead to the measurement of urine protein-to-creatinine ratio (UPCR), to further quantify the level of proteinuria. Note that 1+ protein documented on a urine dipstick in a dilute urine sample is more significant than 1+ protein identified in a concentrated urine sample. UPCR should be interpreted in conjunction with a urine sediment examination, as severe hematuria or pyuria can contribute to an increased UPCR.

Algorithm 13.3 Note 2 Generally, a UPCR >2 is consistent with glomerular protein losses.[18]

Algorithm 13.3 Note 3 Milder increases in UPCR may be secondary to urinary tract inflammation, systemic diseases, steroid administration, or hypertension. Therefore, measuring systemic blood pressure is an important step in investigating proteinuria in the dog.

Algorithm 13.3 Note 4 Confirm or exclude body cavity effusions. If a body cavity effusion is suspected, ultrasonography can be used to confirm this and will also allow for ultrasound-guided fluid aspiration for analysis.

Algorithm 13.3 Note 5 Where an exudate (Table 13.4) is confirmed, third spacing is the likely cause of hypoalbuminemia, and further investigations should focus on identifying the underlying cause of the effusion (e.g., cytology to identify neoplastic cells, fluid cPLI, or bacteria within cells or fluid culture).

Algorithm 13.3 Note 6 Confirm or exclude hepatic dysfunction. Where renal protein losses and proteinaceous effusions have been excluded, a bile acid stimulation test is performed to assess hepatic function (assuming the patient is not icteric). Concurrent assessment of serum urea, cholesterol, glucose, and bilirubin are also recommended as these are additional markers of hepatic function. Elevated bile acids, low urea, hypoglycemia, low cholesterol, or raised bilirubin levels in a hypoalbuminemic patient should increase the suspicion of hepatic dysfunction as the underlying cause. Hepatic biopsies are often necessary to confirm the underlying pathology. Coagulation testing should be performed before performing hepatic biopsies.

Algorithm 13.3 Note 7 Consider intestinal protein losses. After excluding renal losses, effusions, and hepatic dysfunction as the cause of hypoalbuminemia, intestinal losses should be suspected. Not all dogs with intestinal protein loss will have obvious gastrointestinal signs. In cases with mild hypoalbuminemia, a hypoallergenic food trial should be considered in the first instance, but in cases presenting with more severe hypoalbuminemia, imaging of the gastrointestinal tract and pancreas using ultrasound and possibly endoscopic intestinal biopsies should be considered. Where intestinal disease is suspected or confirmed, analysis of cobalamin and folate is recommended. Measurement of serum trypsin-like immunoreactivity (TLI) is also recommended to confirm or exclude exocrine pancreatic insufficiency (EPI).
Although full-thickness intestinal biopsies are more accurate than endoscopic biopsies, severe hypoalbuminemia should be considered a relative contraindication to surgical intestinal biopsies due to the risk of wound dehiscence and subsequent peritonitis as a result of decreased wound healing.

Algorithm 13.3 Note 8 Animals presenting with severe dermal burns or toxic epidermal necrolysis may have significant hypoalbuminemia due to dermal protein exudation. This should be evident from the clinical examination, and further investigations, as described above, may not be necessary.

Hypoglycemia

Hypoglycemia is defined as a blood glucose concentration below 60 mg/dL (3.3 mmol/L) and is caused by either a decrease in glucose production or an increase in glucose utilization.[19] Hypoglycemia is a relatively common finding in severe pancreatitis and may occur as a result of sepsis, malnutrition, anorexia, or concurrent liver disease.
The liver is the main site of gluconeogenesis, and as such, advanced liver dysfunction, with reduced gluconeogenesis and reduced glycogen stores, can lead to hypoglycemia. See chapter 24, Algorithm 24.2, for a summary of the workup of the hypoglycemic patient.

Reduced glucose production

Puppies, especially toy breeds, can develop hypoglycemia after relatively short periods of fasting due to their low glycogen reserves. In contrast, fasting hypoglycemia is rare in healthy adult dogs.

Increased glucose utilization

Artifactual hypoglycemia is very commonly identified due to delayed separation of red blood cells from serum or plasma. In these cases, patients will be asymptomatic despite often quite marked hypoglycemia. Red blood cells continue to metabolize glucose in the blood tube. Therefore, failure to promptly separate the red cells from plasma/serum will lead to artifactual hypoglycemia, which can be marked. Repeat sampling and rapid analysis of glucose levels using a glucometer are recommended in such cases. Erythrocytosis also leads to hypoglycemia by the same mechanism.
Insulin-producing tumors such as insulinomas, oral hypoglycemic agents, and exogenous insulin overdose would all be expected to lead to hypoglycemia. Ingestion of xylitol has also been shown to stimulate inappropriate insulin release with resultant often prolonged hypoglycemia.

ALGORITHM 13.3

Diagnostic approach to hypoalbuminemia.

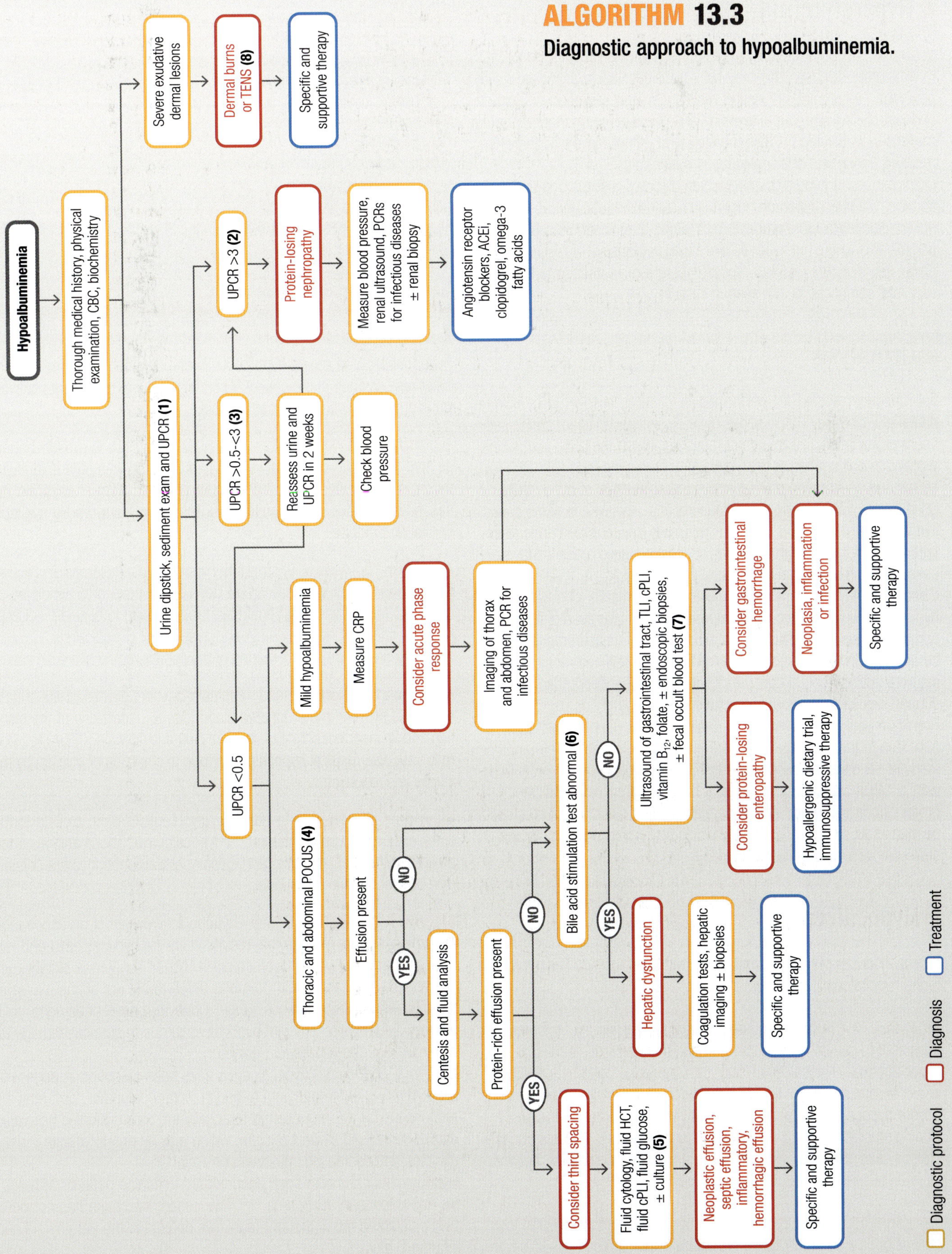

Hyperglycemia

In contrast, hyperglycemia is also a common finding in canine pancreatic inflammatory disease. This may be a transient finding associated with pancreatic inflammation, insulin resistance, and secretion of cortisol and catecholamines, but in around 30% of cases, permanent diabetes mellitus may develop.[20] Close monitoring of glucose levels is, therefore, required during and after episodes of pancreatitis.

Other causes of hyperglycemia include diabetes mellitus and other endocrine diseases (hyperadrenocorticism, pheochromocytoma), drug-induced (glucocorticoids, progestogens, alpha-2 agonists, beta-blockers), and diestrus where the hyperglycemia may be transient or result in newly diagnosed diabetes mellitus. Stress hyperglycemia in dogs tends to be very mild compared to that seen in cats.

Urinalysis

Full urinalysis should be performed in patients suspected of having pancreatic disease. This includes urine dipstick examination, urine sediment examination, refractometer measurement of the USG, and, where proteinuria is identified, a urine protein to creatinine ratio (UPCR). Fluid losses and dehydration often result in the production of hypersthenuric urine (USG >1.030) in dogs with pancreatitis. However, in some cases, isosthenuria (USG 1.008-1.012) or minimally concentrated urine is detected in conjunction with azotemia, suggesting these patients may have concurrent intrinsic renal disease.

Glycosuria may be identified in cases of pancreatitis and can reflect hyperglycemia associated with temporary insulin resistance or the development of diabetes mellitus. Serial blood glucose measurements should be analyzed in such cases to determine if there is a need for long-term insulin administration. If concurrent ketonuria is identified, then this may support diabetic ketosis or ketoacidosis.

Proteinuria has been identified in English Cocker Spaniels with pancreatitis due to the presence of concurrent glomerulonephritis.[2] In another study of 70 dogs of various breeds with acute pancreatitis, proteinuria with a UPCR >2 was considered a negative prognostic indicator.[21] If proteinuria is confirmed and is persistent, then blood pressure should be measured, and an ARB or ACEi would be considered the standard of care once dehydration has resolved.

Hypocalcemia

Potential causes of hypocalcemia are listed in Table 13.3. The approach to the hypocalcemic patient is shown in Algorithm 13.4.

Algorithm 13.4 Note 1 In acute pancreatitis, calcium can become sequestered in saponified fat in and around the pancreas, leading to mild hypocalcemia. Hypocalcemia may be a negative prognostic indicator in canine pancreatitis.[22] Mild hypocalcemia is generally asymptomatic. Severe hypocalcemia can be associated with neuromuscular signs, including muscle twitching, facial rubbing, nervousness, seizures, muscle cramps, and seizures. There may be an inverse correlation between ionized calcium and cPLI in dogs with pancreatitis.[23]

Algorithm 13.4 Note 2 Sample artifact associated with EDTA contamination is a common cause of hypocalcemia. In such cases, severe hyperkalemia and severe hypocalcemia are identified concurrently in an otherwise asymptomatic patient. The first step is to re-evaluate calcium measurement on a fresh blood sample.

TABLE 13.3 Causes of hypocalcemia.

- Immune-mediated hypoparathyroidism
- Surgical damage to parathyroid glands
- Hypoalbuminemia
- Acute and chronic kidney disease
- Pancreatitis
- Eclampsia (postpartum hypocalcemia)
- Sepsis and trauma
- Improper diet (rickets)
- Toxin ingestion, e.g., ethylene glycol
- Sample artifact
- Tumor lysis syndrome
- CPDA excess during transfusion

Algorithm 13.4 Note 3 More than 50% of calcium is protein-bound, so hypocalcemia should always be interpreted in conjunction with serum albumin levels. Ionized calcium provides a more accurate assessment of calcium homeostasis but is not always readily available in clinical practice.

Algorithm 13.4 Note 4 Postpartum hypocalcemia (eclampsia) is sometimes seen in young, small-breed dogs 2-3 weeks after whelping. A history of recent whelping should alert the clinician to consider eclampsia as a cause of hypocalcemia and associated clinical signs. Calcium supplementation and hand-rearing of the pups is required in such cases.

Algorithm 13.4 Note 5 Blood transfusions where excess citrate anticoagulant is present in the donated blood (due to underfilling of the blood bag and an incorrect citrate phosphate dextrose adenine [CPDA] to blood ratio) can also result in hypocalcemia, due to chelation of calcium by the citrate anticoagulant.

Algorithm 13.4 Note 6 In ethylene glycol intoxication, oxalate forms complexes with calcium, leading to hypocalcemia. These animals often present with renal azotemia, and calcium oxalate monohydrate crystals may be identified in their urine.

Algorithm 13.4 Note 7 Primary hypoparathyroidism is an uncommon endocrine disease in dogs that results in severe hypocalcemia and relative or absolute hyperphosphatemia.[24] Ionized calcium is significantly decreased, and parathyroid hormone (PTH) levels are subnormal or at the low end of the reference range. Dogs that have undergone neck surgery can also present with hypocalcemia due to surgical damage to, or removal of, the parathyroid glands.

Both total and ionized hypocalcemia have been identified in dogs with protein-losing enteropathies. Although enteric albumin loss may be responsible for the reduction in total calcium, recent studies have also shown decreased ionized calcium, which may be due to vitamin D deficiencies and decreased intestinal absorption.[25]

Hypocalcemia has also been documented in canine patients with sepsis and secondary to trauma.[26,27] The underlying cause has not been fully elucidated but is thought to involve defects in the parathyroid and vitamin D axis.

ALGORITHM 13.4

Diagnostic approach to hypocalcemia.

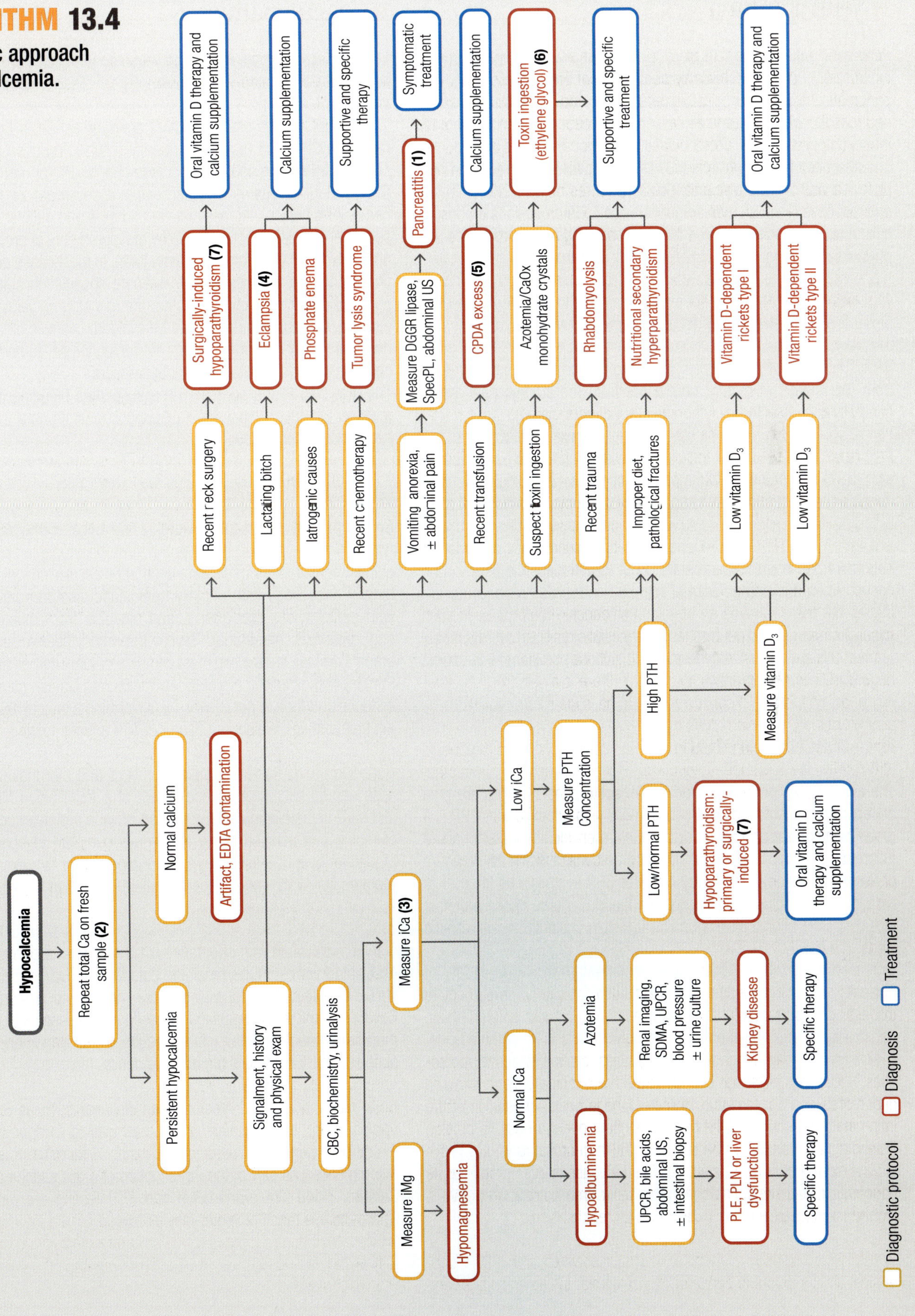

Neutrophilia

Pancreatic inflammation triggers a systemic inflammatory response, which can result in several hematological abnormalities. Dogs with pancreatic disease will usually present with mild to moderate mature neutrophilia, which is generally associated with a nonspecific systemic inflammatory response, and conversely, lymphocyte counts are reduced. The absence of neutrophilia in a dog with suspected pancreatitis should prompt a search for a concurrent condition that would suppress neutrophil response (such as hypoadrenocorticism). Neutrophilia is a nonspecific change associated with a large number of disease processes and physiological responses (Algorithm 13.5).

Algorithm 13.5 Note 1 Fear or exercise can lead to physiological neutrophilia; this is transient and often accompanied by lymphocytosis.

Algorithm 13.5 Note 2 Stress, or steroid-induced neutrophilia, results from the release of mature neutrophils from the storage pool and is generally accompanied by lymphopenia and monocytosis.

Algorithm 13.5 Note 3 An inflammatory neutrophilia can be associated with various systemic inflammatory processes, including infections, neoplasia, and immune-mediated diseases, and may include a left shift.

Algorithm 13.5 Note 4 A regenerative left shift (presence of immature band neutrophils and a neutrophilia count that exceeds the band count) occurs when the storage pool of mature neutrophils has become depleted, but there remains an ongoing demand for neutrophils. In such cases, immature band neutrophils are released from the maturation pool to meet this demand. A regenerative left shift can be identified in some dogs with severe pancreatitis.

C-reactive protein

The acute phase proteins, including C-reactive protein (CRP), are produced in response to any type of tissue injury or inflammation. CRP is a major acute phase protein in dogs and is a nonspecific marker of acute inflammation. Concentrations of CRP increase rapidly within 24-48 hours of tissue injury due to the upregulation of CRP synthesis by the liver in response to stimulus from interleukins 1 and 6. Acute phase proteins, including CRP, should always be interpreted in conjunction with clinical signs.
Increased levels of CRP have been documented in a wide variety of diseases, including canine pancreatitis, inflammatory cerebrospinal disease, discospondylitis, bacterial pneumonia, chronic enteropathies, parvovirus, pyometra, lymphoma, and polyarthritis. In human medicine, CRP is an important prognostic indicator in patients with acute pancreatitis, but in dogs, although CRP correlated with clinical severity of acute pancreatitis and a return to reference range indicated resolution of the inflammatory focus, CRP has not been definitively proven to provide prognostic information.[28] The use of a CRP-to-albumin ratio may prove to be a more promising indicator for the risk of death in dogs with acute pancreatitis, with higher CRP/albumin ratios being associated with a higher risk of death.[29]

Coagulopathies

In severe acute pancreatitis, coagulation abnormalities are common and are mainly associated with consumption in disseminated intravascular coagulation (DIC).
The majority of the clotting factors are synthesized in the liver. Thus, hepatic dysfunction may subsequently result in reduced production of clotting factors and coagulopathy (see chapter 24 for more details).
Coagulation assessment requires the assessment of both primary hemostasis (which includes platelet numbers and platelet function) and secondary hemostasis (assessed by measurements of prothrombin time and activated partial thromboplastin time). In most cases, a combination of tests will be required to fully evaluate coagulation status. Where a coagulopathy is strongly suspected, the use of large veins, such as the jugulars, for venipuncture should be avoided; cephalic or lateral saphenous veins may be better options for venipuncture, as hemorrhage can be more easily controlled with local pressure.
The first step in the approach to a suspected bleeding disorder is to consider whether clinical signs are supportive of a primary or secondary hemostatic disorder (see Algorithm 13.6).

Primary hemostasis

Severe primary hemostatic disorders are uncommonly found in dogs with pancreatic disease because the thrombocytopenia associated with platelet consumption in disseminated intravascular coagulation (DIC) is usually mild. Dogs with primary hemostatic disorders usually present with petechiation, ecchymosis, and bleeding from mucosal surfaces (e.g., epistaxis, hematuria). Severe thrombocytopenia and von Willebrand's disease are the two most common primary hemostatic disorders. Primary hemostasis is evaluated by measuring platelet count in the first instance and then, if necessary, by performing a buccal mucosal bleeding time and von Willebrand Factor (VWF) antigen testing.

Algorithm 13.6 Note 1 Platelet numbers and morphology should be assessed by microscopic assessment of a fresh blood film. Although standard hematological analyzers can provide a platelet count, platelet clumping and poor sampling techniques can lead to underestimation of platelet counts. Assessment of dot plots and a film examination are required in any thrombocytopenic patient to confirm the result.

Algorithm 13.6 Note 2 Platelet values of less than 30-50,000/μL may be associated with spontaneous bleeding and are most commonly associated with immune-mediated platelet destruction. Particular care should be taken when assessing platelet numbers in breeds such as the Cavalier King Charles Spaniel; this breed may present with a hereditary macrothrombocytopenia, which results in thrombocytopenia (large platelets) but without any bleeding tendency.

Algorithm 13.6 Note 3 Vector-borne diseases such as *Babesia* spp., *Ehrlichia* spp., and *Anaplasma* spp. can lead to cytopenias, including thrombocytopenia and bleeding tendencies. A thorough travel history is recommended as part of the investigation of a coagulation abnormality. Capillary blood film examination and PCR testing are recommended where there is a risk of vector-borne disease.

ALGORITHM 13.5

Diagnostic approach to neutrophilia.

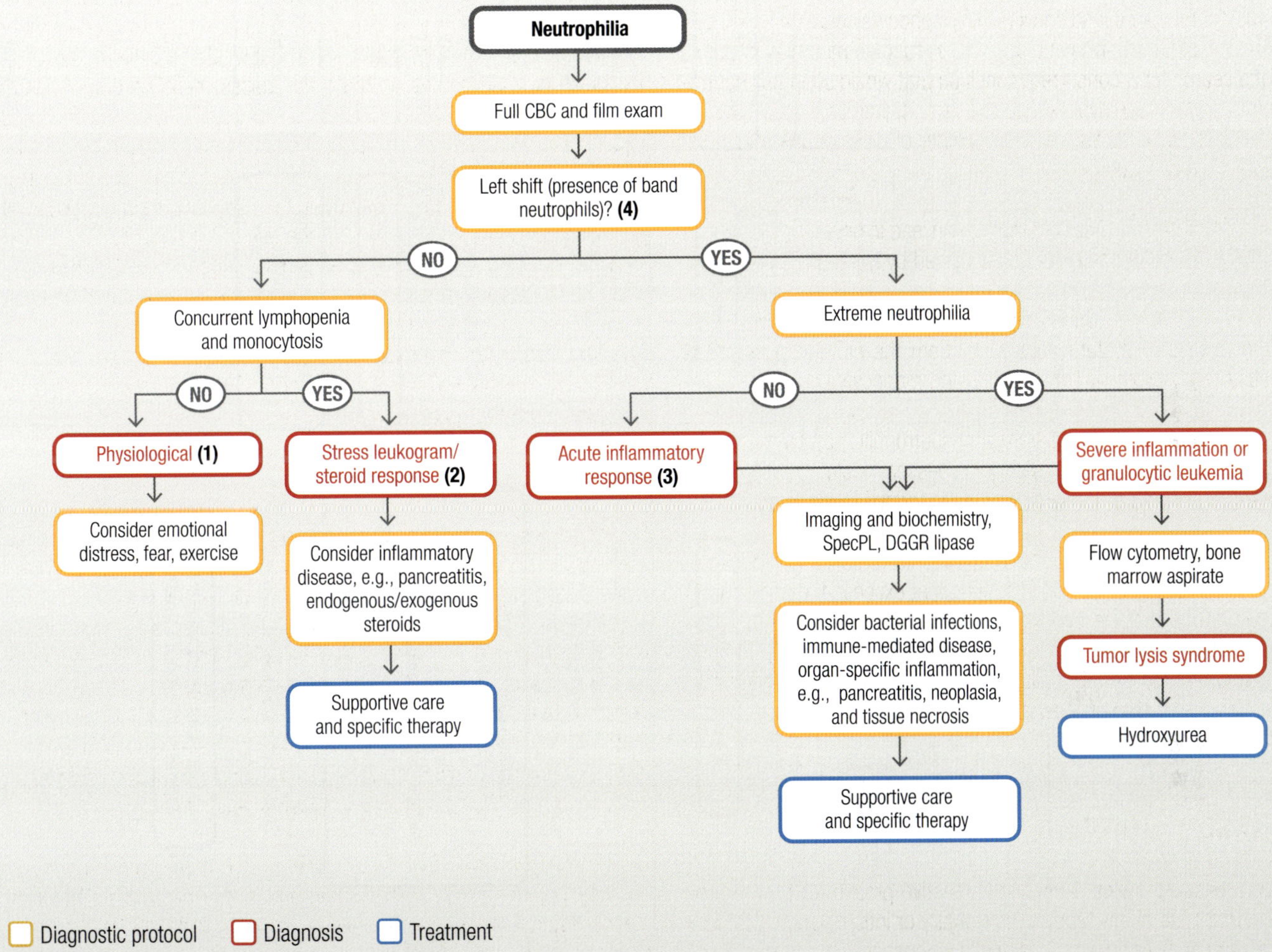

ALGORITHM 13.6

Diagnostic approach to coagulation abnormalities.

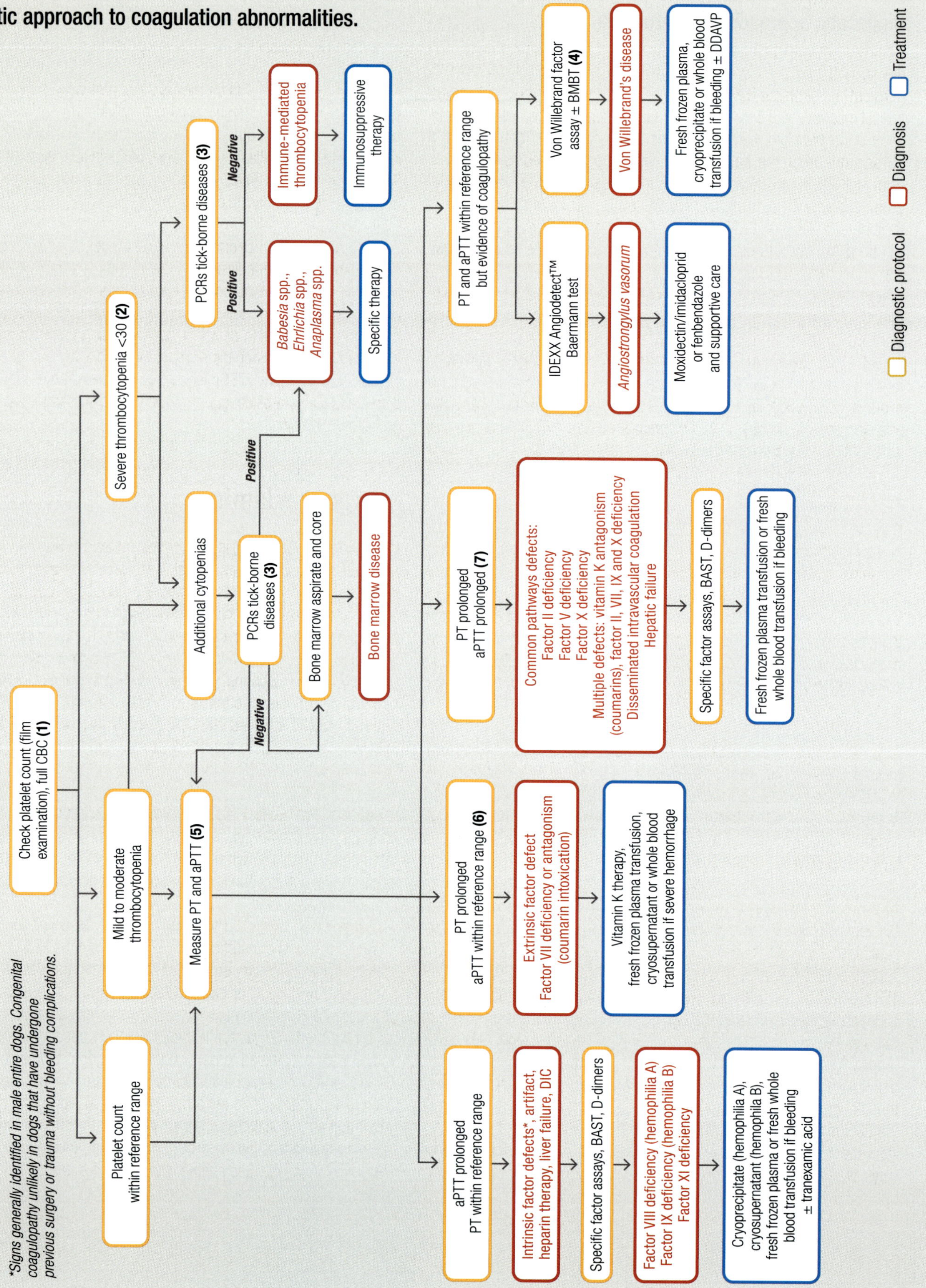

Algorithm 13.6 Note 4 The buccal mucosal bleeding time (BMBT) is a crude indicator of platelet function. It should not be performed in any patient with significant thrombocytopenia as this may result in significant hemorrhage. The dog is placed in lateral recumbency, and the lip is folded back using gauze to expose the buccal mucosa. A Surgicutt or Simplate device is then used to make a small cut on the buccal mucosa, avoiding areas where superficial vessels are obvious. A timer is started from the moment when the device is triggered. Around 15 seconds after the cut is made, filter paper is used to blot blood from just below the incision (taking care not to touch the incision site). Blotting is repeated every 15 seconds until a clot is visualized at the incision site. Normal BMBT in dogs is less than 4.2 minutes. BMBT will be prolonged in animals with functional platelet defects (such as von Willebrand's disease).

Where there is clear evidence to support a primary hemostatic defect (bleeding from mucosal surfaces) but where platelet numbers are not significantly reduced, the clinician should consider a functional platelet defect. The most common functional platelet defect in dogs is von Willebrand's disease (VWD). This is a congenital disease and so would not be expected to be sequelae of pancreatic inflammation; however, proteases released into the circulation during pancreatic inflammation may interfere with VWF activity and lead to coagulation abnormalities.

Secondary hemostasis

Dogs with pancreatitis are more likely to present with disorders of secondary hemostasis due to the consumption of clotting factors in DIC. These disorders of secondary hemostasis usually manifest as hematoma formation or bleeding into tissues or cavities.

The most common acquired secondary hemostatic disorder is coumarin ingestion. Congenital disorders of secondary hemostasis include hemophilia A and B. Other acquired secondary disorders include hepatic failure, disseminated intravascular coagulation, and infection with *Angiostrongylus vasorum*.

Algorithm 13.6 Note 5 Tests used to evaluate secondary hemostasis include prothrombin time (PT). PT evaluates the common pathway (II, V and X) and extrinsic pathway (VII) of coagulation. A reagent is added to the sample, which activates FVII and initiates coagulation. Reference ranges vary depending on the methodology used. Shortened PT values have no diagnostic significance.

Algorithm 13.6 Note 6 Prolongation of PT indicates a disorder of the extrinsic and/or common pathway of coagulation, e.g., coumarin ingestion. Coumarin ingestion leads to prolongation of PT first but also subsequent prolongation of activated partial thromboplastin time (aPTT). aPTT evaluates the intrinsic pathway (factors VIII, IX, XI, and XII) and common pathway (II, V, and X) of coagulation. A reagent is added to the sample, which activates factor XII and thus coagulation. Reference ranges vary depending on the methodology used. Shortened aPTT values have no diagnostic significance. Prolongation indicates a disorder of the intrinsic and/or common pathways, e.g., hemophilia A, due to factor VIII deficiency in dogs.

Activated clotting time (ACT) evaluates the intrinsic and common pathways of coagulation. Whole blood is added to an ACT tube containing diatomaceous earth, and the time for a clot to form at 37°C is noted. It is a good screening test for both congenital and acquired coagulation disorders but is less sensitive than aPTT, as the ACT is only prolonged with severe factor deficiencies. Normal values in dogs are 60-90 seconds.

Algorithm 13.6 Note 7 In the presence of prolonged PT or aPTT and a suspected congenital clotting disorder, individual factor assays can be performed to confirm the underlying diagnosis, e.g., deficiency of FVIII in dogs with hemophilia A or deficiency of FIX in animals with hemophilia B. This type of test is unlikely to prove necessary in dogs with pancreatic disease, as in these cases, coagulation abnormalities are acquired rather than congenital.

Tertiary hemostasis: D-dimers are fibrin degradation products and are a marker of fibrinolysis; as such, they are indirect markers of hypercoagulability. Elevation of D-dimers can be associated with a variety of conditions, including disseminated intravascular coagulation or thromboembolism, both of which may be associated with severe acute pancreatitis, renal or hepatic disease, or neoplasia.

Thromboelastography (TEG): TEG is a patient-side test that provides a global assessment of coagulation, including measuring platelet aggregation and function.

Hypocobalaminemia

Cobalamin (or vitamin B_{12}) is an essential water-soluble vitamin that plays a crucial role in several important physiological processes. Cobalamin is necessary for DNA synthesis and the metabolism of carbohydrates, proteins, and fats. Dogs cannot synthesize cobalamin, so most cobalamin is obtained from dietary sources, then bound to intrinsic factors, and subsequently absorbed in the ileum. Intrinsic factor is produced primarily by the exocrine pancreas in dogs. Consequently, exocrine pancreatic insufficiency often leads to cobalamin deficiency. Any disease that can result in reduced production of intrinsic factors or that reduces cobalamin absorption in the intestine can lead to cobalamin deficiency (Algorithm 13.7).

Algorithm 13.7 Note 1 Causes include pancreatic diseases (exocrine pancreatic insufficiency), intestinal diseases (dysbiosis, chronic enteropathies, intestinal lymphoma), and hereditary disorders (selective cobalamin malabsorption in Border Collie, Giant Schnauzer or Shar Pei).

Algorithm 13.7 Note 2 Hypocobalaminemia is a common finding in exocrine pancreatic insufficiency (EPI) due to impaired digestion and malabsorption of dietary sources. In addition, dogs with EPI may have decreased production of intrinsic factor. EPI can cause dysbiosis and changes in the microbiome, which can further lead to reduced cobalamin absorption from the gastrointestinal tract. Low cobalamin levels in dogs with EPI are considered to be a negative prognostic indicator.[30,31]

Clinical signs of hypocobalaminemia can include weight loss, diarrhea, decreased appetite, and lethargy; neurological signs can rarely occur. Treatment should include oral or parenteral cobalamin supplementation and management of the underlying cause (e.g., pancreatic extract supplementation in EPI). See chapter 20 for more details.

ALGORITHM 13.7

Diagnostic approach to hypocobalaminemia.

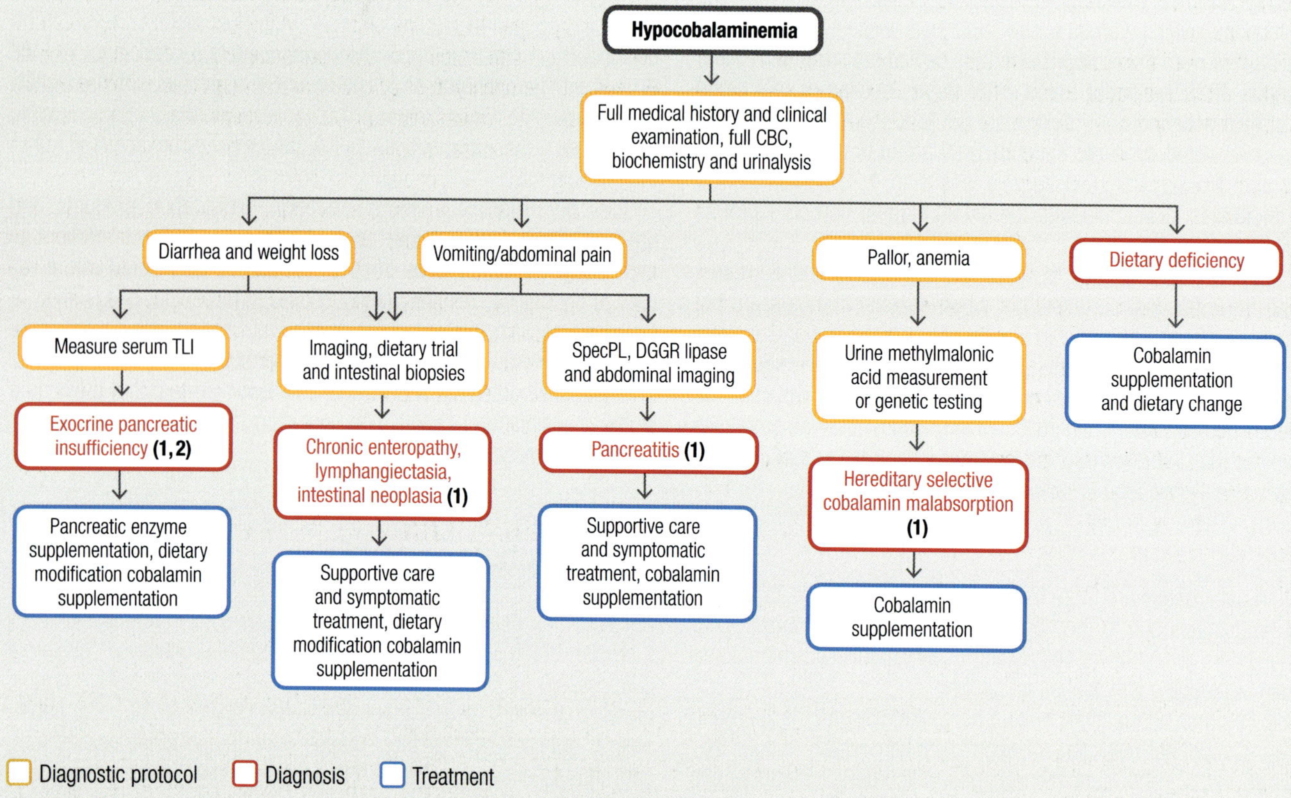

Abdominal effusions

Body cavity effusions can result from a variety of pathophysiological mechanisms, including decreased oncotic pressure, increased hydraulic pressure, increased vascular permeability, or reduced lymphatic flow. A detailed algorithm for the investigation of abdominal fluid is presented in chapter 10 (Algorithm 10.2).

The initial step in effusion analysis is the macroscopic examination of the sample. Gross evaluation of an effusion provides very useful information, e.g., transudates are often clear liquids, while septic effusions are opaque and can have an unpleasant smell, hemorrhagic effusions are red, and chylous effusions are often milky.

Effusions are then classically categorized based on their protein concentrations, total nucleated cell counts (TNCC), and cytological evaluation (Table 13.4). Protein content can be easily and rapidly assessed using a refractometer or in-house chemistry analyzers. Three broad categories of effusion exist: low-protein (pure) transudate, protein-rich (modified) transudate, and exudate. Hemorrhagic and chylous effusions cannot be classified in the same manner and are considered separately.

Mild to moderate abdominal effusions are common in canine acute pancreatitis and may be exudates or protein-rich transudates. Bicavity effusions may also be recognized. If fluid aspiration shows an exudate, it is important to rule out a septic process with analysis. Septic exudates result from rupture of the gastrointestinal tract, penetrating wounds, or following surgery. The pancreas can be inflamed secondary to gastrointestinal rupture, and it would be a mistake, therefore, not to analyze the fluid in a case of suspected acute pancreatitis. Fluid cytology reveals a predominance of degenerate neutrophils and bacteria. The presence of intracellular bacteria confirms a septic effusion, but contemporaneous measurement of blood and fluid glucose can also be useful to aid in the identification of a septic process. Blood glucose >1 mmol/L (20 mg/dL) different from that of fluid glucose has been reported to have a high sensitivity and specificity for septic peritonitis but has subsequently been questioned.[32] Lactate has also been used as a marker of a septic effusion, with fluid lactate levels being higher than blood lactate levels, but neither glucose nor lactate can be considered 100% reliable, and cytological evaluation of the fluid remains the gold standard for diagnosis. Confirmed or suspected septic effusions should be submitted for culture and sensitivity testing.

Nonseptic exudates result from inflammation, including pancreatitis or neoplasia, and contain nondegenerate neutrophils and macrophages and no intracellular bacteria. If pancreatitis is suspected, lipase or canine PLI measurement in the fluid may be diagnostic, and concentrations may be significantly higher than in the blood.[33] Cytological evaluation of the fluid, in conjunction with imaging, is required to confirm a neoplastic process.

Rupture of the urinary tract or biliary system can also result in an abdominal exudate. Urine leakage into the abdominal cavity provokes an inflammatory response. Initially, the fluid may be a transudate, but over time, changes in protein content and cell count due to inflammation lead to the development of an exudate. Where uroperitoneum is suspected, contemporaneous blood and fluid creatinine measurements can be performed. Higher levels of creatinine in fluid, compared to blood, are supportive of uroperitoneum. Measurement of fluid and blood potassium levels can also be diagnostic. Bile peritonitis is often recognized by the color of the fluid (green/brown) and can be confirmed by biochemical analysis, where the fluid bilirubin concentration is more than twice that of blood bilirubin.

Laboratory changes as prognostic indicators in pancreatic disease

Most of the published data continues to question the use of any specific marker as a prognostic indicator in canine acute pancreatitis. However, persistent proteinuria, azotemia, ionized hypocalcemia, and coagulation disorders have all been suggested to be negative prognostic indicators in some studies.[21,22] A clinical scoring system (clinical acute pancreatitis score) can be used to help determine the risk of short-term death in dogs with acute pancreatitis using some of these laboratory changes in conjunction with either the respiratory rate or the presence or absence of systemic inflammatory response syndrome (SIRS).[22] A more recent study has suggested that both blood urea nitrogen and bilirubin may also be negative indicators of short-term survival of dogs with acute pancreatitis.[34] Hypocobalaminemia is a negative prognostic indicator in dogs with EPI.[30,31]

TABLE 13.4 Effusion analysis.

Effusion	Macroscopic appearance	Protein concentration (g/L)	Total nucleated cell count/µL	Cell types
Transudate (protein-poor)	Clear or pale yellow	<20	<1,500	Neutrophils, macrophages, and occasional mesothelial cells
Transudate (protein-rich)	Yellow or blood-tinged	>20	<5,000	Macrophages
Exudate	Turbid color may vary	>20	>5,000	Neutrophils

KEY POINTS

- Nonspecific laboratory changes are commonly identified in dogs with pancreatic disease.
- The most common nonspecific laboratory changes in canine chronic pancreatitis include increased liver enzymes, hyperbilirubinemia, and hypercholesterolemia.
- Some laboratory changes may provide prognostic information, e.g., persistent proteinuria in canine pancreatitis or hypocobalaminemia in EPI.

References

1. Cridge H, Lim SY, Algül H, Steiner JM. New insights into the etiology, risk factors, and pathogenesis of pancreatitis in dogs: potential impacts on clinical practice. *J Vet Intern Med* 36(3):847-864, 2022.
2. Watson P, Coddou F, Blacklaws B, Bazelle J, Day M, Constantino-Casas F. Letter to the editor regarding Immunoglobulin G4-related disease in a dog. *J Vet Int Med* 34(2):542-543, 2020.
3. http://iris-kidney.com/pdf/2_IRIS_Staging_of_CKD_2023.pdf
4. http://www.iris-kidney.com/pdf/4_ldc-revised-grading-of-acute-kidney-injury.pdf
5. Gori E, Lippi I, Guidi G, Perondi F, Pierini A, Marchetti V. Acute pancreatitis and acute kidney injury in dogs. *Vet J* 245:77-81, 2019.
6. Nestor DD, Holan KM, Johnson CA, Schall W, Kaneene JB. Serum alkaline phosphatase activity in Scottish Terriers versus dogs of other breeds. *J Am Vet Med Assoc* 228(2):222-224, 2006.
7. Fahie MA, Martin RA. Extrahepatic biliary tract obstruction: a retrospective study of 45 cases (1983-1993). *J Am Anim Hosp Assoc* 31:478-482, 1995.
8. Mehler SJ, Mayhew PD, Drobatz KJ, Holt DE. Variables associated with outcome in dogs undergoing extrahepatic biliary surgery: 60 cases (1988-2002). *Vet Surg* 33:644-649, 2004.
9. Wilkinson AR, DeMonaco SM, Panciera DL, Otoni CC, Leib MS, Larson MM. Bile duct obstruction associated with pancreatitis in 46 dogs. *J Vet Intern Med* 34(5):1794-1800, 2020.
10. Watson TDG, Barrie J. Lipoprotein metabolism and hyperlipidaemia in the dog and cat: A review. *J Small Anim Pract* 34:479-487, 1993.
11. Xenoulis, PG, Cammarata, PJ, Walzem, RL, Suchodolski, JS, Steiner, JM. Serum triglyceride and cholesterol concentrations and lipoprotein profiles in dogs with naturally occurring pancreatitis and healthy control dogs. *J Vet Intern Med* 34:644–652, 2020.
12. Xenoulis PG, Suchodolski JS, Ruaux CG, Steiner JM. Association between serum triglyceride and canine pancreatic lipase immunoreactivity concentrations in miniature schnauzers. *J Am Anim Hosp Assoc* 46(4):229-234, 2010.
13. Watson PJ, Archer J, Roulois AJ, Scase TJ, Herrtage ME. Observational study of 14 cases of chronic pancreatitis in dogs. *Vet Rec* 167:968-976, 2010.
14. Whitney MS. Evaluation of hyperlipidemias in dogs and cats. *Semin Vet Med Surg Small Anim* 7(4):292-300, 1992.
15. Xenoulis PG, Steiner JM. Lipid metabolism and hyperlipidemia in dogs. *Vet J* 183(1):12-21, 2010.
16. Xenoulis PG, Steiner JM. Canine hyperlipidaemia. *J Small Anim Pract* 56:595-605, 2015.
17. Kaneko JJ. Serum proteins and the dysproteinemias. In Kaneko JJ, Harvey JW, Bruss ML (editors). Clinical Biochemistry of Domestic Animals. San Diego, Academic Press, 1997, pp. 117-138.
18. Lees GE, Brown SA, Elliot J, Grauer GF, Vaden SL. Assessment and management of proteinuria in dogs and cats: 2004 ACVIM forum consensus statement (small animal) *J Vet Intern Med* 19:377-385, 2005.
19. Idowu O, Heading K. Hypoglycemia in dogs: causes, management, and diagnosis. *Can Vet J* 59(6):642-649, 2018.
20. Davison LJ. Diabetes mellitus and pancreatitis – cause or effect? *J Small Anim Pract* 56:50-59, 2015.
21. Gori E, Pierini A, Lippi I, Boffa N, Perondi F, Marchetti V. Urinalysis and urinary GGT-to-urinary creatinine ratio in dogs with acute pancreatitis. *Vet Sci* 6(1):27, 2019.
22. Fabres V, Dossin O, Reif C, Campos M, Freiche V, Maurey C, Pilot-Storck F, Desquilbet L, Benchekroun G. Development and validation of a novel clinical scoring system for short-term prediction of death in dogs with acute pancreatitis. *J Vet Intern Med* 33:499-507, 2019.
23. Cridge H, Wang S, Steiner JM. Serum calcium concentrations are inversely correlated with pancreatic lipase concentrations in dogs. *Am J Vet Res* 84(12), 2023.
24. Bruyette DS, Feldman EC. Primary hypoparathyroidism in the dog. Report of 15 cases and review of 13 previously reported cases. *J Vet Intern Med* 2(1):7-14, 1988.
25. Mellanby RJ, Mellor PJ, Roulois A, Baines EA, Mee AP, Berry JL, Herrtage ME. Hypocalcaemia associated with low serum vitamin D metabolite concentrations in two dogs with protein-losing enteropathies. *J Small Anim Pract* 46(7):345-351, 2005.
26. Luschini MA, Fletcher DJ, Schoeffler GL. Incidence of ionized hypocalcemia in septic dogs and its association with morbidity and mortality: 58 cases (2006-2007). *J Vet Emerg Crit Care* 20(4):406-12, 2010.
27. Holowaychuk MK, Monteith G. Ionized hypocalcemia as a prognostic indicator in dogs following trauma. *J Vet Emerg Crit Care* 21(5):521-530, 2011.
28. Keany, KM, Fosgate, GT, Perry, SM, Stroup, ST, Steiner, JM. Serum concentrations of canine pancreatic lipase immunoreactivity and C-reactive protein for monitoring disease progression in dogs with acute pancreatitis. *J Vet Int Med* 35(5):2187-2195, 2021.
29. Gori E, A Pierini, I Lippi, G Ceccherini, F Perondi, Marchetti V. Evaluation of C-reactive protein/albumin ratio and its relationship with survival in dogs with acute pancreatitis. *New Zealand Vet J* 68(6):345-348, 2020.
30. Soetart N, Rochel D, Drut A, Jaillardon L. Serum cobalamin and folate as prognostic factors in canine exocrine pancreatic insufficiency: An observational cohort study of 299 dogs. *Vet J* 243:15-20, 2019.
31. Batchelor DJ, Noble PJ, Taylor RH, Cripps PJ, German AJ. Prognostic factors in canine exocrine pancreatic insufficiency: prolonged survival is likely if clinical remission is achieved. *J Vet Intern Med* 21(1):54-60, 2007.
32. D'Mello, N. Can measurement of glucose levels in blood and peritoneal fluid be used to diagnose septic peritonitis in dogs? *Vet Evidence* 7(1), 2022.
33. Chartier MA, Hill SL, Sunico S, Suchodolski JS, Robertson JE, Steiner JM. Pancreas-specific lipase concentrations and amylase and lipase activities in the peritoneal fluid of dogs with suspected pancreatitis. *Vet J* 201(3):385-389, 2014.
34. Guglielmini C, Crisi PE, Tardo AM, Di Maggio R, Contiero B, Boari A, Fracassi F, Miglio A. Prognostic role of red cell distribution width and other routine clinico-pathological parameters in dogs with acute pancreatitis. *Animals* 12(24):3483, 2022.

CHAPTER 14

More specific laboratory tests for exocrine pancreatic disease

Harry Cridge
MVB, MS, PG Cert Vet Ed, DACVIM-SAIM, DECVIM-CA, FHEA, MRCVS

Disorders of the exocrine pancreas are commonly encountered in dogs and are often characterized by relatively nonspecific clinical signs. This necessitates the need for advanced diagnostic testing including the use of noninvasive biomarkers. In this chapter, we will first focus on assays to assist in the diagnosis of pancreatitis, followed by assays utilized to diagnose exocrine pancreatic insufficiency (EPI).

Diagnosis of pancreatitis – noninvasive assays

Overview

Traditionally, histopathology was considered the gold standard for the diagnosis of pancreatitis in dogs; however, it is rarely used in clinical practice due to the presence of significant limitations.[1] These limitations include the invasive nature of a biopsy, the potential to miss localized inflammatory lesions, and a lack of standardized criteria for interpretation.[2-4] Thus, clinicians are reliant on a clinical diagnosis comprised of an assessment of patient history, physical examination findings, diagnostic imaging, and noninvasive biomarkers of pancreatic inflammation including catalytic assays, immunologic assays, microRNAs, and other biomarkers.[1] We outline each of these in separate sections below.

Analytical validation of an assay is considered a prerequisite to clinical validation. This includes assessment of linearity, precision, replication, and the effects of interfering substances (e.g., lipemia, hemolysis) on each assay.[5] If an assay has poor analytical performance, then its clinical performance should be interpreted with caution or disregarded.

Catalytic assays measure enzyme activity within a sample by quantification of substrate utilization or product accumulation. This is often linked to a colorimetric reaction. Catalytic assays are considered non-species- and non-organ-specific and are often cheaper than immunologic assays. The lack of substrate specificity may influence test performance, e.g., DGGR lipase assays can detect nonpancreatic sources of lipase, thus decreasing analytical specificity.[6] Due to this reduced analytic specificity, and high background levels of nonpancreatic lipases, ≥3-5× increases in enzyme activity are needed for the results of a catalytic assay to be supportive of a diagnosis of pancreatitis. It is important to note that analytical specificity is influenced by the substrate selected for the assay and additional factors such as the presence of cofactors such as bile acids or colipase, the pH of the assay, or the wavelength used to measure light absorption. Therefore, test performance does vary between assays.

Immunologic assays are considered organ- and species-specific. They utilize antibodies directed against a specific part of an enzyme binding site. This binding is then linked to a radioimmunoassay (RIA) or an enzyme-linked immunosorbent assay (ELISA) to quantify enzyme concentration. It is suspected that assays based on a monoclonal antibody have greater analytical specificity than those based on a polyclonal antibody because monoclonal antibodies only recognize a single epitope of an antigen.[7] Thus, test performance may also vary between immunologic assays.

It is important to note that even when an assay has a high analytical specificity, it cannot be used on its own to diagnose pancreatitis.[1] It is possible to find normal pancreatic lipase concentrations in dogs with a history and imaging findings consistent with pancreatitis. This may be associated with the short half-life of pancreatic lipase (~2 hours), or disease chronicity due to loss of tissue mass (replaced by fibrosis). There is growing evidence that pancreatic lipase concentrations and ultrasonographic abnormalities do not always mirror each other, and this is likely associated with the short half-life of pancreatic lipase, and rapid resolution after injury.[8] Sonographic abnormalities may persist longer. Abnormal pancreatic lipase concentrations can also be seen in disorders other than pancreatitis. This may be related to secondary pancreatic injury or potentially noninflammatory elevations in pancreatic lipase concentration (e.g., portal hypertension).[9] Pancreatic neoplasms are also associated with inflammation and often have increases in pancreatic lipase concentration which may be very marked.[10]

Amylase –Catalytic

Amylase was proposed as a biomarker for acute pancreatitis after experimental studies in dogs, but subsequent studies revealed suboptimal performance, which likely reflects the multiple tissues of origin of amylase.[11] Dogs that have undergone pancreatectomy still have significant serum amylase activity, indicating the presence of amylase from nonpancreatic origin.[12] This high background level impacts test performance. Amylase is also elevated in dogs with renal disease, further minimizing its diagnostic utility.[13,14] Additional data is reported in Table 14.1.

Lipase –Catalytic

Original lipase activity assays were based on hydrolysis of the substrate 1,2 diglyceride (1,2 DiG); however, these assays have now been shown to lack specificity with increased activities being noted in dogs with renal disease, hepatic disease, and also those having undergone laparotomy.[15-17] Since this time, several newer catalytic lipase assays have been developed including those utilizing the substrate 1-2-o-dilauryl-rac-glycero-3-glutaric acid-(6'-methylresorufin) ester (DGGR) or triolein. These assays are thought to be more selective for pancreatic lipase than 1,2 DiG assays.[1,15] However, extrapancreatic lipases can still be detected even by these modern catalytic assays.[6]

It could be argued that the lack of substrate specificity for pancreatic lipase could impact test performance; however, others highlight the level of agreement between modern catalytic lipase assays and immunologic assays to suggest appropriate clinical use.[1,6,7,18-21] Further data is needed before we fully understand the potential impact of the reduced analytical specificity of catalytic assays on clinical performance. Caution is advised until further data exists. Additional data is reported in Table 14.1.

Principle of DGGR-based lipase assays

DGGR-based lipase assays determine lipase activity by quantifying the rate of production of a colored compound called 6'-methylresorufin, which is a downstream product of the effects of lipase on the DGGR substrate. Each DGGR assay needs to be validated individually in the laboratory utilizing the substrate. The sequential reaction is outlined below (Fig. 14.1). Additional data is provided in Table 14.1.

Principle of triolein-based lipase assays

Triolein-based lipase activity is also determined by quantifying the rate of production of a colored compound (blue dye). The blue dye forms when hydrogen peroxide interacts with a diaryl imidazole-type leukopigment. Hydrogen peroxide is a downstream product of triolein hydrolysis by lipase. The sequential reaction is outlined below (Fig. 14.2). Additional data is provided in Table 14.1.

Lipase –Immunologic

Canine pancreas-specific lipase (cPL) immunoassays

The first canine pancreatic lipase immunoreactivity (PLI) assay utilized a radioisotope, but this was subsequently replaced by an enzyme-linked immunosorbent assay (ELISA).[22] Serum PLI concentrations are negligible in dogs with exocrine pancreatic insufficiency (EPI) indicating that nonpancreatic lipases are not detected by the assay.[23] This ELISA was further adapted for commercial use utilizing two monoclonal antibodies, each recognizing a specific epitope of pancreatic lipase.[24] This assay is offered commercially as the Spec cPL assay (IDEXX).

More recently, a patient-side SNAP® cPL test has been developed as a screening assay for pancreatitis.[25] The SNAP® cPL has been shown to have a high level of agreement with the Spec cPL assay.[18,25] The assay is highly sensitive and moderately specific.[18] When discrepancies occur between the SNAP® cPL and Spec cPL assays, they generally occur in the mid-range ("gray zone") between normal and abnormal cPL concentrations. The results of abnormal SNAP® cPL tests should be verified by submitting for a quantitative lipase concentration via the Spec cPL assay. Spec cPL concentrations <200 µg/L are considered normal, Spec cPL concentrations 200-400 µg/L are considered in the "gray zone",

TABLE 14.1 Catalytic assays for the diagnosis of pancreatitis in dogs.

Assay	Advantages	Disadvantages	Sensitivity and specificity	Clinical comments
Amylase	■ Widely available on routine in-house analyzers.	■ Nonspecific biomarker with multiple tissues of origin.[12] ■ Influenced by renal function –elevated in azotemic dogs.[13,14]	■ Varies depending on the cut-off utilized. ■ Sensitivity: 18-54.6%[36,37] ■ Specificity ~50%	■ Both positive and negative results require verification with more sensitive and specific biomarkers. ■ Limited clinical utility.[1] ■ Reported sensitivities and specificities are dependent on study design and diagnostic criteria for pancreatitis and results are not directly comparable between studies.
Lipase (catalytic) *1,2 DiG* *DGGR* *Triolein*	■ Widely available on routine in-house analyzers. ■ More recent assays (DGGR/triolein) have been optimized to detect pancreatic lipase more selectively.	■ Despite the increased selectivity of DGGR relative to 1,2 DiG, DGGR based assays can detect extrapancreatic sources of lipase.[6] ■ Triolein based assays may be affected by hemolysis or lipemia.[38]	■ DGGR based assays: Sensitivity 85.7-93.3%[15,18] Specificity: 53.3-74.3%[15,18] ■ Triolein based assay: Sensitivity: 100%[39] Specificity: 89.5%[39]	■ Clinical performance is dependent on the type of catalytic assay utilized, with DGGR and triolein-based assays preferred over traditional 1,2 DiG assays. ■ Catalytic lipase assays may detect extrapancreatic sources of lipase. ■ Reported sensitivities and specificities are dependent on study design and diagnostic criteria for pancreatitis and results are not directly comparable between studies.

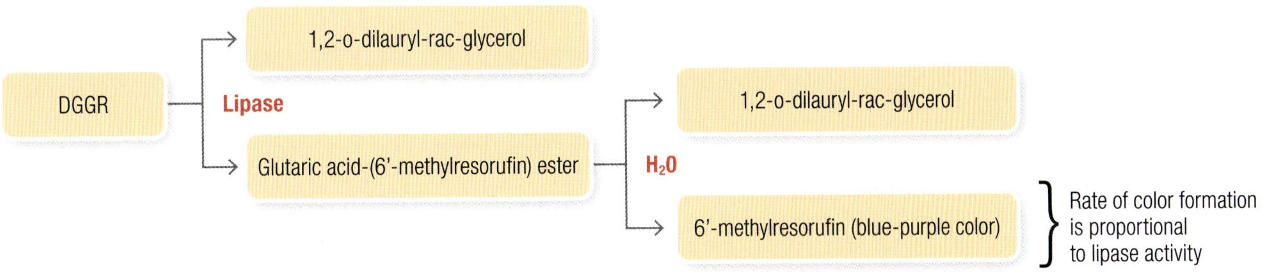

FIG. 14.1 DGGR lipase methodology.

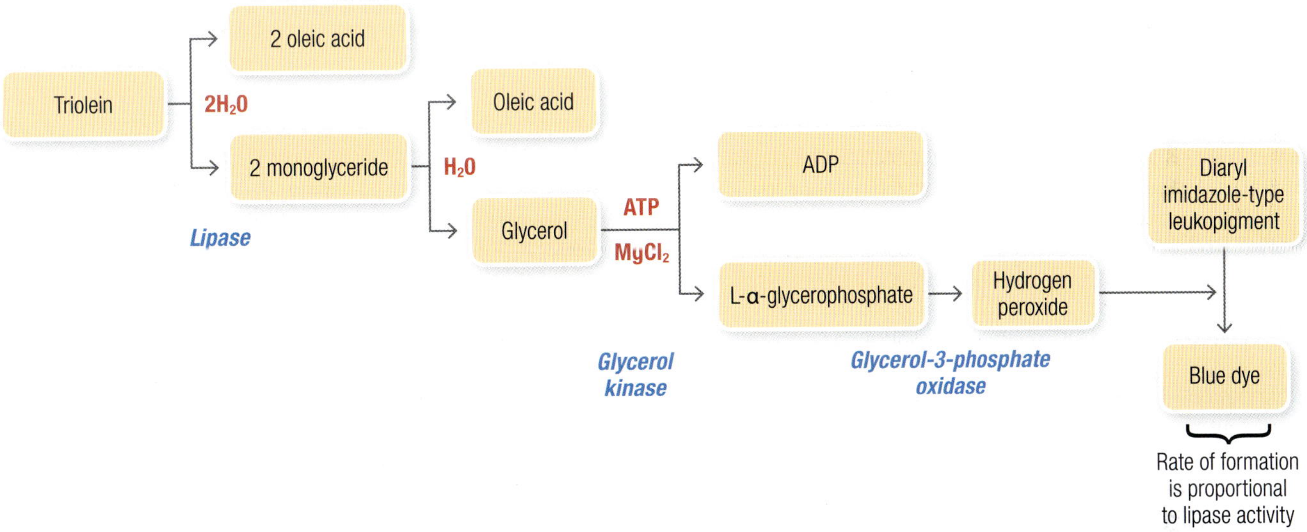

FIG. 14.2 Triolein lipase methodology.

and Spec cPL concentrations >400 μg/L are considered abnormal and consistent with a diagnosis of pancreatitis. Fasting is recommended, although failure to fast has no significant clinical impact on test results in healthy dogs.[26]

The Spec cPL assay is considered the gold standard pancreatic lipase assay to which many other assays are compared. The reported diagnostic sensitivity and specificity of the SNAP® and Spec cPL assays are reported in Table 14.2. These values vary widely based on the diagnostic criteria for pancreatitis utilized, the severity of the disease, and the chronicity of pancreatitis. These assays have higher sensitivities in acute and severe disease, relative to chronic and mild disease; this may be associated with loss of tissue and decreased enzyme leakage in chronic pancreatitis. Nonserum fluids, such as peritoneal fluid have also been investigated in the diagnostic approach to pancreatitis. Peritoneal fluid cPL concentrations have a high sensitivity (100%) and specificity (94.7%) for a diagnosis of pancreatitis.

Other cPL Assays

More recently additional cPL assays have been developed including the patient-side VetScan cPL Rapid Test and the Vcheck cPL, and a send-out alternative commercial cPL test (Laboklin). The VetScan cPL and Laboklin cPL tests use polyclonal antibodies against canine pancreatic lipase, while the antibody type for the VCheck cPL is unknown. Analytical validation concerns were noted with initial versions of the VetScan cPL.[27] Data is limited on the remaining assays. The reliability of these assays in the clinical setting remains unclear. At this time, the author utilizes the Spec cPL and fPL assays due to their analytical validation and long-standing experience with these assays. Additional data is reported in Table 14.2.

Micro RNAs

Micro RNAs are small noncoding RNAs that control gene expression by binding to mRNA.[28] They are tissue-specific and are released into body fluids (including serum) with tissue injury.[28] Micro RNAs 216a and 375 are abundant in the pancreatic tissue of dogs and increase in response to experimental pancreatic injury.[29] Micro RNA 375 has shown the greatest promise as a biomarker for the diagnosis and monitoring of pancreatitis in clinical patients, although more work is needed in this area.[30] Sensitivity and specificity are currently unknown.

TABLE 14.2

Study	Assay	Method of diagnosis	Sensitivity	Specificity
Steiner, et al. 2008[36]	Spec cPL	Histopathology	Spec cPL (>200 µg/L): 72.6% Spec cPL (>400 µg/L): 63.6%	N/A
Neilson-Carley, et al. 2011[40]	Spec cPL	Histopathology	N/A	Spec cPL (>200 µg/L): 95% Spec cPL (>400 µg/L): 97.5%
Trivedi, et al. 2011[41]	Spec cPL	Histopathology	**Mild disease:** Spec cPL (>200 µg/L): 43% Spec cPL (>400 µg/L): 21% **Moderate/severe disease:** Spec cPL (>200 µg/L): 71% Spec cPL (>400 µg/L): 71%	**Mild disease:** Spec cPL (>200 µg/L): 86% Spec cPL (>400 µg/L): 100% **Moderate/severe disease:** Spec cPL (>200 µg/L): 86% Spec cPL (>400 µg/L): 100%
Mansfield, et al. 2012[42]	Spec cPL	Histopathology	N/A	Spec cPL (>200 µg/L): 80% Spec cPL (>400 µg/L): 90%
McCord, et al. 2012[37]	Spec cPL	Clinical assessment	Spec cPL (>200 µg/L): 86.5-93.6% Spec cPL (>400 µg/L): 71.7-77.8%	Spec cPL (>200 µg/L): 66.3-77.0% Spec cPL (>400 µg/L): 80.5-88.0%
Haworth, et al. 2014[43]	Spec cPL	Clinical assessment	Spec cPL (>400 µg/L): 70%	Spec cPL (>400 µg/L): 77%
Cridge, et al. 2018[18]	Spec cPL	Clinical assessment	Spec cPL (>400 µg/L): 81.0-90.9%	Spec cPL (>400 µg/L): 74.1-81.1%
Aupperle-Lellbach, et al. 2020[10]	cPLI (in house)	Histopathology	**Mild disease:** In-house cPLI (>180 µg/L): 75% **Moderate/severe disease:** In-house cPLI (>180 µg/L): 90.9%	In-house cPLI (>180 µg/L): 92.5%
McCord, et al. 2012[37]	SNAP cPL	Clinical assessment	91.5-94.1%	71.1-77.5%
Haworth, et al. 2014[43]	SNAP cPL	Clinical assessment	82%	59%
Cridge, et al. 2018[18]	VetScan cPL	Clinical assessment	73.9-83.3%	76.9-83.8%

Overall interpretation of assays in cases of suspected pancreatitis

The results of diagnostic assays need to be interpreted in the context of the patient's history and diagnostic imaging findings.

Interpretation of the diagnostic assay results and diagnostic imaging findings in dogs and cats with an acute presentation of pancreatitis are shown in Fig. 14.3. Interpretation of diagnostic assay results and diagnostic imaging findings in dogs and cats with suspected chronic pancreatitis are shown in Fig. 14.4.

Miscellaneous assays

Trypsin activation peptide

Trypsin activation peptide (TAP) is cleaved from trypsinogen by enterokinase when trypsin is formed. This reaction should occur in the small intestine, and theoretically negligible amounts should be present in the plasma of healthy dogs, making it a potential biomarker of pancreatitis. In animals with pancreatitis, premature release of TAP within the pancreas increases plasma and urine concentrations. However, there is a wide variation in urine TAP concentration in healthy dogs making interpretation difficult. Plasma TAP can be detected in healthy dogs, and TAP is markedly increased in dogs with necrotizing pancreatitis but also renal disease, which limits its clinical utility.[13] A TAP assay is no longer commercially available.

Trypsin-like immunoreactivity

This is a measure of trypsin and trypsinogen in dogs (see next section). High levels are specific for a diagnosis of pancreatitis in dogs, but the rapid clearance of trypsin from serum reduces its diagnostic sensitivity.[31] Given the low sensitivity, trypsin-like immunoreactivity (TLI) is now predominantly used for a diagnosis of exocrine pancreatic insufficiency (EPI) (low levels).

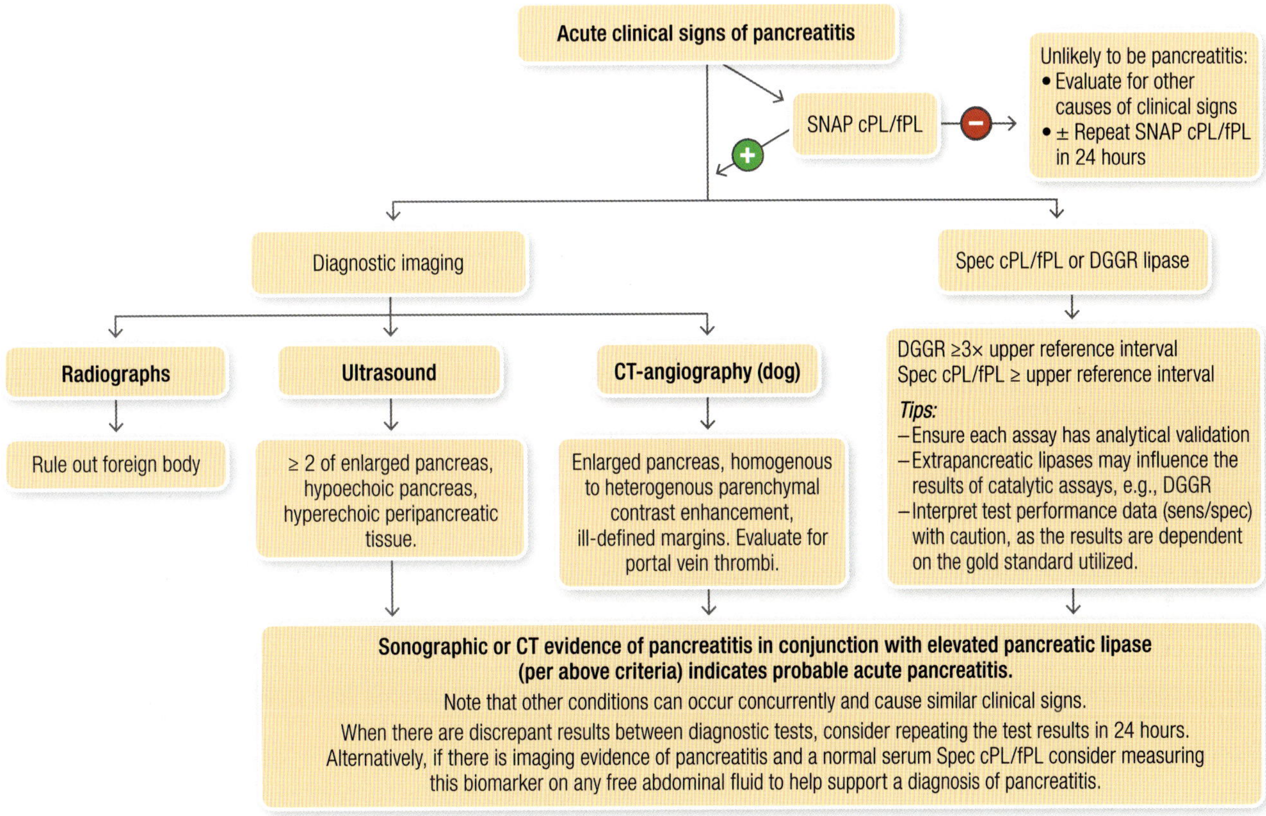

FIG. 14.3 Diagnostic approach to an animal with acute signs of pancreatitis.

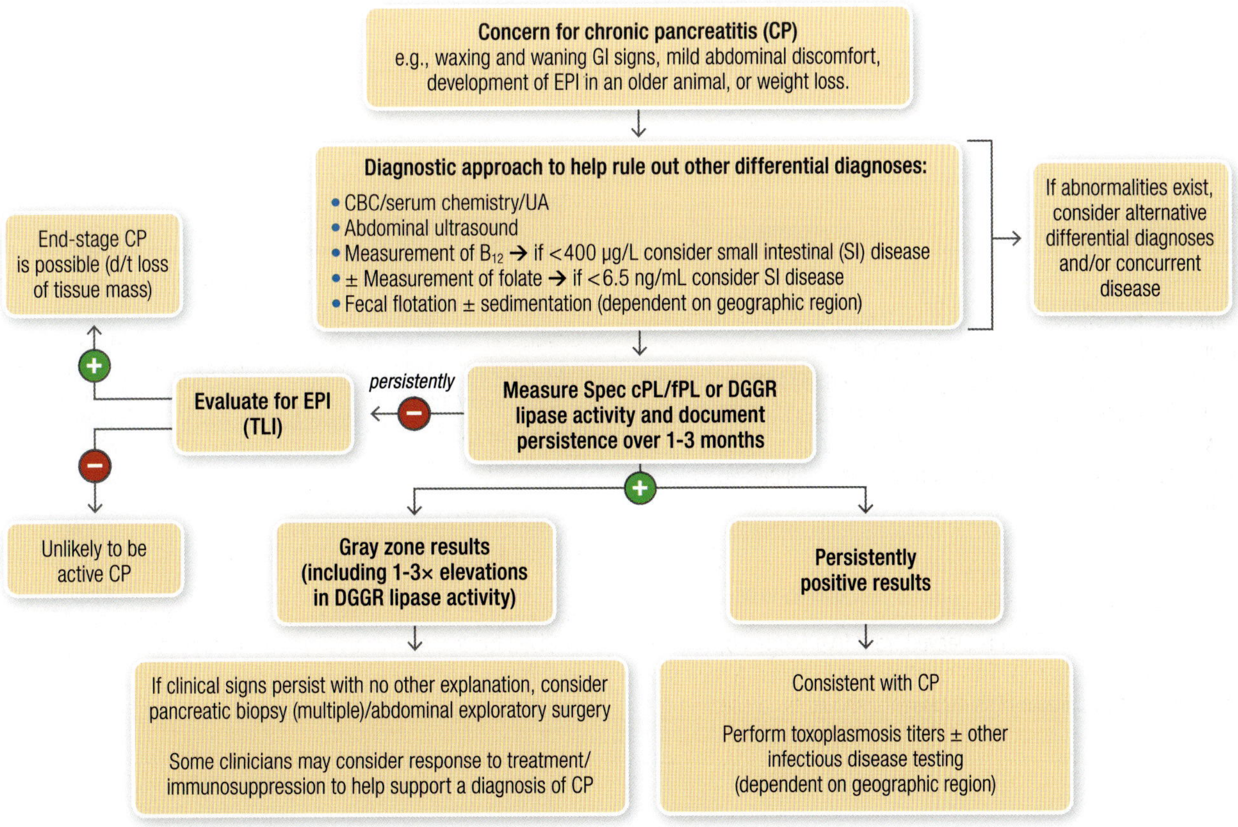

FIG. 14.4 Diagnostic approach to an animal with chronic signs of pancreatitis.

Exocrine pancreatic insufficiency – noninvasive assays

Exocrine pancreatic insufficiency is a functional deficiency of pancreatic enzymes, resulting in maldigestion. It is readily diagnosed based on clinical signs, pancreatic function tests, and response to pancreatic enzyme supplementation.

Trypsin-like immunoreactivity

Trypsin-like immunoreactivity (TLI) is an immunoassay that detects both trypsin and trypsinogen. A low serum TLI concentration is highly sensitive and specific for a diagnosis of EPI in a dog with appropriate clinical signs (weight loss/steatorrhea), particularly with pancreatic acinar atrophy.[32] If no clinical signs are noted, repeat testing is indicated. A persistently low TLI without clinical signs may be suggestive of subclinical disease, and ongoing monitoring is indicated. A gray zone TLI result may occur in a small subset of dogs that go on to develop EPI, and dogs with a gray zone TLI result should be retested in 1-3 months. If clinical signs of maldigestion are present, the dog should also be investigated for other diseases of the small intestine. High TLI values may occur in pancreatitis, and this can make TLI concentrations hard to interpret in dogs with concurrent pancreatitis, or in dogs who develop EPI secondary to chronic pancreatitis. Thus, if an animal is suspected to have EPI and pancreatitis, but has a gray zone TLI, a trial with pancreatic enzymes could be performed. If the stool improved, and they gain weight, the dog likely had some degree of EPI and should be maintained on pancreatic enzymes long-term. Dogs with isolated pancreatic enzyme deficiencies may also have normal TLI concentrations but improve following supplementation with pancreatic enzymes.[33] A flowchart to further assist in the interpretation of TLI results is provided below (Fig. 14.5).

Because the TLI assay is an immunoassay it should not cross-react with digestive enzymes of other species and as such pancreatic enzyme supplementation does not need to be stopped when measuring TLI. Fasting is recommended, although failure to fast has no significant clinical impact on test results in healthy dogs.[26]

Fecal elastase

Elastase is a pancreatic enzyme that can be detected in the feces. A low fecal elastase result (<10 μg/g of feces) from a pooled 3-day sample is consistent with EPI.[34] Fecal elastase may be of particular benefit in dogs with concurrent pancreatitis, where TLI may be falsely elevated, or in dogs with pancreatic duct obstruction where TLI may be misleading. Anecdotal reports suggest both false positive and false negative results.[35]

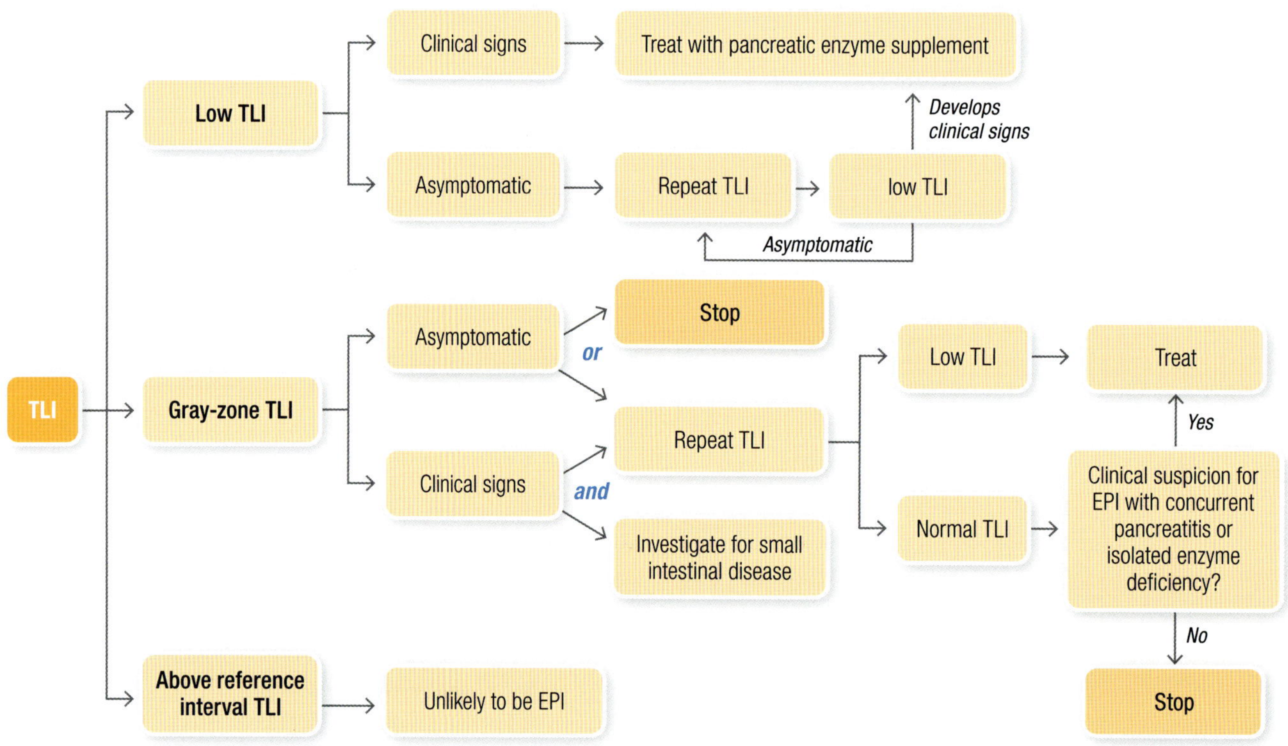

FIG 14.5 Diagnostic interpretation of the TLI assay.

KEY POINTS

- A clinical diagnosis of pancreatitis is based upon a combined assessment of a patient's history, clinical signs, routine bloodwork, a pancreatic lipase assay, and diagnostic imaging results.
- Pancreatic lipase assays may be considered in two broad categories –catalytic and immunologic assays.
- Catalytic assays may detect nonpancreatic sources of lipase, the clinical significance of which is yet to be fully determined.
- Dogs with chronic pancreatitis may have normal pancreatic lipase concentrations, suspected to be due to reduced leakage of lipase from a fibrotic pancreas.
- Micro RNAs offer promise in the future diagnosis of pancreatic disorders.
- Serum TLI is the diagnostic test of choice for diagnosis of exocrine pancreatic insufficiency.

References

1. Cridge H, Twedt DC, Marolf AJ, et al. Advances in the diagnosis of acute pancreatitis in dogs. *J Vet Intern Med* 35:2572-2587, 2021.
2. Newman S, Steiner J, Woosley K, et al. Localization of pancreatic inflammation and necrosis in dogs. *J Vet Intern Med* 18:488-493, 2004.
3. Pratschke KM, Ryan J, McAlinden A, et al. Pancreatic surgical biopsy in 24 dogs and 19 cats: postoperative complications and clinical relevance of histological findings. *J Small Anim Pract* 56:60-66, 2015.
4. Watson PJ, Roulois AJ, Scase T, et al. Prevalence and breed distribution of chronic pancreatitis at post-mortem examination in first-opinion dogs. *J Small Anim Pract* 48:609-618, 2007.
5. Flatland B, Freeman KP, Friedrichs KR, et al. ASVCP quality assurance guidelines: control of general analytical factors in veterinary laboratories. *Vet Clin Pathol* 39:264-277, 2010.
6. Lim SY, Xenoulis PG, Stavroulaki EM, et al. The 1,2-o-dilauryl-rac-glycero-3-glutaric acid-(6'-methylresorufin) ester (DGGR) lipase assay in cats and dogs is not specific for pancreatic lipase. *Vet Clin Pathol* 49:607-613, 2020.
7. Lim SY, Steiner JM, Cridge H. Understanding lipase assays in the diagnosis of pancreatitis in veterinary medicine. *J Am Vet Med Assoc* 260:1249-1258, 2022.
8. Cueni C, Hofer-Inteeworn N, Kummerle-Fraune C, et al. Progression of lipase activity and pancreatic lipase immunoreactivity in dogs hospitalized for acute pancreatitis and correlation with clinical features. *J Vet Intern Med* 37:70-79, 2023.
9. Serrano G, Paepe D, Williams T, et al. Increased canine pancreatic lipase immunoreactivity (cPLI) and 1,2-o-dilauryl-rac-glycero-3-glutaric acid-(6'-methylresorufin) ester (DGGR) lipase in dogs with evidence of portal hypertension and normal pancreatic histology: a pilot study. *J Vet Diagn Invest* 33:548-553, 2021.
10. Aupperle-Lellbach H, Torner K, Staudacher M, et al. Histopathological findings and canine pancreatic lipase immunoreactivity in normal dogs and dogs with inflammatory and neoplastic diseases of the pancreas. *J Vet Intern Med* 34:1127-1134, 2020.
11. Brobst D, Ferguson A, Carter J. Evaluation of serum amylase and lipase activity in experimentally induced pancreatitis in the dog. *J Am Vet Med Assoc* 157:1697-1702, 1970.
12. Simpson K, Simpson J, Lake S, et al. Effect of pancreatectomy on plasma activities of amylase, isoamylase, lipase, and trypsin-like immunoreactivity in dogs. *Res Vet Sci* 51:78-82, 1991.
13. Mansfield CS, Jones BR. Plasma and urinary trypsinogen activation peptide in healthy dogs, dogs with pancreatitis and dogs with other systemic diseases. *Aust Vet J* 78:416-422, 2000.
14. Polzin DJ, Osborne CA, Stevens JB, et al. Serum amylase and lipase activities in dogs with chronic primary renal failure. *Am J Vet Res* 44:404-410, 1983.
15. Graca R, Messick J, McCullough S, et al. Validation and diagnostic efficacy of a lipase assay using the substrate 1,2-o-dilauryl-rac-glycero glutaric acid-(6' methyl resorufin)-ester for the diagnosis of acute pancreatitis in dogs. *Vet Clin Pathol* 34:39-43, 2005.
16. Strombeck DR, Farver T, Kaneko JJ. Serum amylase and lipase activities in the diagnosis of pancreatitis in dogs. *Am J Vet Res* 42:1966-1970, 1981.
17. Bellah JR, Bell G. Serum amylase and lipase activities after exploratory laparotomy in dogs. *Am J Vet Res* 50:1638-1641, 1989.
18. Cridge H, MacLeod AG, Pachtinger GE, et al. Evaluation of SNAP cPL, Spec cPL, VetScan cPL Rapid Test, and Precision PSL assays for the diagnosis of clinical pancreatitis in dogs. *J Vet Intern Med* 32:658-664, 2018.
19. Goodband EL, Serrano G, Constantino-Casas F, et al. Validation of a commercial 1,2-o-dilauryl-rac-glycero glutaric acid-(6'-methylresorufin) ester lipase assay for diagnosis of canine pancreatitis. *Vet Rec Open* 5:e000270, 2018.
20. Morrow L, Graham P. Is the DGGR lipase test as reliable as the Spec cPL test for diagnosing acute pancreatitis in dogs? *Vet Rec* 188:109-110, 2021.
21. Wolfer LA, Howard J, Peters LM. Accuracy of 1,2-o-dilauryl-rac-glycero-3-glutaric acid-(6'-methylresorufin) ester (DGGR)-lipase to predict canine pancreas-specific lipase (cPL) and diagnostic accuracy of both tests for canine acute pancreatitis. *Vet Sci* 9, 2022.
22. Steiner JM, Williams DA. Development and validation of a radioimmunoassay for the measurement of canine pancreatic lipase immunoreactivity in serum of dogs. *Am J Vet Res* 64:1237-1241, 2003.
23. Steiner JM, Rutz GM, Williams DA. Serum lipase activities and pancreatic lipase immunoreactivity concentrations in dogs with exocrine pancreatic insufficiency. *Am J Vet Res* 67:84-87, 2006.
24. Huth SP, Relford R, Steiner JM, et al. Analytical validation of an ELISA for measurement of canine pancreas-specific lipase. *Vet Clin Pathol* 39:346-353, 2010.
25. Beall MJ, Cahill R, Pigeon K, et al. Performance validation and method comparison of an in-clinic enzyme-linked immunosorbent assay for the detection of canine pancreatic lipase. *J Vet Diagn Invest* 23:115-119, 2011.
26. Saver AT, Steiner JM, Hetzel SJ, et al. Effect of withholding food on serum concentrations of cobalamin, folate, trypsin-like immunoreactivity, and pancreatic lipase immunoreactivity in healthy dogs. *Am J Vet Res* 82:367-373, 2021.
27. Steiner JM, Guadiano P, Gomez RR, et al. Partial analytical validation of the VetScan cPL rapid test. *Vet Clin Pathol* 48:683-690, 2019.

28. Condrat CE, Thompson DC, Barbu MG, et al. miRNAs as biomarkers in disease: latest findings regarding their role in diagnosis and prognosis. *Cells* 9, 2020.
29. Rouse R, Rosenzweig B, Shea K, et al. MicroRNA biomarkers of pancreatic injury in a canine model. *Exp Toxicol Pathol* 69:33-43, 2017.
30. Lee D, Yun T, Koo Y, et al. Evaluation of serum miR-216a and miR-375 as biomarkers in dogs with acute pancreatitis. *J Vet Intern Med* 37:92-100, 2023.
31. Simpson KW, Batt RM, McLean L, et al. Circulating concentrations of trypsin-like immunoreactivity and activities of lipase and amylase after pancreatic duct ligation in dogs. *Am J Vet Res* 50:629-632, 1989.
32. Williams DA, Batt RM. Sensitivity and specificity of radioimmunoassay of serum trypsin-like immunoreactivity for the diagnosis of canine exocrine pancreatic insufficiency. *J Am Vet Med Assoc* 192:195-201, 1988.
33. Viviano KR, Ziglioli V. Suspected isolated pancreatic enzyme deficiencies in dogs. *J Vet Intern Med* 27:588-591, 2013.
34. Spillmann T, Wittker A, Teigelkamp S, et al. An immunoassay for canine pancreatic elastase 1 as an indicator for exocrine pancreatic insufficiency in dogs. *J Vet Diagn Invest* 13:468-474, 2001.
35. Steiner JM, Rehfeld JF, Pantchev N. Evaluation of fecal elastase and serum cholecystokinin in dogs with a false positive fecal elastase test. *J Vet Intern Med* 24:643-646, 2010.
36. Steiner JM, Newman S, Xenoulis P, et al. Sensitivity of serum markers for pancreatitis in dogs with macroscopic evidence of pancreatitis. *Vet Ther* 9:263-273, 2008.
37. McCord K, Morley PS, Armstrong J, et al. A multi-institutional study evaluating the diagnostic utility of the spec cPL and SNAP(R) cPL in clinical acute pancreatitis in 84 dogs. *J Vet Intern Med* 26:888-896, 2012.
38. Steiner JM, Gomez R, Suchodolski JS, et al. Specificity of, and influence of hemolysis, lipemia, and icterus on serum lipase activity as measured by the v-LIP-P slide. *Vet Clin Pathol* 46:508-515, 2017.
39. Yuki M, Hirano T, Nagata N, et al. Clinical utility of diagnostic laboratory tests in dogs with acute pancreatitis: a retrospective investigation in a primary care hospital. *J Vet Intern Med* 30:116-122, 2016.
40. Neilson-Carley SC, Robertson JE, Newman SJ, et al. Specificity of a canine pancreas-specific lipase assay for diagnosing pancreatitis in dogs without clinical or histologic evidence of the disease. *Am J Vet Res* 72:302-307, 2011.
41. Trivedi S, Marks SL, Kass PH, et al. Sensitivity and specificity of canine pancreas-specific lipase (cPL) and other markers for pancreatitis in 70 dogs with and without histopathologic evidence of pancreatitis. *J Vet Intern Med* 25:1241-1247, 2011.
42. Mansfield CS, Anderson GA, O'Hara AJ. Association between canine pancreatic-specific lipase and histologic exocrine pancreatic inflammation in dogs: assessing specificity. *J Vet Diagn Invest* 24:312-318, 2012.
43. Haworth MD, Hosgood G, Swindells KL, et al. Diagnostic accuracy of the SNAP and Spec canine pancreatic lipase tests for pancreatitis in dogs presenting with clinical signs of acute abdominal disease. *J Vet Emerg Crit Care (San Antonio)* 24:135-143, 2014.

CHAPTER 15

Pancreatic imaging

Angela Marolf
DVM, DACVR

The pancreas is in the cranial and mid-abdomen caudal to the liver. In dogs, imaging of the pancreas can be challenging due to its thin, lobulated shape and proximity to gas and fluid-filled structures like the stomach and duodenum. The canine pancreas is composed of the right and left lobes connected by a body. The right lobe lies along the medial side of the duodenum and courses cranially to unite with the body. The body lies near the pylorus and portal vein with the left limb extending laterally near the left kidney and spleen (Fig. 15.1). The proximal gastrointestinal tract can become superimposed over the pancreas hindering thorough evaluation.

The pancreas has internal ducts to deliver exocrine secretions to the proximal duodenum to aid in digestion (see chapter 17 for more details). The major pancreatic duct in dogs is the accessory duct which empties onto the minor duodenal papilla. The common bile duct empties onto the major duodenal papilla meaning there are two separate ductal openings for pancreatic juices and bile into the duodenum in most dogs.

Imaging can help diagnose different diseases of the pancreas. In the past, abdominal radiography was performed in dogs suspected of pancreatic disease. Today, ultrasound is the most used modality; however, computed tomography (CT) is becoming more readily utilized in pancreatic imaging. Magnetic resonance imaging (MRI) has been used in people and cats to identify pancreatitis and may be utilized in dogs in the future.

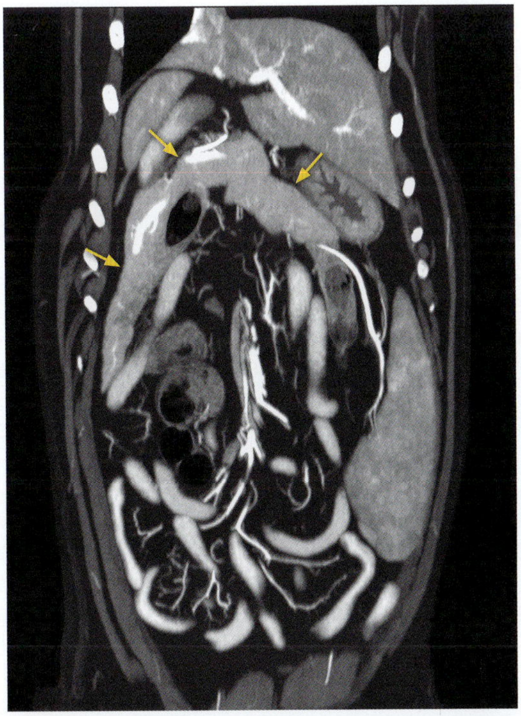

FIG. 15.1 Normal pancreas. CT dorsal plane reconstruction in venous phase highlighting the normal pancreas location and shape within the cranial abdomen (arrows).

Radiographic imaging of the pancreas

The normal pancreas is not usually identified in the cranial abdomen on standard radiographs. To evaluate the normal pancreas, ultrasound or CT are needed. For dogs with clinical signs associated with pancreatic diseases, abdominal radiographs are often initially obtained to evaluate the gastrointestinal tract for the presence of mechanical intestinal obstruction or other causes of vomiting, diarrhea, or inappetence. For dogs suspected of having acute pancreatitis, radiographs can thus be an important method of ruling out other causes of acute abdomen such as intestinal obstruction/perforation, which would have radiographic changes including dilated loops of intestines with or without radiopaque intraluminal foreign material. Acute pancreatitis or other pancreatic diseases may have the following changes noted on radiographs: cranial abdominal decreased serosal detail, a focal mass effect between the stomach and colon, and mild gas dilation of the duodenum. It makes more sense here after describing the findings. These changes are infrequently identified on radiographs and, if present, often indicate a more severe form of pancreatic disease (Fig. 15.2).

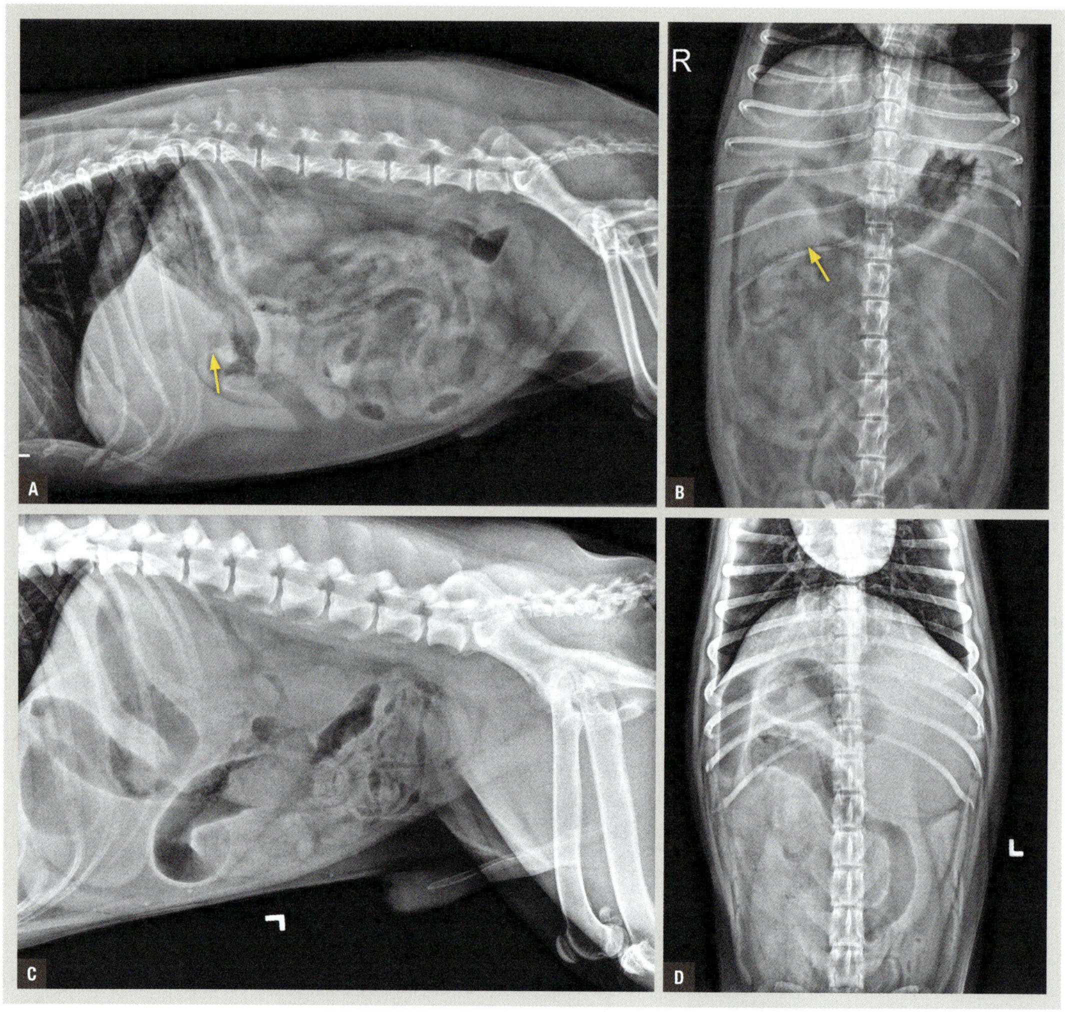

FIG. 15.2 (A) Lateral and (B) ventrodorsal abdominal radiographs showing decreased detail in the cranial abdomen with mild mass effect caudal to the stomach (arrows). (B) On the VD image, there is mild displacement of the adjacent pylorus and colon. This dog had acute pancreatitis based on ultrasound imaging. (C) Lateral and (D) ventrodorsal abdominal radiographs of a dog with small intestinal mechanical obstruction for comparison. On the lateral image, note the multiple gas-dilated intestinal loops with a severely dilated intestine in the mid-abdomen containing radiopaque intraluminal foreign material.

Ultrasound imaging of the pancreas

The normal sonographic appearance of the pancreas is typically isoechoic to mildly hypoechoic to the surrounding mesentery and hypoechoic to the adjacent spleen with smooth margins.[1] The right lobe is located using the right kidney and duodenum as landmarks with the portal vein used as a landmark for the pancreatic body. The left lobe is located using the greater curvature of the stomach and the left kidney as landmarks (Fig. 15.3).[1]

The pancreas should measure less than 10 mm in thickness in normal dogs; however, there can be variation in thickness of the individual right and left lobes and body.[2] Measurements of the pancreatic duct have been obtained for dogs with a general guideline of slightly less than 1.0 mm diameter considered normal.[2] Overlying gas within the stomach and duodenum, or operator experience can limit imaging of the pancreas.

The use of ultrasound-guided fine-needle aspiration or biopsy can be a useful tool in obtaining samples for cytological or histological diagnosis of abnormal tissue identified on imaging. Dogs will usually need effective sedation or general anesthesia for aspirates of the pancreas due to its proximity to other gastrointestinal structures. The complications associated with this procedure are low with a good diagnostic yield.[3]

Pancreatitis

Pancreatitis is the most common exocrine pancreatic disease in dogs.[4] Acute pancreatitis is often easier to identify on ultrasound imaging than chronic pancreatitis. The pathophysiology of acute pancreatitis is usually due to the release of digestive enzymes resulting in inflammation of the pancreatic parenchyma, peripancreatic tissues, surrounding organs, and adjacent vasculature. Pancreatitis can result in pancreatic edema, and in severe cases, necrosis.

Acute pancreatitis

Ultrasound findings in dogs with acute pancreatitis can be divided into pancreatic parenchymal and peripancreatic changes. Pancreatic parenchymal changes include enlargement, irregular margins, and hypoechoic parenchyma. Peripancreatic changes include hyperechoic surrounding mesenteric fat, peripancreatic fluid, and common bile duct dilation.[5] Pancreatic duct dilation is possible. One or more of the above findings can occur, and milder forms of pancreatitis may have slight enlargement of a section of the pancreas, i.e., focal increased thickness in one lobe with normal to mildly hypoechoic pancreatic parenchyma. More severe acute pancreatitis manifests as marked thickening of a segment or the entire pancreas, markedly hypoechoic pancreatic parenchyma with

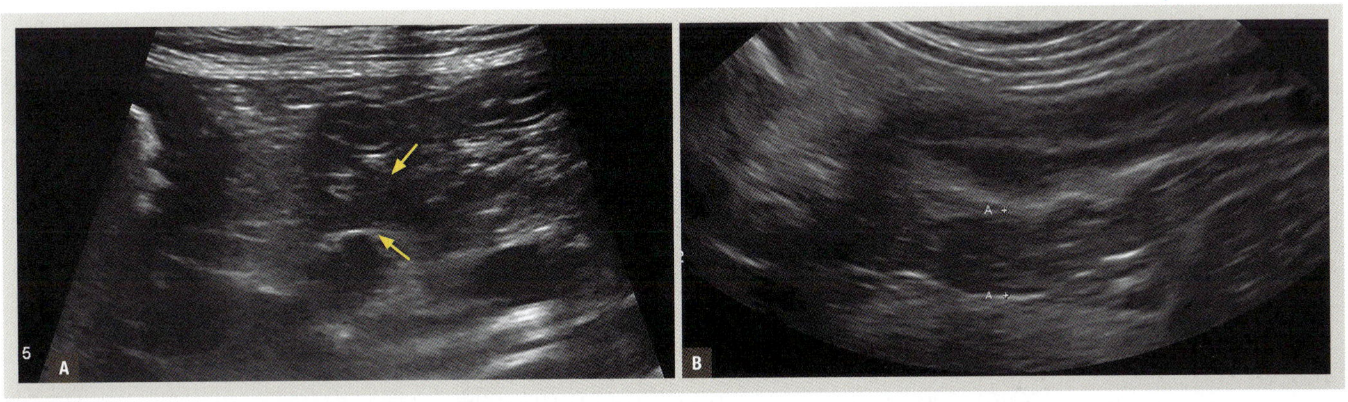

FIG. 15.3 (A) Ultrasound transverse plane imaging of the left pancreatic lobe; the normal pancreas is mildly hypoechoic to the surrounding mesentery (arrows). (B) Ultrasound sagittal plane imaging of the right pancreatic lobe; the normal pancreas is mildly hypoechoic to the surrounding mesentery (calipers). The pancreas measured 7 mm in thickness. The duodenum is located dorsal to the pancreas in the image.

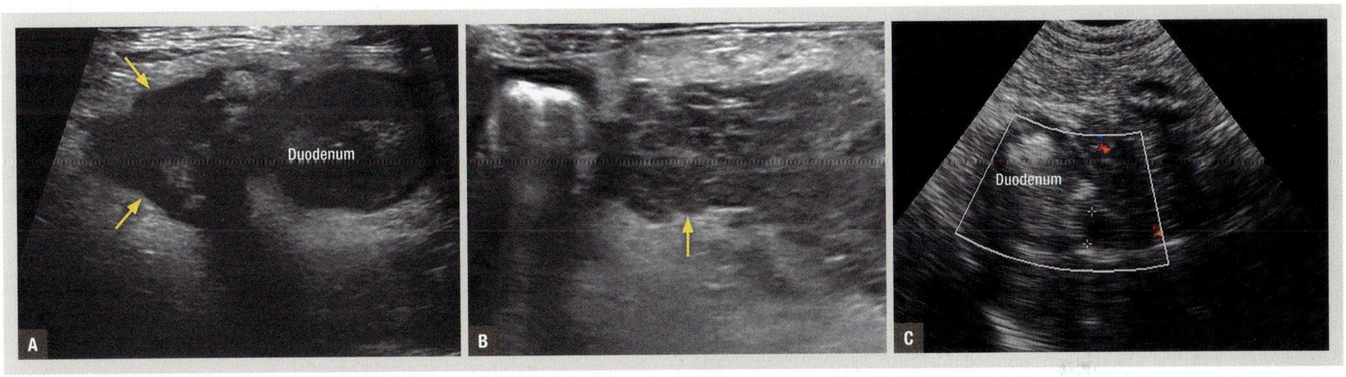

FIG. 15.4 Ultrasound images of different dogs with pancreatitis. (A) Transverse plane image of the right pancreatic lobe. The pancreas is markedly hypoechoic and enlarged (arrows) with hyperechoic surrounding mesentery. The adjacent duodenum is hypoechoic and thickened. (B) Sagittal plane image of the right pancreatic lobe showing hypoechoic thickened parenchyma (arrow) and hyperechoic surrounding mesentery. (C) Transverse plane image of the right pancreatic lobe and dilated common bile duct, which measured 4.8 mm (calipers). The pancreas is hypoechoic. A Doppler box is located over the dilated common bile duct to confirm the lack of blood flow within this structure.

hyperechoic mesentery and free fluid. Secondary extrahepatic biliary duct obstruction due to compression by the thickened pancreas may occur. More severe forms of pancreatitis are more readily detected with ultrasound (Fig. 15.4, Videos 15.1 and 15.2).

Contrast-enhanced ultrasound has been reported as a diagnostic imaging technique to evaluate dogs with acute pancreatitis. This technique showed altered perfusion patterns in dogs with pancreatitis compared to healthy dogs.[6] Serial ultrasound examinations may be beneficial in dogs with suspected acute pancreatitis as initial examination early in the disease process may identify only minimal to no changes in the pancreas and peripancreatic tissues. As disease progresses, imaging changes to the pancreas may become more apparent on ultrasound examination.[7]

Video 15.1

Note the diffusely and markedly hypoechoic pancreas with internal hyperechogenicity and increased size. The surrounding mesentery is hyperechoic. The diffuse nature of the changes and marked hypoechogenic parenchyma indicate a more severe form of pancreatitis.

Video 15.2

Note the pancreatic enlargement, mildly hypoechogenic parenchyma. The surrounding mesentery is hyperechoic. The mildly hypoechogenic parenchyma indicates a more moderate form of pancreatitis.

Chronic pancreatitis

Chronic pancreatitis is difficult to identify with ultrasound imaging and has not been well described in dogs. Chronic changes, such as fibrosis, may be identified ultrasonographically. Possible sonographic changes associated with chronic pancreatitis include normal to small size with a heterogenous echogenicity and/or nodular margins. These changes can be subtle and more challenging to identify with ultrasound imaging. Mineralization may be present and may lead to acoustic shadowing.

Pancreatic abscesses/pseudocysts

Sequelae, such as abscesses and pseudocyst formation, may develop because of pancreatitis (Fig. 15.5). Both are fluid collections with pseudocysts developing a fibrotic capsule over time that may or may not be infected. Abscesses are infected fluid collections. Both structures will be hypoechoic to anechoic fluid with distal acoustic enhancement and

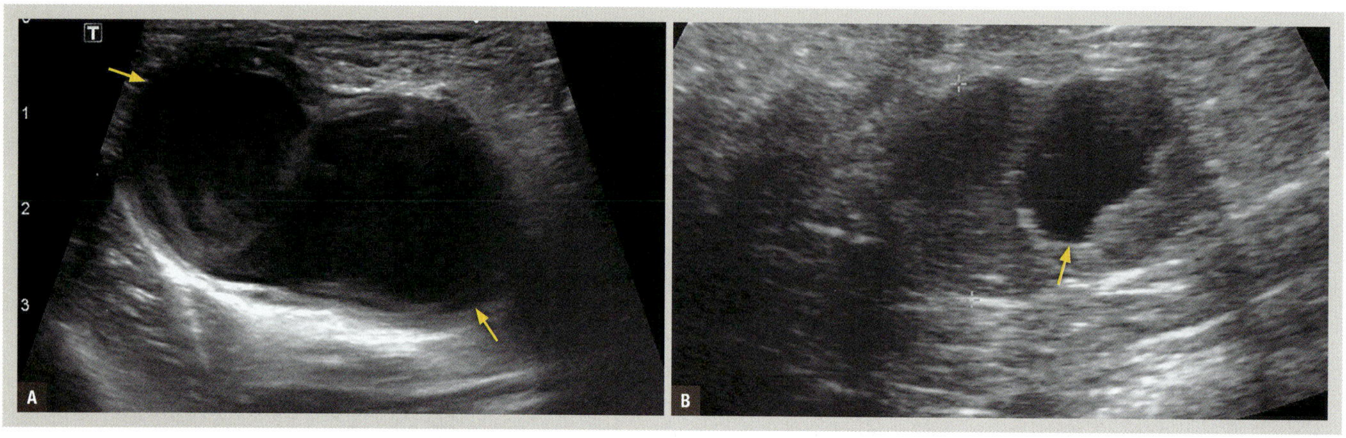

FIG. 15.5 (A) Ultrasound sagittal plane image in the cranial abdomen caudal to the stomach. A large thick-wall, fluid-filled structure (arrows) with internal echogenicity was in the region of the pancreas. Fine-needle aspiration identified suppurative inflammation consistent with a pancreatic abscess. (B) Ultrasound sagittal plane image of the left pancreas. Note the hypoechoic and thickened pancreas, which measured 16 mm (calipers), and the internal anechoic thin-walled cyst at the tip (arrow). This dog was diagnosed with a pancreatic cyst.

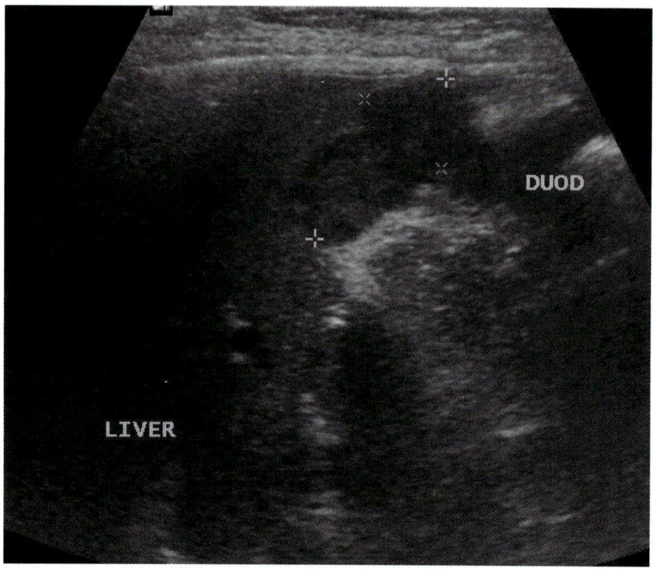

FIG. 15.6 Ultrasound sagittal plane image of the right cranial abdomen. A lobulated mass (outlined by calipers) is in the right limb of the pancreas between the liver (labeled as LIVER) and duodenum (labeled as DUOD). Fine-needle aspirate of the mass confirmed an insulinoma.

varying degrees of thickened walls. Aspiration and cytological analysis and culture of these structures are necessary for definitive diagnosis and determination of further therapeutic recommendations. Leakage or rupture of the abscess or pseudocyst is possible during or after aspiration so attempts to completely drain the abscess or pseudocyst should be attempted.

Pancreatic neoplasia

Pancreatic neoplasia is less common than pancreatitis in dogs.[8] Various kinds of neoplasia can arise in the pancreas including neuroendocrine tumors, such as insulinoma, adenocarcinoma, and metastatic tumors (see chapter 21 for more details). Distinguishing pancreatitis from pancreatic neoplasia with ultrasound may be challenging due to the overlapping features of both diseases (Fig. 15.6, Video 15.3). Regional lymphadenopathy can occur with both pancreatitis and neoplasia and peripancreatic tissue changes are often similar.[8] Fine-needle aspiration or biopsy is often required for definitive diagnosis. Involvement of adjacent organs can occur in both inflammatory disease and neoplasia, and other primary neoplasia can enmesh the pancreas such as liver or bile duct neoplasia.[8] Chronic pancreatitis may begin to appear mass-like on imaging and can be confused with neoplasia. In such cases, a biopsy of both the liver and pancreas is warranted. Diffuse infiltrative disease of the pancreas, liver, and other organs such as the stomach, duodenum, spleen, and lymph nodes may be seen in suppurative, granulomatous, as well as neoplastic disorders.

Video 15.3

Note the lobulated hypoechoic nodule next to the duodenum. This nodule is in the right limb of the pancreas. Fine-needle aspirate of the mass confirmed an insulinoma.

Depending on the size of a pancreatic nodule, the amount of gastrointestinal gas, and the thoracic conformation of the patient, pancreatic neoplasms such as insulinomas and adenocarcinomas may be difficult to detect ultrasonographically. Often, pancreatic neoplasia is focal in nature, hypoechoic to mixed echogenicity, can vary in size, and be in any location along the pancreas.

Computed tomographic imaging of the pancreas

With CT imaging of the pancreas, intravenous iodinated contrast is helpful to assess the pancreatic parenchyma. On CT imaging the pancreas is iso- to hypoattenuating compared to the liver and spleen with homogeneous parenchymal enhancement.[9] The normal pancreas has smooth margins. Normal CT size measurements of the right and left limb and body of the pancreas have been established in dogs.[9] CT imaging is advantageous

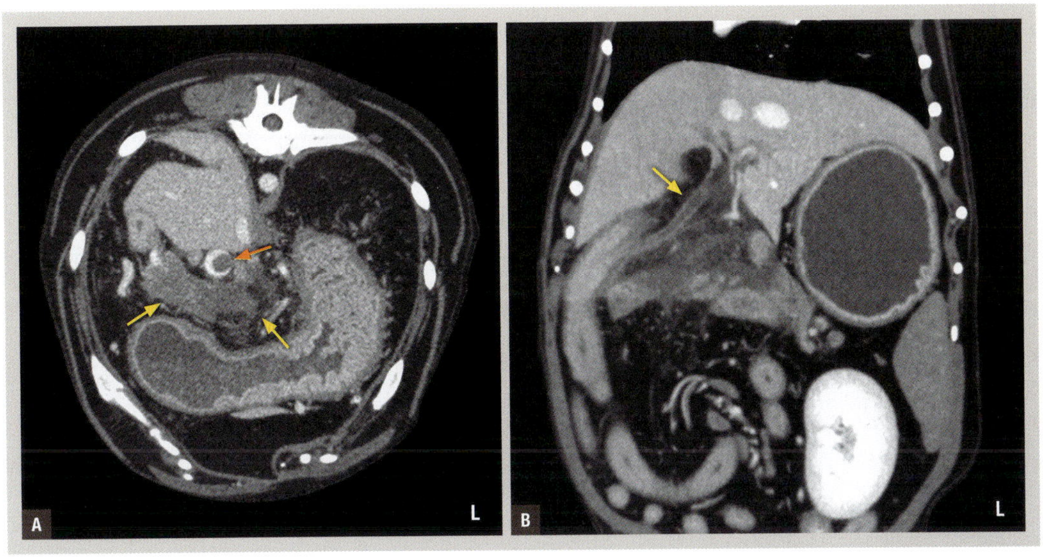

FIG. 15.7 CT transverse and dorsal plane reconstruction images in venous phase. (A) The pancreatic body is minimally contrast-enhancing (yellow arrows) with a visible portal vein thrombus (orange arrow). The surrounding mesenteric fat is abnormal and heterogeneous in attenuation. (B) Portions of the pancreas show heterogeneous contrast enhancement. The common bile duct is dilated (arrow). This dog was diagnosed with severe pancreatitis. "L" designates laterality.

as the entire pancreas can be evaluated due to the lack of superimposition of other organs. This global view of the pancreas and portal vein ensures complete evaluation in dogs with suspected pancreatitis or other pancreatic disease. Due to increased availability, CT is becoming more readily used for the assessment of pancreatitis in dogs.[9] Intravenous iodinated contrast can be used to assess the pancreatic parenchyma for contrast enhancement changes. The common bile duct can be traced to its entrance on the major duodenal papilla, allowing for the identification of extrahepatic biliary duct dilation. Additionally, the adjacent vasculature, particularly the portal vein, can be reviewed for evidence of thrombosis. Typically, ultrasound is an appropriate first-line diagnostic imaging choice for evaluating the pancreas. If ultrasound is inconclusive or there is lack of improvement of clinical signs after treatment, a CT examination would be a useful next-tier diagnostic imaging test.

Acute pancreatitis and sequelae

CT imaging features of acute pancreatitis are similarly divided into pancreatic parenchymal and peripancreatic changes (Fig. 15.7). Parenchymal changes include enlargement, irregular margins, and alterations in parenchymal enhancement. Decreases in pancreatic contrast enhancement cause a more heterogeneous enhancement pattern often associated with areas of decreased pancreatic perfusion or necrosis. Peripancreatic changes include mesenteric fat stranding, free fluid, lymphadenopathy, and portal vein thrombosis. Heterogeneous pancreatic contrast enhancement has been linked with portal vein thrombosis indicating more severe pancreatitis and a poorer prognosis in dogs.[10] Dogs with milder forms of pancreatitis often have mild thickening of the pancreas with normal homogeneous contrast enhancement. Sequelae are readily identified with CT imaging, abscesses, and pseudocysts are hypoattenuating, and the walls surrounding pseudocysts and abscesses may contrast enhance. Imaging-guided sampling can be performed with ultrasound or CT if pancreatic abnormalities are identified. Chronic pancreatitis has not been well described in CT imaging; however, similar imaging features would be expected as in ultrasound such as normal to small size, irregular margins, heterogenous attenuation, and contrast enhancement with or without mineralization.

Pancreatic neoplasia

Due to the global view provided by CT imaging, pancreatic nodules, and masses are more easily identified with CT imaging. CT angiography can be helpful in diagnosing pancreatic neoplasia due to altered contrast enhancement of the nodule or mass compared to the adjacent parenchyma. CT angiography may improve the diagnosis of insulinomas in dogs as these can appear as an enhancing discrete mass in the arterial phase.[11] Little is reported on CT imaging of pancreatic adenocarcinoma in dogs. Lymphadenopathy and other peripancreatic changes can be identified with CT imaging; however, a biopsy is still recommended for definitive diagnosis.

TABLE 15.1 Typical ultrasound features of pancreatic diseases.

Disease	Echogenicity	Focal/ diffuse	Size
Acute pancreatitis	Hypoechoic	Either	Enlarged
Chronic pancreatitis	Mixed	Either	Normal to small
Pancreatic cyst/abscess	Anechoic with distal enhancement	Focal	Variable
Pancreatic neoplasia	Hypoechoic to mixed	Usually focal	Variable

Summary

Diagnostic imaging is integral in evaluating dogs with suspected pancreatic disease, both for ruling out other causes of presenting clinical signs and to demonstrate pancreatic pathology. Ultrasound is most utilized, and there can be an overlap in imaging features of different disease processes in the pancreas. Please review Table 15.1, which compares ultrasound features of different pancreatic diseases. CT is becoming more readily available which increases its utility in diagnosing pancreatic diseases. CT could be considered when ultrasound imaging is not definitive or clinical signs are worsening or recurrent.

KEY POINTS

- The pancreas is a thin lobulated organ in the cranial abdomen of dogs.
- Ultrasound imaging of the pancreas can be challenging due to superimposition of the gas-filled gastrointestinal tract.
- Ultrasound changes associated with acute pancreatitis include pancreatic enlargement, changes in pancreatic echogenicity, and hyperechoic mesentery and hypoechoic fluid.
- Sequelae such as pancreatic abscesses or pseudocysts are fluid-filled, hypoechoic to anechoic structures with acoustic enhancement.
- Ultrasound changes associated with pancreatic neoplasia include hypoechoic to mixed echoic nodule/mass in any location of the pancreas. There may be overlapping features between neoplasia and pancreatitis.
- Computed tomography utilizes intravenous contrast to evaluate the pancreatic parenchyma and eliminates the superimposition of adjacent structures.
- CT imaging features of acute pancreatitis include pancreatic enlargement, changes in pancreatic parenchymal contrast enhancement, peripancreatic/mesenteric inflammation, fluid, and portal vein thrombosis.
- CT evidence of heterogeneous pancreatic contrast enhancement and portal vein thrombosis indicate a more serious form of pancreatitis.

References

1. Mattoon JS, Nyland TG. Pancreas. In Mattoon JS, Nyland TG, editors. Small animal diagnostic ultrasound, 3rd edition, St. Louis, Elsevier, 2015, p 439.
2. Penninck DG, et al. Ultrasonographic measurement of the pancreas and pancreatic duct in clinically normal dogs. *Am J Vet Res* 74(3):433, 2013.
3. Cordner LP, et al. Cytologic findings and diagnostic yield in 92 dogs undergoing fine needle aspiration of the pancreas. *J Vet Diagn Invest* 27(2):236-240, 2015.
4. Newman SJ, et al. Histologic assessment and grading of the exocrine pancreas in the dog. *J Vet Diagn Invest* 18(1):115, 2006.
5. Penninck DG. Gastrointestinal tract. In Penninck DG, d'Anjou Ma, editors. Atlas of small animal ultrasonography 2nd edition. Ames, Iowa, Blackwell Publishing, 2015, p 259.
6. Rademacher N, et al. Contrast-enhanced ultrasonography of the pancreas in healthy dogs and in dogs with acute pancreatitis. *Vet Radiol Ultrasound* 56(1):58-64, 2016.
7. Leoni F, et al. Ultrasonographic monitoring in 38 dogs with clinically suspected acute pancreatitis. *Vet Sci* 7(4):180, 2020.
8. Bennett PF, Hahn KA, Toal RL, et al. Ultrasonographic and cytopathological diagnosis of exocrine pancreatic carcinoma in the dog and cat. *J Am Anim Hosp Assoc* 37:466-473, 2001.
9. Caceres AV, et al. Helical computed tomographic angiography of the normal canine pancreas. *Vet Radiol Ultrasound* 47(3):270, 2006.
10. French JM, et al. Computed tomographic angiography and ultrasonography in the diagnosis and evaluation of acute pancreatitis in dogs. *J Vet Int Med* 33(1):79, 2019.
11. Coss P, et al. The appearance of canine insulinoma on dual phase computed tomographic angiography. *J Small Anim Pract* 62(7):540-546, 2021.

CHAPTER 16

Pancreatic biopsy

Laura J. Owen
BVSc, AFHEA,
DECVS, MRCVS

Indications for pancreatic biopsy

A pancreatic biopsy can be performed as a sole procedure to confirm a suspected diagnosis of acute or chronic pancreatitis or to investigate a pancreatic mass further. However, it is more commonly performed as part of an exploratory celiotomy to investigate nonspecific clinical signs, e.g., lethargy, inappetence, abdominal pain, vomiting, and/or diarrhea, or when multiorgan abdominal pathology is suspected.

The decision to biopsy the pancreas is usually based upon the inclusion of pancreatic disease in the list of differential diagnoses for that patient rather than solely on the results of preoperative diagnostic testing. The sensitivity and specificity of available serum biochemical tests are variable, resulting in false positive and false negative results. Ultrasonography of the pancreas is challenging and often does not correlate with clinical disease or histopathological analysis of the tissue. A recent study showed only a weak-moderate correlation of ultrasonographic findings with pancreatic lipase concentration and clinical diagnosis of pancreatitis;[1] thus, the normal appearance of the pancreas on imaging does not obviate the need for biopsy.

The potential risks of pancreatic biopsy should be included for consideration as part of this decision-making process, particularly with respect to the potential to worsen pathology in this organ, either as a direct result of tissue handling during the biopsy procedure or due to the general anesthesia required for surgical intervention (e.g., hypotension-induced pancreatic ischemia). Thus, when there is a high degree of suspicion for acute pancreatitis, a biopsy is often avoided, and appropriate medical management is instigated instead.

Anatomy of the pancreas

The pancreas consists of right and left lobes, connected by a central body; the right lobe is closely associated with the descending duodenum, and the left lobe is situated within the dorsal leaf of the omentum adjacent to the greater curvature of the stomach. The arterial supply to the pancreas derives from three sources; the cranial pancreaticoduodenal artery, a terminal branch of the gastroduodenal artery entering the body of the pancreas; the pancreatic artery (a branch of the splenic artery in 80% of dogs and the cranial mesenteric artery in 20%) supplying the left pancreatic limb; and the caudal pancreaticoduodenal artery, arising from the cranial mesenteric artery and supplying the caudal aspect of the right pancreatic limb. The cranial and caudal pancreaticoduodenal arteries anastomose within the right limb of the pancreas and supply branches to the duodenum along its length. Venous drainage occurs via the pancreaticoduodenal vein (right limb) and the splenic vein (body and left limb). Lymphatic drainage is to multiple local lymph nodes. Two pancreatic ducts are present in the dog, facilitating drainage of pancreatic secretions into the duodenum. The accessory pancreatic duct is the larger of the two in this species and enters the duodenum at the minor duodenal papilla (located in the mid-descending duodenum). The smaller pancreatic duct exits at the major duodenal papilla immediately adjacent to the common bile duct and approximately 3-6 cm distal to the pylorus.

Open vs. laparoscopic approach

Pancreatic biopsy is performed under general anesthesia via either a ventral midline celiotomy or laparoscopy. The chosen approach in an individual dog will depend upon the availability of equipment and surgical expertise, concurrent procedures being performed, financial limitations, client choice, and other factors. Advantages and disadvantages of these two approaches are detailed in Table 16.1.

Perioperative antibiotics are not administered unless indicated for concurrent procedures. Appropriate analgesia is provided on an individual basis and will usually include opioid administration and/or local anesthesia blocks, e.g., transversus abdominis plane (TAP) block or local infiltration/splash block. Administration of nonsteroidal anti-inflammatories is avoided in dogs with suspected pancreatitis. See chapter 23 for more details on analgesia.

TABLE 16.1 Comparison of open vs. laparoscopic approach for pancreas biopsy in dogs.

Ventral midline celiotomy *Key advantages*	**Laparoscopy** *Key advantages*
Enables complete examination and palpation of all organs	Minimally invasive, low morbidity
Easy access to all abdominal organs for sampling/procedures	Magnification of lesions
Familiar approach	Quicker return to normal function
Facilitates concurrent procedures if needed	Reduced wound-healing complications

Ventral midline celiotomy

The length of the incision required for an open surgical biopsy is dependent upon the full list of procedures/biopsies to be performed on that patient. Access to the pancreas requires only a cranial abdominal incision (xiphoid to umbilicus), but this may need to be extended more caudally to fully examine all the abdominal organs (in a true "exploratory laparotomy") or to access more caudally located organs for biopsy or additional procedures.

A midline abdominal incision (of the desired length) is performed using standard surgical instruments or monopolar diathermy. The falciform fat, immediately visible on entry, reduces access to the cranial abdominal organs and should be excised to improve visualization. A self-retaining abdominal retractor, e.g., Balfour or Gosset retractor, is also desirable to improve exposure.

Mini laparotomy

An alternative to a standard midline laparotomy, where limited abdominal exposure is required, is the use of a circumferential wound retraction device, e.g., Surgisleeve™ (Medtronic) or Alexis™ (Applied Medical). These retractors exert a 360° radial force along the edges of the incision, maximizing the area of abdominal exposure (perfect for smaller incisions), reducing tissue trauma, and protecting the surrounding tissues from contamination (infection/neoplasia) and desiccation. Evaluation of these retractors in dogs has demonstrated their utility for achieving biopsy of the stomach, small intestine, liver, pancreas, and mesenteric lymph nodes in patients in which full exploration of the abdominal organs is not required, based on preoperative imaging results.[2] Multiple-sized wound retraction devices are commercially available, making them suitable for any size of the patient, and adjustment of their exact placement can facilitate access to particular organs on an individual basis.

Laparoscopic approach

A two- or three-port laparoscopic approach is used for pancreatic biopsy in the dog, dependent upon the specific biopsy technique to be utilized and the need to manipulate or grasp other organs to achieve appropriate visualization/access. The latter will vary according to the size of the dog, the size of other organs, and the body condition score.

A subumbilical telescope port is placed as the first point of access to the abdominal cavity, using a modified Hasson or a Veress needle technique. This location avoids the falciform fat and allows cannula placement through the avascular linea alba. The abdomen is insufflated to a pressure of 8-10 mmHg with medical grade carbon dioxide (CO_2). Under direct visualization, additional instrument cannulas are placed in paramedian locations as required to access and biopsy the pancreas.[3]

Biopsy technique

Open surgical biopsy

The entire pancreas (left and right lobes and body) is explored and examined grossly for abnormalities by performing a duodenal maneuver (Fig. 16.1) and retracting the stomach and omentum ventrally. Gentle palpation can be performed, but visual inspection is often sufficient for examination purposes. Assuming the pancreas is of uniform appearance, the distal tip of the right lobe is usually selected for biopsy due to its relative accessibility, distance from the pancreatic and biliary ducts, and lack of adjacent major blood vessels. It is common practice to obtain only a single biopsy specimen from the pancreas due to concerns about inducing or worsening pancreatitis; however, histopathological lesions are not necessarily uniformly distributed despite a diffuse gross appearance, resulting in biopsies that may not be diagnostic.[4] Given the low rate of complications attributed to pancreatic biopsy, this current approach may benefit from re-evaluation.

Several methods of pancreatic biopsy have been reported in dogs. Two well-described traditional open surgical techniques are suture fracture, and blunt dissection with ligation. In one comparative study of these procedures used for partial pancreatectomy, no adverse clinical events occurred in either group.[5] More recently, the use of a pretied ligature loop, harmonic scalpel, and vessel-sealing device has also been reported. These latter techniques are equally applicable to open surgery and laparoscopy.

Suture fracture technique

The suture fracture technique is limited in applicability to the edges of the pancreas; ideally, the right or left distal tip. To perform the procedure on the right pancreatic limb, the pancreas is exposed and stabilized by a surgical assistant retracting the duodenum medially and ventrally (duodenal maneuver). A window is created in the avascular

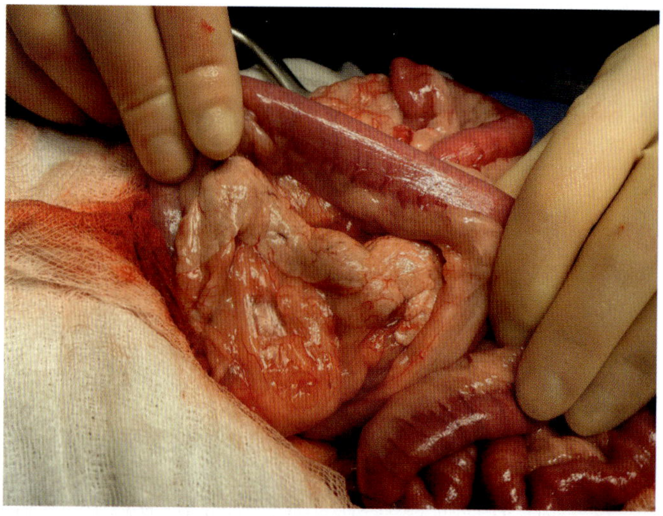

FIG. 16.1 Image demonstrating exposure of the right limb of the pancreas via the duodenal maneuver.

mesoduodenum to allow access to the pancreatic tissue (Fig. 16.2A). An absorbable suture (monofilament or multifilament) is passed around an accessible portion of the distal tip of the pancreas and is tightened securely, ligating the pancreatic ducts and vessels and crushing the parenchyma (Fig. 16.2B); the same procedure can be performed with hemostatic clips if desired. The portion of the pancreas distal to the ligature/clips is excised using a number 11 blade (Fig. 16.2C). Care must be taken whilst handling the biopsy specimen so as not to cause a crush artifact, particularly in light of the small sample size. Atraumatic forceps, e.g., Debakey forceps, are suitable for tissue handling but should still be used cautiously. A sterile suture card can be a useful conduit for the transfer of the sample into a formalin pot (Fig. 16.2D). Closure of the mesoduodenum is performed following the biopsy procedure to avoid intestinal herniation through the defect.

Blunt dissection technique

This technique is applicable to any area of the pancreas, providing the major ducts and blood vessels are spared. It is more technically challenging and is associated with increased hemorrhage compared with the suture fracture technique, which makes the latter the more popular choice when a specific biopsy location is not required.

The mesoduodenum is incised as above if the right pancreatic limb is to be biopsied. Other areas are exposed with appropriate retraction of adjacent organs. A curved Halsted mosquito forceps is used to bluntly dissect between lobules of pancreatic tissue, exposing the ducts and vessels running within the parenchyma. These are individually ligated with suture or hemostatic clips, and the pancreatic tissue excised distal to the ligatures using a number 11 blade.

Laparoscopic biopsy

To visualize the right limb of the pancreas, located in the paravertebral gutter, the dog should be tilted to the left (≥30 degrees). A blunt probe can be used to locate the duodenum, retracting other small intestinal loops to the left, and atraumatic laparoscopic graspers can manipulate the duodenum ventromedially to expose and stabilize the right limb of the pancreas. The left limb is more challenging to inspect laparoscopically; this requires cranial elevation of the stomach and omentum and may be facilitated by placing the patient in a reverse Trendelenburg position. The pancreas is examined for the presence/absence of adhesions, edema, hemorrhage, and necrosis; these findings have been shown to correlate with experimentally induced acute pancreatitis in dogs.[6] A biopsy is subsequently performed.

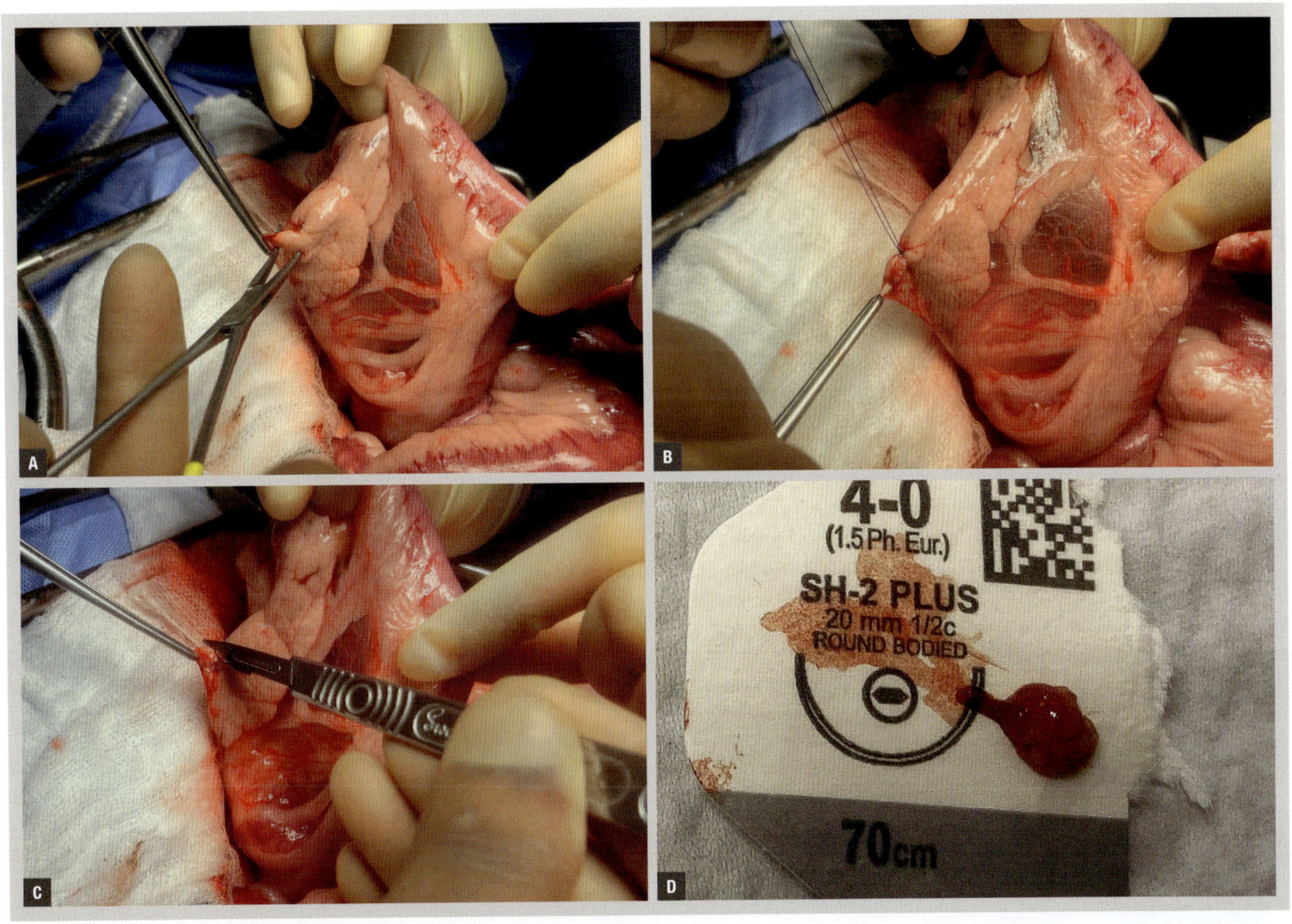

FIG. 16.2 Suture fracture biopsy technique. (A) Creation of a window in the mesoduodenum to gain access to the pancreatic tissue for biopsy. (B) Placement of a suture around the pancreatic tissue to crush the parenchyma and ligate vessels/ducts. (C) Excision of the biopsy sample using a number 11 blade. Be careful handling the edge of the sample with Debakey forceps to avoid crush artifacts. (D) Placement of the biopsy specimen on a small piece of sterile card to facilitate transfer to a formalin pot, avoiding iatrogenic tissue injury.

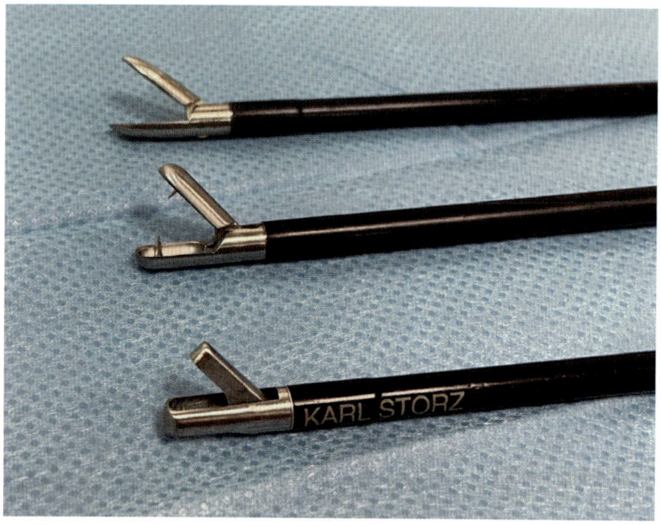

FIG. 16.3 Image of laparoscopic cup and punch biopsy forceps.

Laparoscopic pancreatic biopsies can be performed with a selection of instrumentation. The chosen technique in an individual case is likely to depend upon factors such as the availability of instruments, the potential for the use of the same instrument for concurrent procedures (to minimize expense), and the surgeon's preference.

Cup/punch biopsy technique

Following appropriate visualization of the pancreas (most commonly the distal tip of the right limb), a laparoscopic biopsy forceps (cup or punch biopsy forceps [Fig. 16.3]) is inserted through the instrument cannula and used to grasp a section of pancreatic tissue along the free edge of the organ. The forceps are held closed for 30 seconds to achieve hemostasis and are then removed with a sharp tug to assist in separating the tissue (Video 16.1). Once exteriorized, the forceps are opened, and a hypodermic needle is used to transfer the biopsy to a formalin pot gently. The use of other instrumentation to manipulate the sample is not recommended due to the risk of creating crush artifacts and compromising the histopathology results. The technique is repeated to obtain a second sample if required. The pancreas is examined for hemorrhage, and the scope and cannulas are removed. If hemorrhage is observed, this can be controlled by applying pressure with the blunt probe for 1-2 minutes or the use of hemostatic agents.

The laparoscopic punch biopsy of the pancreas has been evaluated in healthy adult cats and was found to provide high-quality tissue samples for histology in all cases, measuring approximately 5×4 mm, with no adverse events relating to the procedure.[7] Laparoscopic biopsy of the pancreas has also been evaluated in both healthy and clinically affected dogs, with no clinically significant complications noted.[8-10]

Video 16.1

Video demonstrating a laparoscopic pancreatic biopsy in a dog using punch forceps.

Pretied ligature loop/hemostatic clips

This technique requires three laparoscopic ports. The pretied ligature loop is laid over the free edge of the pancreas. Laparoscopic graspers are placed through the loop to grasp and elevate a portion of the pancreatic free edge. The pretied ligature loop is tightened around this section of tissue, and the pancreatic biopsy is excised with laparoscopic scissors, leaving a 5 mm cuff of tissue distal to the suture to prevent dislodgement. The suture is cut, and the free end is removed from the abdomen.[3,11,12]

A similar technique can be achieved by placing hemostatic clips to delineate the area of the pancreas to be biopsied, with excision of the tissue performed with laparoscopic scissors as above.[12]

Harmonic scalpel and vessel-sealing devices

Harmonic scalpel (HS) and vessel-sealing devices use energy in the form of high-frequency ultrasonic vibrations and electrical current, respectively, to provide hemostasis and/or cutting of tissue. The advantages of this technology are thus reduced hemorrhage and ease of use, whilst the key disadvantages are collateral thermal injury to tissues and cost.

Experimentally, when compared to a laparoscopic wedge biopsy technique performed using hemostatic clips in normal dogs, hemorrhage was noted from only three pancreatic biopsy sites obtained using the HS technique, compared to seven using the standard wedge technique.[8] Coagulation necrosis was noted in all samples obtained via HS technique and affected up to 25% of the sample;[8] thus, attainment of a larger biopsy specimen may be indicated when using HS to allow for adequate histological analysis of unaffected pancreatic tissue. Increased inflammation and fibrin deposition were also noted on histopathology of the remaining pancreas after HS biopsy, and thus, potential caution was advised in using this technique.[8] This concern is yet to be corroborated in clinical patients.

The use of a vessel-sealing device has been reported during open surgery for the excision of insulinomas in dogs but not as yet for pancreatic biopsy.[13] The potential for collateral damage to tissue in a small biopsy sample is potentially greater with vessel-sealing devices compared to the harmonic scalpel due to the increased distance of lateral thermal spread when comparing these devices; thus, tissue sample size should be considered.[14] When used for larger resections of pancreatic tissue, vessel-sealing devices have been shown to be safe and effective options with the benefits of reduced hemorrhage and surgical time, with no increase in complication rate compared to standard techniques.[13,15] Further investigation is required to ascertain the utility of both devices for obtaining smaller biopsy samples in clinical patients.

Processing of biopsy samples and interpretation of results

Pancreatic biopsy samples are fixed in formalin and submitted to the laboratory for histopathological examination. The culture of pancreatic biopsies is rarely indicated.

A positive histological diagnosis is taken as evidence of the disease process, and treatment can be instigated as appropriate. The absence of a positive histological diagnosis from pancreatic biopsies is reported to occur in over 50% of cases, with dogs more likely to have a negative result than cats.[16] In addition, a separate study of dogs undergoing postmortem analysis reported pancreatic lesions to be often localized, despite a uniform gross appearance;[4] thus, whilst a negative result in dogs may be a true finding, it may also occur as a result of a nonrepresentative sample and as such, does not rule out pancreatitis or other pancreatic disease. Pancreatic biopsy results should, therefore, be interpreted alongside other diagnostic tests performed and include an assessment of the clinical picture rather than in isolation.

Postoperative care

Analgesia is provided as indicated, based upon the full extent of abdominal procedures performed and any underlying disease requirements. Opioids are used in combination with lidocaine or ketamine; nonsteroidal anti-inflammatory drugs are avoided in dogs with suspected pancreatitis. An epidural or epidural catheter may be considered to provide prolonged analgesia in dogs with acute pancreatitis. More details on analgesia can be found in chapter 23. Intravenous fluid therapy is continued until oral food and water intake has resumed. A low-fat or readily digestible diet may be offered after recovery from anesthesia. Consideration should be given to placing a feeding tube, e.g., an esophagostomy tube, at the time of the biopsy procedure if the dog is considered unlikely to eat in the immediate postoperative period. Maropitant may be administered if nausea or inappetence are noted. Standard instructions for exercise restriction for 7-10 days are given to owners of dogs undergoing open surgical biopsy. No exercise restriction is required for those undergoing a laparoscopic procedure.

Complications of pancreatic biopsy

Whilst inevitably, some degree of injury to adjacent pancreatic tissue will occur during the biopsy procedure, based on current evidence, the potential for induction of pancreatitis or worsening of clinical signs due to pancreatic biopsy appears to be low.

In 27 healthy adult Beagles, cPLI was not increased intraoperatively by surgical sampling of the pancreas; this was, unfortunately, a nonsurvival study, and did not continue to investigate in the postoperative period.[17]

In a separate experimental study, no clinical complications were noted in 12 healthy adult dogs undergoing multiple laparoscopic pancreatic biopsies.[8] In a clinical study of dogs and cats undergoing pancreatic biopsy, major complications were reported in six of 43 dogs and cats; however, only one was considered to relate to the biopsy procedure itself (inappropriate crush technique potentially resulting in leakage of pancreatic enzymes and peritonitis), with others associated with concurrent intestinal biopsies or pre-existing underlying disease.[16]

Overall, clinical experience and literature review would suggest that both intraoperative and postoperative complications are rare following pancreatic biopsy and that it is a safe technique to perform in most dogs.

KEY POINTS

- Pancreatic biopsy is most commonly performed as part of a general diagnostic workup in dogs with clinical signs referable to the gastrointestinal tract or abdominal cavity.
- Biopsy is avoided in dogs with suspected acute pancreatitis due to the potential to worsen clinical signs.
- Ultrasound imaging of the pancreas and biochemical testing have a poor correlation with histopathological diagnosis.
- Surgical biopsies are generally taken from the tip of the right pancreatic limb, avoiding the vascular supply and ductal tissue unless a specific gross lesion is detected.
- Gentle handling of the pancreas is advised to avoid inducing inflammation in this organ. Delicate handling of the biopsy sample avoids crush artifacts.
- Suture fracture is the most commonly applied open surgical technique; this has been demonstrated to be both safe and effective whilst requiring no specialist equipment.
- Histopathological results should be interpreted in light of the clinical signs and single location biopsy site.
- Complications of pancreatic biopsy are rare, and consideration should be made to performing multiple biopsies in the future, as histopathological change may not be uniform throughout the tissue.

References

1. Cridge H, Sullivant AM, Wills RW, et al. Association between abdominal ultrasound findings, the specific canine pancreatic lipase assay, clinical severity indices, and clinical diagnosis in dogs with pancreatitis. *J Vet Intern Med* 34:636-643, 2019.
2. Shamir SK, Singh A, Mayhew PD, et al. Evaluation of minimally invasive small intestinal exploration and targeted abdominal organ biopsy with the use of a wound retraction device in dogs: 27 cases (2010-2017). *J Am Vet Med Assoc* 255:78-84, 2019.
3. Buishand FO, van Nimwegen SA, Kirpensteijn J. Laparoscopic surgery of the pancreas. In Fransson BA, Mayhew PD (editors). Small Animal Laparoscopy and Thoracoscopy 1st edition. Fransson and Mayhew, 2015, pp. 167-178.
4. Newman S, Steiner J, Woosley K, et al. Localization of pancreatic inflammation and necrosis in dogs. *J Vet Intern Med* 18:488-493, 2004.
5. Allen SW, Cornelius LM, Mahaffey EA. A comparison of two methods of partial pancreatectomy in the dog. *Vet Surg* 18(4):274-278, 1989.
6. Kim HW, Oh YI, Choi JH, et al. Use of laparoscopy for diagnosing experimentally induced acute pancreatitis in the dog. *J Vet Sci* 15(4):551-556, 2014.
7. Cosford KL, Shmon CL, Myers SL, et al. Prospective evaluation of laparoscopic pancreatic biopsies in 11 healthy cats. *J Vet Intern Med* 24:104-113, 2010.
8. Barnes RF, Greenfield CL, Schaeffer DJ, et al. Comparison of biopsy samples obtained using standard endoscopic instruments and the harmonic scalpel during laparoscopic and laparoscopic-assisted surgery in normal dogs. *Vet Surg* 35:243-251, 2006.
9. Webb CB, Trott C. Laparoscopic diagnosis of pancreatic disease in dogs and cats. *J Vet Intern Med* 22:1263-1266, 2008.
10. Harmoinen J, Saari S, Rinkinen M et al. Evaluation of pancreatic forceps biopsy by laparoscopy in healthy beagles. *Vet Ther* 3(1):31-36, 2002.
11. Cornell K. Pancreas. In Tobias KM, Johnston SA. (editor). Veterinary Surgery: Small Animal Vol. 2 1st edition. St Louis, Elsevier Saunders, pp. 1659-1673, 2012.
12. Mayhew PD. Techniques for laparoscopic and laparoscopic-assisted biopsy of abdominal organs. *Compend Contin Educ Vet* 31:170-176, 2009.
13. Wouters EGH, Buishand FO, Kik M, et al. Use of a bipolar vessel-sealing device in resection of canine insulinoma. *J Small Anim Pract* 52:139-145, 2011.
14. Druzijanic N, Pogorelic Z, Perko Z, et al. Comparison of lateral thermal damage of the human peritoneum using monopolar diathermy, harmonic scalpel and LigaSure. *Can J Surg* 55(5):317-321, 2012.
15. Hartwig W, Duckheim M, Strobel O, et al. LigaSure for pancreatic sealing during distal pancreatectomy. *World J Surg* 34:1066-1070, 2010.
16. Pratschke KM, Ryan J, McAlinden A, et al. Pancreatic surgical biopsy in 24 dogs and 19 cats: postoperative complications and clinical relevance of histological findings. *J Small Anim Pract* 56:60-66, 2015.
17. Cordner AP, Armstrong J, Newman SJ, et al. Effect of pancreatic tissue handling on serum pancreatic enzyme levels in clinically healthy dogs. *J Vet Diagnostic Invest* 22:702-707, 2010.

Introduction to the anatomy and physiology of the exocrine pancreas

Ran Nivy
DVM, DECVIM-CA (Internal Medicine)

Asaf Berkowitz
DVM, Dip. ACVP

Anatomy of the pancreas in dogs

The pancreas in dogs is a pinkish-gray organ that nestles craniodorsally in the abdomen, surrounded by abdominal viscera on all sides. The lobules of exocrine cells, supported by interstitial connective tissue, comprise the exocrine pancreas and create its nodular to crenated appearance (Fig. 17.1). Embedded within this tissue are aggregates of hormone-secreting cells ("islets of Langerhans") which form the endocrine part of the pancreas and account for only 1-2% of the pancreatic weight.[1,2]

The characteristic, symmetric V-shaped canine pancreas consists of the pancreatic body (*corpus pancreatis*), the longer right lobe/limb (*lobus pancreatis dexter*), and the shorter, albeit thicker, left lobe/limb (*lobus pancreatis sinister*). The former runs cranially towards the pylorus before it follows the descending duodenum, to which it is attached within the mesoduodenum, while the latter runs dorsally along the deep leaf of the greater omentum. Rarely, an accessory pancreas (a rare asymptomatic embryopathy) is found in the dog, in the wall of the gallbladder, the caudal part of the great mesentery, and the intestines.[1-3]

Many organs within the abdominal cavity, including the liver, segments of small and large intestines, the stomach, spleen, and the kidneys, lie in close relation to the pancreas (Fig. 17.1), although the degree of gastrointestinal distension, the presence of ascites and other physiological and pathological processes can change these anatomical relationships. The right pancreatic lobe is related to the sublumbar fat, containing the ureter and ventral surfaces of the right kidney and the caudate process of the caudate liver lobe. Additionally, it is related ventrally to the ileum, jejunal loops, the cecum, and the ascending colon. The left pancreatic lobe is related dorsally to the caudate liver lobe and ventrally to the transverse colon, while its distal end lies near the left kidney and the spleen. Furthermore, the left lobe is also anatomically related to major blood vessels such as the portal vein, caudal vena cava, and the aorta.

The pancreatic body lies caudomedially to the pylorus, while the portal vein courses through the *incisura pancreatis* at the concave notch of the pancreatic body.[1,2] These anatomical relationships might bear clinical implications in cases of pancreatitis since the local inflammatory process can spread peripherally and affect adjoining organs. The occurrence of gastrointestinal inflammation, edema and ulceration, ileus, colonic strictures, and portal vein thrombosis are a few of the complications which might partly be accounted for by these anatomical proximities.

An elaborate network of intra- and interlobular ductules converge into one or two ducts, which drain exocrine pancreatic secretions from acinar cells and empty into the proximal duodenum. Most dogs have two pancreatic ducts. The larger accessory duct constitutes the main draining duct of the exocrine pancreas in the dog and opens at the minor duodenal papilla. The pancreatic duct, which some dogs lack, opens at the major duodenal papilla, on the opposite side of the proximal descending duodenum, next to the bile duct. The musculature of the pancreatic duct and the adjacent bile duct jointly form the sphincter of Oddi.[1,2]

Several arteries supply the pancreas. The cranial pancreatoduodenal artery, a branch of the hepatic artery, supplies the right lobe, while the splenic and caudal pancreaticoduodenal arteries supply the left lobe. Venous drainage of the pancreas empties into the portal vein and supplies the liver with pancreas-derived hepatotropic factors such as insulin.[4] Lymphatic fluid is drained into many groups of lymph nodes, including the duodenal, hepatic, splenic, and mesenteric lymph nodes. Correspondingly, these lymph nodes might become enlarged in dogs with pancreatitis or when metastases spread from the pancreas through the lymphatic system.[1,2]

A complex neural network connects the pancreas to the central nervous system (extrinsic innervation) and the enteric and pancreatic nervous system (intrinsic innervation).[5,6] Spinal sensory and vagal sensory afferent nerves convey nociceptive signals and mediate physiological processes, while neurotransmitters from the enteric-nervous system facilitate pancreatic secretion, nociception,

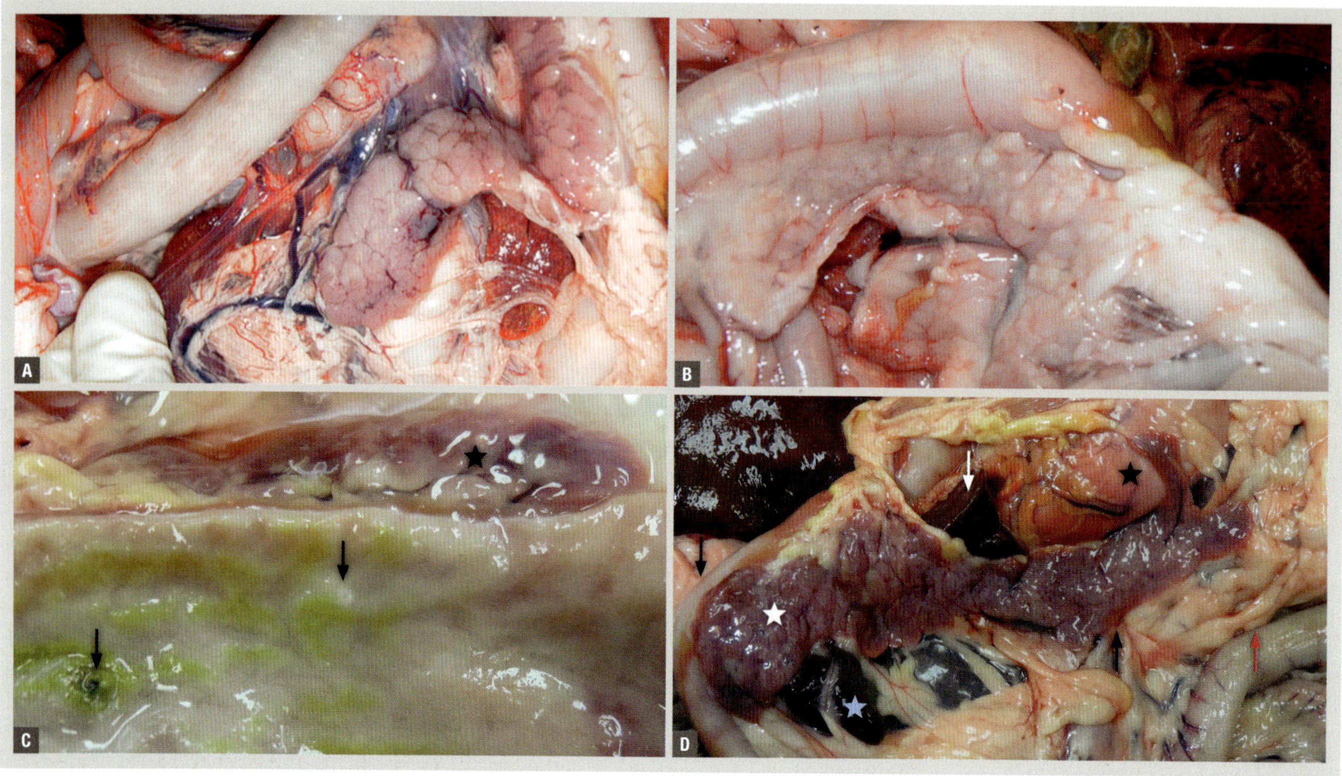

FIG. 17.1 (A) A normal canine pancreas exhibiting a uniform pink hue and a lobular pattern. Each lobule is supported by a delicate fibrovascular stroma. (B) Pancreatic nodular hyperplasia, a common finding in older dogs, of no clinical significance. (C) In dogs, the accessory duct constitutes the main draining duct of the exocrine pancreas and opens at the minor duodenal papilla (right arrow) which abuts upon the pancreatic right limb (black star). The pancreatic duct, which some dogs lack, opens at the major duodenal papilla (left arrow), on the opposite side of the proximal descending duodenum and next to the bile duct. (D) Postmortem image of a pancreas, demonstrating its proximity to many organs in the cranial abdomen (the dark pinkish discoloration of the pancreas is the result of postmortem changes). White arrow: liver; left black arrow: duodenum; black star: gastric wall; right black arrow: pancreatic left lobe; white star: pancreatic right lobe; light blue star: liver (covered with omentum); red arrow: jejunum.

and inflammation.[7] Parasympathetic and sympathetic fibers play a pivotal role in neuronal regulation of the pancreas by mediating a plethora of digestive, hormonal, hemodynamic, and inflammatory processes. They originate from the dorsal vagal trunk (cranial nerve X) and the solar (celiac) and cranial mesenteric plexuses (T5-T12), respectively.[1,2] Parasympathetic stimulation induces the secretion of digestive enzymes and fluid from acinar cells, as well as the release of glucagon and insulin from endocrine cells. Conversely, the sympathetic system inhibits insulin secretion while stimulating glucagon secretion and induces vasoconstriction of pancreatic vessels, thereby reducing blood flow and inhibiting pancreatic exocrine secretion. In addition to homeostatic activities, neuron-derived neuropeptides and neurotransmitters play a role in states of disease by propagating or ameliorating inflammation, participating in the development of diabetes mellitus, and potentially contributing to the progression of pancreatic ductal adenocarcinoma.

Pancreatic physiology: fluid components, regulation and protective mechanisms

The exocrine and endocrine pancreas jointly regulate energy balance through the secretion of digestive enzymes and hormones, including the exclusive secretion of insulin and glucagon. Any interference in the secretion or production of pancreatic digestive enzymes engenders a state of malnutrition, failure to thrive, and weight loss, rendering the exocrine pancreas an indispensable organ in the process of digestion and, consequently, survival. However, the secretory reserve of the exocrine pancreas is large, and ≥90% of exocrine function could be lost before clinically significant complications occur.[8]

Digestion commences, to a minor degree, in the mouth through the breakdown of carbohydrates by amylase (a negligible process in dogs), continues in the stomach through the actions of pepsin and gastric lipase, and is completed in the small intestines by pancreas-derived digestive enzymes and small intestinal brush-border enzymes. The alkaline pancreatic juice consists of a mixture of digestive enzymes, which are secreted by pancreatic acini, and sodium bicarbonate from ductal cells. Digestive enzymes enable the breakdown of food into smaller molecules which are either directly absorbed in the small intestines or are further digested by intestinal brush border enzymes. Carbohydrates are digested by pancreatic amylase, while trypsin, chymotrypsin, elastase, and carboxypeptidase facilitate the digestion of proteins and peptides. Lipids are digested through the action of pancreatic lipases, cholesterol elastase, and phospholipases (Table 17.1). Digestion of lipids is greatly enhanced in the presence of bile salts which emulsify lipid globules into smaller particles, thereby increasing the surface area of lipid aggregates upon which pancreatic lipases can work. Pancreatic fluid also contains ribonucleases and deoxyribonucleases, which act on nucleic acids, in addition to intrinsic factor, which facilitates the absorption of vitamin B_{12} in the ileum, and whose main site of production in the dog is the pancreas.[9]

TABLE 17.1 Major constituents of exocrine pancreatic juice.

		Comments	Function
Digestive enzymes	Amylase	Secreted in its active form	Digestion of starch
	Trypsin Chymotrypsin Elastase Carboxypeptidase	Secreted in an inactive form; activation by intestine-derived enterokinase (trypsin) or trypsin itself (all enzymes)	Digestion of proteins and peptides
	Lipases Cholesterol elastase Phospholipases	Secreted as active enzymes, lipase activity is optimized by a pancreas-derived coenzyme called colipase; bile acids markedly increase the efficacy of lipolytic enzymes by emulsifying lipid globules	Digestion of lipids, including triglycerides, cholesterol, and phospholipids
	Ribonucleases and deoxyribonucleases	Active enzymes	Nucleic acid digestion
Sodium bicarbonate		Secreted with water from ductular cells	Neutralizes hydrochloric acid in chyme, thereby facilitating the actions of digestive enzymes; prevention of intestinal mucosal damage by acidic gastric content
Intrinsic factor		The pancreas is a major source of production in dogs, in addition to the stomach	Mediates transportation and absorption of vitamin B_{12} in the ileum
Antimicrobial proteins		Might constitute up to 10% of proteins in pancreatic juice; antibacterial properties of pancreatic juice are independent of its pancreatic proteolytic activity; regulation and signaling pathways of their secretion differ from those of digestive enzymes	Limit bacterial overgrowth and colonization by pathogenic bacteria; prevent ascending infections

Additionally, the actions of pancreatic enzymes also help inhibit bacterial proliferation and exert a trophic effect on the intestinal mucosa.

Sodium bicarbonate and water constitute a major component of pancreatic juice and are secreted by epithelial cells of ductular origin, which stem from the acini. The copious amount of sodium bicarbonate in pancreatic fluid serves to neutralize the hydrochloric acid in the chyme upon passage from the stomach into the duodenum, thereby facilitating the actions of pancreatic enzymes, which require a neutral pH. Acid neutralization also serves to protect the duodenal mucosa from the deleterious effects of gastric juice and ulcer formation. This flow of alkali is augmented by the secretion of sodium bicarbonate from Brunner's glands in the proximal duodenum and sodium bicarbonate from bile fluid.

Three phases of pancreatic secretion exist, which closely resemble the three phases of gastric secretion with which they share similar mechanisms. During the "cephalic phase", sensory signals (i.e., sight, smell, and taste), as well as mastication (prior to swallowing), trigger pancreatic secretion. The second "gastric phase" is triggered by gastric distension and plays a minor part in pancreatic secretion, while the third, "intestinal phase", which is stimulated by the passage of acidic chyme from the stomach into the proximal duodenum, is the most significant stimulus for pancreatic secretion. A complex system of hormonal and neural pathways regulates these phases and includes a variety of peptides and neurotransmitters of pancreatic, gastrointestinal, and vagal origin. Among them are the stimulatory hormones secretin, cholecystokinin (CCK), and motilin, the endocrine hormone insulin that plays a permissive role in their actions, and the inhibitory hormones somatostatin, peptide YY, and pancreatic polypeptide. Secretin and CCK are two of the most potent stimulants of pancreatic secretion and account for 70-80% of the total secretion of pancreatic enzymes postfeeding (Fig. 17.2). Both are polypeptide hormones of duodenal and jejunal origin. Secretin is released and activated in response to the passage of hydrochloric acid from the stomach to the duodenum, while CCK is secreted in response to the presence of protein breakdown products (proteoses and peptones) and long-chain fatty acids in the chyme. Following secretion, they are conveyed to the pancreas in the blood, where their principal activity is to stimulate the secretion of bicarbonate from ductular cells (secretin and CCK) and digestive enzymes (CCK).

Vagal stimulation facilitates pancreatic secretion through the actions of acetylcholine, gastrin-releasing peptide, and vasoactive intestinal peptide, while peptides from the enteric and pancreatic nervous systems, including nitric oxide and 5-HT, play a dual role in the regulation of pancreatic secretion.[7,10] Collectively, these intricate pathways enable the coordinated digestion of food through the timely secretion of pancreatic fluid.

Pancreatic fluid possesses proteolytic and lipolytic activities, which are vital for the dog's survival, but detrimental when inappropriately exposed to tissues outside the intestinal lumen. Therefore, several protective mechanisms exist to prevent autodigestion of the pancreas by digestive enzymes. Firstly, most of the digestive enzymes (except for amylase and lipase that are secreted in their active form) are synthesized and stored within acinar cells as inactive proenzymes packed within membrane-bound zymogen granules (i.e., trypsinogen, chymotrypsinogen, and procarboxypeptidase). Their activation entails release into the duodenum, where trypsinogen is converted into its active form, trypsin, by enterokinase (an enzyme secreted by the small intestinal mucosa upon passage of chyme from the stomach). Trypsin then cleaves other trypsinogen molecules, as well as chymotrypsinogen and procarboxypeptidase, into their enzymatically active forms. The activity of lipases is

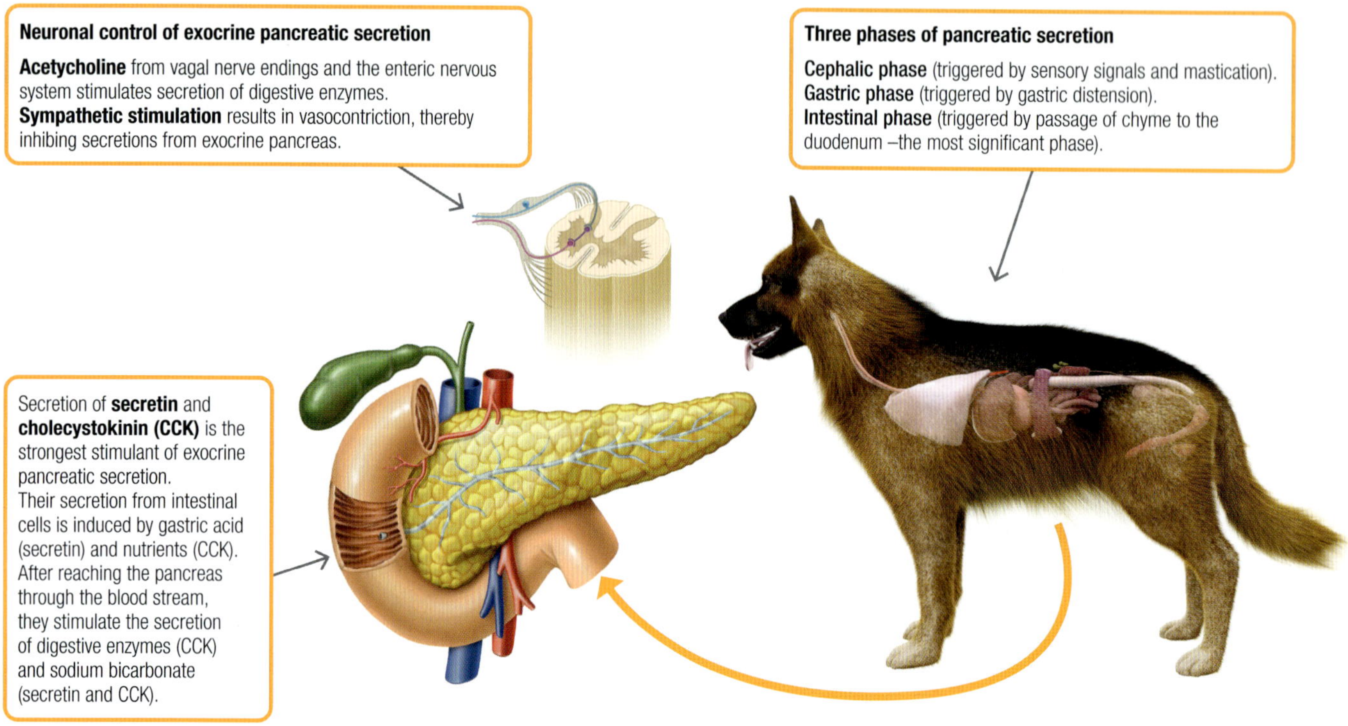

FIG. 17.2 Regulation of exocrine pancreatic secretion.

also confined to the small intestines since it relies on such cofactors as bile acids and colipase. The former are directly secreted to the duodenum from the gallbladder, while the latter is produced and secreted by the pancreas in an inactive form to the duodenum before its activation by trypsin.

Compartmentalization of zymogen granules within pancreatic acinar cells, which prevents any interaction with lysosomal hydrolases that can potentially activate them, is another protective mechanism against autodigestion. Thirdly, the alkaline environment within pancreatic ducts is suboptimal for the activity of many pancreatic enzymes. Calcium is also required for trypsin activation and is in very low concentration within cells. Lastly, a protein called pancreatic secretory trypsin inhibitor (PSTI, also known as serine peptidase inhibitor Kazal type 1, SPINK1) is synthesized and stored by the same secretory cells in the pancreas that synthesize digestive enzymes and precludes activation of trypsinogen, and consequently the activation of other proteolytic enzymes, both intracellularly in pancreatic acinar cells, and extracellularly in pancreatic acini and ducts.[11] When these protective mechanisms fail because of colocalization of lysosomal hydrolases and zymogens within acinar cells, mutations in the trypsin molecule which make it resistant to PSTI, or mutation/depletion of PSTI itself, autodigestion of the pancreas and acute pancreatitis ensue.

KEY POINTS

- The canine pancreas lies craniodorsally in the abdomen, in close proximity to the stomach, segments of small and large intestines, several liver lobes, the spleen, kidneys and the portal vein.
- These anatomical relationships might lead to gastrointestinal inflammation and ulceration, ileus, colonic stricture, and portal vein thrombosis when pancreatic-derived enzymes and inflammation spread locally.
- Complex intrinsic and extrinsic neuronal networks control pancreatic exocrine and endocrine secretions, regulate pancreatic blood flow, convey nociceptive signals, and mediate inflammation.
- Consumption of food initiates a series of neuronal and hormonal processes which promote pancreatic exocrine secretion.
- The hormones secretin and cholecystokinin are potent stimulants of pancreatic exocrine secretion.
- Digestive enzymes enable the breakdown of food into smaller molecules which are either directly absorbed in the small intestines or are further digested by intestinal brush border enzymes.
- Exocrine pancreatic secretions also contain intrinsic factor, which enables the absorption of vitamin B_{12} in the ileum, and antimicrobial proteins which limit bacterial overgrowth.
- Most digestive enzymes are synthesized and stored as inactive proenzymes to prevent autodigestion of the pancreas.
- Suboptimal cytosolic pH and calcium concentration, and lack of important enzymatic co-factors also prevent pancreatic autodigestion.
- The PSTI/SPINK1 protein preferentially precludes the activation of trypsinogen, and consequently other pro-enzymes whose activation is mediated by trypsin, in the pancreas.

References

1. Evans HE. The digestive apparatus and abdomen. In Evans HE, Miller ME, editors. Miller's Anatomy of the Dog, 3rd edition, Philadelphia, W.B. Saunders Company, 1993, pp. 458-460.
2. Konig HE, Sautet J, Liebich Konig HG. Digestive system. In HE, Liebich HG, editors. Veterinary Anatomy of Domestic Mammals, Stuttgart, Schattauer GmbH, 2004, p. 340.
3. Barron CN. Ectopic pancreas in the dog; a report of three cases. *Acta Anat (Basel)* 36:344-352, 1959.
4. Starzl TE, Porter KA, Kashiwagi N. Portal hepatotrophic factors, diabetes mellitus and acute liver atrophy, hypertrophy and regeneration. *Surg Gynecol Obstet* 141:843-858, 1975.
5. Xiaofan Ding JC, Wenwen Zeng. Neuroimmune regulation in the pancreas. *Fundamental Res* 8:19-22, 2022.
6. Travagli RA, Browning KN. Central autonomic control of the pancreas. In Llewellyn-Smith IJ, Verberne AJM, editors. Central Regulation of Autonomic Functions. Oxford University Press, 2011.
7. Hansen MB. The enteric nervous system II: gastrointestinal functions. *Pharmacol Toxicol* 92:249-257, 2003.
8. Westermarck E, Wiberg M. Exocrine pancreatic insufficiency in the dog: historical background, diagnosis, and treatment. *Top Companion Anim Med* 27:96-103, 2012.
9. Batt RM, Horadagoda NU, McLean L, Morton DB, Simpson KW. Identification and characterization of a pancreatic intrinsic factor in the dog. *Am J Physiol* 256:517-523, 1989.
10. Chey WY. Neural hormonal regulation of exocrine pancreatic secretion. *Pancreatology* 1:320-335, 2001.
11. Watson P. Pancreatitis in dogs and cats: definitions and pathophysiology. *J Small Anim Pract* 56:3-12, 2015.

CHAPTER 18

Acute pancreatitis

Sue Yee Lim
DVM, PhD

Jörg M. Steiner
med.vet., Dr.med.vet., PhD, DACVIM, DECVIM-CA, AGAF

Disease definition

Acute pancreatitis is the most common exocrine pancreatic disease in dogs, has a high morbidity rate, and has an estimated mortality rate of two- to three-fold of what is observed in people when accounting for death by euthanasia. The overall mortality rate in human acute pancreatitis patients has been estimated at 1-3%, and acute pancreatitis accounts for nearly 300,000 hospitalizations in the United States. The incidence of pancreatitis on postmortem in dogs has been reported to range from 60-92%, and most patients had acute to chronic changes, with only a small subset of patients having acute changes exclusively.[1] The term acute, chronic, or acute on chronic pancreatitis refers to its histopathological classification and not clinical presentation. The clinical appearance of these patients often overlaps regardless of their histopathological findings, as dogs with recurrent acute pancreatitis can mimic a patient with chronic disease, and patients with chronic pancreatitis may have low-grade gastrointestinal signs that worsen acutely. Acute pancreatitis is characterized histopathologically by the presence of neutrophilic inflammation, edema, necrosis, and peripancreatic saponification that are potentially completely reversible.[1] Chronic pancreatitis is characterized by lymphocytic inflammation with permanent, irreversible, and typically progressive fibrosis and acinar cell atrophy.[1] (See chapter 19 for more details on chronic pancreatitis).

Etiology

In people, gallstones and chronic alcohol use are the most common causes of acute pancreatitis.[2] Other triggers of local and systemic inflammation include hypertriglyceridemia, hereditary pancreatitis associated with mutations in the cationic trypsinogen gene, various drugs, endoscopic retrograde cholangiopancreatography, trauma, obesity, diabetes, and infection. Mutations in other genes in humans, such as the serine protease inhibitor Kazal type 1 (SPINK) gene, which encodes for pancreatic secretory trypsin inhibitor (PSTI), and the cystic fibrosis transmembrane conductance regulator gene, predispose to acute pancreatitis in the presence of other environmental risk factors.

The risk factors in dogs are less clear, and often, pancreatitis in dogs is idiopathic because the underlying cause cannot be determined. Many factors have been identified as potential risk factors for acute pancreatitis in dogs, including diet, drugs and toxins, endocrinopathies, hypertriglyceridemia, hypercalcemia, hereditary/breed predisposition, and other miscellaneous causes. It must be noted that many of these factors are temporally associated with pancreatitis, yet true causation has not been definitively established.

Dietary factors

Dogs reported to have been given human foods, dog treats, unusual food items, and getting into the trash have an increased risk of acute pancreatitis or an increased serum concentration of canine pancreatic lipase immunoreactivity (cPLI).[3,4] A high-fat diet has also been associated with the development of acute pancreatitis. However, in a current study, most dogs with increased cPLI concentrations were fed a commercial adult maintenance diet with a variable fat content.[4] It is unknown which of these dogs also received concurrent human foods and/or dog treats. At this time, it is unclear if dogs exposed to a high-fat diet will develop pancreatitis at some point in their life or at what dietary fat level the risk of pancreatitis increases. Anecdotally, there are dogs with pancreatitis that have controlled gastrointestinal signs when fed a low-fat diet and often will relapse with dietary indiscretion. The association of a high-fat diet is further complicated by the dietary effect on lipid metabolism and obesity, both of which are also considered risk factors for pancreatitis.

Drugs/toxins

Drug or toxin-associated acute pancreatitis is rare in people and poses great clinical challenges. More than 100 drugs and toxins have been potentially associated with human acute pancreatitis, but only a few have a true cause-and-effect relationship demonstrated. L-asparaginase is one of these. It is used for the treatment of acute lymphoblastic leukemia in people and lymphoma and leukemia in dogs. Unfortunately, L-asparaginase-associated pancreatitis is a well-known treatment-limiting toxicity in people. The exact pathophysiology is unknown but is thought to be associated with reduced protein synthesis, which will further injure organs with a high protein turnover rate, such as the pancreas.[5] Genetics may also play a role as patients with certain gene mutations have an increased risk of asparaginase-associated pancreatitis. Acute pancreatitis has been reported in one dog receiving L-asparaginase, but this has not been confirmed in a larger cohort of dogs receiving L-asparaginase for lymphoid malignancies. The rare reports of acute pancreatitis in dogs receiving L-asparaginase when compared to people could be due to a myriad of reasons such as dose and frequency of administration and genetics.

Some studies have suggested an association between antiepileptic drugs and acute pancreatitis in dogs, particularly potassium bromide and phenobarbital.[6] Dogs treated with potassium bromide and/or phenobarbital were reported to have an increased risk for elevated serum cPLI concentrations. It is unknown how many of these dogs actually had clinical pancreatitis. One confounding factor is that long-term administration of phenobarbital and/or potassium bromide can lead to hypertriglyceridemia, which is a risk factor for pancreatitis itself. Therefore, it is important to monitor fasting triglyceride concentrations in patients receiving long-term antiepileptic therapy to recognize their increased risk for potential pancreatitis. A recent study reported that only a small percentage (2%) of dogs with elevated serum cPLI concentrations had exposure to antiepileptic drugs.[4] Acute pancreatitis has also been reported in two case reports of dogs receiving dual immunosuppressive therapy with azathioprine and prednisone for a variety of immune-mediated diseases. Azathioprine, and not prednisone, was thought to be the cause of acute pancreatitis in those dogs because of improvement in clinical signs after discontinuation of this drug. Although acute pancreatitis is infrequently reported with potassium bromide, phenobarbital, or azathioprine administration, a clinician should evaluate these patients for pancreatitis if they develop acute gastrointestinal signs while receiving these drugs and should also consider stopping these drugs, if possible, in animals that present with acute pancreatitis while on them.

Corticosteroids have long been considered a potential cause of acute pancreatitis in people, but the incidence is rare, and a cause-and-effect relationship is unproven. Therefore, they are no longer considered to cause human acute pancreatitis. In fact, corticosteroids are used for the treatment of autoimmune pancreatitis in people. There have been some case series in which some dogs developed clinical pancreatitis following the use of steroids, but a cause-and-effect relationship is doubtful. However, one study reported that dogs receiving prednisolone at an immunosuppressive dose (4 mg/kg/day) for 2-3 weeks developed an increase in cPLI concentrations without clinical signs nor histopathological changes associated with acute pancreatitis.[7] Importantly, only one of six dogs in that study developed an increase in cPLI concentrations that is consistent with pancreatitis. Other medications and drugs that are less commonly reported as potential causes of acute pancreatitis in dogs include organophosphates, potentiated sulfonamides, furosemide, clomipramine, atovaquone/proguanil (malorone), and N-methylglucamine (meglumine).[8] Given that drug or toxin-associated acute pancreatitis is equally infrequent in dogs and people, these reactions should be considered idiosyncratic. A thorough drug history should be obtained in all dogs with acute pancreatitis, and medications with known or suspected association with acute pancreatitis should be replaced with alternatives if possible.

Endocrinopathies

The three most common endocrinopathies associated with acute pancreatitis are hyperadrenocorticism, diabetes mellitus, and hypothyroidism.[3,4,9] All three endocrinopathies are associated with hypertriglyceridemia, which is an independent risk factor for acute pancreatitis. In a cohort of hospitalized dogs with acute pancreatitis, 12% had a pre-existing or subsequent diagnosis of hyperadrenocorticism.[9] Also, 4-8% of dogs with acute pancreatitis or increased cPLI concentrations have hypothyroidism.[4,9] Dogs with diabetes mellitus are more likely to have pancreatitis, which increases the hazard of death.[3,10] The relationship between pancreatitis and diabetes mellitus is complex and can be bidirectional. Several mechanisms that support diabetes mellitus as an inciting factor for pancreatitis include glucose toxicity, the development of autoantibodies or anti-insulin antibodies, or the development of hypertriglyceridemia.[8] Conversely, some argue that pancreatitis is an inciting factor for diabetes through mechanisms including pancreatic inflammation causing islet cell damage, initiation of autoimmune injury, insulin resistance, and the action of cytokines and adipokines.[8] However, a single, isolated, acute episode of pancreatitis is unlikely to cause permanent diabetes mellitus. The pancreatic beta-cells are more likely to be affected with severe chronic inflammation (see chapter 19 for more details on chronic pancreatitis).

Hypertriglyceridemia

Hypertriglyceridemia is the third most common cause of acute pancreatitis in people, and it typically occurs with primary (familial) lipid disorders and in the presence of secondary conditions such as uncontrolled diabetes mellitus. Hypertriglyceridemia is also a risk factor for acute pancreatitis in dogs.[3] Triglycerides themselves are not toxic to pancreatic acinar cells, but the breakdown of excess triglycerides to free fatty acid by pancreatic lipase can injure pancreatic acinar cells.[11] Miniature Schnauzers often have concurrent hypertriglyceridemia and pancreatitis and have been the focus of several clinical studies.[12] Miniature Schnauzers with a history of pancreatitis are five times more likely to be hypertriglyceridemic compared to those without a history of pancreatitis.[13] Those with severe hypertriglyceridemia (≥862 mg/dL) are also 4.5 times more likely to have an elevated cPLI concentration when compared to those with normal serum triglyceride concentrations.[12] The exact cause of hypertriglyceridemia in Miniature Schnauzers is unknown but is thought to be hereditary. Given that the prevalence of hypertriglyceridemia in dogs with acute pancreatitis is generally low, it is likely that hypertriglyceridemia is a risk factor for acute pancreatitis. Therefore, controlling hypertriglyceridemia is important as a therapeutic target for dogs with pancreatitis.

Breed and hereditary predisposition

The Miniature Schnauzer is the most commonly affected breed for acute pancreatitis in the USA.[3,12,14] There are two potential reasons for Miniature Schnauzers to be predisposed to acute pancreatitis. Firstly, Miniature Schnauzers often have hypertriglyceridemia, and this is associated with an increased risk of pancreatitis. Secondly, Miniature Schnauzers have been reported to have mutations in the SPINK gene, which encodes for PSTI.[15] This inhibitor plays an important role in ameliorating pancreatic autodigestion when premature zymogen activation occurs within the acinar cells. The role of SPINK gene mutations in the pathogenesis of acute pancreatitis in Miniature Schnauzers is currently unclear as these mutations are not only nonfunctional but also have been reported in Miniature Schnauzers without acute pancreatitis.[16] Yorkshire Terriers also commonly have pancreatitis, but together with diabetes mellitus.[9,14] Other terrier breeds, Poodles, Miniature Poodles, Dachshunds, Cocker Spaniels, Alaskan Malamutes, and Laikas are also predisposed breeds. In a recent study, dogs with an increased risk of elevated serum cPLI concentrations were Greyhounds, Pointers, Fox Terriers, Eskimo dogs, black and tan Coonhounds, Staffordshire Terriers, Cardigan Welsh Corgis, soft-coated Wheaten Terriers, Brussels Griffons, and Miniature Pinschers.[4] Interestingly, the same study concluded that Poodles, Pugs, and Shih Tzus are at a lower risk of developing increased serum cPLI concentrations.[4]

Miscellaneous risk factors

Older, neutered, and overweight dogs are more likely to have pancreatitis.[3,9,14] Multiple studies have reported recent surgical and anesthetic events in dogs with acute pancreatitis.[3,9] The development of pancreatitis could be due to direct tissue manipulation and/or hypoperfusion. Splanchnic hypoperfusion can cause reperfusion injury, which triggers local and systemic inflammation. Prior or current infections, such as ehrlichiosis, babesiosis, and schistosomiasis, have also been reported to be associated with pancreatitis.[8] Other diseases closely related with pancreatitis include gallbladder pathology (including gallbladder mucocele, cholecystitis) and pancreatic neoplasia, though pancreatic neoplasia is rare in dogs.

Pathophysiology

The pathophysiology of acute pancreatitis in dogs is not fully understood, and much of our current understanding is extrapolated from studies in humans or experimental studies. Pancreatitis can develop through trypsin-dependent or trypsin-independent pathways, and many mechanisms have been proposed to initiate pancreatic acinar cell injury.[8] These include colocalization of zymogen and lysosomal granules, high intracellular calcium concentrations, low acinar cell pH, impaired autophagy, endoplasmic reticulum stress with maladaptive unfolded protein response, mitochondrial dysfunction, and oxidative stress.

The trypsin-dependent pathway is better understood and involves the premature activation of digestive zymogens (such as trypsinogen to trypsin) within the pancreatic acinar cells.[8,17] Under physiologic conditions, zymogen and lysosomal granules are physically separated within the pancreatic acinar cells (Fig. 18.1). Digestive zymogens are released apically into the pancreatic ducts and channeled to the duodenum where they are activated by enterokinase on the brush border of duodenal epithelial cells. During inflammation, there is apical blockage, which leads to colocalization and fusion of zymogen and lysosomal granules within the acinar cells. This allows the lysosomal enzymes to activate zymogens. Usually, PSTI within the acinar cell will immediately inhibit trypsin if premature activation occurs. However, this protective mechanism is overwhelmed if more than 10% of the trypsin is activated, resulting in acinar cell damage. The trypsin-independent pathway is less well understood and includes activation of nuclear factor kappa beta (NF-KB), which occurs alongside the trypsin-dependent pathway.

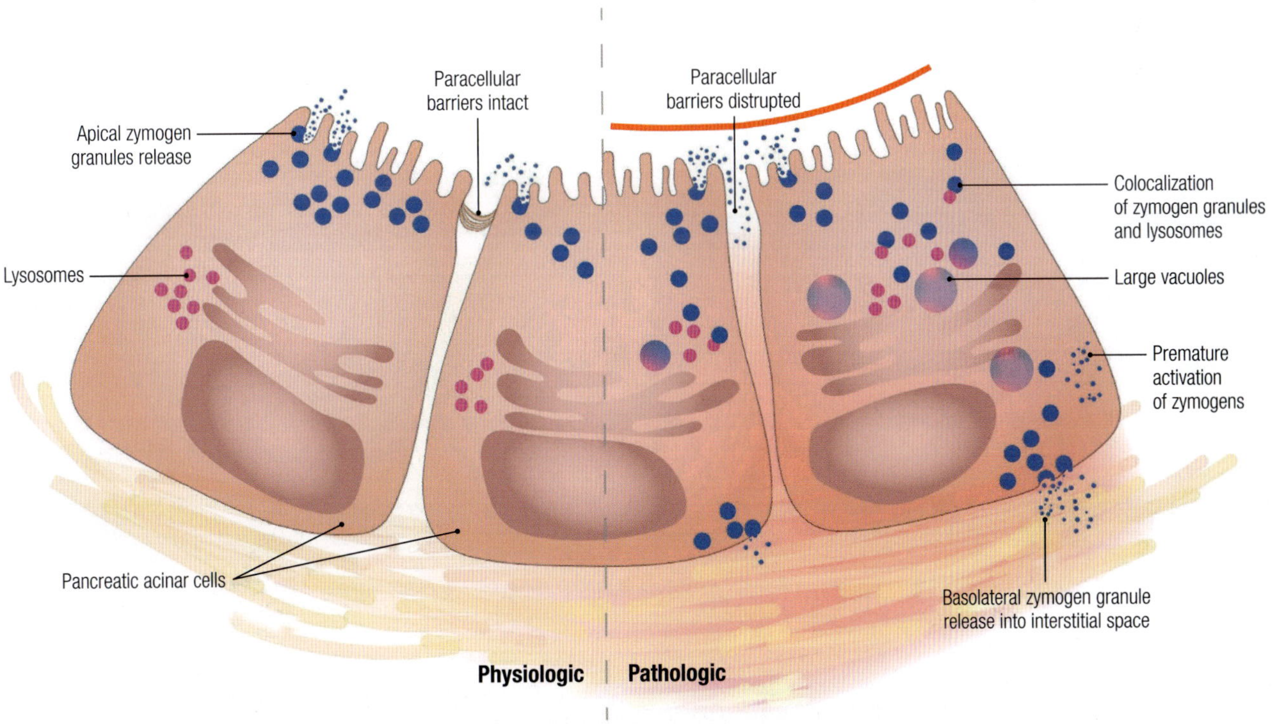

FIG. 18.1 Colocalization theory. Under physiologic conditions (left), lysosomal and zymogen granules are physically separated within the pancreatic acinar cells. Digestive zymogens (trypsinogen) are released apically into the pancreatic ducts for further activation in the gastrointestinal tract. During inflammation (right), there is apical blockage (red line), which leads to colocalization and fusion of zymogen and lysosomal granules within the acinar cells. This allows the lysosomal enzyme to prematurely activate zymogens within the pancreatic acinar cells. Modified with permission from Cridge H, Lim SY, Algül H, et al. New insights into the etiology, risk factors, and pathogenesis of pancreatitis in dogs: Potential impacts on clinical practice. *J Vet Intern Med* 36(3):847-864, 2022. Available from: doi: 10.1111/jvim.16437.

Acute pancreatitis can range from a mild, self-limiting disease to moderate-to-severe when systemic inflammation is present. Patients with moderate-to-severe pancreatitis can develop a systemic inflammatory response syndrome (SIRS), multiorgan dysfunction (MODS), and acute lung injury. Neutrophils play a key role in the systemic inflammatory response in acute pancreatitis.[18] When the pancreas is inflamed, it releases chemokine CXCL-2 (also known as macrophage inflammatory protein-2), which recruits neutrophils into the pancreas (Fig. 18.2). Neutrophil extravasation into the pancreas is dependent on the rolling, activation, adhesion, and migration of neutrophils within the capillaries (Fig. 18.3).[8] Activated neutrophils within the pancreas cause further injury by releasing their granules, forming neutrophil extracellular traps, and causing further recruitment of macrophages.[18] These activated neutrophils can reverse migrate into the circulation, adding to other circulating neutrophils and causing inflammation in distant organs, such as the kidneys and lungs. The neutrophil extravasation pathway is potentially amenable to therapeutic intervention.

Diagnosis

Although histopathology is considered the "gold standard" for the diagnosis of acute pancreatitis, it has major shortcomings due to the heterogeneous distribution of inflammation,[1] invasiveness, and cost, and in the majority of cases, it is not clinically justified. If the clinician has undertaken an exploratory laparotomy for other reasons (for example,

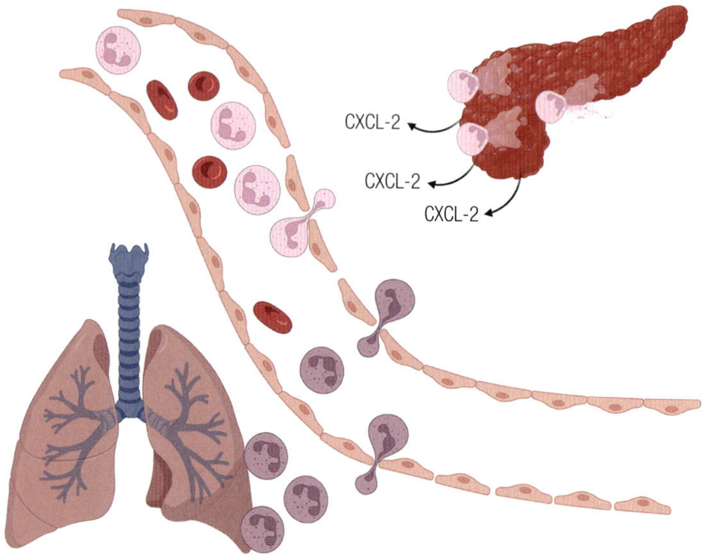

FIG. 18.2 When the pancreas is inflamed, it releases chemokine CXCL-2, which recruits neutrophils into the pancreas. Activated neutrophils within the pancreas cause further injury by releasing their granules, forming neutrophil extracellular traps, and recruiting macrophages. These activated neutrophils can reverse migrate into the circulation, causing inflammation in distant organs such as the kidneys and lungs. Created with BioRender.com (2023).

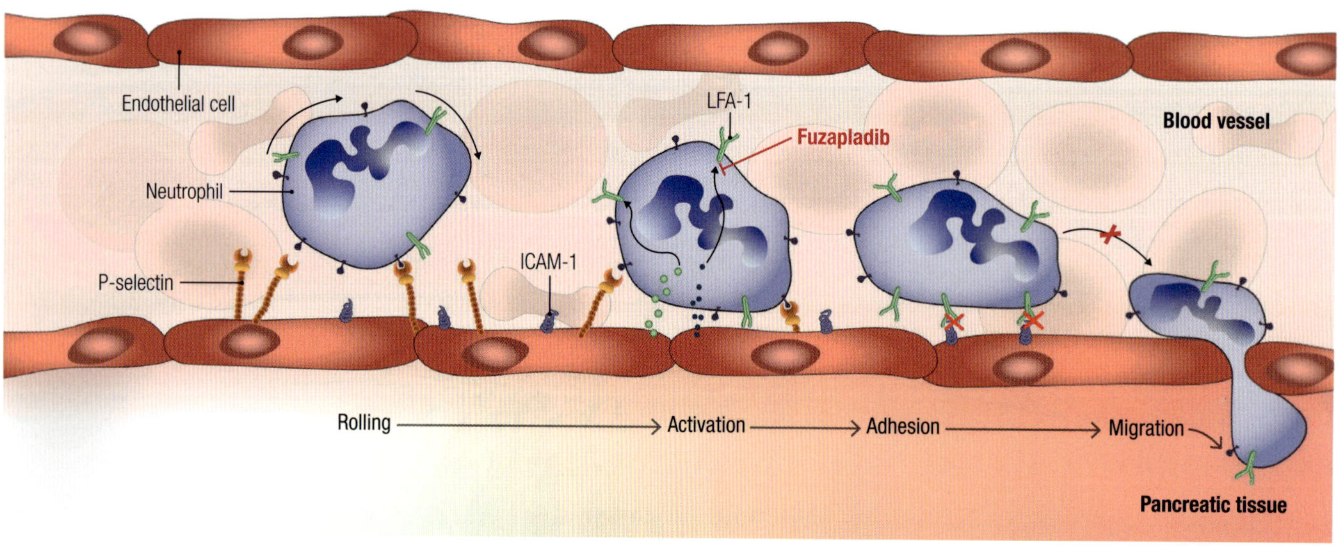

FIG. 18.3 Neutrophil extravasation into the pancreas is dependent on the rolling, activation, adhesion, and migration of neutrophils within the capillaries. During acute inflammation, endothelial P-selectin can mediate the initial capture of neutrophils from the bloodstream and activate the rolling phase. The rolling phase allows the immunoglobulin-like cell adhesion molecule 1 (ICAM-1) expressed on the endothelial cells to bind with leukocyte function antigen-1 (LFA-1) on neutrophils. This will cause neutrophils to adhere and migrate into the pancreas. Fuzapladib inhibits LFA-1, which prevents neutrophil adhesion on endothelial surfaces and subsequent migration into the pancreas as well as extrapancreatic organs. Reproduced with permission from Cridge H, Lim SY, Algül H, et al. New insights into the etiology, risk factors, and pathogenesis of pancreatitis in dogs: Potential impacts on clinical practice. *J Vet Intern Med* 36(3):847-864, 2022. Available from: doi: 10.1111/jvim.16437.

suspected intestinal foreign body), then the pancreas should at least be visually assessed and could be carefully biopsied (see chapter 16 for more details on pancreatic biopsy techniques). However, in the majority of cases, the diagnosis of acute pancreatitis in dogs is based on a global assessment of clinical data, which includes history, clinical signs, physical examination findings, clinicopathologic (including measurement of pancreatic lipase), and diagnostic imaging findings. A summary of the diagnostic approach to an animal with signs suggestive of acute pancreatitis can be found in Fig. 14.3.

Clinical presentation

Dogs with acute pancreatitis can present with nonspecific clinical signs, such as dysrexia, lethargy, vomiting, nausea, diarrhea, hematemesis, hematochezia, polyuria, and polydipsia[4,14] (see chapters 1-6 for differential diagnoses of these presenting signs). Many dogs will have a prior history of self-limiting gastrointestinal upset before being presented to a veterinarian.[4] Physical examination findings may include dehydration, icterus, hyper- or hypothermia, with variable degrees of perceived abdominal pain[4,14] (see chapters 8 and 11 for differential diagnoses of icterus and abdominal pain). The severity of pancreatitis can vary from mild to severe, depending on the degree of local and/or systemic inflammation. A patient with localized inflammation is usually hemodynamically stable and may be managed with at-home symptomatic care. Conversely, a systemically inflamed patient often presents with signs of SIRS, is usually hemodynamically unstable, and requires in-hospital intensive care. It is important to be able to recognize this distinction early and to monitor for clinical progression, as pancreatitis is a dynamic disease with potential systemic consequences, such as acute lung injury, SIRS, MODS, or disseminated intravascular coagulation (DIC).

Clinicopathological findings

Minimum database

A minimum database (i.e., complete blood count, serum or plasma chemistry profile, and urinalysis) should be obtained for all patients with suspected pancreatitis. The main purpose of the minimum database is to rule out other potential causes of the acute gastrointestinal signs shown by a patient with suspected pancreatitis. Typical findings in acute pancreatitis are discussed below and in more detail with algorithms for differential diagnoses in chapter 13.

Complete blood count findings are often nonspecific and may reflect changes secondary to dehydration, such as an increased PCV or plasma proteins. Local pancreatic and systemic inflammation can cause mild to moderate leukocytosis, characterized by neutrophilia with a left shift and toxic changes. If a stress leukogram (helpful mnemonic "SMILED": segmented (neutrophils) and monocytes are increased, lymphocytes and eosinophils are decreased) is not observed in a sick patient with gastrointestinal signs, a baseline cortisol concentration should be obtained to rule out hypoadrenocorticism as a reason for the lack of inflammatory response. A baseline cortisol of ≤2 µg/dL has a high sensitivity (99-100%) but a lower specificity (63-78%) for the diagnosis of hypoadrenocorticism.[19] Therefore, a baseline cortisol concentration of ≥2 µg/dL rules out hypoadrenocorticism. However, a baseline cortisol concentration of ≤2 µg/dL is compatible with, but not confirmatory, hypoadrenocorticism, and a follow-up adrenocorticotropic hormone (ACTH) stimulation test should be performed. A mild thrombocytopenia may be observed in dogs with pancreatitis due to a consumptive process. However, when severe thrombocytopenia is observed, this can indicate DIC, and further coagulation testing (see below) should be performed.

Serum chemistry finding changes are also nonspecific and may include hyperglycemia or hypoglycemia, azotemia, hypercalcemia or hypocalcemia, hyperphosphatemia, elevated liver enzyme activities (often ALP>ALT), hyperbilirubinemia, hypercholesterolemia, hypertriglyceridemia, and in some chemistry panels, hyperlipasemia.[14]

Urinalysis will often show variable specific gravities depending on the hydration status and pre-existing renal health of the dog. A patient that has prerenal azotemia from dehydration should show a concentrated urine specific gravity (>1.030), while a patient with renal azotemia is usually unable to concentrate their urine (<1.030) even when dehydrated. A patient can certainly have a combination of prerenal and renal azotemia, and sustained prerenal azotemia can also lead to acute kidney injury, which will reduce concentrating ability. A urine dipstick may be positive for protein, bilirubin (some amount of bilirubinuria is normal for dogs), glucose, and ketones. A follow-up urine protein to creatinine ratio (UPCR) may not be necessary as proteinuria can occur as a physiological response to systemic inflammation. A urine dipstick should be rechecked for the presence of persistent protein when systemic inflammation improves, and a UPCR should only be measured if the proteinuria is persistent.

Coagulation testing

Dogs with acute pancreatitis can present with severe systemic inflammation, as evidenced by increased inflammatory cytokines such as IL-6 and TNFα. These patients are also hypercoagulable and are at an increased risk of developing microthrombi.[20] It is important to recognize occult DIC and start antithrombotic therapy earlier in the disease before it progresses to overt DIC.[21] In dogs at risk of DIC that are evaluated with a combination of six coagulation parameters, a cutoff of ≥3 abnormal coagulation parameters from the following list identified overt DIC with high sensitivity and specificity: increased prothrombin time, increased activated thromboplastin time, increased D-dimer concentration, decreased antithrombin activity, decreased fibrinogen concentration and decreased platelet count.[21] This accurately predicts mortality as dogs diagnosed with overt DIC diagnosed with this method had a mortality rate of 63% versus 13% in dogs not in overt DIC.[21]

C-reactive protein

C-reactive protein is an IL-6-dependent acute phase protein that increases in various inflammatory conditions and is, therefore, useful as a nonspecific marker for inflammation. C-reactive protein increases in experimental and naturally-occurring pancreatitis in dogs and is helpful in assessing the degree of systemic inflammation.[22] Repeated measurements of C-reactive protein can be used to track the improvement or worsening of systemic inflammation and may be helpful in monitoring response to treatment.[22]

Pancreatic lipase testing

Under physiologic conditions, most pancreatic lipase (~99%) is secreted from the pancreatic acinar cells through their apical membrane into the pancreatic duct and travels to the duodenum for the digestion of dietary fat.[23] Less than 1% is released into circulation through the basolateral membrane. During pancreatitis, this apical secretion is blocked, resulting in pancreatic lipase being released through the basolateral membrane into circulation. Hence, the measurement of serum pancreatic lipase can be used as a noninvasive diagnostic test for pancreatitis. In the clinical setting, there are two common methods of measuring serum lipase –immunological and catalytic methods. The immunological method can be further divided into quantitative and semiquantitative assays.

The Spec cPL test (Idexx Laboratories) is an example of a quantitative immunological assay that is measured at a reference laboratory. This test specifically measures the concentration of pancreatic lipase in serum using two sets of monoclonal antibodies produced against recombinant canine pancreatic lipase. The principle of this test is explained in Fig. 18.4. Various validation studies have shown this assay to be precise, linear, stable, and reproducible (for more details, see chapter 14 and Table 14.2). It is unaffected by hemolysis, icterus, or lipemia. This is useful because dogs with acute pancreatitis are often icteric and may have variable degrees of hypertriglyceridemia. This assay is not affected by extrapancreatic lipases and is, therefore, analytically specific to detecting pancreatic lipase.[24] A Spec cPL concentration of <200 µg/L makes acute pancreatitis unlikely while a concentration of ≥400 µg/L is suggestive of pancreatitis. Spec cPL concentrations between 200-400 µg/L are considered equivocal. Depending on the criteria for diagnosis of pancreatitis and the severity of pancreatitis, it generally has a high diagnostic sensitivity and specificity for pancreatitis in dogs (Table 14.2).[23] The SNAP cPL test (Idexx Laboratories) is also an example of a semiquantitative immunological assay. This test is commonly used as a patient-side point-of-care test. This test has a higher sensitivity (74-100%) compared to a specificity of 59-78%. Using the "SPin & SNout" rule may be helpful for a practitioner to remember that a very SPecific test is generally useful for ruling IN a disease, while a very SeNsitive test is generally useful for ruling OUT a disease. Generally, increasing the cutoff for a test will increase its specificity but reduce its sensitivity. A SNAP cPL that is normal correlates with a Spec cPL concentration of <200 µg/L. Therefore, acute pancreatitis is unlikely, and other disease processes should be considered. A SNAP cPL that is abnormal correlates with a Spec cPL concentration of ≥200 µg/L (which includes the equivocal and the positive results) and is compatible with but not confirmatory of pancreatitis, and a follow-up Spec cPL test should be performed. There are other immunological assays such as the VetScan cPL Rapid Test (Zoetis), Vcheck cPL (Bionote USA Inc), and cPLI ELISA (Laboklin GmbH & Co KG). More information on these assays is available in a recent review article and chapter 14.[25]

Catalytic lipase assays measure serum lipase activity by the rate at which substrates are converted to a colored product. The higher the serum lipase activity, the more intense the color change and the higher the measured value. The serum lipase activity assays commonly included in chemistry profiles lack the specificity for pancreatic lipase and can be elevated in a myriad of nonpancreatic diseases. A synthetic compound (1,2-o-dilauryl-rac-glycero-3-glutaric acid-(6'-methylresorufin) ester [DGGR]) was introduced as a substrate that is more pancreatic lipase specific. This assay is unaffected by sample freezing, glycerol, anticoagulants, or carboxyl ester lipase, but it is variably affected by hemoglobin and lipemia. Depending on the criteria for the diagnosis of pancreatitis, severity of pancreatitis, and cutoff values of the assay used, the reported diagnostic sensitivity and specificity are generally high (see chapter 14 and Table 14.1).[23] However, this assay may be affected by extrapancreatic lipases such as hepatic and/or lipoprotein lipases.[24] Although pancreatic lipase accounts for most of the serum lipase activity, extrapancreatic lipases can contribute up to 25% of serum lipase activity in healthy dogs. However, as detailed in Fig. 14.3, further investigations of pancreatitis are indicated if DGGR is elevated significantly (suggested cutoff >3 times above the reference range) in an animal with compatible clinical signs.

The emergence of various pancreatic lipase assays has provided ease to the diagnosis of acute pancreatitis in dogs. While these assays are convenient, they should not be used in isolation. Several studies have reported increased serum lipase concentrations or activities in various extrapancreatic diseases, such as renal, gastrointestinal, cardiac, or endocrine diseases, neoplasia, infections, intervertebral disc disease, portal hypertension, and chronic use of corticosteroids.[25] In addition, pancreatic inflammation and an increase of serum concentrations of pancreatic lipases can occur in any dog with an acute abdomen, whether that be peritonitis or an intestinal obstruction due to a foreign body, conditions which often present clinically in a similar way to dogs with just

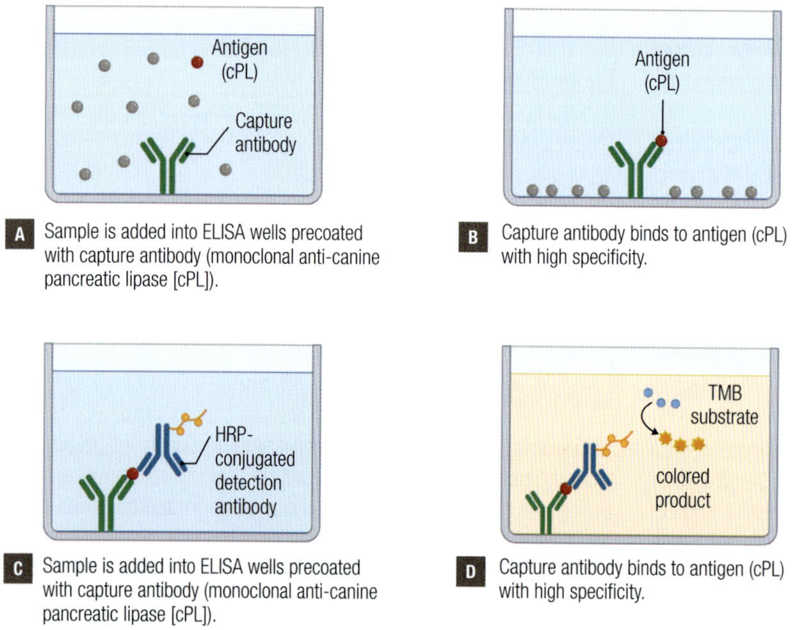

FIG. 18.4 Principle of Spec cPL ELISA (**A**) sample is added into ELISA wells precoated with capture antibody (green), (**B**) the capture antibody binds to the antigen (red dot; cPL) with high specificity, (**C**) horseradish peroxidase (HRP)-conjugated detection antibody (blue) binds to the immobilized antigen, and (**D**) HRP binds to tetramethylbenzidine (TMB) substrate (blue dots) and catalyzes an enzymatic color reaction that is detected spectrophotometrically at 650 nm. Modified with permission from Lim SY, Steiner JM, Cridge H. Understanding lipase assays in the diagnosis of pancreatitis in veterinary medicine. *J Am Vet Med Assoc* 260(11):1249-1258, 2022. Available from: doi/10.1111/jvim.12609. Created with BioRender.com (2023).

acute pancreatitis, so diagnostic imaging and integration of all diagnostic information is imperative to allow the most effective treatment.

Diagnostic imaging

Abdominal radiography

Abdominal radiography is generally not considered to be useful for the diagnosis of acute pancreatitis. However, abdominal radiography can be helpful to rule out conditions such as a foreign body obstruction, intussusception, or pneumoperitoneum, which present with similar clinical signs as do dogs with acute pancreatitis but will require immediate surgical intervention. Radiographic changes associated with pancreatitis are variable and are usually subtle and localized to the right cranial abdomen (see chapter 15 and Fig. 15.2).[26] Other radiographic findings could be associated with secondary gastric stasis or functional ileus.

Abdominal ultrasound

Abdominal ultrasound is useful as a noninvasive diagnostic modality to image the pancreas. Details of pancreatic ultrasonography with figures and videos can be found in chapter 15. Abdominal ultrasound is highly dependent on the skill and experience of the operator and the equipment available. Thus, the diagnosis of pancreatitis with ultrasound is challenging, and criteria to differentiate acute from acute on chronic pancreatitis have not been described. The sensitivity of ultrasound in detecting acute pancreatitis was historically reported to be 68%.[14] With modern ultrasound technology, this sensitivity has increased to 89% in one publication.[27] It should also be pointed out that the diagnostic success of abdominal ultrasound is dependent on various factors, including the severity of the disease, the quality of the imaging equipment, the expertise of the ultrasonographer, as well as the level of suspicion of the ultrasonographer. Thus, there are no definitive values for either the sensitivity or specificity of abdominal ultrasound for diagnosing acute pancreatitis in dogs. However, it is important not to overinterpret ultrasonographic findings as they only correlate weakly, at best, with cPLI concentrations and moderately with a clinical diagnosis of pancreatitis.[27,28] Additionally, ultrasonographic severity does not correlate with the clinical severity of pancreatitis.[27] False negatives may also occur as the development of ultrasonographic changes may lag behind the clinical presentation and abnormal pancreatic lipase concentration.[28] Therefore, it remains important to include a quantitative pancreatic lipase assay in addition to performing ultrasound in all dogs evaluated for pancreatitis. Similarly, because improvement in ultrasonographic changes does not correlate with clinical signs or pancreatic lipase concentration, the routine use of repeat ultrasound to monitor and guide treatment cannot be recommended at this time[27] except in specific situations such as monitoring pancreatic fluid accumulation or monitoring for complications when patients are not responding to supportive treatment or have worsening abdominal pain.

Other imaging tools

Contrast-enhanced computed tomography is the most common diagnostic imaging modality for diagnosing acute pancreatitis in people. Magnetic resonance imaging and contrast-enhanced ultrasound have also been reported in both people and dogs. While these advanced diagnostic modalities provide a superior cross-sectional study of the pancreas, their use in veterinary medicine is limited due to cost and the need for general anesthesia that could potentially further exacerbate pancreatic microcirculatory derangements. (See chapter 15 for more details of pancreas CT in dogs).

Cytology

Fine-needle aspiration of the pancreas for cytology is considered safe and should be helpful in differentiating inflammatory from neoplastic lesions of the pancreas. However, it is not routinely performed in dogs. In one study, 74% of dogs undergoing pancreatic FNA had a diagnostic yield that correlated well with histopathology.[29] Most of these dogs either had inflammation or neoplasia.[29] However, it is important to remember that the disease can be heterogenous and that pancreatic inflammation often accompanies underlying pancreatic neoplasia. Thus, finding evidence of neoplasia on cytology is definitive, and cytology is highly specific, but a negative result does not exclude it. Finding evidence of acute pancreatitis on cytology confirms inflammation but does not rule out underlying neoplasia or chronic disease, and sensitivity is limited.

Management

Acute pancreatitis in dogs can vary in clinical severity. Therefore, it is important to determine which patients will benefit from in-hospital intensive care versus at-home symptomatic care. It is also important to identify and manage comorbidities, such as aspiration pneumonia, functional ileus, and hyperglycemia. Recently, a new drug (fuzapladib) has received conditional FDA approval as a specific treatment for acute pancreatitis in dogs in the USA. Apart from this drug, the management of acute pancreatitis is supportive rather than specific, with the most important considerations being pain management, effective fluid and electrolyte therapy, and nutritional support. Identifying an underlying cause or existing risk factors that can be managed and close monitoring and management of complications is also essential.

Novel specific treatment for acute pancreatitis in dogs

Fuzapladib sodium hydrate is a leukocyte function antigen-1 (LFA-1) inhibitor that prevents the extravasation of circulating neutrophils into the pancreatic tissue (Fig. 18.3) and has been approved for the treatment of pancreatitis in dogs in Japan. Data from a proof-of-concept study showed that fuzapladib improved survival in an experimental model (bile infusion) of pancreatitis in dogs (personal communication, 2023). Subsequent pilot randomized clinical trials have shown clinical scores and C-reactive protein improvement in dogs treated with fuzapladib. This medication has received conditional FDA approval in the United States. It is not yet available in Europe. Fuzapladib is administered at 0.4 mg/kg/day IV q24h for 3 days. A multicenter randomized clinical trial in the US has also shown promising results, but further clinical studies are needed and underway.[30]

Pain management

Published studies in dogs suggest between 33% and 70% of dogs with acute pancreatitis have abdominal pain on clinical examination at presentation.[14,28] Pain is commonly severe in people with acute pancreatitis, and the same is assumed for dogs, although their pain is often under-recognized.[4] This could be due to our inability to detect pain or due to the patient's temperament. Dogs with severe pain due to acute pancreatitis manifest their pain by displaying a praying stance, crouched appearance, or guarding/tensing of the abdomen on palpation.[14] Dogs with suspected acute pancreatitis should be assumed to be in pain until demonstrated otherwise and analgesics administered appropriate to their degree of pain. Details of pain assessment, appropriate analgesics, and suggested protocols are found in chapter 23.

Opioids should be used in all but the mildest cases of acute pancreatitis. Pain should be assessed after administration to ensure that treatment has been effective, and thereafter every 2 to 4 hours, depending on the duration of action of the analgesics being used and the severity of pain. These authors will initially administer a full μ-agonist such as methadone or fentanyl (see chapter 23)[31,32] for dogs with moderate to severe pain and then de-escalate to a partial μ-agonist, such as buprenorphine when pain is managed. When escalation of pain control is necessary, a multimodal approach, using drugs targeting different pain pathways, may be helpful while minimizing the side effects associated with increased opioid use, such as respiratory compromise, obtundation, functional ileus, and nausea. Obtunded animals are at risk of aspiration pneumonia due to a lack of protective laryngeal reflexes. Delayed gastric emptying time and intestinal ileus are common clinical signs seen in dogs with acute pancreatitis, and this can be exacerbated by full μ-agonists. Gastric stasis can lead to regurgitation, which increases the risk of aspiration pneumonia. Encouraging patients to resume voluntary enteral feeding when gastric stasis or functional ileus are present is also challenging. Constipation is also a common sequela of intestinal ileus. A multimodal approach may be utilized with a combination of opioids with continuous infusion of systemic local anesthetics (e.g., lidocaine), NMDA antagonist (e.g., ketamine), or α2-adrenoceptor agonists (e.g., dexmedetomidine). The authors will typically use the "FLK" protocol, which includes fentanyl, lidocaine, and ketamine administered initially with a loading dose followed by continuous rate infusion. Epidural or local ganglion blocks are also options in intractable pain, as discussed in chapter 23. Adjustment of pain management should be tailored to an individual patient and can be done stepwise by increasing the dose of a single agent and subsequently adding a second agent and increasing the dose of the second agent before reaching for a third agent. The same concept can be used when de-escalating pain management.

Transdermal fentanyl patches are approved for use in people. They are attached to the skin and deliver a controlled dose of fentanyl over time through the skin using a reservoir patch. Transdermal fentanyl patches can also be used in dogs, but uptake is variable because of skin thickness, residual hair, body temperature, peripheral circulation, and hydration status. Even in dogs that are normothermic and euhydrated, the absorption of fentanyl from a patch is slow and can take 12-24 hours before effective plasma concentrations are achieved. A patch can typically last for 3-5 days. The authors will use a transdermal fentanyl patch when planning to discharge a patient with acute pancreatitis that is euhydrated. The patch will be applied, and parenteral pain management will be continued for an additional 8-10 hours until effective plasma concentrations of fentanyl are expected to have been achieved. The patient is reassessed at the end of that period before being released. This is to ensure that the fentanyl patch alone is adequate to provide pain management before a patient is discharged. It is imperative to provide adequate discharge instructions when a patient goes home with a fentanyl patch, as it can be hazardous when humans (particularly children) are exposed to the patch. Patients will also commonly be discharged with other adjunct pain management, such as gabapentin or acetaminophen/codeine. See chapter 23 for more details on home management of pain in pancreatitis. Unlike in cats, tramadol is not useful in dogs because this species lacks the ability to metabolize tramadol to its active metabolite.

While nonsteroidal anti-inflammatory drugs (NSAIDs) are widely used for short and long-term pain management in dogs, pancreatitis is considered a side effect of their use in people. Also, NSAIDs do not provide sufficient analgesic effects in patients with pancreatitis. Additionally, the most common side effects of NSAIDs include vomiting, diarrhea, and anorexia, all of which can worsen the clinical picture of a patient with acute pancreatitis. NSAIDs are also contraindicated in hypovolemic patients. Thus, the risks of using NSAIDs outweigh their benefits, and their use should be avoided in dogs with acute pancreatitis.

Intravenous fluid therapy

Vomiting, diarrhea, and dysrexia can result in dehydration and hypovolemia in dogs with acute pancreatitis. In addition to the systemic effects of dehydration, the pancreas is particularly susceptible to altered blood flow.[33] Disturbed pancreatic microcirculation is an important step in the transformation of acute self-limiting pancreatitis to severe, necrotizing pancreatitis. Disturbed pancreatic microcirculation is usually multifactorial and can occur because of hypovolemia, increased vascular permeability, and microthrombi caused by hypercoagulability.[33] Therefore, patients with acute pancreatitis generally require intravenous fluid therapy. While aggressive fluid resuscitation has been recommended in the past, a landmark study in people showed that aggressive compared to moderate fluid therapy increases the risk of fluid overload without improving the primary outcome of preventing moderate-to-severe pancreatitis.[34] Both normal saline and lactated Ringer's solution are recommended by the human pancreatitis guidelines,[35] but a recent study in a large number of patients showed that lactated Ringer's prevented moderate-to-severe pancreatitis more effectively than normal saline.[36] There is no evidence supporting the use of colloids or fresh frozen plasma in acute pancreatitis in either humans or dogs. A patient's hydration status should be evaluated to estimate the fluid volume required to correct dehydration and compensate for ongoing losses. This should be given in conjunction with maintenance fluid requirements. A patient's hydration status should be reassessed, and fluid therapy should be adjusted every few hours. As is the case in people, it is important to not fluid-overload dogs with pancreatitis as they can develop edema or third-spacing in addition to worsening of any hypoalbuminemia.

Early nutritional support

Traditionally, early nutrition was not part of the recommendation in people or dogs with acute pancreatitis. The idea of "resting the pancreas" aimed to avoid further pancreatic enzyme release that was postulated to worsen autodigestion of the pancreas and surrounding tissues. However, it has since been established that early enteral feeding in severe acute pancreatitis in humans not only reduces infectious complications but also reduces overall mortality in some studies.[37] Acute pancreatitis is a hypermetabolic state with increased protein catabolism, marked inflammation, and deranged glucose metabolism.[2] Patients with acute pancreatitis often have impaired nutrient digestion and absorption that may further exacerbate a negative energy balance.[2] While parenteral nutrition has been historically recommended, many randomized clinical trials in people have shown that patients receiving oral/enteral feeding have better outcomes compared to those receiving parenteral nutrition.[2] Fasting or parenteral nutrition leads to enteral starvation. This results in intestinal atrophy, loss of epithelial barrier function, increased gut inflammatory protein expression, and dysbiosis favoring gram-negative proinflammatory bacteria. This leads to the translocation of bacteria and their endotoxins, pancreatic enzymes that are usually confined to the lumen of the intestinal tract, and cytotoxic and inflammatory mediators through a gut wall, which may also be compromised by local peritonitis. Consequently, sepsis and MODS may ensue.[2] A study in people also showed that those receiving immediate oral refeeding versus delayed oral refeeding had a shorter hospital stay, lower health care costs, and lower rate of relapse and complications.[38] However, stepwise increasing versus immediate full calories were equally tolerated without a difference in hospital stay. Although enteral feeding distal to the pylorus was recommended in the past, nasogastric tube feeding is now considered equally safe in humans and is more feasible in the clinical setting compared to nasojejunal tube placement.[2] In a prospective pilot study in dogs with severe acute pancreatitis, early esophageal feeding given within 12-24 hours of admission was well tolerated and safe and showed a more rapid reduction in clinical severity compared with dogs receiving parenteral nutrition.[39] Dogs receiving parenteral nutrition also had more catheter-associated complications. The effect of a low-fat diet versus a conventional fat diet was not investigated as all dogs were fed a low-fat diet (19 g/1000 kCal) in that study.

Extrapolating from the management of people with acute pancreatitis and the pilot study in dogs, it makes sense to provide early nutrition in dogs with acute pancreatitis. Voluntary oral feeding is most desirable but may not be achievable in a sick patient. Vomiting, nausea, gastric stasis, and ileus must be addressed for a dog to resume voluntary feeding. If these clinical signs are appropriately managed, a patient may commence voluntary feeding. Appetite stimulants such as capromorelin can be used but only if the animal is not nauseous and is showing an interest in food (Table 18.1).[40] However, if the patient does not resume voluntary feeding and has not been eating for more than 48-72 hours a nasoesophageal or nasogastric tube should be placed under light sedation (butorphanol 0.2-0.3 mg/kg IV). A nasoesophageal tube may theoretically be preferred over a nasogastric tube as it does not traverse the lower esophageal sphincter, thus preventing gastroesophageal reflux. However, it does not provide the ability to remove gastric contents that accumulate with gastric stasis. An abdominal FAST scan may be helpful in identifying gastric stasis. An esophagostomy tube may be preferred, particularly in animals that need more prolonged nutritional support. However, general anesthesia and endotracheal intubation are necessary. See chapter 22 for more details on feeding in acute pancreatitis.

It is unnecessary to feed a patient its full resting energy requirement initially (RER; 70 x body weight [kg]$^{0.75}$). The authors typically start feeding ⅓ of the daily RER on the first day. With the improvement of intestinal motility and enteral health, the patient will be able to tolerate a higher

TABLE 18.1 Select drugs for management of acute pancreatitis in dogs.

Drug		Type	Dose	Remarks
Analgesics	*See chapter 23 for details*			
Antiemetic/ antinausea drugs	Maropitant	NK_1 antagonist	1 mg/kg IV SC q24h	■ More effective as an antiemetic, less antinausea effects when compared to ondansetron. ■ Has the potential advantage of reducing visceral pain.
	Ondansetron	5-HT_3 antagonist	0.5-1 mg/kg IV, SC, PO q8-12h	■ Extra-label use in dogs. Has antinausea effects in addition to its antiemetic effects. ■ Poor oral bioavailability.
Prokinetic agents	Cisapride	5-HT_4 agonist	0.5-1 mg/kg IV q8h	■ Extra-label use in dogs. Accelerates gastric emptying time and increases lower esophageal sphincter tone. ■ Caution: can crystallize with many injectable substances.
	Erythromycin	Macrolide antibiotic with motilin-like properties	0.5-1 mg/kg IV q8h	■ Extra-label use in dogs. Accelerates gastric emptying time and increases lower esophageal sphincter tone. ■ Used at a 10 times lower dose than used for antimicrobial activity.
	Metoclopramide	D_2 antagonist centrally, mild 5-HT_3 antagonist peripherally	*CRI dose:* 1-2 mg/kg/day IV	■ Extra-label use in dogs. Weak antiemetic, more useful as a prokinetic drug when administered as a continuous infusion. ■ Increases lower esophageal sphincter tone.
Appetite stimulants	Capromorelin	Ghrelin agonist	3 mg/kg PO q24h	■ Best if used consistently instead of intermittently.
	Mirtazapine	Tetracyclic antidepressant	*Variable anecdotal doses:* a) 3.75-30 mg/dog (not mg/kg) PO q24h, do not exceed 30 mg/dog PO q24h b) 0.5-1.3 mg/kg PO q24h	■ Extra-label use in dogs. Can cause serotonin syndrome (such as hyperexcitability). May have the additional benefit of improving gastric emptying and colonic transit time. There is no effect on small intestinal transit time.
Gastric acid suppressant: note only to be used for bleeding gastric ulcers or reflux esophagitis	Omeprazole	Proton pump inhibitor	1 mg/kg PO or IV q12h	■ Extra-label use in dogs. Not useful when given q24h. ■ Oral preparation can cause gastrointestinal signs such as vomiting and diarrhea in a subset of patients.

volume of food at one time. Trickle and slow bolus feeding can be used, and this is usually determined by the amount of diet to be fed. Currently, a low-fat diet is recommended in people, especially those with hypertriglyceridemia, as the cause of their pancreatitis. Tight regulation of triglyceride concentration after presentation with acute pancreatitis is associated with a lower risk of recurrence of hypertriglyceridemia-induced pancreatitis in people,[41] so it might be wise to feed a low-fat diet to dogs with marked hypertriglyceridemia on admission. However, it is unknown if a low-fat diet is truly necessary for all patients and, if so, what level of fat should be aimed at in dogs with acute pancreatitis. Randomized clinical trials are much needed to help answer these questions. Readers are encouraged to visit Today's Veterinary Practice website (https://todaysveterinarypractice.com/nutrition/step-by-step-guide-to-making-an-enteral-nutrition-plan) for information to formulate a nutritional plan for a sick patient in the hospital.

If a patient has persistent hypertriglyceridemia postdischarge, a long-term low-fat diet, in addition to addressing the underlying etiology of hypertriglyceridemia, is important. Some patients may require additional therapies such as omega-3 fatty acid supplementation, fibrates, and/or statins.

Other supportive therapy

It is important to control the vomiting and nausea that are commonly associated with acute pancreatitis (Table 18.1). Maropitant (NK1 antagonist) and ondansetron (5-HT3 antagonist) are efficacious antiemetics that act both centrally and peripherally. Both drugs are equally effective in controlling vomiting, but ondansetron is more effective in controlling nausea. Maropitant may also have the added advantage of reducing visceral pain, although this is unproven in dogs (see chapter 23). In one single study, ondansetron was suggested to have poor oral bioavailability in dogs and thus may not be as effective orally as when administered parenterally.[42] Metoclopramide (D2 antagonist centrally, mild 5-HT3 antagonist peripherally) is a weak antiemetic in dogs and may be more useful as a prokinetic drug. Many dogs with severe forms of acute pancreatitis have a functional ileus. The decision to start a prokinetic drug should be guided by physical examination findings, such as lack of gut sounds or the presence of regurgitation. Diagnostic imaging evidence of functional ileus can also help support the use of prokinetics. Inappropriate use of prokinetics will result in gastrointestinal spasms, which can be equally painful anecdotally, particularly in dogs with pancreatitis. Commonly used prokinetic drugs include cisapride, erythromycin, and metoclopramide. Cisapride and erythromycin are useful prokinetic drugs for gastric stasis, gastroesophageal reflux, and reflux esophagitis by accelerating gastric emptying time and increasing lower esophageal sphincter tone. Metoclopramide, when used as a continuous infusion, is helpful in stimulating motility of the upper gastrointestinal tract without stimulating gastric, pancreatic, and biliary secretions. It also prevents gastroesophageal reflux and reflux esophagitis by increasing the lower esophageal sphincter tone.

Acid suppressants are not considered the standard of care for acute pancreatitis in dogs as there is no clear benefit or indication. However, if a patient has clinical evidence of gastroduodenal ulceration and erosion (i.e., substantial hematemesis, melena) or esophagitis (e.g., hard swallowing, persistent regurgitation), then acid suppressants may be indicated. Omeprazole given twice daily (1 mg/kg PO q12h) is more potent in increasing gastric pH compared to once daily administration or histamine type-2 receptor antagonists (e.g., cimetidine, famotidine) given once or twice daily.

A recent scoping review of corticosteroid treatment for acute pancreatitis in several species concluded that using corticosteroids reduces the duration of hospitalization and serum C-reactive protein concentration, though the data they based this conclusion on was very weak.[43] Also, there are mixed results when it comes to improvement in clinical scores and mortality rates.[44] Because of these mixed results and the lack of robust randomized clinical trials, the routine use of corticosteroids as a standard of care in acute pancreatitis is not recommended at this time. While corticosteroids are potent anti-inflammatory drugs, they are also procoagulative, thus increasing the risk of DIC in severe acute pancreatitis and, dependent on the dose, immunosuppressive. Therefore, the risks and benefits of using corticosteroids should be individualized to the patient and its comorbidities.

The routine use of antibiotics is not recommended for acute pancreatitis because it is generally a sterile inflammation. With the emergence of antibiotic-resistant infections, it becomes paramount to uphold antibiotic stewardship. It can be challenging to distinguish sepsis secondary to bacterial translocation as sterile inflammation from acute pancreatitis often results in pyrexia and an inflammatory leukogram. Accompanying signs of poor gastrointestinal health (e.g., melena, hematochezia) with a history of prolonged enteral fasting can increase the suspicion of bacterial translocation. The authors of this chapter will only start intravenous antibiotics (broad-spectrum, such as ampicillin with or without sulbactam) when there is persistent pyrexia with melena and/or hematochezia with an inflammatory leukogram with toxic changes or some other clinical data that strongly suggest a bacterial infection. Administration of antibiotics by mouth should be avoided since most antibiotics will worsen gastrointestinal signs and may have questionable absorption secondary to poor gastrointestinal health.

Other comorbidities, including aspiration pneumonia, hyperglycemia, and DIC, should be managed as they occur. Aspiration pneumonia is a common sequela in patients with acute pancreatitis, especially when vomiting and regurgitation are present. If a hospitalized patient develops pyrexia, tachypnea, or dyspnea, with variably increased lung sounds, a three-view chest radiograph or point-of-care lung ultrasound should be performed for investigation of potential aspiration pneumonia, which would then require appropriate antibiotic administration together with supportive care such as regular coupage.

Some dogs with acute pancreatitis may develop transient insulin exhaustion or resistance, resulting in transient hyperglycemia or diabetic ketosis. Intermittent regular insulin (0.1 unit/kg IM q4h if blood glucose >250-300 mg/dL) can be administered, and blood glucose can be rechecked every 4 hours. In some cases, particularly where the pancreatitis is acute or chronic, the dog may become permanently diabetic and require long-term insulin.

Parenteral antithrombotic agents such as heparin (unfractionated or low molecular weight) should be started in patients with occult/overt DIC, and monitoring response to therapy is important to determine successful therapy. A positive response will be normalization of prothrombin time, activated thromboplastin time, D-dimer concentration, antithrombin activity, fibrinogen concentration, and platelet count.

Many dogs with uncomplicated acute pancreatitis will clinically improve, and those that are successfully discharged should continue to receive pain management and other supportive therapies at home. More details of at-home pain management can be found in chapter 23. Long-term feeding of a low-fat diet may only be necessary in those cases associated with hypertriglyceridemia or with chronic or recurrent disease, but prospective studies are needed to assess this more conclusively.

Prognosis

Acute pancreatitis is a common disease in dogs and is associated with significant morbidity and mortality. Dogs with mild, localized, uncomplicated acute pancreatitis are often hemodynamically stable and can be managed successfully with supportive at-home care. Conversely, a patient with risk factors (e.g., hypertriglyceridemia, concurrent endocrinopathy) and local (i.e., pancreatic necrosis) and/or systemic (e.g., SIRS, MODS, DIC, acute lung and/or kidney injury, myocarditis, and others) complications require close monitoring and in-hospital intensive care. The development of systemic complications will also result in a higher mortality rate. While the treatment of acute pancreatitis in the past has been mostly supportive, a new specific treatment is now available in Japan and the USA, which requires further clinical trials. Other supportive therapies should address pain management, intravenous fluid administration, and early oral/enteral feeding. It is important to recognize the presence of nausea, ileus, aspiration pneumonia, hyperglycemia, and coagulopathy that can accompany acute pancreatitis in dogs.

KEY POINTS

- Pancreatitis is the most common exocrine pancreatic disease in dogs and can either be acute or chronic.
- The severity of acute pancreatitis can range from mild to moderate to severe, which is often associated with systemic complications. Moderate to severe acute pancreatitis is associated with high morbidity and even significant mortality.
- It is challenging to identify the etiology of acute pancreatitis in dogs in most cases.
- A systematic and global patient assessment is important for an accurate diagnosis of acute pancreatitis.
- Treatment is largely supportive and nonspecific. Pain management, intravenous fluid therapy with lactated Ringer's solution, and early oral/enteral nutrition are important.
- The neutrophil extravasation cascade is an important pathway to local and systemic inflammation, and manipulation of this pathway with drugs may be the future of treatment.

References

1. Newman SJ, Steiner JM, Woosley K, et al. Histologic assessment and grading of the exocrine pancreas in the dog. *J Vet Diagn Invest* 18(1): 115-118, 2006. doi: 10.1177/104063870601800119.
2. Rinninella E, Annetta MG, Serricchio ML, et al. Nutritional support in acute pancreatitis: from physiopathology to practice. An evidence-based approach. *Eur Rev Med Pharmacol Sci* 21(2):421-432, 2017.
3. Lem KY, Fosgate GT, Norby B, et al. Associations between dietary factors and pancreatitis in dogs. *J Am Vet Med Assoc* 233(9):1425-1431, 2008. doi: 10.2460/javma.233.9.1425.
4. Cridge H, Scott N, Steiner JM. Risk factors and clinical Presentation in dogs with increased serum pancreatic lipase concentrations - A descriptive analysis. *Animals (Basel)* 12(12):1581, 2022. doi: 10.3390/ani12121581.
5. Flores-Calderon J, Exiga-Gonzalez E, Moran-Villota S, et al. Acute pancreatitis in children with acute lymphoblastic leukemia treated with L-asparaginase. *J Pediatr Hematol Oncol* 31(10):790-793, 2009. doi:10.1097/MPH.0b013e3181b794e8.
6. Gaskill CL, Cribb AE. Pancreatitis associated with potassium bromide/phenobarbital combination therapy in epileptic dogs. *Can Vet J* 41(7):555-558, 2000.
7. Ohta H, Kojima K, Yokoyama N, et al. Effects of immunosuppressive prednisolone therapy on pancreatic tissue and concentration of canine pancreatic lipase immunoreactivity in healthy dogs. *Can Vet J* 82(4):278-286, 2018.
8. Cridge H, Lim SY, Algül H, et al. New insights into the etiology, risk factors, and pathogenesis of pancreatitis in dogs: potential impacts on clinical practice. *J Vet Intern Med* 36(3):847-864, 2022. doi: 10.1111/jvim.16437.
9. Cook AK, Breitschwerdt EB, Levine JF, Bunch SE, Linn LO. Risk factors associated with acute pancreatitis in dogs: 101 cases (1985-1990). *J Am Vet Med Assoc* 203(5):673-679, 1993.
10. Mattin M, O'Neill D, Church D, et al. An epidemiological study of diabetes mellitus in dogs attending first opinion practice in the UK. *Vet Rec* 174(14):349, 2014. doi.org/10.1136/vr.101950.
11. Yang AL, McNabb-Baltar J. Hypertriglyceridemia and acute pancreatitis. *Pancreatology* 20(5):795-800. 2020. doi: 10.1016/j.pan.2020.06.005.
12. Xenoulis PG, Suchodolski JS, Ruaux CG, et al. Association between serum triglyceride and canine pancreatic lipase immunoreactivity concentrations in miniature schnauzers. *J Am Vet Med Assoc* 46(4):229-234, 2010. doi: 10.5326/0460229.
13. Xenoulis PG, Levinski MD, Suchodolski JS, et al. Serum triglyceride concentrations in Miniature Schnauzers with and without a history of probable pancreatitis. *J Vet Intern Med* 25(1):20-25, 2011. doi: 10.1111/j.1939-1676.2010.0644.x.
14. Hess RS, Saunders HM, Van Winkle TJ, et al. Clinical, clinicopathologic, radiographic, and ultrasonographic abnormalities in dogs with fatal acute pancreatitis: 70 cases (1986-1995). *J Am Vet Med Assoc* 213(5):665-670, 1998.
15. Bishop MA, Xenoulis PG, Levinski MD, et al. Identification of variants of the SPINK1 gene and their association with pancreatitis in Miniature Schnauzers. *Am J Vet Res* 71(5):527-533, 2010. doi:10.2460/ajvr.71.5.527.
16. Furrow E, Armstrong PJ, Patterson EE. High prevalence of the c.74A>C SPINK1 variant in miniature and standard Schnauzers. *J Vet Intern Med* 26(6):1295-1299, 2012. doi:10.1111/j.1939-1676.2012.01013.x.
17. Mansfield C. Pathophysiology of acute pancreatitis: potential application from

experimental models and human medicine to dogs. *J Vet Intern Med* 26(4):875-887, 2012. doi: 10.1111/j.1939-1676.2012.00949.x.

18. Wan J, Ren Y, Yang X, et al. The role of neutrophils and neutrophil extracellular traps in acute pancreatitis. *Front Cell Dev Biol* 8:565758, 2020. doi: 10.3389/fcell.2020.565758.
19. Lathan P. Laboratory diagnosis of thyroid and adrenal disease. *Vet Clin North Am Small Anim Pract* 53(1):207-224, 2023. doi: 10.1016/j.cvsm.2022.08.005.
20. Nielsen L, Holm J, Rozanski E, et al. Multicenter investigation of hemostatic dysfunction in 15 dogs with acute pancreatitis. *J Vet Emerg Crit Care (San Antonio)* 29(3):264-268, 2019. doi: 10.1111/vec.12840.
21. Goggs R, Mastrocco A, Brooks MB. Retrospective evaluation of 4 methods for outcome prediction in overt disseminated intravascular coagulation in dogs (2009-2014): 804 cases. *J Vet Emerg Crit Care (San Antonio)* 28(6):541-550, 2018. doi: 10.1111/vec.12777.
22. Lim SY, Nakamura K, Morishita K, et al. Serial evaluation of specific canine pancreatic lipase immunoreactivity and C-reactive protein in dogs with cerulein-induced acute pancreatitis. Proceedings of ACVIM Forum 2015, 3-6 June 2015, Indiana, USA.
23. Lim SY, Steiner JM, Cridge H. Understanding lipase assays in the diagnosis of pancreatitis in veterinary medicine. *J Am Vet Med Assoc* 260(11): 1249-1258, 2022. doi/10.1111/jvim.12609.
24. Lim SY, Xenoulis PG, Stavroulaki EM, et al. The 1,2-o-dilauryl-rac-glycero-3-glutaric acid-(6'-methylresorufin) ester (DGGR) lipase assay in cats and dogs is not specific for pancreatic lipase. *Vet Clin Pathol* 49(4):607-613, 2020. doi: 10.1111/vcp.12906.
25. Cridge H, Twedt DC, Marolf AJ, et al. Advances in the diagnosis of acute pancreatitis in dogs. *J Vet Intern Med* 35(6):2572-2587, 2021. doi: 10.1111/jvim.16292.
26. Stieger-Vanegas SM, Frank PM. Peritoneal Space. In Thrall DE (editor). Textbook of veterinary diagnostic radiology. St. Louis, Elsevier, 2018, pp.764-791.
27. Cridge H, Sullivant AM, Wills RW, et al. Association between abdominal ultrasound findings, the specific canine pancreatic lipase assay, clinical severity indices, and clinical diagnosis in dogs with pancreatitis. *J Vet Intern Med* 34(2):636-643, 2020. doi: 10.1111/jvim.15693.
28. Cueni C, Hofer-Inteeworn N, Kümmerle-Fraune C, et al. Progression of lipase activity and pancreatic lipase immunoreactivity in dogs hospitalized for acute pancreatitis and correlation with clinical features. *J Vet Intern Med* 37(1):70-79, 2023. doi: 10.1111/jvim.16591.
29. Cordner AP, Sharkey LC, Armstrong PJ, McAteer KD. Cytologic findings and diagnostic yield in 92 dogs undergoing fine-needle aspiration of the pancreas. *J Vet Diagn Invest* 27(2):236-240, 2015. doi: 10.1177/1040638715574862.
30. Steiner JM, Lainesse C, Noshiro Y, Domen Y, Sedlacek H, Bienhoff SE, et al. Fuzapladib in a randomized controlled multicenter masked study in dogs with presumptive acute onset pancreatitis. *J Vet Intern Med*, 2023 (Online ahead of print). doi: 10.1111/jvim.16897.
31. Monteiro BP, Lascelles BDX, Murrell J, et al. 2022 WSAVA guidelines for the recognition, assessment and treatment of pain. *J Small Anim Pract* 64(4):177-254, 2023. doi: 10.1111/jsap.12200.
32. Mansfield C, Beths T. Management of acute pancreatitis in dogs: a critical appraisal with focus on feeding and analgesia. *J Small Anim Pract* 56(1):27-39, 2015. doi: 10.1111/jsap.12296.
33. Gardner TB, Vege SS, Pearson RK, et al. Fluid resuscitation in acute pancreatitis. *Clin Gastroenterol Hepatol* 6(10):1070-1076, 2008. doi: 10.1016/j.cgh.2008.05.005.
34. de-Madaria E, Buxbaum JL, Maisonneuve P, et al. Aggressive or moderate fluid resuscitation in acute pancreatitis. *N Engl J Med* 387(11):989-1000, 2022. doi: 10.1056/NEJMoa2202884.
35. Crockett SD, Wani S, Gardner TB, et al. American Gastroenterological Association Institute guideline on initial management of acute pancreatitis. *Gastroenterology* 154(4):1096-1101, 2018. doi: 10.1053/j.gastro.2018.01.032.
36. Lee PJ, Culp S, Kamal A, et al. Lactated Ringer's use in the first 24 hours of hospitalization is associated with improved outcomes in 999 patients with acute pancreatitis. *Am J Gastroenterol*, 2023. Online ahead of print. doi: 10.14309/ajg.0000000000002391.
37. Al-Omran M, Albalawi ZH, Tashkandi MF, et al. Enteral versus parenteral nutrition for acute pancreatitis. *Cochrane Database Syst Rev* 2010(1):CD002837, 2010. doi:10.1002/14651858.CD002837.pub2.
38. Ramirez-Maldonado E, Lopez Gordo S, Pueyo EM, et al. Immediate oral refeeding in patients with mild and moderate acute pancreatitis: A multicenter, randomized controlled trial (PADI trial). *Ann Surg* 274(2):255-263, 2021. doi: 10.1097/SLA.0000000000004596.
39. Mansfield CS, James FE, Steiner JM, et al. A pilot study to assess tolerability of early enteral nutrition via esophagostomy tube feeding in dogs with severe acute pancreatitis. *J Vet Intern Med* 25(3):419-425, 2011. doi: 10.1111/j.1939-1676.2011.0703.x.
40. Plumb DC. Plumb's Veterinary Drugs. Available from: https://app.plumbs.com/drugs [Accessed 12th October 2023].
41. Charlesworth A, Steger A, Crook MA. Acute pancreatitis associated with severe hypertriglyceridaemia; A retrospective cohort study. *Int J Surg* 23(Pt A):23-27, 2015. doi: 10.1016/j.ijsu.2015.08.080.
42. Saynor DA, Dixon CM. The metabolism of ondansetron. *Eur J Cancer Clin Oncol* 25 Suppl 1:S75-77, 1989.
43. Bjornkjaer-Nielsen KA, Bjornvad CR. Corticosteroid treatment for acute/acute-on-chronic experimental and naturally occurring pancreatitis in several species: a scoping review to inform possible use in dogs. *Acta Vet Scand* 63(1):28, 2021. doi:10.1186/s13028-021-00592-0.
44. Okanishi H, Nagata T, Nakane S, et al. Comparison of initial treatment with and without corticosteroids for suspected acute pancreatitis in dogs. *J Small Anim Pract* 60(5):298-304, 2019. doi: 10.1111/jsap.12994.

CHAPTER 19

Chronic pancreatitis

Panagiotis G. Xenoulis
DVM, DrMedVet, PhD

Jörg M. Steiner
MedVet, DrMedVet, PhD, DACVIM, DECVIM-CA (Internal Medicine), AGAF

Pancreatitis is the most common disorder of the exocrine pancreas in dogs.[1] Although both acute and chronic pancreatitis occur in dogs, acute pancreatitis has traditionally been believed to be more common and clinically important in this species, but more recent data suggests that chronic pancreatitis is far more common than acute disease, albeit less frequently diagnosed.[1] Also, chronic pancreatitis has generally been considered less clinically significant than acute disease, although several complications and concurrent diseases can affect the outcome and long-term prognosis of patients with chronic pancreatitis.[1,2] In addition, acute-on-chronic episodes are believed to be common and can lead to significant morbidity and mortality. A clinical diagnosis of chronic pancreatitis can be challenging because the disease is often subclinical or is associated with mild, nonspecific clinical signs and blood work abnormalities. Consequently, many cases of chronic pancreatitis likely remain undiagnosed.[1,2]

Classification and definitions

A standardized classification system for pancreatitis does not exist in veterinary medicine. In general, canine pancreatitis can be divided into acute and chronic forms based on the presence (chronic form) or absence (acute form) of permanent histopathologic changes such as fibrosis and acinar atrophy (Fig. 19.1).[3-5] Other histopathologic findings (e.g., pancreatic cell necrosis, peripancreatic fat necrosis, predominant type of cell infiltration) and clinical criteria are often used to further classify the disease process in dogs.[3-5] Chronic pancreatitis can be defined as a continuous, usually progressive inflammation of the pancreas characterized by permanent damage, such as acinar atrophy and/or fibrosis that can lead to irreversible impairment of both exocrine and endocrine pancreatic function.[3-5]

Clinically, both acute and chronic pancreatitis can be mild or severe.[1,2] Some animals show histopathologic evidence of both acute and chronic disease concurrently (e.g., fibrosis and concurrent pancreatic cell necrosis); these are typically classified as acute-on-chronic cases.[1-4] The term chronic active pancreatitis has also been used to describe the simultaneous presence of fibrosis and pancreatic cell necrosis.

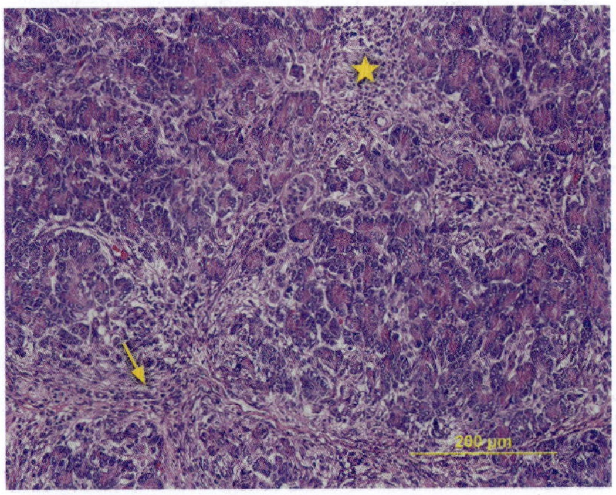

FIG. 19.1 Histologic section of the pancreas from a dog with chronic pancreatitis. Extensive fibrosis (arrow) and lymphocytic infiltration (star) areas are noted. Hematoxylin and eosin stain; magnification ×40. Courtesy of Dr. S. Newman.

Prevalence

The exact prevalence of chronic pancreatitis in dogs is unknown. The majority of data originates from necropsy studies, which do not accurately reflect all clinically important diseases. Chronic pancreatitis has traditionally been thought to be much less common than acute pancreatitis in dogs. One study examined 73 pancreata from dogs presented for postmortem examination, with 64% showing histologic evidence of inflammation.[3] Surprisingly, the most common lesions detected were lymphocytic infiltration (72%), fibrosis (60%), and a combination of both lesions (47%), findings that are suggestive of chronic disease.[3] Another study evaluated pancreata from 200 unselected canine postmortem examinations from first opinion practices in the UK.[5] In that study, the prevalence of chronic pancreatitis was 34%, and 15% of those were classified histologically as moderate or marked.[5] These results indicate that chronic pancreatitis may be more common in dogs than previously believed. However, it should be noted that postmortem studies tend to overestimate the prevalence of chronic disease, which causes permanent histological changes, and the clinical significance of these findings remains to be determined.

Etiology

Little is known about the etiology of chronic pancreatitis in dogs, and most cases are considered idiopathic because an underlying initiating factor cannot be identified.[1] It is unclear whether chronic pancreatitis exists as a distinct disease entity or whether it results from recurrent attacks of acute pancreatitis, but it is likely that both scenarios occur in dogs. Factors that have been associated with the development of pancreatitis in dogs are summarized in Table 19.1. Whether or not all these factors can specifically lead to the development of chronic pancreatitis remains to be determined. Some of these factors may lead to chronic pancreatitis or repeated bouts of acute pancreatitis.

In humans, the major causes of chronic pancreatitis are environmental insults (such as alcohol abuse or smoking tobacco products) and genetic factors (hereditary pancreatitis, including mutations of the cationic trypsinogen gene, serine peptidase inhibitor Kazal type 1 (SPINK1) gene, cystic fibrosis transmembrane conductance regulator (CFTR) gene, and others). In dogs, a breed predisposition for pancreatitis has been reported for several breeds, including Miniature Schnauzers, Yorkshire Terriers, Cavalier King Charles Spaniels, Cocker Spaniels, Boxers, and Border Collies, suggesting a possible genetic component.[5,6] Early studies in Miniature Schnauzers with pancreatitis failed to identify any cationic or anionic trypsinogen gene mutations. Subsequent studies in the same breed identified variants of the SPINK1 gene that cosegregated with pancreatitis, but a later study found no association of these SPINK1 variants with pancreatitis.[7,8] CFTR variants have also been reported in dogs, although a clear association with pancreatitis is lacking.

TABLE 19.1 Factors that have been associated with the development of pancreatitis in dogs (acute and chronic).

Nutritional factors	■ High-fat diets (>90 g of fat/1000 Kcal) ■ Dietary indiscretion ■ Obesity
Drugs	■ Organophosphates ■ L-Asparaginase ■ Azathioprine ■ Potassium bromide ■ Antimonate salts ■ Others
Infectious agents	■ Babesiosis ■ Ehrlichiosis ■ Leishmaniosis ■ Leptospirosis ■ Heterobilharziosis
Endocrinopathies	■ Diabetes mellitus ■ Hypothyroidism ■ Hyperadrenocorticism
Breed predisposition	■ Miniature Schnauzers ■ Yorkshire and other terriers ■ Boxers ■ English Cocker Spaniels ■ Cavalier King Charles Spaniels ■ Collies
Other factors	■ Hypertriglyceridemia ■ Ischemia ■ Duct obstruction ■ Trauma/surgery ■ Hypercalcemia ■ Genetic associations (SPINK1 gene?)

A rare subtype of chronic pancreatitis in humans is autoimmune chronic pancreatitis, which is divided into two types (types 1 and 2) associated with distinct histopathologic features and a distinct clinical course. In dogs, a form of pancreatitis that might resemble type 1 autoimmune pancreatitis (now known as IgG4-related disease) has been reported in English Cocker Spaniels in the UK.[9,10] This disease tends to affect multiple organs in humans, including kidneys and tear and salivary ducts, and there is some evidence of this also in English Cocker Spaniels. However, further studies are needed to confidently prove whether the disease in dogs truly is autoimmune.

Hypertriglyceridemia has been associated with frequent episodes of pancreatitis in humans (hypertriglyceridemic pancreatitis), and such a relationship has also been suggested in dogs. This is more often reported to cause recurrent acute pancreatitis (see chapter 18 for more details) but can become chronic in humans with concurrent risk factors, and the same may be true in dogs. Studies in Miniature Schnauzers, a breed that is commonly affected by primary hypertriglyceridemia, have suggested that severe hypertriglyceridemia is a potential risk factor for pancreatitis in this breed.[11,12]

Signalment

Dogs of any age, breed, or sex can develop pancreatitis. However, older animals appear to be more likely to develop chronic disease. As mentioned above, breed predispositions for chronic pancreatitis have been reported for Miniature Schnauzers, Yorkshire Terriers, Cavalier King Charles Spaniels, Cocker Spaniels, Boxers, and Border Collies.[5,6] Breed predispositions might be affected by the geographic region of the canine population due to genetic and environmental differences and different bloodlines.

Diagnosis

Diagnosis of chronic pancreatitis is clinically challenging due to the low level of suspicion, the presence of mild, sporadic, and nonspecific clinical signs, and the relatively low sensitivity of noninvasive diagnostic methods for detecting chronic pancreatitis in the absence of an acute exacerbation. Histopathology is currently the gold standard for the diagnosis of chronic pancreatitis but is rarely performed antemortem. Therefore, many chronic pancreatitis cases are misdiagnosed as another differential diagnosis, which is associated with similar clinical signs (e.g., food-responsive enteropathy, other inflammatory chronic enteropathies, chronic liver disease). In addition, diagnosing acute-on-chronic episodes of pancreatitis (as opposed to true acute pancreatitis) is clinically impossible during the acute episode. Therefore, maintaining a high level of suspicion and using the most sensitive and specific tests available (and knowing their limitations) is crucial for a diagnosis of chronic pancreatitis.

Clinical picture

Acute and chronic pancreatitis are difficult to differentiate clinically because they usually lead to similar clinical signs. Thus, the gold standard for differentiation is still considered to be histopathology, even though the collection of a biopsy is rarely in the best interest of the patient. Chronicity of clinical signs may be an indication of chronic disease. However, clinical signs might be a consequence of concurrent disease (e.g., chronic enteropathy) and not chronic pancreatitis. In addition, an acute episode of pancreatitis may develop in an animal that has underlying chronic disease. Therefore, acute exacerbation of chronic pancreatitis is often misdiagnosed as acute pancreatitis.

Most cases of chronic pancreatitis are considered to be mild, and many remain subclinical unless an acute exacerbation occurs. Often, the clinician needs to specifically ask the owner for the presence of mild clinical signs that might be considered normal by the owner (e.g., occasional hyporexia, a change in behavior, or occasional vomiting). When present, clinical signs are nonspecific and usually transient and are indistinguishable from several other gastrointestinal and other diseases, such as food-responsive enteropathy, inflammatory bowel disease, gastrointestinal hypomotility, and many others. Therefore, it is common for dogs with chronic pancreatitis to be misdiagnosed. Some dogs with chronic pancreatitis may respond to a dietary change if the new diet is low in fat, further complicating the differentiation of chronic pancreatitis and food-responsive enteropathy.

Clinical signs in dogs with chronic pancreatitis are usually mild and sporadic unless an acute episode occurs. In a study of 61 dogs with histopathologically confirmed chronic pancreatitis, clinical signs included lethargy (80%), decreased appetite (70%), vomiting (63%), diarrhea (36%), and abdominal pain (27%).[13] The combination of vomiting and cranial abdominal pain, which is considered especially suggestive of acute pancreatitis in dogs, is not as common in dogs with chronic pancreatitis. Some animals may also develop weight loss.

Other clinical signs may be present in animals with chronic pancreatitis but may be a consequence of concurrent disease (e.g., polyuria/polydipsia in animals with diabetes mellitus; diarrhea, weight loss, polyphagia, and a poor haircoat in animals with exocrine pancreatic insufficiency [EPI]).[2]

In cases of acute exacerbation of the disease, a clinical presentation similar to that of acute pancreatitis is typically seen (see chapter 18, for example, severe lethargy, anorexia, vomiting, dehydration, shock) and differentiation between a single episode of acute pancreatitis and an exacerbation of chronic pancreatitis is clinically impossible. In a dog that has been known to have chronic pancreatitis based on history, chronic clinical signs, and specific testing, acute-on-chronic episodes of pancreatitis are to be expected, and these episodes may not be considered as single episodes of acute pancreatitis. Recognition of underlying chronic disease is important because although both acute-on-chronic cases and true acute episodes are managed in the same manner in the short term, recognition of potential long-term sequelae (exocrine pancreatic insufficiency and diabetes mellitus) and long-term management is indicated for chronic cases.

Clinical examination findings are usually unremarkable in dogs with chronic pancreatitis without an acute exacerbation. In some cases, abdominal pain may be detectable upon abdominal palpation, which is often focal in the cranial abdomen. In some cases of dogs with autoimmune pancreatitis (IgG4-related disease), dry eye/dry mouth and/or anal sac disease might be present and should alert the clinician of the possibility of autoimmune disease.

Routine clinical pathology

In many cases of chronic pancreatitis, the minimum database consisting of a complete blood count, serum biochemistry profile, and urinalysis is normal. During an episode of acute-on-chronic pancreatitis, any findings described for acute pancreatitis might be seen (see chapters 13 and 18 for more details).

Laboratory tests for pancreatitis

Pancreatic lipase immunoreactivity

Pancreatic lipase is produced exclusively by pancreatic acinar cells. Immunoassays for the specific measurement of pancreatic lipase have been developed and analytically validated for dogs.[14] Pancreatic lipase immunoreactivity (PLI) assays are currently considered the most sensitive and specific serum tests for diagnosing pancreatitis in dogs. The main advantage of PLI assays over traditional lipase activity assays is based on the fact that, in contrast to the traditional activity assays for lipase, which indiscriminately measure activities of lipases of multiple cellular origins, immunoassays that are used to measure pancreatic lipase concentrations in serum (i.e., PLI assays) exclusively quantify lipase of pancreatic acinar cell origin based on its unique three-dimensional structure.[15] Therefore, PLI assays have inherent advantages over the traditional serum lipase activity assays that make them more suitable for specific evaluation of the exocrine pancreas in dogs. See chapter 14 for more details on cPLI tests.

Both clinical[17] and histopathological[18-20] studies concerning cPLI for canine pancreatitis have been published, and all generally agree that serum cPLI is the most sensitive and specific serum marker for pancreatitis in dogs to date. It needs to be noted that most of the published studies have included acute pancreatitis cases. However, the sensitivity of cPLI is believed to be lower in mild or chronic pancreatitis. This is expected because the main lesions in chronic pancreatitis (i.e., fibrosis, atrophy, and lymphocytic infiltration) are not associated with increased leakage of pancreatic enzymes into the vascular space. In an observational study, serum cPLI concentrations had a sensitivity of 26-58% for chronic pancreatitis. However, in the same study, serum amylase and lipase activities had even lower sensitivities.[2] Therefore, chronic pancreatitis cannot be ruled out on the basis of a single normal serum cPLI concentration. Repeated testing might increase the sensitivity, particularly if performed during clinically acute flare-ups, and is recommended in cases where chronic pancreatitis is suspected clinically. The serial measurement of serum cPLI concentrations may be useful for monitoring dogs with chronic pancreatitis, as concentrations are expected to mirror ongoing acinar cell damage, which would be more pronounced at times of more severe inflammation or an acute exacerbation.

A rapid, in-clinic, semiquantitative, visually-read test for the estimation of canine pancreatic lipase in serum is also available –the SNAP cPL (see chapter 14 for more details).[21] The main use of this diagnostic tool is to rule out pancreatitis (i.e., a normal result makes a diagnosis of pancreatitis very unlikely), and thus, the sensitivity of the SNAP cPL is more important than its specificity. Although not specifically investigated, similar to the quantitative assay, the clinical accuracy of the SNAP cPL should be expected to be lower for chronic pancreatitis than for acute disease.

Serum amylase and lipase activities

Serum amylase and lipase activities have long been considered markers for pancreatitis in dogs, but several studies have shown that they are not good markers for spontaneous canine pancreatitis due to their low sensitivity and specificity (see chapter 14 for more details).[15] Many tissues other than the exocrine pancreas synthesize amylases and lipases, and traditional catalytic assays are not able to differentiate amylases and lipases according to their tissue of origin. In one study, about 50% of dogs with an increased serum activity of either amylase or lipase had no histopathologic evidence of pancreatitis.[15] Even large increases in amylase and lipase activities can result from nonpancreatic disorders and should always be followed by the use of more specific and sensitive tests.[15] Therefore, pancreatitis cannot be diagnosed or ruled out based on serum amylase and/or lipase activities alone. In one study that included chronic pancreatitis cases, the sensitivity of serum amylase and lipase activities was <30% when a cutoff or 3 times the upper limit was used.[2] Therefore, chronic pancreatitis cannot be ruled out on the basis of normal serum amylase or lipase activity.

More recently, developed colorimetric lipase activity assays, such as those based on DGGR as a substrate, have been reported to show better performance than traditional catalytic assays. This substrate is claimed to be more specific for pancreatic lipase than traditional catalytic assays, but such increased analytical specificity was not found in humans. Some studies have compared DGGR-based assays with PLI assays and have suggested similar performance between the two.[22] A study in 142 dogs found high agreement between one specific DGGR-based lipase assay and the Spec cPL assay, with the best agreement ($\kappa = 0.80$) for a cutoff of this DGGR-based lipase activity assay of >216 U/L.[22] However, it should be noted that an agreement of 0.8 is not very high for two assays that supposedly measure the same analyte. There are various DGGR-based assays for the measurement of serum lipase activity, and they differ dramatically due to changes in added compounds (e.g., colipase, bile acids), assay conditions (e.g., pH), and the analyzer being used requiring each to be validated individually. See chapter 14 for more details on the methodology of this assay. None of the currently available DGGR-based assays have been shown to be consistently any more specific for the measurement of pancreatic lipase than more traditional serum lipase activity assays. A recent experimental study in both dogs and cats showed that DGGR is not only hydrolyzed by pancreatic lipase but also by lipoprotein lipase and hepatic lipase.[23] These extrapancreatic lipases may contribute to a lack of analytic specificity in this assay.[23] In the same study, no significant effect of hepatic or lipoprotein lipase was shown for serum cPLI concentrations.[23] Different studies have reported very different results for the specificity of this assay, which are summarized in chapter 14. The sensitivity and specificity of DGGR have not been systematically evaluated in dogs with chronic pancreatitis, but as leakage of pancreatic lipase from acinar cells is usually less pronounced, the lack of specificity for measuring pancreatic lipase and the associated increase in cutoff value makes an elevated value above the cutoff value less likely.

In a recent study, DGGR lipase activity was found to have limited utility in monitoring the clinical progression of chronic pancreatitis in dogs.[26] Increased activity was considered to be associated with emergency visits likely representing acute exacerbations but could not differentiate disease severity.

Serum trypsin-like immunoreactivity

Assays for serum trypsin-like immunoreactivity (TLI) are species-specific immunoassays that measure trypsinogen and trypsin in serum. The assay was originally developed to diagnose exocrine pancreatic insufficiency (EPI) in which it is expected to be low (see chapters 14 and 20 for more details). It would also be expected to be elevated in pancreatitis but the sensitivity of serum cTLI concentration for the diagnosis of canine acute pancreatitis is low (36-47%), probably due to its short half-life.[15] Also, although there was strong evidence that trypsinogen is exclusively of pancreatic origin, it is believed that there might be some extrapancreatic expression under certain conditions and also that TLI is cleared by glomerular filtration in dogs. Increased serum cTLI concentrations have been seen in dogs with renal failure and also in those with chronic enteropathies, limiting its usefulness for the diagnosis of pancreatitis.[15] Importantly, the measurement of serum TLI is the test of choice for the diagnosis of EPI. In cases of chronic pancreatitis, serum TLI may be used periodically to evaluate pancreatic function because it is expected to decline over time. Some animals with chronic pancreatitis will eventually develop EPI. Measuring serum TLI concentrations in dogs with chronic pancreatitis will help to monitor the functional decline of the pancreas and diagnose EPI early if it occurs. Having said this, patients that do not show weight loss and/or loose stools do not need to be tested as subclinical EPI does not require pancreatic enzyme replacement therapy (PERT). Finally, it has been suggested that low serum TLI concentrations may be masked by concurrent chronic inflammation (leading to an increase in serum TLI).

Nonspecific clinicopathologic abnormalities in chronic pancreatitis

Several nonspecific clinicopathological abnormalities might be present in dogs with chronic pancreatitis (please refer to chapter 13 for a more detailed discussion). However, for many of them, it is not known for sure if they are the result of chronic pancreatitis *per se* or concurrent diseases. One such abnormality that might be of importance is serum cobalamin. Some dogs with chronic pancreatitis have hypocobalaminemia and might benefit from cobalamin supplementation. The reason for this finding is not known and might be related to decreased pancreatic function and/or concurrent small intestinal disease. Also, dogs with autoimmune chronic pancreatitis often have proteinuria as part of a more generalized immune-mediated condition leading to glomerulonephritis. Therefore, measuring a urine protein:creatinine ratio is useful in dogs with chronic pancreatitis, especially in those predisposed to immune-mediated disease, such as English Cocker Spaniels. Kidney function might also be affected in some cases, so measuring serum creatinine and/or SDMA might be useful.

Diagnostic imaging

Diagnosis or exclusion of chronic pancreatitis is not possible based on abdominal imaging alone, but ultrasound can be of clinical utility. See chapter 15 for more details on pancreatic imaging.

Abdominal radiography

In the majority of dogs with chronic pancreatitis, abdominal radiographs are normal.[15]

Abdominal ultrasound

Abdominal ultrasound is considered the imaging modality of choice for the investigation of chronic pancreatitis in dogs.[15] Both the quality of ultrasound machines and the overall expertise of ultrasonographers have greatly advanced over the last two decades, and ultrasonography is now routinely used for the investigation of dogs suspected of having pancreatitis. However, abdominal ultrasonography is highly dependent on the skill and experience of the ultrasonographer, the level of suspicion for pancreatitis, and the equipment available. Importantly, diagnostic accuracy is dependent on the severity of the disease, with the sensitivity of ultrasound being higher with more severe disease, whereas chronic pancreatitis is often mild.

The vast majority of studies evaluating abdominal ultrasound for the diagnosis of pancreatitis have enrolled dogs with acute pancreatitis (or acute-on-chronic episodes). Less is known about ultrasonographic changes in dogs with chronic pancreatitis, and these are considered to be far less obvious than in those with acute disease. This is to be expected because ultrasound relies on edema, necrosis, and inflammation to produce tissue interfaces, and these lesions are not a main feature of chronic pancreatitis except in acute flare-ups. Therefore, it is important to note that a normal pancreas on ultrasound examination does not rule out chronic pancreatitis in dogs. The only finding in dogs with chronic pancreatitis that is recognized with some frequency is a mottled appearance of the pancreas with hyperechoic areas, representing pancreatic fibrosis. However, the frequency of this finding has not been systematically studied to date. The sensitivity of abdominal ultrasound for chronic pancreatitis (not during acute exacerbations) is considered low and was reported at 56% in one study when considering any abnormal finding on ultrasound (which would be expected to significantly reduce the specificity).[2]

It should also be noted that, at least in acute pancreatitis, there may be a delay in the appearance of imaging findings in comparison to the actual disease process, which means that repeat ultrasonography 24-48 hours after initial presentation is recommended.[27] This applies to chronic pancreatitis cases that present with an acute exacerbation of the disease, but it remains unknown whether this also applies to low-grade chronic disease. Also, there is currently no convincing evidence that repeated ultrasonography is useful for disease monitoring and response to treatment in dogs with chronic pancreatitis.

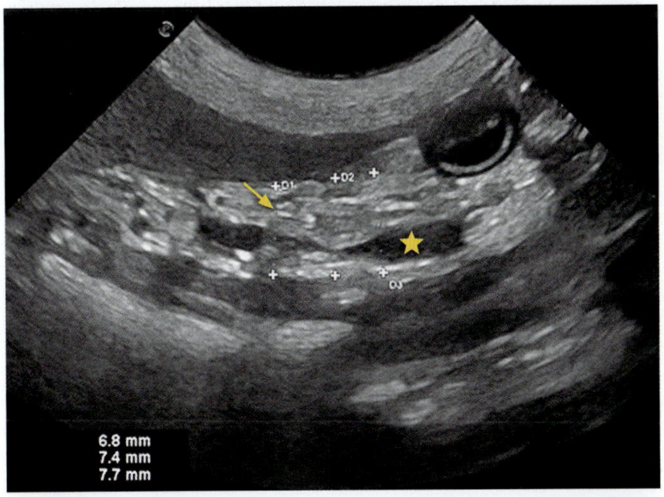

FIG. 19.2 Ultrasonographic image from a dog with chronic pancreatitis showing a diffuse increase in the echogenicity of the pancreas (arrow), which is believed to represent pancreatic fibrosis. Dilation of the pancreatic duct (star) is also evident. Courtesy of Dr. M. Barbagianni.

The most important ultrasonographic findings suggestive of pancreatitis in dogs with acute-on-chronic disease include hypoechoic areas within the pancreas, increased echogenicity of the surrounding mesentery (because of necrosis of the peripancreatic fat), and enlargement and/or irregularity of the pancreas (Fig. 19.2).[15]

Pathology

Histopathologic examination of pancreatic tissue is considered the gold standard for a definitive diagnosis of pancreatitis in dogs. However, pancreatic biopsies are not advised or taken in most clinical cases of chronic pancreatitis because of the associated morbidity, which is difficult to justify when the results may not change treatment or prognosis. As in human medicine, one justification for biopsy may be to rule out neoplasia if that is a concern. In addition, if the dog is already undergoing a laparotomy or laparoscopy for another reason, the clinician should remember to inspect the pancreas visually. Taking a small biopsy from the tip of a pancreatic limb is considered relatively safe but may not be representative of the disease (see below). More details on pancreatic biopsies are found in chapter 16. Histopathology is also the only way to differentiate acute from chronic disease definitively. The presence of permanent histopathologic changes (such as fibrosis and/or acinar atrophy) is considered suggestive of chronic pancreatitis. Acute pancreatitis is characterized by the absence of such permanent histopathologic changes. The predominant inflammatory cellular infiltrate (neutrophils and macrophages or lymphocytes and plasma cells) is often used to describe pancreatitis as suppurative or lymphocytic, respectively, and a significant degree of necrosis is usually used to characterize pancreatitis as necrotizing.

Certain gross pancreatic lesions identified during surgery, laparoscopy, or necropsy are highly suggestive of pancreatitis and are preferred sites for the collection of a tissue specimen. Gross pancreatic lesions suggestive of chronic pancreatitis are fibrosis, adhesions to adjacent tissues, including the small intestine, and, late in the disease process, a small pancreas, which may be difficult to find. However, gross pathologic lesions may not always be apparent in dogs with pancreatitis, and in some cases, they might be difficult to differentiate from nodular hyperplasia or neoplasia. In dogs with acute or chronic disease, findings may include peripancreatic fat necrosis, pancreatic hemorrhage or congestion, and a dull granular capsular surface (Fig. 19.3).

Several limitations are associated with pancreatic histopathology as a definitive diagnostic tool for pancreatitis. First, determining the clinical significance of histopathologic findings may be challenging, especially when the disease is mild, which, as noted, is common with chronic pancreatitis. At the same time, exclusion of pancreatitis based on histopathology is difficult because inflammatory lesions of the pancreas are often highly localized and can easily be missed. Therefore, multiple sections of the pancreas must be evaluated in order to increase the likelihood of finding microscopic lesions, although this is only feasible in postmortem sections.

Cytology

Fine-needle aspiration (FNA) of the pancreas, followed by cytological examination of the aspirated material, is a minimally invasive technique that can be used to help diagnose pancreatitis and differentiate pancreatic neoplasia. It should be performed either under ultrasonographic

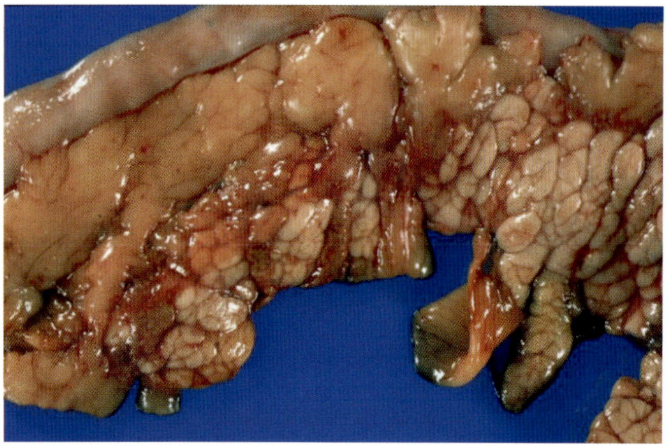

FIG. 19.3 Gross appearance of the pancreas postmortem from a dog with acute or chronic pancreatitis. Note the irregular appearance indicative of pancreatic fibrosis. There also appears to be edema and some bleeding, findings that are more commonly seen with acute or chronic disease. Courtesy of Dr. S. Newman.

guidance (in which case specimen collection is quite demanding) or during laparotomy.

In the only published study in dogs, ultrasound-guided pancreatic aspiration was described retrospectively in 92 dogs and was found safe. Aspirated material was reported to be diagnostic in 74% of the samples obtained.[28] In the same study, there was a 91% agreement with histopathology in the small number of dogs for which histopathology was also available. However, pancreatic cytology is expected to be less useful in dogs with chronic pancreatitis as fibrosis replaces acinar tissue and inflammation is more highly localized. Furthermore, fibrosis, a hallmark of chronic disease, cannot be determined based on the evaluation of cytology samples. Therefore, the authors do not currently recommend using pancreatic cytology to diagnose chronic pancreatitis in dogs.

Treatment of chronic pancreatitis

Treatment of the cause

The etiology of chronic pancreatitis remains unknown in the majority of cases in dogs, and therefore, a specific treatment is not possible in most of these cases. It is expected that better characterization of this disease in the future will allow for the development of new and specific treatments for different forms of pancreatitis that are currently being classified as idiopathic. Until then, the presence of possible risk factors should be investigated in all animals with chronic pancreatitis. If any of these factors are present, they should be removed or treated. Dogs should be investigated for the presence of factors such as hypertriglyceridemia, hypercalcemia, concurrent endocrine diseases, obesity, certain toxicities (e.g., zinc), evidence of certain infectious diseases (e.g., babesiosis), and inflammatory diseases of the intestine and the hepatobiliary system. Important information should be extracted from the medical history of the animal, including drugs administered (especially potassium bromide, phenobarbital, and azathioprine), diet offered (especially high-fat diets), and recent surgery or trauma. Concurrent diseases that may have an etiologic association with pancreatitis, such as IBD or diabetes mellitus, should also be investigated.

A subset of dogs with chronic pancreatitis may have immune-mediated disease. A condition similar to IgG4-related disease in humans has been described in English Cocker Spaniels. Diagnosis is difficult, but concurrent dry eye and proteinuria might increase the index of suspicion and support the use of immunosuppressives (see below).

Nutrition

The most important nutritional aspects in dogs with chronic pancreatitis include the type of diet and managing potential hyporexia or anorexia. The ideal type of diet in dogs with chronic pancreatitis is unknown but should be selected on the basis of concurrent diseases that need to be nutritionally managed (e.g., diabetes mellitus, chronic enteropathy, chronic kidney disease, etc). A low-fat diet in dogs has been traditionally recommended in acute and chronic pancreatitis cases. However, clear scientific evidence for such a recommendation is lacking, and this recommendation is mainly based on older studies that show that diets very high in fat content (>90 g/1000 Kcal) can cause pancreatitis. The same is true for humans, for whom low-fat diets were traditionally recommended but for whom evidence-based information is lacking. Low-fat diets are definitely indicated in dogs with hypertriglyceridemia, which has been shown to be a risk factor for pancreatitis in dogs. Despite the lack of compelling scientific evidence, the authors currently recommend feeding a low-fat diet (<25 g/1000 Kcal) in dogs with chronic pancreatitis unless other conditions necessitate a different nutritional approach. However, moderate-fat diets might be appropriate too. Limited evidence indicates that low-fat diets might help reduce abdominal pain in dogs with pancreatitis. Monitoring of clinical signs and serum Spec PL concentrations may help determine the response after a dietary change. Importantly, treats need to be considered, as well as the main diet, when assessing fat intake. More details on dietary management of chronic pancreatitis are found in chapter 22.

Finally, appetite stimulants might also be useful in dogs with chronic pancreatitis that are anorectic or hyporexic. Capromorelin is likely the most effective treatment option for dogs (3 mg/kg PO q24h), but this compound is currently not available in Europe. Mirtazapine (1.1-1.3 mg/kg PO q24h; not exceeding 30 mg/dog/day) is also a good option. Mirtazapine might also have antiemetic properties.

Analgesic therapy

Pain is believed to accompany virtually all cases of chronic and, even more commonly, acute-on-chronic pancreatitis in dogs, even when pain is not clinically apparent. Pain induces several physiologic responses, including a decrease in appetite, a decreased gastrointestinal tone, decreased regional blood flow to several abdominal organs (including the pancreas), tachycardia, and a catabolic state. Therefore, analgesic therapy is important, even in dogs with chronic pancreatitis. More details on analgesic therapy in pancreatitis are found in chapter 23.

Pain in dogs with chronic pancreatitis can range from mild to severe. In hospitalized patients, opioid administration (e.g., buprenorphine, fentanyl, hydromorphone) is often necessary for the management of pain in acute pancreatitis, and the intravenous route is usually preferred because it provides fast relief. Multimodal pain management might be indicated in some dogs with severe pain because it seems to be more effective and associated with fewer side effects due to lower doses of each of the drugs that are being administered. Lidocaine and ketamine are commonly used together with opioids.

In dogs with chronic pancreatitis that are not hospitalized, analgesic options are more limited. Tramadol can be used, but the evidence for efficacy in dogs is very limited (see chapter 23). Acetaminophen (see chapter 23 for dose recommendations) has been recommended by some, but the authors of this chapter do not recommend the use of acetaminophen for dogs or cats with chronic pancreatitis. Other drugs that target neurogenic pain, such as gabapentin, may also be tried. See chapter 23 for more details on these and adjunctive physical therapies for chronic pain. Maropitant, which targets substance P, might also have analgesic effects in chronic pancreatitis cases. Nonsteroidal anti-inflammatory drugs (NSAID) should ideally be avoided in chronic pancreatitis in dogs because of the potential to increase the risk of intestinal ulceration and also the high prevalence of concurrent renal disease in some breeds. However, in some countries, metamizole is a popular analgesic drug for canine and human patients with pancreatitis as it is not a traditional NSAID and has not been implicated in causing pancreatitis. Importantly, the use of metamizole is illegal in many countries, and the veterinarian should carefully check licensing in their jurisdiction.

Antiemetic therapy

Some dogs with chronic pancreatitis experience nausea and/or sporadic vomiting. Nausea is hard to detect in dogs and might be clinically evident as anorexia. Therefore, antiemetic therapy might be useful in dogs with chronic pancreatitis that have anorexia and/or show occasional vomiting. Maropitant (1-2 mg/kg, q24h, PO) is a very potent and safe antiemetic that is often used as a first-line antiemetic in dogs with pancreatitis. There is also evidence that maropitant has analgesic properties, making this drug very attractive for use in pancreatitis patients. Furthermore, recent evidence in experimental models of pancreatitis has suggested that maropitant may also have anti-inflammatory properties. Ondansetron (0.1-0.2 mg/kg, q12h, PO) is also a good option. Finally, mirtazapine, which is often used as an appetite stimulant, also has antiemetic properties.

Immunosuppressive drugs

Some chronic pancreatitis cases are believed to have an autoimmune component (such as has been reported in a small number of English Cocker Spaniels in the UK).[9,10] In these cases, immunosuppressive treatment would seem logical. However, there are no published clinical trials evaluating immunosuppressive treatment in dogs with chronic pancreatitis. In addition, it is currently impossible to know which animals have autoimmune chronic pancreatitis and would likely benefit from immunosuppressive treatment.

Glucocorticoids were once believed to cause pancreatitis in both humans and dogs. However, the scientific basis for this hypothesis is weak, and in humans, glucocorticoids are no longer considered a risk factor for pancreatitis and are, in fact, used to treat cases of autoimmune pancreatitis. Although prednisolone was recently reported to be beneficial in a retrospective study in dogs with acute pancreatitis,[29] studies in dogs with chronic pancreatitis are not available. However, prednisolone might be of benefit in dogs with suspected immune-mediated pancreatitis.

Cyclosporine might also be of benefit in chronic pancreatitis cases in which an autoimmune component is suspected, but controlled studies in dogs are lacking, and to date, only a single case report has been published in a dog with chronic pancreatitis with poorly controlled diabetes mellitus. In cats, a recent retrospective, uncontrolled study showed that cyclosporine treatment reduced supranormal serum Spec fPL concentrations in cats with presumed CP but did not affect the improvement of clinical signs.[30]

Anecdotally, treatment with glucocorticoids or cyclosporine has been used in some dogs with chronic pancreatitis that did not respond well to other treatments with mixed outcomes. Therefore, it might be recommended that if a dog with chronic pancreatitis does not respond well to other symptomatic treatments, prednisolone (2 mg/kg/day for up to 6 weeks, then tapering) or cyclosporine (5 mg/kg, q24h for 3-6 weeks, then tapering) may be trialed. During treatment, clinical signs and serum Spec cPL concentration should be closely monitored to check for potential improvement. If an improvement is evident, immunosuppressive treatment may continue at the lowest effective dose. If the dog has concurrent proteinuria (often recognized in affected English Cocker Spaniels), then this should also be monitored during treatment.

Much work needs to be done before immunosuppressive treatments can be recommended for routine use in dogs with chronic pancreatitis.

Pancreatic enzymes

There has been a suggestion in humans that pancreatic enzymes, when given at a high dose, improve pain associated with chronic pancreatitis. Several experimental and clinical studies tried to explain this observation, and this led to the negative feedback theory, based on which replacing endogenous secretion with exogenous pancreatic enzymes will reduce endogenous secretion in response to meals, blunt the increase in ductal and parenchymal pressure, and reduce pain. Several meta-analysis studies in humans generally conclude that the available studies do not support the hypothesis that pancreatic enzyme supplementation was useful for treating abdominal pain associated with chronic pancreatitis. Some studies may have shown some improvement in some markers of digestion, but in those studies, a large percentage of patients also had EPI in addition to chronic pancreatitis. Further studies using direct comparisons of different formulations and outcomes are needed to definitively show if there is any benefit in pancreatic enzyme administration in chronic pancreatitis in human patients.

There are no studies on the use of pancreatic enzymes in dogs with chronic pancreatitis. Some clinicians have used pancreatic enzymes in such cases, but, to the authors' knowledge, there has never been any suggested benefit in dogs except for the treatment of EPI in end-stage disease. Therefore, until further evidence is available, the authors currently do not recommend the use of pancreatic enzyme treatment in dogs with chronic pancreatitis unless they have progressed to clinical EPI.

Complications of chronic pancreatitis

Diabetes mellitus

Extension of inflammation from the exocrine to the endocrine portion of the pancreas can lead to progressive destruction of the islets of Langerhans, impaired β-cell function, and, subsequently, diabetes mellitus. Chronic pancreatitis is a well-known cause of diabetes mellitus in humans, and this relationship has also been suggested in dogs.[2,15] Insulin therapy is necessary in cases of chronic pancreatitis complicated by diabetes mellitus, and good glycemic control may be difficult to achieve in these animals as long as pancreatic inflammation is present.

Exocrine pancreatic insufficiency

Chronic pancreatitis is a well-recognized and common cause of EPI in humans and is believed to be responsible for approximately half of

EPI cases in dogs. In another small study, 5 of 14 dogs with chronic pancreatitis also had EPI, suggesting that chronic pancreatitis is a common cause of EPI in dogs.[2] Thus, EPI must be considered a potential long-term complication of chronic pancreatitis in dogs. In some animals, chronic pancreatitis may result in EPI and diabetes mellitus, and animals with both of these conditions are more likely to have chronic pancreatitis as the underlying cause.

Pancreatic complications

Pancreatic fluid accumulations have been infrequently reported in dogs with chronic pancreatitis. Clinical signs of pancreatic complications do not differ from those of pancreatitis and may persist despite treatment of pancreatitis. Ultrasonography and ultrasound-guided fine-needle aspiration can be very useful for diagnosing, differentiating, and managing pancreatic complications. However, differentiation of a pancreatic mass effect due to pancreatitis from one due to a pancreatic complication can be difficult. Histopathology may be required for definitive diagnosis and differentiation of pancreatic complications in some cases, and this would be a justification for pancreatic biopsy. Surgical treatment might be indicated in some cases to resolve large pancreatic abscesses or remove necrotic masses.

Pancreatic cancer

It has been suggested that humans with chronic pancreatitis may be at increased risk for the development of pancreatic cancer. However, such a relationship has not yet been described for dogs. Furthermore, pancreatic adenocarcinoma is rather rare in dogs (see chapter 21 for more details of pancreatic neoplasia).

KEY POINTS

- Chronic pancreatitis is more common than acute pancreatitis, although less frequently diagnosed.
- The etiology of chronic pancreatitis is not fully understood, although several causes have been proposed.
- Histopathology is currently the gold standard for the diagnosis of chronic pancreatitis but is rarely performed antemortem.
- Several laboratory tests have been developed to aid in the diagnosis of chronic pancreatitis, like pancreatic lipase immunoreactivity (PLI), serum amylase and lipase activities, and serum trypsin-like immunoreactivity (TLI).
- Diagnostic imaging techniques and fine-needle aspiration also help in the diagnosis of chronic pancreatitis.
- The treatment of chronic pancreatitis comprises treating the inciting cause, plus analgesic and antiemetic therapy, immunosuppressive drugs, and supplementation with pancreatic enzymes, as needed.

References

1. Xenoulis PG, Suchodolski JS, Steiner JM. Chronic pancreatitis in dogs and cats. *Compend Contin Educ Vet* 30(3):166-180, 2008.
2. Watson PJ, Archer J, Roulois AJ, et al. Observational study of 14 cases of chronic pancreatitis in dogs. *Vet Rec* 167(25):968-976, 2010.
3. Newman SJ, Steiner JM, Woosley K, et al. Localization of pancreatic inflammation and necrosis in dogs. *J Vet Intern Med* 8(4):488-493, 2004.
4. Newman SJ, Steiner JM, Woosley K, et al. Histologic assessment and grading of the exocrine pancreas in the dog. *J Vet Diagn Invest* 18(1):115-118, 2006.
5. Watson PJ, Roulois AJ, Scase TJ, et al. Prevalence and breed distribution of chronic pancreatitis at post-mortem examination in first-opinion dogs. *J Small Anim Pract* 48(11): 609-618, 2007.
6. Lem KY, Fosgate GT, Norby B, et al. Evaluation of associations between dietary factors and spontaneous pancreatitis in dogs. *J Am Vet Med Assoc* 233(9):1425-1431, 2008.
7. Bishop MA, Xenoulis PG, Steiner JM. Association between this SPINK1 variant and clinically detectable pancreatitis. *J Vet Intern Med* 27(3):427-428, 2013.
8. Furrow E, Armstrong PJ, Patterson EE. High prevalence of the c.74A>C SPINK1 variant in miniature and standard Schnauzers. *J Vet Intern Med* 26(6):1295-1299, 2012.
9. Watson PJ, Roulois AJ, Scase TJ, et al. Characterization of chronic pancreatitis in English Cocker Spaniels. *J Vet Intern Med* 25(4):797-804, 2011.
10. Coddou MF, Constantino-Casas F, Scase TJ, et al. Chronic inflammatory disease in the pancreas, kidneys, and salivary glands of English Cocker Spaniels and dogs of other breeds shows similar histological features to human IgG4-related disease. *J Comp Pathol* 177:18-33, 2020.
11. Xenoulis PG, Suchodolski JS, Ruaux CG, et al. Association between serum triglyceride and canine pancreatic lipase immunoreactivity concentrations in miniature schnauzers. *J Am Anim Hosp Assoc* 46(4):229-234, 2010.
12. Xenoulis PG, Levinski MD, Suchodolski JS, et al. Association of insulin resistance with hypertriglyceridemia in healthy Miniature Schnauzers. *J Am Vet Med Assoc* 238(8):1011-1016, 2011.
13. Bostrom BM, Xenoulis PG, Newman SJ, et al. Chronic pancreatitis in dogs: a retrospective study of clinical, clinicopathological, and histopathological findings in 61 cases. *Vet J* 195(1):73-79, 2013.
14. Steiner JM, Teague SR, Williams DA. Development and analytic validation of an enzyme-linked immunosorbent assay for the measurement of canine pancreatic lipase immunoreactivity in serum. *Can J Vet Res* 67(3):175-182, 2003.

15. Xenoulis PG. Diagnosis of pancreatitis in dogs and cats. *J Small Anim Pract* 56(1):13-26, 2015.
16. Huth SP, Relford RL, Steiner JM, et al. Analytical validation of an ELISA for measurement of canine pancreas-specific lipase. *Vet Clin Pathol* 39(3):346-353, 2010.
17. McCord K, Morley PS, Armstrong J, et al. A multi-institutional study evaluating the diagnostic utility of the spec cPL and SNAP(R) cPL in clinical acute pancreatitis in 84 dogs. *J Vet Intern Med* 26(4):888-896, 2012.
18. Steiner JM, Newman SJ, Xenoulis PG, et al. Sensitivity of serum markers for pancreatitis in dogs with macroscopic evidence of pancreatitis. *Vet Ther* 9(4):263-273, 2008.
19. Trivedi SR, Marks SL, Kass PH, et al. Sensitivity and specificity of canine pancreas-specific lipase (cPL) and other markers for pancreatitis in 70 dogs with and without histopathologic evidence of pancreatitis. *J Vet Intern Med* 25(6):1241-1247, 2011.
20. Aupperle-Lellbach H, Torner K, Staudacher M, et al. Histopathological findings and canine pancreatic lipase immunoreactivity in normal dogs and dogs with inflammatory and neoplastic diseases of the pancreas. *J Vet Intern Med* 34(3):1127-1134, 2020.
21. Beall MJ, Cahill R, Pigeon KE, et al. Performance validation and method comparison of an in-clinic enzyme-linked immunosorbent assay for the detection of canine pancreatic lipase. *J Vet Diagn Invest* 23(1):115-119, 2011.
22. Kook PH, Kohler N, Hartnack S, et al. Agreement of serum Spec cPL with the 1,2-o-dilauryl-rac-glycero glutaric acid-(6'-methylresorufin) ester (DGGR) lipase assay and with pancreatic ultrasonography in dogs with suspected pancreatitis. *J Vet Intern Med* 28:863-870, 2014.
23. Lim SY, Xenoulis PG, Stavroulaki EM, et al. The 1,2-o-dilauryl-rac-glycero-3-glutaric acid-(6'-methylresorufin) ester (DGGR) lipase assay in cats and dogs is not specific for pancreatic lipase. *Vet Clin Pathol* 49(4):607-613, 2020.
24. Graca R, Messick JB, McCullough S, et al. Validation and diagnostic efficacy of a lipase assay using the substrate 1,2-0-dilauryl-rac-glycero glutaric acid-(6' methyl resorufin)-ester for the diagnosis of acute pancreatitis in dogs. *Vet Clin Pathol* 34(1):39-43, 2005.
25. Hope A, Bailen EL, Shiel RE, et al. Retrospective study evaluation of DGGR lipase for diagnosis, agreement with pancreatic lipase and prognosis in dogs with suspected acute pancreatitis. *J Small Anim Pract* 62(12):1092-1100, 2021.
26. Kuzi S, Adlersberg D, Aroch I, et al. Utility of 1,2-o-dilauryl-rac-glycero glutaric acid-(6'-methylresorufin)-ester-lipase for monitoring dogs with chronic pancreatitis. *J Vet Intern Med* 37(2):437-445, 2023.
27. Puccini Leoni F, Pelligra T, Citi S, et al. Ultrasonographic monitoring in 38 dogs with clinically suspected acute pancreatitis. *Vet Sci* 7(4):180, 2020.
28. Cordner AP, Sharkey LC, Armstrong PJ, et al. Cytologic findings and diagnostic yield in 92 dogs undergoing fine-needle aspiration of the pancreas. *J Vet Diagn Invest* 27(2):236-240, 2015.
29. Okanishi H, Nagata T, Nakane S, et al. Comparison of initial treatment with and without corticosteroids for suspected acute pancreatitis in dogs. *J Small Anim Pract* 60(5): 298-304, 2019.
30. Hoeyrup N, Spillmann T, Toresson L. Cyclosporine treatment in cats with presumed chronic pancreatitis –A retrospective study. *Animals (Basel)* 11(10):2993, 2021

CHAPTER 20

Exocrine pancreatic insufficiency

Daniel Batchelor
BVSc, PhD, DSAM, DECVIM-CA, SFHEA, MRCVS

Disease definition/etiology

Exocrine pancreatic insufficiency (EPI) is present when the production of digestive enzymes from the pancreas is inadequate, leading to maldigestion and associated characteristic clinical signs. The pancreas has a large reserve capacity, and clinical signs of maldigestion are typically present when an estimated 90% or more of pancreatic function has been lost.

EPI is an important disorder in canine gastroenterology because it requires specific management (enzyme supplementation), without which clinical signs will persist regardless of other empirical treatments or well-designed therapeutic trials. Therefore, understanding the etiology and diagnosis of EPI in dogs is important for veterinarians. EPI should be considered and excluded early in the investigation when dogs are presented with weight loss or chronic/recurrent gastrointestinal signs.

EPI can be caused by several disease processes, including pancreatic acinar atrophy and chronic pancreatitis, which are prevalent in some breeds and potentially under-recognized. German Shepherd dogs (GSD), Rough Collies, Cavalier King Charles Spaniels (CKCS), and Chow Chows are predisposed to developing EPI, but it can be seen in numerous other breeds. In the United Kingdom, 60% of dogs with EPI are GSD. Conversely, some breeds seem rarely to develop EPI: Boxers, Golden Retrievers, Labradors, Rottweilers, and Weimaraners are underrepresented in the population of dogs with EPI and may be in some way protected from it. There is a reported female predisposition in EPI, although the reason for this is not known.

Pancreatic acinar atrophy

Pancreatic acinar atrophy (PAA) is almost always the reason for EPI when diagnosed in GSD or Rough Collies. In PAA, selective destruction of acinar cells, which produce the digestive enzymes, occurs. Islet cells are spared, and endocrine function is normal. Bicarbonate production by the pancreas is also normal.

Although it occurs in young dogs, PAA is not a congenital disease but an acquired one: affected dogs are born with a histologically normal pancreas and develop PAA and EPI later, typically showing signs between 1-4 years of age. It is most likely an autoimmune disease, evidenced by genetic susceptibility to disease and compatible findings on histopathology during the progression from normal to end-stage, including a gradual loss of acinar structure associated with lymphocytic inflammation (Figs. 20.1 and 20.2).[1] However, immunosuppression does not seem to prevent the development of EPI in susceptible dogs.[2] Dogs begin to show signs when the destruction of acinar tissue has progressed to the late stage, when the pancreas is grossly abnormal, appearing thin and transparent, with prominent ductal structures. On histology, acinar tissue is either absent or much reduced (sometimes replaced by adipose tissue), ducts are prominent, there is no fibrosis, and the endocrine tissue is well preserved.[3] The progression from subclinical lymphocytic inflammation to the clinical phase of PAA appears to be highly variable and unpredictable, and it remains unknown which factors affect progression. Dogs can, in fact, remain in the subclinical phase for years or even lifelong.[2]

PAA has been shown to be hereditary in GSD, Rough Collies, and Eurasian dogs, and inheritance likely involves several genes. Pedigree analysis suggests an autosomal recessive mode of inheritance, but a test mating showed that PAA is not a monogenic disease: this test mating between two affected GSD produced six puppies, of which only two became affected, with the other four never developing EPI before dying of unrelated causes, aged 8-13 years, each with a normal pancreas on necropsy.[4] Subsequent investigations, including linkage studies and genome-wide association studies, have confirmed that EPI is a genetically complex disorder in GSD.[5] We know that alleles of the major histocompatibility complex are involved in at least two breeds, GSD and Pembroke Welsh Corgis,[6,7] but it is unknown whether there are different genetic causes in different families, multiple genetic variants that interact, or both genetic and environmental influences on the expression of the disease.

Chronic pancreatitis

Chronic pancreatitis (CP) can lead to EPI because of progressive destruction of glandular tissue.[8,9] Based on postmortem studies, the prevalence of CP is very high in dogs, present in around 34% of cadavers,[10] and although

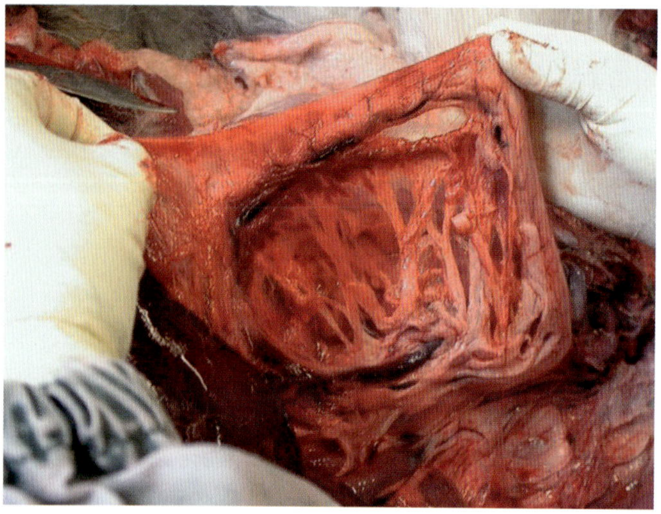

FIG. 20.1 Gross postmortem image of a German Shepherd dog with pancreatic acinar atrophy. Note marked atrophy of the pancreas in comparison with fig. 20.2. (Picture published with permission from the Department of Pathology, Queen's Veterinary School Hospital, University of Cambridge).

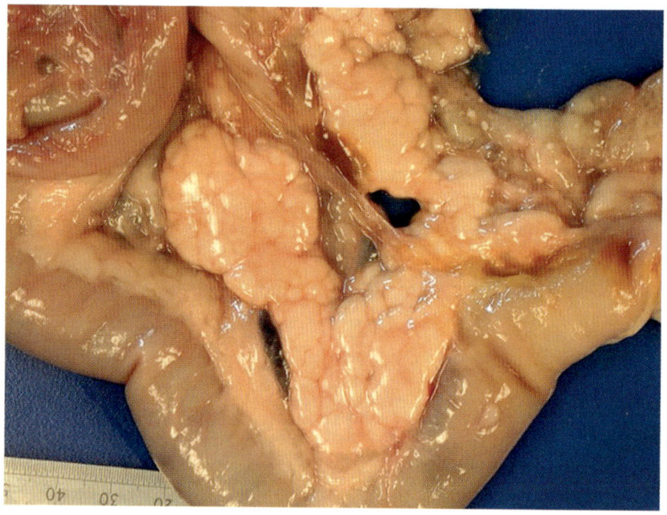

FIG. 20.2 For comparison with fig. 20.1, gross postmortem from a Cavalier King Charles Spaniel with pancreatitis but with normal pancreatic mass and exocrine function. Note the large amount of pancreatic tissue adjacent to the duodenum. (Picture published with permission from the Department of Pathology, Queen's Veterinary School Hospital, University of Cambridge).

diagnosis can be challenging, CP is now increasingly recognized antemortem. In CP, the pancreas is usually firm, nodular, and reduced in size and may be adhered to adjacent structures. On histopathology, the hallmark findings are fibrosis and a lymphocytic or lymphoplasmacytic inflammatory infiltrate with disorganized acini.[1,11]

CP can occur in any breed, but CKCS, English Cocker Spaniels, Boxers, and Collies have been shown to be at increased risk among dogs in the United Kingdom,[9,10] and in the USA, dogs with CP were more likely to be pure-bred, particularly those classified by the American Kennel Club as toy and nonsporting breeds.[12] Of these breeds, CKCS are known to be predisposed to EPI,[13] so presumably the cause of EPI in CKCS is CP (Fig. 20.3). This is in keeping with the higher median age at diagnosis of EPI in CKCS (6 years) than in GSD and Rough Collies, in which the presumed etiology is PAA (3 years). Pathogenesis of CP, including the degree of fibrosis and regeneration of damaged tissue, is probably different in different breeds, and this may be the reason why CP appears to be associated with EPI in CKCS but not in Boxers.

In contrast to PAA, endocrine tissue is typically also damaged in CP, so dogs with EPI caused by CP often develop diabetes mellitus (or at least are at risk for developing it). Because of the large reserve capacity of the pancreas, diabetes mellitus and EPI only occur when functional mass of the pancreas is drastically reduced. Whether EPI or diabetes mellitus develops first seems to vary; either may occur first, with the other often developing within the following year. Breed differences in the ability to regenerate tissue are again likely present, with Boxers being a good example: Boxers have a reduced risk of diabetes mellitus, as well as their reduced risk of EPI, despite their predisposition to CP.[14]

CP should be suspected if EPI is diagnosed in an older dog that is not a Rough Collie or GSD or if EPI and diabetes mellitus are both diagnosed in the same animal. Awareness of the possible presence of CP as a cause of diabetes mellitus or EPI in a dog is important because the clinical signs of polyphagia and weight loss are common to both; if a diabetic dog continues to lose weight despite adequate glycemic control, EPI should be considered.

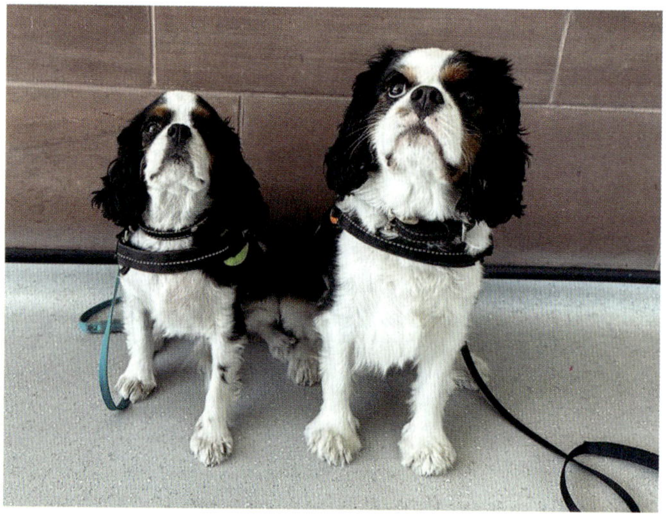

FIG. 20.3 The dog on the left is a 2 ½-year-old Cavalier King Charles Spaniel with EPI, as well as juvenile hypothyroidism. The other dog is his unaffected littermate. Signs had been going on for several months before diagnosis, highlighting the importance of maintaining an index of suspicion for EPI in dogs with compatible signs. In the absence of a biopsy, the reason for EPI is unknown in this dog. This breed is predisposed to both chronic pancreatitis and EPI, although dogs with chronic pancreatitis are typically older than this at the onset of EPI. (Photo courtesy of James Barton).

Other causes of EPI

Pancreatic hypoplasia/juvenile pancreatic atrophy

Case reports exist of very young dogs (up to 6 months of age) diagnosed with EPI and often concurrent diabetes mellitus.[15-18] On biopsy or necropsy, investigators have typically found a pancreas markedly smaller than normal, with atrophic acinar tissue and reduced number and size of islets in those dogs with endocrine dysfunction. This pancreatic hypoplasia has been reported in various breeds, including a series of Greyhounds with EPI and diabetes mellitus in which the median age at diagnosis was 12 weeks.[17]

Congenital isolated lipase deficiency

Cases are reported of young dogs with signs of EPI but normal serum trypsin-like immunoreactivity.[19,20] When measured, pancreatic lipase immunoreactivity was low or low-normal, and dogs responded well to pancreatic enzyme supplementation. A congenital defect in pancreatic lipase production leading to EPI is suspected in these dogs. This condition is distinct from PAA, but some of the reported dogs were GSD or Rough Collies, so isolated lipase deficiency may be over-represented in breeds predisposed to EPI.

Other

EPI can, in principle, be caused by pancreatic neoplasia, although the incidence of this is unknown and probably rare. Experimentally, ligation of the pancreatic duct will lead to the syndrome of EPI, so pathological causes of pancreatic duct obstruction such as a stricture or tumor could cause EPI.

Clinical presentation/features

Typical clinical signs of EPI are consistent with malabsorption and include increased appetite, weight loss, and increased fecal volume with poorly digested, loose, pulpy, or greasy feces. Watery diarrhea is not typical. Dogs may be coprophagic. Nervousness and aggression have been reported and are hypothesized to be associated with abdominal discomfort, although a breed effect cannot be excluded. In retrospective studies,[21,22] loose stools were present in the vast majority (95-96%) of dogs with EPI. Classical signs were not always present: polyphagia was present in only about half of dogs, and some were inappetent. Vomiting was present in 11-24%. Most dogs (84-87%) were underweight at diagnosis. CP is a potentially under-recognized cause of EPI. Signs that could alert the veterinarian to the presence of CP can include an older dog presenting with low-grade intermittent gastrointestinal signs (typically anorexia, vomiting, and diarrhea, which may be large bowel in character with blood and mucus). Some dogs may instead show intermittent anorexia and abdominal pain (e.g., stretching, adopting the prayer position, or apparent back pain), more typical of pancreatitis (see chapters 18 and 19).[11] Because EPI only develops when around 90% of functional pancreatic tissue has been destroyed, these signs may occur for months or years before the onset of EPI. It is also possible that signs could be relatively mild and either missed or not considered important, and EPI may already have developed by the time CP is recognized. CP, and therefore actual or imminent EPI, should be suspected when diabetes mellitus is diagnosed in an older dog of a predisposed breed such as a CKCS or an English Cocker Spaniel. If concurrent EPI and diabetes mellitus are diagnosed in an older dog, CP is likely.

Clinicopathological findings

EPI is diagnosed by recognizing signs of maldigestion and malabsorption, or signs compatible with CP (see above), and confirmed by a pancreatic function test, most commonly the serum trypsin-like immunoreactivity (TLI) assay.

Routine screening

Hematology is usually normal in EPI, although lymphopenia and eosinophilia have been reported. On serum biochemistry, no specific changes are found; mild increases in alanine aminotransferase (ALT) activity may be seen (reflecting a reactive hepatopathy), and serum cholesterol concentration is sometimes reduced. Serum lipase concentration can be increased in dogs with CP, but serum amylase or lipase concentrations are not useful for diagnosing EPI.

Pancreatic function tests

Trypsin-like immunoreactivity

Serum TLI is the most commonly used pancreatic function test. It is well-established, comparatively inexpensive, unaffected by concurrent intestinal disease, and simple to perform. The reference interval is typically 5-40 µg/L, with an abnormally low value of <2.5 µg/L considered highly diagnostic for EPI in the presence of compatible clinical signs. The published sensitivity and specificity for the test are both 100%.[23] The low serum concentration correlates with the dramatic loss of enzyme-producing acinar cells in PAA (see chapter 14 for more details). Clinical signs of EPI are not seen in dogs with PAA and serum TLI in the "gray zone" between 2.5 and 5 µg/L, and treatment with pancreatic enzymes is not needed. Another cause for gastrointestinal signs should be suspected in these dogs, and many have normal TLI on repeat testing. Recently, it has been suggested that there has been a shift in the assay and dogs with a cTLI up to 10 µg/L could have clinical EPI. Readers should be alert to changes in their laboratory ranges and, if in doubt, trial pancreatic enzymes.

The TLI test performs extremely well in the context of EPI caused by PAA and deserves its status as an often-cited example of a highly sensitive and specific test in small animal practice. Things become more difficult in the context of EPI caused by CP, where concurrent pancreatic inflammation can increase serum TLI into the normal range or even above.[8,9,24] Where CP is suspected to be the underlying cause of EPI (e.g., older dog, non-GSD, non-Rough Collie), blood sampling to establish the presence of EPI by TLI assay should be done when the dog has shown no gastrointestinal signs for at least 7 days, and may need to be performed more than once.[11] In dogs with CP, it is not possible to definitively exclude EPI using serum tests, so if a dog with CP begins to lose weight, a treatment trial with pancreatic enzymes is recommended, even if serum TLI is repeatedly normal.

Other pancreatic function tests

Because of the advantages of the TLI assay, other function tests are rarely performed and are not recommended. Measurement of fecal proteolytic activity can be unreliable and false positives can occur. More recently, a fecal elastase assay was developed, but this test is associated with an unacceptable number of false positives.[25] Serum pancreatic lipase immunoreactivity (PLI) is not recommended as a test for EPI.[26]

Cobalamin measurement

Measurement of serum cobalamin is recommended in all dogs with EPI: hypocobalaminemia is very prevalent in dogs with EPI (affecting >80% of dogs in some studies). This is not surprising, considering the important role of pancreatic intrinsic factor in cobalamin absorption and the probable severe reduction in intrinsic factor in dogs with EPI. If serum cobalamin is adequate at the time of diagnosis, it should be monitored every 6 months in case deficiency develops later.

Diagnosis of subclinical EPI

PAA can be diagnosed in the subclinical phase before the destruction of acinar tissue is extensive enough to lead to clinical signs. In one study, dogs with a serum TLI concentration in the range between 2.5 and 5 µg/L, which is a subnormal result but above the accepted cutoff for a diagnosis of EPI, were followed with repeat measurement of serum TLI.[27] These dogs did not have clinical signs suggestive of EPI when first seen. On repeat testing, TLI returned to normal in about half of the dogs. In the other half, TLI remained <5 µg/L, usually remaining above 2.5 µg/L, although a few progressed to clinical EPI. Some dogs underwent pancreatic biopsy, and all of these had partial PAA.

Therefore, a single measurement of TLI in the range of 2.5-5 µg/L in a dog without clinical signs of EPI has questionable value, but repeated measurements in this range are suggestive of subclinical EPI and partial PAA. These dogs should be monitored, but the progression of PAA varies widely, and the subclinical phase may last for years –the dog may in fact die of another cause without ever developing EPI.[2]

Diagnostic imaging findings

Diagnostic imaging is not mandatory for the diagnosis of EPI as the diagnosis can be confirmed by pancreatic function testing on a serum sample. However, ultrasonographic reference values for pancreas size have been established.[28] In a retrospective study of 34 dogs with clinical or subclinical EPI, the mean pancreatic thickness was lower than these reference values, but the pancreas was otherwise ultrasonographically normal in two-thirds of the dogs.[29] Abnormal ultrasound appearance of the intestine (dilation of intestinal loops, liquid intestinal content, reduced peristalsis, and hyperechogenicity of the mucosa) was found in 85% of dogs with EPI, showing that these findings should not be misinterpreted as a primary intestinal disease. Whether these abnormalities resolve after treatment for EPI remains to be investigated.

Ultrasound is frequently used in the investigation of CP but has low sensitivity for detecting the low-grade inflammation and fibrosis characteristically present in CP.

Other diagnostic procedures

Biopsy

A pancreas biopsy would be required if a definitive diagnosis of the underlying reason for EPI were desired, but this invasive procedure does not change the treatment, so it is usually not recommended. If the affected dog is a GSD or Rough Collie, PAA is highly likely, and a pancreatic biopsy cannot be justified. In a dog with suspected end-stage chronic pancreatitis, obtaining a histological diagnosis is also very unlikely to change the treatment, which is symptomatic and described below. Confirmation of disease, if wanted, can be obtained postmortem when the dog dies. A biopsy might be justified if neoplasia is suspected as the underlying cause of EPI (which is unusual), and it can be performed carefully via celiotomy or laparoscopy (see chapter 16), but it must be remembered that pancreatic lesions can be unevenly distributed, so results can vary, depending on which part of the pancreas was sampled.

The procedure is relatively safe as long as tissue handling is gentle and careful dissection of the sample is done. In practice, a pancreatic biopsy is rarely performed because the procedure is quite invasive, and the results would not alter management in most cases.

Genetic testing

Although progress has been made in determining the genetic basis of EPI in dogs, its inheritance is complex, and no genetic test is available.

Treatment

Pancreatic enzyme supplementation

The most important aspect of the management of EPI is the provision of pancreatic enzymes with every meal. Suitable options include enteric-coated enzyme preparations, uncoated enzyme powder, or raw pancreas. Raw pancreas, usually porcine or bovine in origin, can be sourced from abattoirs in some countries and stored frozen for several months before feeding. Owner education is important to ensure correct dosing: enzymes must be present with all food given, or the dog will be unable to digest that food. Manufacturers' instructions must also be followed: for example, some capsulated enzymes must be emptied out of the capsule onto the food, and owners do not always realize this.

Choosing an enteric-coated product is rational, as degradation by gastric acid is likely to reduce enzyme efficacy, especially lipase, but the literature does not strongly support using one enzyme product over another. In a controlled study, dogs with EPI received either an enteric-coated enzyme product or an identical preparation without the enteric coating.[30] Clinical disease severity scores decreased in both groups, with no difference noted between groups. Body weight increased in both groups, but dogs gained weight more quickly on the enteric-coated preparation. This suggests a possible benefit of using an enteric-coated product. However, the control uncoated enzyme preparation used in this study is not a commercially available product. In another study, dogs with EPI received either powdered enzymes or raw chopped pancreas.[31] No difference between groups was found. In a more recent clinical trial with a crossover design, dogs received either a novel microencapsulated enteric-coated enzyme product or a commercially available uncoated product.[32] Differences between groups were not detected, although the study had low power. In conclusion, the optimal enzyme product has not been determined, and good results can be obtained with any available high-quality source of active enzymes. An enteric-coated product might be slightly preferred, but in practice, the choice of enzyme preparation is usually decided by availability, practicality, and cost. However, commercial enzyme products are classed as nutraceuticals rather than drugs, and producers are therefore not compelled to prove efficacy. Switching to a different enzyme preparation is recommended if a dog responds poorly to a chosen product.

Even with supplementation, digestion does not return to normal in dogs with EPI. The dose of enzyme needed to control signs frequently increases over time, and the dose may need to be higher than the label dose. This can sometimes be an unacceptable financial burden to owners, with the cost of treatment a common reason for euthanasia in dogs with EPI. The mean amount of raw pancreas fed in one study was 87 g/meal.[31] Attempts have been made to improve the efficacy of oral pancreatic enzymes by using acid-blocking drugs. These are of no known benefit and are not recommended.

Enzyme therapy is generally safe, although high doses of powdered enzyme have been associated with gingival bleeding, presumably a local effect: this is usually successfully managed by reducing the dose or changing the product used.[33]

Diet

Feeding a high-quality, digestible diet with moderate fat content is probably a suitable starting point for most dogs with EPI caused by PAA. Historically, low-fat diets have been recommended, as fat digestion is difficult to normalize with oral enzymes, but feeding higher fat to dogs with EPI can improve weight gain and fecal quality.[34] Humans with EPI due to end-stage chronic pancreatitis are encouraged to eat more fat rather than less to improve their weight gain; in fact, low-fat diets are used only as a last resort in humans with EPI.

Prospective studies have often only been small studies from which it is difficult to draw firm conclusions, but to date no single dietary strategy seems to show a clear benefit over any other.[35,36] Similarly, in retrospective studies, no clear benefit of fat restriction or fat supplementation has been demonstrated, and the ideal diet seems to vary widely between individuals.[21,22] In practice, an empirical approach is recommended, monitoring response and altering dietary strategy accordingly to find the diet that suits that individual best. In dogs with CP, a fat-restricted diet likely becomes more important (see below).

Cobalamin

Hypocobalaminemia is common in dogs with EPI and is associated with a poorer prognosis.[21,22] Cobalamin is a cofactor for nucleic acid synthesis and, therefore, essential for normal cell turnover, especially in rapidly dividing cells, such as enterocytes. Therefore, measurement of cobalamin is important in all dogs diagnosed with EPI, and correction of deficiency using either oral or injectable cobalamin supplementation is recommended. Oral supplementation is now preferred: it is very effective,[37] and as well as being more convenient, a clinical trial showed that oral cobalamin supplementation appeared to be more effective than injectable, leading to a decrease in serum methylmalonic acid whereas injectable cobalamin did not.[38] The recommended oral cobalamin dose is 0.25 mg once daily (0.5 mg every other day works just as well) for dogs <10 kg, 0.5 mg once daily for dogs 10-20 kg, and 1 mg once daily for dogs >20 kg. Treatment is usually required lifelong, and supplementation is considered adequate if serum cobalamin is >400 ng/L.

Managing EPI caused by chronic pancreatitis

In dogs with EPI caused by CP, considerations for enzyme and cobalamin replacement are the same as for PAA. In CP, fat-restricted diets may be beneficial in reducing postprandial pain associated with recurrent bouts of pancreatitis. It is unpredictable in dogs (and humans) with EPI due to chronic pancreatitis whether the bouts of pancreatitis will continue or eventually stop due to loss of tissue mass. In those with recurrent bouts, additional analgesia should be provided, typically paracetamol, although opioids or gabapentin can be used as needed (see chapter 23 for more details of analgesia in acute and chronic pancreatitis). Dogs with CP, EPI, and diabetes mellitus (end-stage pancreas) should have their diabetes managed as normal and do not seem to be any more difficult to manage than other dogs with diabetes mellitus, nor have a worse prognosis. However, insulin requirements may increase after starting oral enzymes.

Antibiotics

Antibiotics have previously sometimes been recommended as part of the management of EPI in dogs, usually oxytetracycline, metronidazole, or tylosin. The theory is that the presence of undigested food particles in EPI, coupled with a relative absence of bacteriostatic substances in pancreatic juice, can predispose dogs to small intestinal bacterial overgrowth. However, evidence exists that enzyme replacement alone can reduce bacterial numbers in the small intestine[39,40] and antibiotics do not seem to positively influence the treatment response in EPI.[21,22] In the era of antimicrobial stewardship, antibiotics are not recommended as routine therapy in EPI.

Treatment of subclinical EPI

Supplementation of enzymes is not required when clinical signs are absent. Attempts to prevent the autoimmune destruction of acinar tissue using azathioprine did not show any clear benefit.[2] Therefore, the use of immunosuppressive treatment to prevent progressive pancreatic destruction in PAA is not recommended. In any case, dogs with subclinical EPI may not progress to clinical EPI during their lifetime.

In dogs with CP, diagnosis of EPI is more difficult, as mentioned earlier. In dogs with CP, it is recommended that the veterinarian should encourage the owner to monitor for subtle clinical signs of EPI and should be proactive in supplementing enzymes if signs of EPI occur (e.g., weight loss, increased appetite).

Prognosis

Prognosis is cautiously optimistic in EPI, with most dogs responding favorably to enzyme supplementation (although not all do). For dogs that do respond, a long period of successful remission is expected, with most dogs ultimately dying of old age or other diseases.

Initial response

It appears from several studies that around 60% of dogs will respond well, with a further 20% having a partial response.[21,22,31,41] Unfortunately, around 20% of dogs show a poor response. The reasons for this treatment failure in some dogs are unknown.

Long-term survival

Around 20-25% of dogs are euthanized within the first year of treatment, either because of a poor response to enzyme supplementation or the significant cost of ongoing treatment. However, prolonged survival is expected for dogs that respond well: the median survival time is ~5 years in published studies.[21,22]

Predictors of survival

Severe hypocobalaminemia is consistently associated with a worse prognosis. In one study, dogs were more likely to be euthanized if they were male, or were inappetent at the time of diagnosis, or (predictably) if they did not receive any enzyme replacement therapy.[22] Other factors studied (such as diet, type of enzyme preparation used, use or non-use of antibiotics) do not seem to affect the prognosis.

KEY POINTS

- EPI is a condition in which the production of digestive enzymes from the pancreas is inadequate, leading to maldigestion of food.
- Typical clinical signs include weight loss despite a ravenous appetite, and stools are usually poorly formed but not watery.
- EPI is common in some breeds (especially German Shepherd dogs, Rough Collies, Chow Chows, and Cavalier King Charles Spaniels).
- In many dogs, the disease is caused by progressive atrophy of the pancreas, with signs developing when 90% or more of the pancreas has been lost (usually between 1 and 4 years of age).
- EPI can also result from end-stage chronic pancreatitis, which can affect dogs of any age. They are usually older by the time they develop EPI and will also be at risk for developing diabetes mellitus.
- The diagnosis is usually quite straightforward using a blood test.
- Based on current evidence, recommended treatment for EPI includes pancreatic enzyme supplementation with every meal, a highly digestible diet that does not need to be fat-restricted (unless the dog also has chronic pancreatitis), and, for most dogs, cobalamin supplementation.
- Lifelong treatment is required.
- Most dogs respond well to treatment and can survive for a long time, but a subset of dogs do not respond well.

References

1. Westermarck E, Wiberg ME. Exocrine pancreatic insufficiency in the dog: historical background, diagnosis, and treatment. *Top Companion Anim Med* 27:96-103, 2012.
2. Wiberg ME, Westermarck E. Subclinical exocrine pancreatic insufficiency in dogs. *J Am Vet Med Assoc* 220:1183-1187, 2002.
3. Hill FW, Osborne AD, Kidder DE. Pancreatic degenerative atrophy in dogs. *J Comp Pathol* 81:321-330, 1971.
4. Westermarck E, Saari SAM, Wiberg ME. Heritability of exocrine pancreatic insufficiency in German Shepherd Dogs. *J Vet Intern Med* 24:450-452, 2010.
5. Clark LA, Cox ML. Current status of genetic studies of exocrine pancreatic insufficiency in dogs. *Top Companion Anim Med* 27:109-112, 2012.
6. Evans JM, Tsai KL, Starr-Moss AN, et al. Association of DLA-DQB1 alleles with exocrine pancreatic insufficiency in Pembroke Welsh Corgis. *Anim Genet* 46(4):462-465, 2015.
7. Tsai KL, Starr-Moss AN, Venkataraman GM, et al. Alleles of the major histocompatibility complex play a role in the pathogenesis of pancreatic acinar atrophy in dogs. *Immunogenetics* 65(7):501-509, 2013.
8. Watson PJ. Exocrine pancreatic insufficiency as an end stage of pancreatitis in four dogs. *J Small Anim Pract* 44:306-312, 2003.
9. Watson PJ, Archer J, Roulois AJ, et al. Observational study of 14 cases of chronic pancreatitis in dogs. *Vet Rec* 167:968-976, 2010.
10. Watson PJ, Roulois AJ, Scase T, et al. Prevalence and breed distribution of chronic pancreatitis at post-mortem examination in first-opinion dogs. *J Small Anim Pract* 48:609-618, 2007.
11. Watson PJ. Chronic pancreatitis in dogs. *Top Companion Anim Med* 27:33-139, 2012.
12. Bostrom BM, Xenoulis PG, Newman SJ, et al. Chronic pancreatitis in dogs: A retrospective study of clinical, clinicopathological, and histopathological findings in 61 cases. *Vet J* 195:73-79, 2013.
13. Batchelor DJ, Noble PJ, Cripps PJ, et al. Breed associations for canine exocrine pancreatic insufficiency. *J Vet Intern Med* 21:207-214, 2007.
14. Davison LJ, Herrtage ME, Catchpole B. Study of 253 dogs in the United Kingdom with diabetes mellitus. *Vet Rec* 156:467-71, 2005.
15. Boari A, Williams DA, Bergamini PF. Diagnosis and management of concurrent exocrine pancreatic insufficiency (EPI) and diabetes mellitus (DM) in a young Rottweiler dog. *European Journal of Comparative Gastroenterology* 1:29-31, 1997.
16. Kang JH, Na KJ, Chang D, et al. Juvenile diabetes mellitus accompanied by exocrine pancreatic insufficiency in a dog. *J Vet Med Sci* 70(12):1337-1340, 2008.
17. Brenner K, Harkin KR, Andrews GA, et al. Juvenile pancreatic atrophy in Greyhounds: 12 cases (1995-2000). *J Vet Intern Med* 23:67-71, 2009.
18. Alvarez MS, Herreria-Bustillo V, Font Utset A, et al. Juvenile diabetes mellitus and concurrent exocrine pancreatic insufficiency in a Labrador Retriever: long-term management. *J Am Anim Hosp Assoc* 51:419-423, 2015.
19. Xenoulis PG, Fradkin JM, Rapp SW, et al. Suspected isolated pancreatic lipase deficiency in a dog. *J Vet Intern Med* 21:1113-1116, 2007.
20. Viviano KR, Ziglioli V. Suspected isolated pancreatic enzyme deficiencies in dogs. *J Vet Intern Med* 27:588-591, 2013.
21. Batchelor DJ, Noble PJ, Taylor RH, et al. Prognostic factors in canine exocrine pancreatic insufficiency: prolonged survival is likely if clinical remission is achieved. *J Vet Intern Med* 21:54-60, 2007.
22. Soetart N, Rochel D, Drut A, et al. Serum cobalamin and folate as prognostic factors in canine exocrine pancreatic insufficiency: An observational cohort study of 299 dogs. *Vet J* 243:15-20, 2019.
23. Williams DA, Batt RM: Sensitivity and specificity of radioimmunoassay of serum trypsin-like immunoreactivity for the diagnosis of canine exocrine pancreatic insufficiency. *J Am Vet Med Assoc* 192:195-201, 1988.
24. Keller ET. High serum trypsin-like immunoreactivity secondary to pancreatitis in a dog with exocrine pancreatic insufficiency. *J Am Vet Med Assoc* 196(4):623-626, 1990.
25. Steiner JM, Rehfeld JF, and Pantchev N. Evaluation of fecal elastase and serum cholecystokinin in dogs with a false positive fecal elastase test. *J Vet Intern Med* 24:643-646, 2010.
26. Steiner JM, Rutz GM, Williams DA. Serum lipase activities and pancreatic lipase immunoreactivity

concentrations in dogs with exocrine pancreatic insufficiency. *Am J Vet Res* 67:84-87, 2006.

27. Wiberg ME, Nurmi AK, Westermarck E. Serum trypsin-like immunoreactivity measurement for the diagnosis of subclinical exocrine pancreatic insufficiency. *J Vet Intern Med* 13:426-432, 1999.
28. Penninck DG, Zeyen U, Taeymans ON, et al. Ultrasonographic measurement of the pancreas and pancreatic duct in clinically normal dogs. *Am J Vet Res* 74:433-437, 2013.
29. Pelligra T, Puccinelli C, Marchetti V, et al. Ultrasonographic findings of exocrine pancreatic insufficiency in dogs. *Vet Sci* 9:407, 2022.
30. Mas A, Noble PJM, Cripps PJ, et al. A blinded randomised controlled trial to determine the effect of enteric coating on enzyme treatment for canine exocrine pancreatic efficiency. *BMC Vet Res* 8:127, 2012.
31. Wiberg ME, Lautala HM, Westermarck E. Response to long-term enzyme replacement treatment in dogs with exocrine pancreatic insufficiency. *J Am Vet Med Assoc* 213:86-90, 1998.
32. Parambeth JC, Fosgate GT, Suchodolski JS, et al. Randomized placebo-controlled clinical trial of an enteric coated micro-pelleted formulation of a pancreatic enzyme supplement in dogs with exocrine pancreatic insufficiency. *J Vet Intern Med* 32:1591-1599, 2018.
33. Rutz GM, Steiner JM, Williams DA. Oral bleeding associated with pancreatic enzyme supplementation in three dogs with exocrine pancreatic insufficiency. *J Am Vet Med Assoc* 221:1716-1718, 2002.
34. Biourge V, Fontaine J. Exocrine pancreatic insufficiency and adverse reaction to food in dogs: a positive response to a high-fat, soy isolate hydrolysate-based diet. *J Nutrition* 134:2166S-2168S, 2004.
35. Westermarck E, Junttila JT, Wiberg ME. Role of low dietary fat in the treatment of dogs with exocrine pancreatic insufficiency. *Am J Vet Res* 56:600-605, 1995.
36. Westermarck E, Wiberg M. Effects of diet on clinical signs of exocrine pancreatic insufficiency in dogs. *J Am Vet Med Assoc* 228:225-229, 2006.
37. Toresson L, Steiner JM, Spodsberg E, et al. Effects of oral cobalamin supplementation on serum cobalamin concentrations in dogs with exocrine pancreatic insufficiency: A pilot study. *Vet J* 269:105619, 2021.
38. Chang C-H, Lidbury JA, Suchodolski JS. Effect of oral or injectable supplementation with cobalamin in dogs with hypocobalaminemia caused by chronic enteropathy or exocrine pancreatic insufficiency. *J Vet Intern Med* 36:1607-1621, 2022.
39. Simpson KW, Batt RM, Jones D, et al. Effects of exocrine pancreatic insufficiency and replacement therapy on the bacterial flora of the duodenum in dogs. *Am J Vet Res* 51:203-206, 1990.
40. Westermarck E, Myllys V, Aho M. Effect of treatment on the jejunal and colonic bacterial flora of dogs with exocrine pancreatic insufficiency. *Pancreas* 8:559-562, 1993.
41. Hall EJ, Bond PM, Mclean C, et al. A survey of the diagnosis and treatment of canine exocrine pancreatic insufficiency. *J Small Anim Pract* 32:613-619, 1991.

CHAPTER 21

Neoplasia of the exocrine pancreas in dogs

Antonio Giuliano
DVM, MS, PgCert(CT), GpCert(SAM), DECVIM-CA (Oncology), DACVIM (Oncology), MRCVS

Jane Dobson
MA BVetMed, DVetMed, DECVIM-CA (Internal Medicine, Oncology, Radiation Oncology) MRCVS

Tumors affecting the exocrine pancreas are rare in dogs, with an estimated incidence of around 0.01%, 17.8 per 100,000, and 3 in 4300 dogs.[1,2] By comparison, the estimated incidence of pancreatic carcinoma in people is around 8.2 per 10,000 in men and 5.4 per 10,000 in women.[3] The exocrine portion of the pancreas comprises mainly the acinar and tubular pancreatic cells but also blood vessels and stroma. Both the epithelial and the mesenchymal components of the pancreas are subjected to neoplastic transformation. However, carcinoma is by far the most common cancer type in both people and dogs. Occasionally, secondary invasion of the pancreas by gastric or intestinal tumors has been reported.[4] Anecdotally, metastasis from other primary tumors or involvement of the pancreas from gastrointestinal lymphoma has been reported (data not published, personal communication, Penny Watson).

As in human patients, carcinoma of the exocrine pancreas in dogs can be broadly divided into acinar and ductal carcinoma.[5] While the cell of origin of acinar and ductal carcinoma is not completely understood, histologically, acinar carcinoma resembles acinar cells, and well-differentiated tumors can produce zymogens, while ductal carcinoma morphologically carries ductal structure appearance.[6] In people, acinar cell carcinoma is very rare and represents only 1% of all pancreatic carcinomas, while pancreatic ductal carcinoma represents more than 90% of all pancreas malignancies.[7,8] According to the cell type of origin and a variety of other histologic morphologic characteristics, clinically important subclassifications of exocrine pancreatic neoplasia have been identified in humans.[9] The histologic characteristics of exocrine pancreatic neoplasia in domestic animals vary greatly: tubular, acinar, or solid types with various degrees of fibroplasia have been described.[10] However, despite the limited studies available in veterinary medicine, in contrast to people, the most common type of pancreatic carcinoma seems to be poorly differentiated solid or acinar carcinoma in dogs.[1] The relationship between the histological subtype of pancreatic carcinoma and biological behavior in dogs remains unclear. In a small case series, an unusual form of pancreatic carcinoma referred to as hyalinizing pancreatic adenocarcinoma has also been reported. This rare form of pancreatic carcinoma is characterized by the buildup of homogenous eosinophilic extracellular material in tumor stroma and tubular lumina with well-granulated epithelial cells with modest cellular atypia, indicative of low-grade malignancy. This rare subtype of pancreatic carcinoma could carry a better prognosis than other reported pancreatic adenocarcinomas in some cases.[11]

Etiology

Exocrine pancreatic carcinoma is extremely rare in young compared to old dogs, with an average age of 9-11 years. No proven gender or breed predisposition has been reported.[1,12] There are known hereditary predispositions in people, and the BRCA2 gene may be the most prevalent inherited genetic condition linked to pancreatic cancer, with 7-10% of patients thought to have a hereditary germline deficiency.[13] However, no germline defects or genetic predispositions have been identified in dogs. The most important risk factors for pancreatic carcinoma in people are considered cigarette smoking, heavy alcohol consumption, pancreatitis, and obesity.[12,14,15] Contrary to people, there are no recognized risk factors associated with the development of pancreatic carcinoma in dogs, although since dogs share an environment with humans (and thus passive smoking) and have a high prevalence of obesity, it would be interesting to investigate these and other potential risk factors.

KRAS is a proto-oncogene that is mutated in many different cancer types and is implicated in the PI3K and MAPK pathways.[16,17] Around 57% of human ductal pancreatic carcinomas include mutations in KRAS codons 12, 13, and 61, but carcinomas with such mutations rarely occur in pancreatic acinar cells. Similarly, to people, mutations in exons 12 and 13 of the KRAS gene have not been found in canine acinar cell carcinomas.[16-18]

Clinical features and biological behavior

Canine pancreatic carcinoma is a locally aggressive neoplasia with a high rate (>70%) of local, distant and transcelomic metastases. The most common metastatic sites are the regional lymph nodes, liver, duodenum, jejunum, and lungs, with occasionally reported metastasis to the adrenal gland, lumbar vertebra, and brain.[1,12,19,20] Pancreatic carcinoma often presents with diffuse infiltration of the whole pancreas, followed by large solitary masses located on the right or the body of the pancreas, while the left lobe is less commonly affected.[1,12] The most common clinical signs are anorexia, lethargy, vomiting, diarrhea, abdominal pain, occasional jaundice, and seizures.[1,12] Rarely, some dogs can be asymptomatic and a mass in the pancreas is found incidentally.[12] Clinical signs related to pancreatitis are common, and occasionally hypoglycemia and subcutaneous steatitic/panniculitis, polyarthritis, and osteomyelitis have also been reported.[1,21,22,23] These are rare clinical signs also reported in people and are likely related to the significant release of pancreatic enzymes into the bloodstream, causing necrosis and hydrolysis of adipocytes and secondary inflammation.[22]

Clinical pathology findings and diagnostic imaging

The incidence of clinical pathological abnormalities has been rarely investigated. Pancreatic enzymes, including cPLI, TLI, and DGGR lipase, are often elevated in pancreatic carcinoma, but the elevations of liver enzymes, CRP, and an inflammatory leukogram are also reported.[1,12]
Ultrasound is often used in the investigation of suspected pancreatitis or pancreatic masses. Abdominal ultrasound is more likely to identify pancreatic carcinoma, while radiographs are less sensitive. Ultrasound is also useful for identifying abdominal metastases, invasion of organs, and carcinomatosis. Pancreatic carcinoma often presents with a mass of heterogenous echogenicity that can be cavitated, while in the case of diffuse infiltration, the pancreas can appear enlarged, hypoechoic, or even with a normal appearance.[12,19]

Ultrasound alone cannot differentiate a pancreatic cyst/pseudocyst, abscess, regenerative nodules, or severe/necrotic pancreatitis from pancreatic carcinoma, and fine-needle aspiration is often needed for further evaluation (Fig. 21.1). Cytology of pancreatic lesions/masses is also considered relatively safe.[24,25] Insulinoma or other neuroendocrine tumors cannot be differentiated based on ultrasound appearance alone, but cytology is often useful to differentiate from pancreatic carcinoma. Other clinical signs of hypoglycemia paired with high normal serum insulin are often characteristic of insulinoma and absent in pancreatic carcinoma.

Ultrasound-guided fine-needle aspiration (FNA) is often used to achieve a diagnosis, and the presence of atypical carcinoma cells with various criteria of malignancy is often confirmatory of pancreatic carcinoma.[24] However, if only the necrotic area is sampled, pancreatic abscess, necrotic pancreatitis, or severe pancreatitis can be difficult to differentiate from necrotic pancreatic carcinoma. In cases where metastases to the draining lymph nodes or liver are present, FNA of the metastases could be more reliable in reaching a final diagnosis. However, where a final diagnosis cannot be achieved by FNA, a biopsy is often needed. Ultrasound-guided Tru-Cut needle biopsy is rarely used in dogs, while exploratory laparotomy followed by tumor resection or biopsy and histopathology is more likely to be used to achieve a final diagnosis.[12]

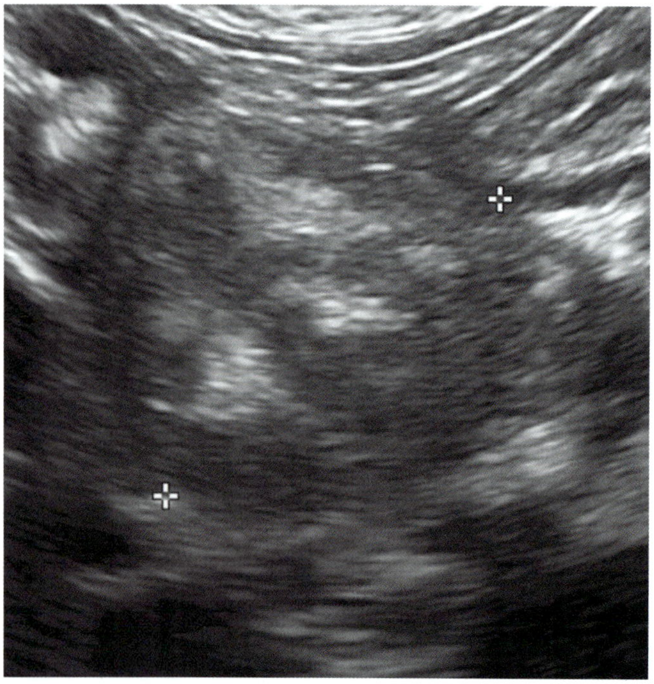

FIG. 21.1 Ultrasound appearance of the pancreas of an 11-year-7-month-old Cockerpoo with a history of weight loss, hyporexia, vomiting, marked elevation of serum lipase and jaundice. The pancreas was markedly enlarged with a hypoechoic and heterogeneous parenchyma. There were also multiple hypoechoic nodules within the mesentery and extension of abnormal pancreatic tissue into the left peritoneal space. Cytology of fine-needle aspirates of the pancreatic mass, liver nodules, and mesenteric mass were diagnostic of pancreatic carcinoma. Photo courtesy of the Diagnostic Imaging Department, Queen's Veterinary School Hospital, University of Cambridge.

Treatment and prognosis

In people, pancreatic carcinoma carries a very poor prognosis and is one of the leading causes of cancer-related death worldwide.[26,27] In the USA, the 5-year survival rate for those with pancreatic cancer is only 9%.[24] Despite advances in surgery and adjuvant therapy as part of multimodal treatment, the survival rate has not improved. Surgery is the most effective treatment for pancreatic carcinoma in people. However, most patients with pancreatic cancer only show symptoms when the disease has progressed to an advanced stage.[28] Therefore, only a small percentage of patients can be considered candidates for surgery since pancreatic carcinoma typically has already local or systemic metastases at the time of diagnosis.[29] Surgical excision is the only curative option for pancreatic carcinoma in people, but the prognosis is dismal even after a successful surgical excision due to high recurrence and metastatic rate.[30] These findings have prompted multimodal therapies as the gold standard, and numerous clinical trials have demonstrated some efficacy of adjuvant chemotherapy in extending disease-free and overall survival in individuals with resectable disease, especially regimens containing 5-fluorouracil, gemcitabine, and combination regimens (e.g., FOLFIRINOX: folinic acid, 5-fluorouracil, irinotecan, and oxaliplatin).[30-33] Unfortunately, even in people, there are no approved or standard-of-care target treatments for pancreatic carcinoma. However, with the increased use of single tumor molecular profiles in recent years, some pancreatic cancers with specific targetable mutations can be treated with certain tyrosine kinase inhibitors in a case-by-case scenario. Immunotherapy with monoclonal antibodies against checkpoint inhibitors (such as PD-L1 or PD-1) has become the standard of care in humans for many cancer types, including melanoma, lung, and colon cancer as others.[34] Immunotherapy with monoclonal antibodies against PD-L1 has not been successful with pancreatic carcinoma, but pembrolizumab, a PD-1 checkpoint inhibitor, has been found to be effective and has been FDA-approved for patients with advanced pancreatic cancer whose tumors are mismatched repair-deficient or have microsatellite instability.[34]

In dogs, similarly to people, surgery is rarely curative due to the advanced disease at presentation and high recurrence and metastatic rate.[1,12] Even though neoadjuvant and adjuvant combination chemotherapy has improved survival in people, chemotherapy treatment is rarely performed in dogs with pancreatic carcinoma, and the benefit of conventional chemotherapy in both adjuvant and macroscopic/metastatic disease is largely unknown in this species. There is anecdotal evidence for the use of gemcitabine for the treatment of dogs with pancreatic carcinoma, but the benefit in terms of response rate and survival time is also unknown. Two case reports in cats and a small case series in dogs suggest that toceranib phosphate could have some benefit in pancreatic carcinoma.[12,35,36] In a case series of eight dogs treated with toceranib in microscopic and macroscopic disease, a toceranib-specific median survival time of 89 days (14-506 days) was achieved. Four cases were evaluated for objective response; one achieved a partial response for 56 days, two stable diseases for 302 and 506 days, and one progressive disease.[35]

The prognosis for canine exocrine pancreatic carcinoma remains very poor, with the most recent publication evaluating the prognosis showing a median survival time of 8 days (0-56 days).[12] However, it is also true that most dogs with pancreatic carcinoma are diagnosed late in their disease when significant clinical signs are present and often even euthanized at diagnosis.[12] It is possible that early diagnosis and treatment could result in a better outcome.

KEY POINTS

- Tumors of the exocrine pancreas are rare in dogs.
- The most common pancreatic tumor in dogs is solid or acinar pancreatic carcinoma.
- Clinical signs are often confused with signs of pancreatitis.
- Canine pancreatic carcinoma is a locally aggressive neoplasia with a high rate (>70%) of local, distant, and transcelomic metastases.
- The most common metastatic sites are the regional lymph nodes, liver, duodenum, jejunum, and lungs.
- Most canine pancreatic tumors are diagnosed at an advanced stage when surgery is not feasible, and the prognosis remains very poor.
- There are no effective medical treatments for advanced-stage pancreatic carcinoma in dogs.
- Toceranib phosphate could be beneficial in some cases.

References

1. Aupperle-Lellbach H, Törner K, Staudacher M, Müller E, Steiger K, Klopfleisch R. Characterization of 22 canine pancreatic carcinomas and review of literature. *J Comp Pathol* 173, 2019.
2. Priester WA. Data from eleven United States and Canadian colleges of veterinary medicine on pancreatic carcinoma in domestic animals. *Cancer Res* 34(6), 1974.
3. Jemal A, Bray F, Center MM, Ferlay J, Ward E, Forman D. Global cancer statistics. *CA Cancer J Clin* 61(2), 2011.
4. Lamb CR, Simpson KW, Boswood A, Matthewman LA. Ultrasonography of pancreatic neoplasia in the dog: a retrospective review of 16 cases. *Vet Rec* 137(3), 1995.
5. Stelow EB, Shaco-Levy R, Bao F, Garcia J, Klimstra DS. Pancreatic acinar cell carcinomas with prominent ductal differentiation: Mixed acinar ductal carcinoma and mixed acinar endocrine ductal carcinoma. *Am J Surg Pathol* 34(4), 2010.
6. Grimont A, Leach SD, Chandwani R. Uncertain beginnings: acinar and ductal cell plasticity in the development of pancreatic cancer. *Cell Mol Gastroenterol Hepatol* 13(2), 2022.
7. Hu JX, Lin YY, Zhao CF, Chen WB, Liu QC, Li QW, Gao F. Pancreatic cancer: A review of epidemiology, trend, and risk factors. *World J Gastoentrol* 27(27), 2021.
8. Orth M, Metzger P, Gerum S, Mayerle J, Schneider G, Belka C, Schnurr M, Lauber K. Pancreatic ductal adenocarcinoma: Biological hallmarks, current status, and future perspectives of combined modality treatment approaches. *Radiat Oncol* 14 (1), 2019.
9. Azadeh B, Campbell F. Pathology of exocrine neoplasms of the pancreas. *Surgery* 25 (2), 2007.
10. Kiupel M, Capen C, Miller M, Smedley R. Histological classification of tumors of the endocrine system of domestic animals. *International Histological Classification of Tumors of Domestic Animals*, 1994.
11. Dennis MM, O'Brien TD, Wayne T, Kiupel M, Williams M, Powers BE. Hyalinizing pancreatic adenocarcinoma in six dogs. *Vet Pathol* 45(4), 2008.
12. Pinard CJ, Hocker SE, Weishaar KM. Clinical outcome in 23 dogs with exocrine pancreatic carcinoma. *Vet Comp Oncol* 19(1), 2021.
13. Midha S, Chawla S, Garg PK. Modifiable and non-modifiable risk factors for pancreatic cancer: A review. *Cancer Letters* 381 (1), 2016.
14. Duell EJ, Lucenteforte E, Olson SH, Bracci PM, Li D, Risch HA, et al. Pancreatitis and pancreatic cancer risk: A pooled analysis in the International Pancreatic Cancer Case-Control Consortium (PanC4). *Ann Oncol* 23(11): 2964-2970, 2012.
15. Rawla P, Sunkara T, Gaduputi V. Epidemiology of pancreatic cancer: global trends, etiology and risk factors. *World J Clin Oncol* 10(1), 2019.

16. Crozier C, Wood GA, Foster RA, Stasi S, Liu JHW, Bartlett JMS, Coomber BL, Sabine VS. KRAS mutations in canine and feline pancreatic acinar cell carcinoma. *J Com Pathol* 155(1), 2016.
17. Oliveira-Cunha M, Hadfield KD, Siriwardena AK, Newman W. EGFR and KRAS mutational analysis and their correlation to survival in pancreatic and periampullary cancer. *Pancreas* 41(3), 2012.
18. Forbes SA, Beare D, Gunasekaran P, Leung K, et al. COSMIC: exploring the world's knowledge of somatic mutations in human cancer. *Nucleic Acids Res* 43(D1), 2015.
19. Bennett PF, Acvim D, Hahn KA, Toal RL, Legendre AM. Ultrasonographic and cytopathological diagnosis of exocrine pancreatic carcinoma in the dog and cat. *J Am Anim Hosp Assoc* 37, 2001.
20. Chang SC, Liao JW, Lin YC, Liu CI, Wong, ML. Pancreatic acinar cell carcinoma with intracranial metastasis in a dog. *J Vet Med Sci* 69(1), 2007.
21. Brown PJ, Mason KV, Merrett DJ, Mirchandani S, Miller RI. Multifocal necrotising steatites associated with pancreatic carcinoma in three dogs. *J Small Anim Pract* 35(3), 1994.
22. Gear RNA, Bacon NJ, Langley-Hobbs S, Watson PJ, Woodger N, Herrtage ME. Anniculitis, polyarthritis and osteomyelitis associated with pancreatic neoplasia in two dogs. *J Small Anim Pract* 47(7), 2006.
23. Roberto GB, Magro AL, Seki MC, Tranquilim MV, Ziliotto L. Exocrine pancreatic carcinoma with hypoglycemia in a dog. *Acta Scientiae Veterinariae* 44(1), 2016.
24. Cordner AP, Sharkey LC, Armstrong PJ, McAteer KD. Cytologic findings and diagnostic yield in 92 dogs undergoing fine-needle aspiration of the pancreas. *J Vet Diagn Invest* 27(2), 2015.
25. Hecht S, Henry G. Sonographic evaluation of the normal and abnormal pancreas. *Clin Tech Small Anim Pract* 22(3), 2007.
26. Rahib L, Smith BD, Aizenberg R, Rosenzweig AB, Fleshman JM, Matrisian LM. Projecting cancer incidence and deaths to 2030: the unexpected burden of thyroid, liver, and pancreas cancers in the United States. *Cancer Res* 74(11), 2014.
27. Siegel RL, Miller KD, Jemal A. Cancer statistics, 2019. *CA Cancer J Clin* 69(1), 2019.
28. Khachfe HH, Habib JR, Nassour I, Al Harthi S, Jamali FR. Borderline resectable and locally advanced pancreatic cancers: A review of definitions, diagnostics, strategies for treatment, and future directions. *Pancreas* 50(9), 2021.
29. Ansari D, Tingstedt B, Andersson B, Holmquist F, Sturesson C, Williamsson C, Sasor A, Borg D, Bauden M, Andersson R. Pancreatic cancer: yesterday, today and tomorrow. *Future Oncology* 12(16), 2016.
30. Qian Y, Zheng S, Jia C. The role of modified FOLFIRINOX regimen in unresectable advanced pancreatic cancer: A retrospective clinical study. *J Clin Oncol* 35(15_suppl), 2017.
31. Neoptolemos JP, Stocken DD, Tudur Smith C, Bassi C, Ghaneh P, Owen E, Moore M, Padbury R, Doi R, Smith D, Büchler MW. Adjuvant 5-fluorouracil and folinic acid vs observation for pancreatic cancer: Composite data from the ESPAC-1 and -3(v1) trials. *Br J Cancer* 100(2), 2009.
32. Neoptolemos JP, Moore MJ, Cox TF, Valle JW, *et al.* Effect of adjuvant chemotherapy with fluorouracil plus folinic acid or gemcitabine vs observation on survival in patients with resected periampullary adenocarcinoma: the ESPAC-3 periampullary cancer randomized trial. *J Am Med Assoc* 308(2), 2012.
33. Oettle H, Neuhaus P, Hochhaus A, Hartmann JT, Gellert K, Ridwelski K, Niedergethmann M, Zülke C, Fahlke J, Arning MB, Sinn M, Hinke A, Riess H. Adjuvant chemotherapy with gemcitabine and long-term outcomes among patients with resected pancreatic cancer: The CONKO-001 randomized trial. *J Am Med Assoc* 310(14), 2013.
34. Ludford K, Ho WJ, Thomas JV, Raghav KPS, et al. Neoadjuvant pembrolizumab in localized microsatellite instability high/deficient mismatch repair solid tumors. *J Clin Oncol* 41(12):2181-2190, 2023.
35. Musser ML, Johannes CM. Toceranib phosphate (Palladia) for the treatment of canine exocrine pancreatic adenocarcinoma. *BMC Vet Res* 17(1), 2021.
36. Pinard CJ, Stegelmeier AA, Bridle BW, Mutsaers AJ, Wood D, Wood GA, Woods JP, Hocker SE. Evaluation of lymphocyte-specific PD -1 receptor expression and cytokines in blood and urine in canine urothelial carcinoma patients. *Vet Comp Oncol* 20(2), 2021.

CHAPTER 22

Nutrition for acute and chronic pancreatitis and exocrine pancreatic insufficiency

Daniel L. Chan
DVM, DACVECC, DECVECC, DACVIM (Nutrition), FHEA, MRCVS

In addition to its central role in the endocrine system, the pancreas has an exocrine component that is vital for proper digestion. The pancreas synthesizes and secretes a host of digestive enzymes responsible for carbohydrate, protein, and fat digestion. When the pancreas is affected by conditions such as acute or chronic inflammation or permanently by exocrine pancreatic insufficiency, nutritional management has important implications. This chapter will discuss the nutritional considerations when the pancreas is affected by disease and outline nutritional plans for dogs with these conditions. Although understanding the physiology of pancreatic function, the pathophysiology of pancreatitis (both acute and chronic), and exocrine pancreatic insufficiency are important to appreciate the implications for nutritional management, these are beyond the scope of this chapter, so the reader is referred elsewhere for more detail (see chapters 17, 18, 19 and 20).

Nutritional considerations in dogs with acute pancreatitis

Historically, based on the previous poor evidence base for nutritional recommendations in acute pancreatitis in both dogs and people, the standard nutritional approach was to withhold food ("allowing pancreatic rest") to reduce pancreatic autodigestion by decreasing pancreatic stimulation and digestive enzyme release.[1-3] This was also thought to be the means of addressing clinical signs such as abdominal pain, nausea, and vomiting. However, a better (although still incomplete) understanding that the initiating events of spontaneous acute pancreatitis involve intracellular premature activation of proteolytic enzymes rather than pancreatic secretion of digestive zymogens has altered our approach to this condition.[4] As a result, avoidance of feeding as a means to decrease pancreatic stimulation is unwarranted as this not only contributes to underfeeding but also further compromises the patient by potentially impairing gastrointestinal barrier function.[5-9] In dogs with experimentally induced pancreatitis, enteral nutrition was associated with a reduction of bacterial translocation and improved intestinal barrier function.[8,9] In people with acute pancreatitis (AP), enteral nutrition has been associated with fewer infectious complications, shorter hospitalization, and even decreased mortality when compared with parenteral nutrition.[10,11] For these reasons, the main nutritional consideration for dogs with acute pancreatitis is to explore feeding (in particular enteral feeding) as soon as possible. This is not to say that there are no challenges with introducing enteral feeding in dogs with acute pancreatitis (e.g., protracted vomiting, abdominal pain, persistent nausea), but the alternative of withholding nutrition does not ameliorate the condition and delays recovery.[12,13]

Nutritional plan for dogs with acute pancreatitis

Management of abdominal pain, nausea, and continuation of diagnostics can proceed whilst formulating an initial nutritional plan for the patient. Complete cessation of vomiting may also not be a prerequisite for initiation of enteral feeding.[13,14] Although the definition of "early enteral nutrition" is not standardized in veterinary medicine, the concept of feeding sooner (e.g., within 48 hours of hospitalization) rather than delayed until there is a resolution of vomiting, does appear to be feasible and convey some positive results in some but not all studies in dogs with acute pancreatitis, parvovirus, and acute hemorrhagic gastroenteritis.[12-15] A small pilot study in dogs with severe acute pancreatitis was terminated early because of positive results in dogs fed enterally (within 24 hours of enrollment) compared with dogs fed parenterally.[13] In this study, dogs were fed despite the presence of vomiting, and the frequency of vomiting decreased with the initiation of feeding, suggesting that early enteral feeding is not only tolerated but could speed up the resolution of vomiting in dogs with acute pancreatitis.[13] The authors hypothesized that clinical improvement may have resulted

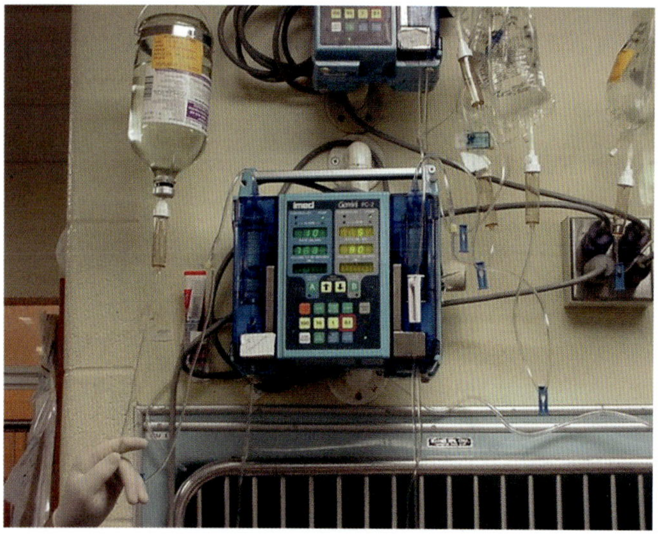

FIG. 22.1 Effective nutritional management of dogs with acute pancreatitis often requires placement of esophagostomy feeding tubes.

from improved gastrointestinal perfusion or motility, although these effects have yet to be confirmed.

A subsequent retrospective study in dogs with acute pancreatitis similarly identified that feeding within 48 hours of hospitalization was also associated with a more rapid return to voluntary eating and resolution of gastrointestinal signs.[12] Although definitive evidence is still lacking, a sensible approach with dogs with acute pancreatitis is to attempt initiation of enteral feeding within 48 hours of hospitalization. If there is no voluntary eating within 48 hours, a feeding tube is recommended to enable more effective nutritional support. Although more invasive than nasoesophageal feeding tubes, the author recommends esophagostomy feeding tubes (Fig. 22.1) as dogs with acute pancreatitis that do not show interest in voluntary eating within 48 hours of treatment often require more direct nutritional support. Such cases typically require 5 to 7 days of assisted feeding, and esophagostomy tubes are more appropriate and effective.

However, a recent retrospective study reported the tolerability of nasoesophageal feeding tubes in dogs and cats managed at home.[16] In this study, the authors reported that 29 dogs with various diseases were managed with gastroesophageal feeding tubes in the home environment for a median of 5 days (range 1-17 days), suggesting that some dogs with pancreatitis could theoretically be managed with nasoesophageal tubes beyond the period of hospitalization.[16] However, the study did not report the amount of calories provided nor if dogs maintained weight being fed in this manner. Therefore, it is unknown if dogs are nutritionally effectively managed this way. Nonetheless, if the clinical expertise or equipment is lacking to place an esophagostomy tube, placement of a gastroesophageal tube may be considered, although recognizing this is not ideal.

It is worth noting that the common approach of feeding dogs with acute pancreatitis low-fat diets once enteral feeding is initiated is not based on direct evidence relating to treatment outcomes but only on historical or temporal associations with the initiation or trigger of acute pancreatitis.[4] While some authors recommend restricting fat in the diet to 20% of metabolizable energy (ME),[17] this author reserves this approach to dogs exhibiting hyperlipidemia. Otherwise, a highly digestible diet with moderate fat content (34-51% of metabolizable energy [ME]) is appropriate in most dogs with acute pancreatitis. When initiating feeding, most dogs should be gradually fed, starting with 33% of resting energy requirements (RER) on the first day and aiming to achieve 100% RER by the third day. If this amount of calories is well tolerated and the dog is not maintaining weight, the RER may be exceeded by 10-20% (see chapter 3 for details of calculating RER).

Feeding via feeding tubes has been reported using bolus feeding from three to four times a day and as continuous infusions. Both methods have been successfully used. As both esophageal and nasoesophageal feeding tubes utilize the upper gastrointestinal tract, bolus feeding better approximates normal feeding. In dogs with apparently altered GI motility and who are not tolerating bolus feeding, a continuous infusion, so-called "trickle feeding", may be attempted. Rates for trickle feeding have been reported to range from 2-20 mL/kg/h. A summary of nutritional considerations for dogs with pancreatic diseases is listed in Table 22.1.

Parenteral nutritional support of dogs with acute pancreatitis

Although the preferred route of nutritional support in dogs with pancreatitis is to use the enteral route, there may be rare occasions when these patients do not tolerate enteral feedings despite the appropriate use of analgesia, prokinetics, and antiemetics. When these patients cannot be consistently fed near their resting energy requirements (RER), they will be at increased risk of becoming malnourished, which may delay their recovery. In such cases, there is a need to consider feeding these patients parenterally. In many of these cases, a combination of small amounts of enteral feeding and supplemental parenteral feeding can be an effective strategy as there will be benefits to some enteral feeding in supporting enterocytes and promoting gastrointestinal motility and

TABLE 22.1 Summary of nutritional consideration in dogs with exocrine pancreatic diseases.

Condition	Feeding tube required?	Fat-restricted diet?	Other nutritional measures required?
Canine acute pancreatitis	Commonly if not voluntarily eating within 48 hours of treatment	Sometimes if accompanied by hypertriglyceridemia	No
Canine chronic pancreatitis	Uncommonly required	Commonly required	No
Canine exocrine pancreatic insufficiency	Rarely required	Sometimes if not responding to pancreatic enzyme supplementation or secondary to chronic pancreatitis	Pancreatic enzyme supplementation, cobalamin supplementation

perfusion. In such cases, the dog's energy and substrate needs are met with the combination of parenteral and enteral nutrients.[18] Formulation and compounding of parenteral nutrition solutions require special skills and expertise more likely found in specialist centers.

However, short-term use of ready-made three-in-one commercial solutions (containing amino acids, dextrose, and lipid emulsions) can be implemented (Fig. 22.2). Generally, patients with acute pancreatitis that require parenteral nutrition (i.e., when enteral nutrition is contraindicated) can be safely supported with parenteral formulations containing lipids as long as they do not have hypertriglyceridemia, at least in people.[19] When dogs have persistent hypertriglyceridemia, these three-in-one solutions may not be suitable due to the relatively high lipid content, and bespoke formulation without lipids may be required. Alternatively, there are commercially available two-in-one solutions of amino acids and dextrose or sorbitol that could be used in such cases (Fig. 22.3).

Additionally, dogs with acute pancreatitis may have persistent hyperglycemia not related to pre-existing diabetes mellitus, and this is likely due to a combination of insulin resistance and endocrine pancreatic dysfunction. There is some evidence that hyperglycemia itself could negatively impact the outcome in people with pancreatitis.[20] Therefore, formulation for such patients may require lower dextrose content and higher amino acid content (e.g., 8 g protein/100 Kcal compared with typical 4-5 g protein/100 Kcal). The optimal composition of parenteral nutritional formulation for dogs with pancreatitis with and without persistent hypertriglyceridemia or hyperglycemia has not been established. The reader is referred elsewhere for guidance in formulating parenteral nutrition solutions suitable for such patients.[21]

Nutritional considerations for dogs with chronic pancreatitis

Dogs with chronic or recurrent pancreatitis tend to have less severe systemic involvement and typically do not require prolonged hospitalization. However, many of these dogs already have some evidence of negative nitrogen balance due to recurrent bouts of anorexia and, in dogs with chronic pancreatitis, developing exocrine insufficiency, so nutritional considerations remain important. Many of these dogs can eat voluntarily and are less dependent on feeding tubes to aid in their recovery. As many of these dogs have evidence of dyslipidemia (e.g., persistent increased fasting triglycerides), long-term fat restriction is indicated.

A target level of fat restriction to elicit a benefit in this population has not been defined, but some authors empirically recommend a 50% reduction in fat ME compared with the dog's normal diet.[22] Commercial therapeutic diets for dogs with these levels of fat restriction are limited, and the dry extruded forms tend to have lower fat content. If commercial diets fail to control hyperlipidemia, nutritionally balanced fat-restricted homemade diets can be formulated by veterinary nutritionists. While fed low-fat diets, dogs with persistent dyslipidemia may benefit from omega-3 fatty acid supplementation found in fish oils.[23-24] Although omega-3 fatty acids are themselves lipids, they improve the regulation of lipid metabolism and, therefore, appear beneficial in dogs with dyslipidemias. Suggested dosing of concentrated fish oils ranges from 220-330 mg/kg/day.[23-24] This is approximately 1 gram of fish oil capsule per 4.5 kg body weight.

Exocrine pancreatic insufficiency

Pathophysiology

With severe loss of exocrine pancreatic function (about 90%), animals develop exocrine pancreatic insufficiency (EPI). With the loss of digestive enzymatic function and reduced secretion of bicarbonate and other substances, dogs lose the ability to properly digest and assimilate nutrients such as fats, proteins, and carbohydrates. As a result, animals with EPI suffer from maldigestion and malabsorption. These animals develop significant malnutrition typified by weight loss, poor body and muscle condition, diarrhea, and sometimes steatorrhea, and these signs are accompanied by polyphagia.[25] The etiology and pathophysiology of EPI are discussed in detail elsewhere (chapter 20).

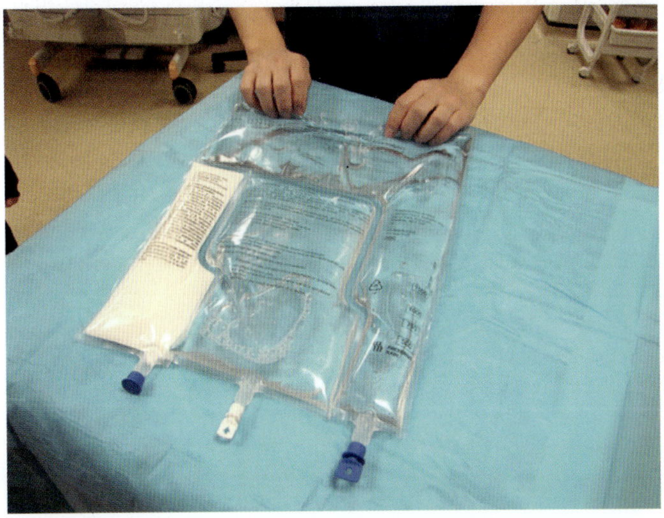

FIG. 22.2 In rare occasions when animals with pancreatitis cannot tolerate enteral feeding despite medical management, parenteral nutrition can be used to provide nutritional support.

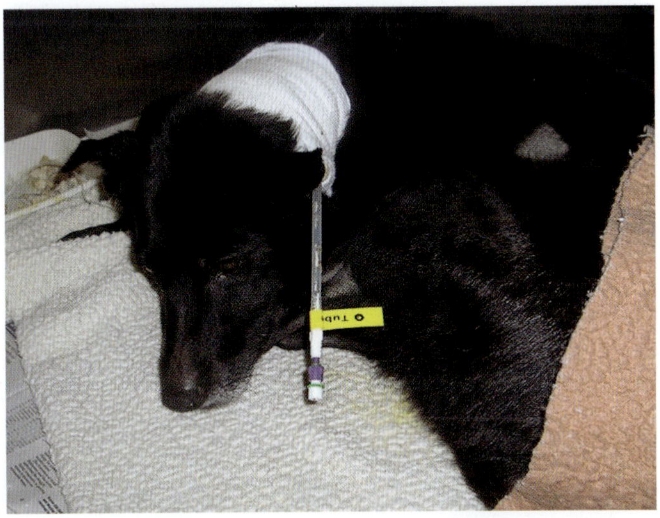

FIG. 22.3 Dogs with acute pancreatitis with hyperlipidemia and an intolerance for enteral feeding may be supported with lipid-free parenteral solutions.

Nutritional considerations for dogs with exocrine pancreatic insufficiency

Due to the poor nutritional status of dogs with EPI, a nutritional strategy to complement medical management is key to a successful outcome. Lifelong dietary pancreatic enzyme supplementation is the key aspect of nutritional management in animals with EPI. It is important to recognize that whilst enzyme supplementation is the best-known approach, it does not completely restore digestion and assimilation, and dogs may still have some degree of diarrhea and steatorrhea. In addition to enzyme supplementation, management of steatorrhea may include a recommendation to feed diets that are reduced in fat.[26] However, it must be recognized that restricting fat in the diet of dogs with poor body conditions makes it particularly challenging to improve their nutritional status. Whilst the ideal diet for dogs with EPI has not been established, a highly digestible and high protein content with moderately reduced fat content may be advised in combination with pancreatic enzyme supplementation.

Nutrition plan for dogs with exocrine pancreatic insufficiency

The cornerstone of nutritional management in dogs with EPI is pancreatic enzyme supplementation. Extracts from bovine or porcine pancreas are commercially available. These supplements are best administered in powdered or tablet form, and there is no need to preincubate the food with the pancreatic enzyme. Some owners choose to add raw pancreas to the food. However, there are well-described risks of feeding animals raw meat diets, and clients should be made aware of these risks.[27]
Dosing of pancreatic enzymes is largely empiric and adjusted to effect based on response. As a starting guide, one teaspoon of the powdered supplement per 10 kg of body weight is added to every meal. It is important to stress to the owner that the enzymes should be added to every meal. The use of a fat-restricted diet may not be necessary in some cases, and it is advised to consider changing the diet only after a period of 3-4 weeks after the introduction of the pancreatic supplement. The benefits of using fat-restricted diets appear to be inconsistent and may be due to individual variations. There is some suggestion that fat-restricted diets are more important in dogs with EPI due to end-stage chronic pancreatitis (see chapters 19 and 20). Cobalamin supplementation, either parenterally or orally, is thought to be beneficial in these cases, many of which will be deficient. The supplementation of fat-soluble vitamins does not appear to be necessary once animals are fed complete and balanced diets with pancreatic enzyme supplementation.

Role of appetite stimulants in dogs with pancreatic disease

While it is not uncommon for dogs with both acute and chronic pancreatitis to be hyporexic, it is preferable to use more effective means of nutritional support such as feeding tubes rather than relying on appetite stimulants. Although there has been some progress in the development of appetite stimulants with fewer side effects (e.g., capromorelin), their effectiveness in maintaining lean body tissue and aiding the recovery of dogs with diseases remains unproven. Attempts to use appetite stimulants early in disease management tend to delay the implementation of more effective nutritional support methods. A better strategy, perhaps, is to use appetite stimulants once animals are in the recovery phase, as this can enhance food intake and aid in their recovery. Further research is warranted to establish the role of appetite stimulants in the management of diseased animals.

KEY POINTS

- Nutritional support plays an important role in managing dogs with acute and chronic pancreatitis and in exocrine pancreatic insufficiency.
- In most cases, enteral nutrition (either voluntarily consumed or via tube feeding) is the preferred route and imparts the greatest benefits.
- Cessation of vomiting does not appear to be a requirement before initiation of enteral feeding in acute pancreatitis.
- Fat restriction of diets appears to be of greater importance in dogs with chronic, recurrent pancreatitis or those with obvious dyslipidemia seen with either acute or chronic pancreatitis.
- Parenteral nutrition should be reserved for those animals who cannot tolerate enteral feeding and, ideally, should be given a small amount of enteral food to support the gut wall barrier.
- The mainstay dietary approach with dogs with exocrine pancreatic insufficiency is lifelong supplementation of pancreatic enzymes with every meal.

References

1. Petrov MS. Gastric feeding and "gut rousing" in acute pancreatitis. *Nutr Clin Pract* 29(3):287-290, 2014.
2. Simpson K, Lamb C. Acute pancreatitis. *In Practice* 17(10):328-337, 1995.
3. Williams DA. Diagnosis and management of pancreatitis. *J Small Anim Pract* 35:445-454, 1994.
4. Cridge H, Lim SY, Algul H, et al. New insights into the etiology, risk factors, and pathogenesis of pancreatitis in dogs: Potential impacts on clinical practice. *J Vet Intern Med* 36:847-864, 2022.
5. Nathens AB, Curtis JR, Beale RL, et al. Management of the critically ill patient with severe acute pancreatitis. *Crit Care Med* 32:2524-2536, 2004.
6. Ioannidis O, Lavrentieva A, Botsios D. Nutrition support in acute pancreatitis. *J Pancreas* 9:375-390, 2008.
7. Curtis CS, Judsk KA. Nutrition support in pancreatitis. *Surg Clin North Am* 87: 1403-1415, 2007.
8. Qin HL, Su ZD, Gao Q, Lin QT. Early intrajejunal nutrition: bacterial translocation and gut barrier function of severe acute pancreatitis in dogs. *Hepatobiliary Pancreat Dis Int* 1:150-154, 2002.
9. Wang G, Wen J, Xu L, Zhou S, Gong M, Wen P, Xiao X. Effect of enteral nutrition and ecoimmunonutrition on bacterial translocation and cytokine production in patients with severe acute pancreatitis. *J Surg Res* 183(2):592-597, 2013.
10. Petrov M, Kukosh M, Emelyanov N. A Randomized controlled trial of enteral versus parenteral feeding in patients with predicted severe acute pancreatitis shows a significant reduction in mortality and in infected pancreatic complications with total enteral nutrition. *Digestive Surg* 23:336-345, 2006.
11. Petrov MS, Whelan K. Comparison of complications attributable to enteral and parenteral nutrition in predicted severe acute pancreatitis: a systematic review and meta-analysis. *Br J Nutr* 103:1287-1295, 2010.
12. Harris JP, Parnell NK, Griffith EH, et al. Retrospective evaluation of the impact of early enteral nutrition on clinical outcomes in dogs with pancreatitis: 34 cases (2010-2013). *J Vet Emerg Crit Care* 27(4):425-433, 2017.
13. Mansfield CS, James CE, Steiner JM, et al. A pilot study to assess tolerability of early enteral nutrition via esophagostomy tube feeding in dogs with severe acute pancreatitis. *J Vet Intern Med* 25:419-425, 2011.
14. Mohr AJ, Leisewitz AL, Jacobson LS, et al. Effect of early enteral nutrition on intestinal permeability, intestinal protein loss, and outcomes in dogs with severe parvoviral enteritis. *J Vet Intern Med* 17:791-798, 2003.
15. Will K, Nolte I, Zentek J. Early enteral nutrition in young dogs suffering from haemorrhagic gastroenteritis. *J Vet Med Series A* 52(7):371-376, 2005.
16. Dumont R, Lemetayer J, Desquilbet L, et al. Tolerability of naso-esophageal feeding tubes in dogs and cats at home: Retrospective review of 119 cases. *J Vet Intern Med* 37(6):2315-2321, 2023.
17. Mansfield CS. Acute pancreatitis in dogs: advances in understanding, diagnostics and treatment. *Top Companion Anim Med* 27:123-32, 2012.
18. Chan DL, Freeman LM, Labato M, et al. Retrospective evaluation of partial parenteral nutrition in dogs and cats. *J Vet Intern Med* 16:440-445, 2002.
19. Gianotti L, Meier R, Lobo DN, et al. ESPEN Guidelines on Parenteral Nutrition: Pancreas. *Clin Nutr* 28:428-435, 2009.
20. Yang X, Zhang R, Jin T, et al. Stress hyperglycemia is independently associated with persistent organ failure in acute pancreatitis. *Dig Dis Sci* 67:1879-1889, 2022.
21. Chan DL. Parenteral Nutrition in Small Animals. In Chan D (editor). Nutritional Management of Hospitalized Small Animals. Chichester, West Sussex, Wiley Blackwell, 2015, pp.100-116.
22. Villaverde C, Hervera M. Nutritional management of exocrine pancreatic diseases. In Fascetti, Delaney, Larsen, Villaverde (editors). Applied Veterinary Clinical Nutrition 2nd edition. Hoboken, John Wiley & Sons, 2024, pp. 299-317.
23. Bauer JE. Evaluation and dietary consideration in idiopathic hyperlipidemia in dogs. *J Am Vet Med Assoc* 206(11):1684-88, 1995.
24. LeBlanc CJ, Bauer JE, Hosgood G, et al. Effect of dietary fish oil and vitamin E supplementation on hematologic and serum biochemical analytes and oxidative status in young dogs. *Vet Ther* 6(4):325-340, 2005.
25. Westermarck E, Wiberg ME. Effects of diet on clinical signs of exocrine pancreatic insufficiency in dogs. *J Am Vet Med Assoc* 228:225-229, 2006.
26. Westermarck E, Junttila JT, Wiberg ME. Role of low dietary fat in the treatment of dogs with exocrine pancreatic insufficiency. *Am J Vet Res* 56:600-605, 1995.
27. Davies RH, Lawes JR, Wales AD. Raw diet for dogs and cats: a review of particular reference to microbiological hazards. *J Small Anim Pract* 60(6):329-339, 2019.

CHAPTER 23

Analgesia in acute and chronic pancreatitis

Ian Self
BSc. BVSc, CertVA, DECVAA, PGCertVetEd, PGCert, MAPP, MAcadMedEd FHEA, FRCVS

Disease definition and etiology

Pain is commonly recognized as one of the cardinal clinical signs of pancreatitis in dogs and cats. The International Association of Pain (IASP) definition of pain has recently been changed and is: "An unpleasant sensory and emotional experience associated with, or resembling that associated with actual or potential tissue damage".[1] The definition is expanded upon by the addition of six keynotes and the etymology of the word pain for contextual content, and of particular relevance to veterinary practitioners is the note that "inability to communicate does not negate the possibility that a human or a nonhuman animal experiences pain". Thus, the emphasis is on the veterinary professional to both recognize and treat pain associated with pancreatitis.

The importance of pain has also been emphasized by the WSAVA, which produced the Global Pain Management Guidelines in 2022.[2] In the document, it is argued that pain should be considered equally alongside other clinical signs when assessing a case: "Pain is the fourth vital sign and should be incorporated into the TPR (temperature, pulse, respiration) assessment of every patient", and this is particularly important when deciding on the approach to pancreatitis in dogs and cats. It is considered likely by the author that pain in animals is worse than similar pain in humans as animals are "locked in" to their pain with no concept of the possibility of analgesia.

Irrespective of the ethical obligations of veterinary professionals to relieve suffering, untreated pain leads to several adverse physiological effects, including the release of cortisol, poor immune function, and initiation of a catabolic state.[3] Pain management in pancreatitis cases should, therefore, be a primary treatment goal.

Clinical presentation and features

Clinical signs of acute or chronic pancreatitis are varied and often nonspecific and share similar features with other abdominal conditions, as discussed elsewhere in this book, particularly in chapters 18 and 19. However, one of the major clinical signs is abdominal pain, which is often severe and refractory to treatment in cases of acute pancreatitis and apparently low-grade but refractory with a "waxing and waning" pattern in cases of chronic pancreatitis.[4] This offers challenges in the analgesic treatment of the condition, as acutely presenting patients may require hospitalization for adequate intervention. Conversely, cases of chronic pancreatitis are a challenge in terms of recognizing the subtle and nonspecific signs of pain and recognizing how severe this pain is, and there are limited analgesic agents available for the long-term control of chronic pain in the home setting.

Despite the variety of presenting signs, pain is a consistent symptom. In a questionnaire sent to Italian veterinarians in first opinion practice, pancreatitis was highlighted as the most frequent cause of abdominal visceral pain (19% of respondents). Pain recognition was based on posture, gait, and movement changes (32%) and physiological changes (31%), and pancreatitis and peritonitis were considered the most painful abdominal conditions. In the same study, 97% of respondents believed that their knowledge regarding pain management required improvement, emphasizing the need for more continuing education in the subject.[5]

Clinically, abdominal pain is diffuse and difficult to localize and may be confused with spinal/back pain. The range of signs exhibited by animals is incredibly diverse and can range from changes in behavior, including altered bowel and urinary habits, to alterations in mood, including withdrawal and aggression, and nausea and vomiting associated with autonomic nervous system activation.[6] In acute cases, patients often appear hunched and reluctant to move. They occasionally exhibit the prayer position/lordosis associated with cranial abdominal pain (Fig. 23.1).[7] However, this is not specific to pancreas pain, and the author will commonly also see patients who exhibit this position with renal pain. Physiological changes are common, although the underlying disease may produce these. Finally, reaction to abdominal palpation, when tender areas are examined, will help confirm the origin of the pain.

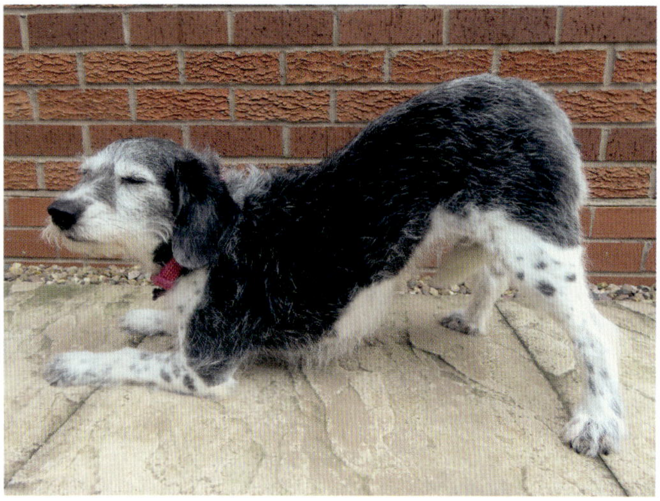

FIG. 23.1 "Prayer position" typically exhibited by dogs experiencing cranial abdominal pain.

Clinicopathological findings

Abdominal viscera are innervated by nociceptors that respond to mechanical, chemical, or thermal activation as with somatic nociceptors. Inflammation of the pancreas is likely to lead to stretch in the capsule as well as inflict pressure on organs in the vicinity of the organ. Premature activation of proteases within the pancreas leads to altered cellular pH and alterations in intracellular calcium concentrations (nociceptive), which initiates neutrophil migration into the pancreas, ultimately leading to cell necrosis and an exacerbation of inflammation. In severe cases, there may also be localized peritonitis. As well as the direct effects, hypoventilation is often recognized in acute pancreatitis as deep diaphragmatic excursions are painful, leading to a typical pattern of fast and shallow respiration without adequate alveolar ventilation.

Pain originating from abdominal organs is poorly localized because innervation is by a sparse number of nociceptors supplied by C fibers (slow transmission, high-activation threshold fibers[3]). In addition, large overlapping receptive fields exhibit a graded response to stimulation. Multiple mechanoreceptors are also present in the walls of hollow viscera and solid organ capsules that respond to distension.

Another feature of abdominal pain is somatic-visceral convergence.[8] This refers to nociceptive input from visceral structures such as the pancreas projected as pain into more distal somatic structures that share the same segmental innervation, obfuscating the true source of pain. This typically leads to difficulties in distinguishing renal or spinal pain from that caused by pancreatitis. Visceral pain is also associated with marked autonomic activation, including changes in body temperature, blood pressure, heart rate, nausea, and GI disturbances such as diarrhea and nausea/vomiting.

The motivational, affective, and behavioral aspects of severe pancreatic pain should also be considered.[3] Fear and anxiety increase pain perception. Many labile connections exist between pain pathways and neuroendocrine and limbic systems (pain, pleasure, autonomic components). In addition, the cortex responds to pain, giving rise to the behavioral component, which may be assessed by validated small animal pain scales (see below).

The final source of pain, which the author has seen in many cases, is pain originating from the esophagus. Many patients with acute pancreatitis will present with overt vomiting or esophageal reflux with resultant lesions of esophagitis apparent on endoscopic examination. In extreme cases, there may also be aspiration pneumonia. Both conditions are painful and should be addressed in addition to the primary source of discomfort.

Other diagnostic procedures

Pancreatic pain can be challenging to diagnose and localize, but basic principles should always apply. Alterations in behavior, abnormal gait/posture, reaction to abdominal palpation, and signs of autonomic response should always raise the suspicion of pain. Owner reports of changes in the dog's routine at home should also raise the index of suspicion that pain may be present, and an excellent way of confirming this is to see the response to a test dose of a suitable analgesic agent, which often results in a return to normal behavior for the duration of the treatment.

Once diagnosed with acute or chronic pancreatitis, every patient should receive analgesia even if they are not showing obvious pain symptoms because of the difficulties inherent in diagnosis and monitoring of visceral pain, as discussed above.

Of additional use when monitoring response to analgesia is the use of pain scales. Several validated pain scoring systems allow an attempt to quantify acute pain and adjust analgesia accordingly, although pain scoring should never override clinical examination and decision-making. In particular, companion animals that are expected to be painful but score low on pain scales should always be given the "benefit of doubt", and analgesia should be administered.

The author uses the Glasgow Short Form scales (canine and feline) for acute pancreatitis cases. One of the steps in the scale, developed for surgical pain, is palpation of an area "at least 5 cm from the wound" to detect allodynia (perception of a nonpainful stimulus as pain). As this is difficult in cases of pancreatic pain, the author palpates over both sides of the thorax at approximately the level of the tenth rib to see if the patient reacts. Assessing chronic pancreatitis pain is much more challenging, and the author favors client-specific outcome measures and the Helsinki Chronic Pain Index as tools to guide intervention. The available scales are shown in Table 23.1.

As well as addressing pain, treating pancreatitis cases should always consider the patient's quality of life. Mostly, this will involve discussions with the owner regarding prognosis and "suffering", but these conversations can be guided by the use of validated quality of life scales such as the Vetmetrica HRQOL (health-related quality of life) system (http://www.newmetrica.com/).[11]

TABLE 23.1 Validated pain scales suitable for monitoring pain in pancreatitis patients.

Acute pain scales	Chronic pain scales
■ Glasgow Short Form – canine	■ Canine Brief Pain Inventory (CBPI) ■ Helsinki Chronic Pain Index (HCPI) ■ Client questionnaire of behavioral and lifestyle changes[9] ■ Client-Specific Outcome Measures (CSOM)[10]

While it should rarely be a first-line treatment, euthanasia on humane grounds is always an option, especially in the cases of severe, unresponsive pain, despite the interventions listed below. Although a disappointing outcome for all concerned, this still remains the ultimate way of controlling pain in some cases.

Treatment of pancreatitis pain

Introduction and evidence

Analgesic therapy should be aggressive and immediate in any case of suspected pancreatitis, even in those patients not exhibiting overt pain behaviors.[12] The WSAVA has recently published guidelines for the recognition and treatment of pain, and the reader is advised to consult this document for additional details.[2] Another useful resource is the World Health Organization (WHO) analgesic ladder, recently modified by Anekar et al., 2023.[13] The diagram below (Fig. 23.2) shows the modified ladder, indicating the type of pharmacological analgesic agents suitable for various pain presentations. The modification adds invasive and minimally invasive interventions (e.g., epidural analgesia) as a fourth step and emphasizes the fact that the ladder is bidirectional and that once adequate pain control has been achieved, it is appropriate to decrease the level of intervention.

In veterinary medicine, there is a paucity of controlled studies examining the benefits and risks associated with commonly used analgesic agents in the management of acute or chronic pancreatitis. Therefore, most recommendations are extrapolated from human guidelines and based on experience in the management of this condition. Several published guidelines exist for the management of pancreatitis in humans, and the reader is referred to references 14 and 15 as examples. Another overriding consideration when choosing analgesic therapies is the side effect profile in relation to the physiological status of the patient, and these considerations are discussed under the relevant analgesic class below.

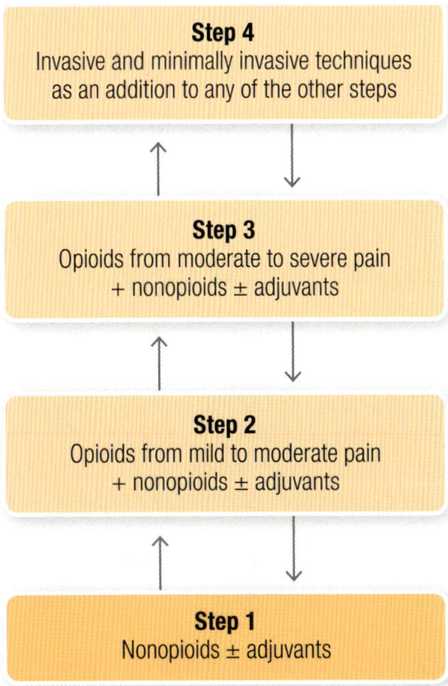

FIG. 23.2 Diagram showing the modified WHO analgesic ladder, representing different analgesic interventions appropriate for different pain levels.

Analgesic protocols for acute and chronic pancreatitis

It should always be appreciated that the intensity of pain felt will vary between individuals, and as such, there are no set analgesia protocols suitable for all patients. Constant evaluation of the treatment is necessary, using pain scoring techniques to guide decision-making. Acute pancreatitis can generally be managed with opioids, lidocaine (dogs only), ketamine and other centrally acting agents, epidural and other local analgesic techniques, intravenous paracetamol (dogs only), and physical therapies. Oral therapies may need to continue in these cases for some time after discharge. Chronic pancreatitis pain can be managed with oral opioids, oral paracetamol, and potentially nonsteroidal anti-inflammatory drugs, depending on the patient's cardiovascular, hepatic, and renal status (see below). A range of additional agents have been reported for use, and these are discussed below. Suggested doses are found in any veterinary formulary, and opioids are shown in Table 23.2.

Referral to specialized pain management clinics is also an option for any pancreatitis case. Such clinics will work with the patient and the referring clinician to ensure that a suitable pain management protocol is in place and will be in a position to offer advanced analgesic techniques where appropriate to aid recovery of the patient.

TABLE 23.2 Opioids commonly used for the control of acute pancreatic pain.

Opioid	Loading dose	Maintenance dose	Comments/side effects
Methadone	0.1-0.5 mg/kg IV/IM depending on response	Repeat every 4 hours or as needed. Infuse at 0.1-0.2 mg/kg/h	May cause nausea. Care with prolonged infusion –preservative
Morphine	0.1-0.5 mg/kg IV/IM depending on response	Repeat every 4 hours or as needed. Infuse at 0.1-0.2 mg/kg/h	May cause nausea and histamine release. Preservative-free favored for IV infusions
Pethidine (meperidine)	3-5 mg/kg IM	Repeat every 90 minutes as needed	Must not be given IV –serious risk of histamine release
Fentanyl	0.002-0.005 mg/kg IV	CRI dose of 3-10 µg/kg/h IV	May cause bradycardia, and initial bolus may cause temporary apnea
Remifentanil	Limited data – suggest use of fentanyl as a loading drug as above	CRI dose of 5-20 µg/kg/h IV	May cause bradycardia. No hepatic metabolism, so theoretical drug of choice in hepatic disease

Acute pancreatitis

While not a fixed protocol, the author favors hospitalization for acute pancreatitis cases to gain control of the pain, which is often extreme and difficult to manage. The approach to pain control is stepwise based on the WHO analgesic ladder and pain scale assessment, but the degree of pain often necessitates initial opioid therapy, using full mu agonists such as methadone, pethidine, fentanyl, or morphine given as intermittent boluses or as a constant rate IV infusion. Unless contraindicated (severe hepatic disease), the author also administers paracetamol, usually at a dose of 15 mg/kg IV three times daily. If, on assessment, this is not providing adequate analgesia, the next step is typically to add in ketamine and/or lidocaine infusions as part of the "MLK" constant rate infusion –see below. In cases where there is still not adequate pain control, the application of local anesthetic techniques should be considered.

In humans, epidural analgesia is an alternative for a full mu opioid agonist administered via the intravenous route or given alongside systemic opioids as part of a multimodal approach.[14] In dogs, placing an epidural catheter or a single epidural administered under general anesthesia should be considered where adequate pain control is not achieved using systemic analgesics. An epidural catheter allows the use of 0.1 mg/kg preservative-free morphine to be administered every 24 hours as required.

Other local anesthetic techniques reported in the literature for treating pancreatitis pain include ganglion blocks in humans[16] and erector spinae blocks in a dog.[17] In refractory pancreatic pain cases, the author has administered a local analgesic agent in the vicinity of the celiac plexus ganglion under ultrasound guidance with excellent clinical response, effectively resetting the pain threshold and allowing other systemic agents to "take over" pain control. This procedure should always be carried out in an anesthetized patient by a suitably trained individual due to the proximity of major blood vessels near the ganglion.

Home management after acute pancreatitis

Following adequate analgesia in hospitalized patients, it is always necessary to maintain analgesic therapy after discharge, as typically, patients will remain painful for several weeks before resolution. Usually, this consists of paracetamol and/or oral opioids such as transmucosal buprenorphine or oral tapentadol (unlicenced oral opioid). In addition, tramadol has previously been used for this purpose, but current evidence points to a lack of efficacy, and the author does not recommend its use – see later discussion. Some authors advocate the use of nonsteroidal anti-inflammatory agents, but it must always be remembered that patients must be fully rehydrated with normal renal and hepatic function and no evidence of gastric mucosal damage before these agents are considered suitable due to their side effect profile. The decision to use NSAIDs should be taken on a case-by-case basis and should not be administered during acute flare-ups.

Management of chronic pancreatitis

While many patients may not exhibit the overt signs of pain, it should always be considered likely that chronic pancreatitis will present with a waxing and waning degree of discomfort, which will require ongoing analgesic management, often aided using repeated pain scale evaluation. Owner cooperation is vital, and any reported change in behavior should be a red flag for inadequate pain control.

Unfortunately, there is still a lack of suitable agents for the control of chronic pancreatic pain despite the prevalence of the condition, and as discussed, treatment plans should be formulated based on the presentation and comorbidities of the patient. Initially, the author will use oral paracetamol administered three times daily at a dose of 15 mg/kg, dropping to twice daily if adequate analgesia is obtained. The dose can be increased should the patient appear uncomfortable, and the normal recommendation is to give 30 mg/kg three times daily in the case of flares for up to 5 days, but always to seek professional help in these circumstances as it may be necessary to hospitalize and treat aggressively as outlined above.

There are anecdotal reports of chronic pancreatic pain responding to neuropathic pain treatments such as gabapentin or pregabalin (see discussion below). The author regularly adds these agents into an analgesic regime if the patient exhibits poorly controlled pain and will also add memantine, a centrally-acting analgesic effective in some chronic pain states. However, only one agent at a time is added so the effect of the agent on pain control can be assessed.

In addition to pharmacological intervention, low-fat diets and suitable environmental stimulation and enrichment are vital to maintaining the quality of life of the patients, including ensuring good interaction between pet and owner to strengthen the bonds that will comfort a chronically ill pet. Our animal companions are comforted by stroking, petting, careful nursing, and gentle handling. It must be remembered that pain is an unpleasant experience, and taking care of a patient's emotional needs will decrease the experience of pain and allow the animal to cope.

Other physical therapies should also be explored. For example, Lindley (2019)[18] advocates the use of acupuncture, arguing that visceral pain can create myofascial pain in epaxial and abdominal muscles supplied by the same nerves as the viscera, and it is possible that these "trigger points" will maintain pain states in between pancreatitis flare-ups.

Pharmacological agents used in the management of pancreatitis

Opioids

Despite minor side effects, there are very few contraindications to opioid use, and these should be used to provide analgesia even in cardiovascularly compromised patients with acute pancreatitis. Most are controlled drugs with associated legal requirements and exert their effects via opioid receptors, the most important from an analgesia perspective being the mu receptor, agonism of which results in profound analgesia.

There is some controversy in veterinary medicine about the use of opioids for analgesia in pancreatitis cases. Firstly, some opioids, such as morphine, may cause vomiting and histamine release. However, this vomiting is usually seen in nonpainful animals, especially those receiving morphine as a premedicant prior to anesthesia, and can be easily controlled with antiemetics such as ondansetron. According to human trials, Stigliano et al. (2017)[15] stated, "there is no credible clinical evidence to avoid the use of morphine in treating the pain associated with acute pancreatitis". However, Leppäniemi et al. (2019)[14] recommend that in humans the use of hydromorphone is encouraged instead of morphine, although hydromorphone is not commonly used in veterinary medicine, methadone would be a sensible alternative (see details below). A further controversy exists concerning the sphincter of Oddi. It has traditionally been cited that full mu opioids such as morphine and methadone may cause contraction of the sphincter of Oddi with resultant restriction of outflow along the pancreatic duct, although there is no evidence in animals that this is of clinical concern. In addition, the sphincter of Oddi in dogs only controls flow through the bile duct with a separate pancreatic duct, and therefore, this argument is irrelevant.[19]

The notes below outline the most important features of selected opioids.

- Methadone: in Europe, methadone is licensed for use in dogs and is a full mu agonist. It is also an N-methyl-D-aspartate (NMDA) receptor antagonist, which is involved in developing central sensitization that can lead to chronic (pathological) pain states. It is unlikely to cause vomiting (unlike morphine) and is commonly used in acutely painful patients, providing excellent, titratable analgesia. The onset of action is 10-15 minutes by IV or IM injection, with a duration of action of up to 4 hours in dogs and up to 6 hours in cats. Methadone can be administered by IV or IM injection. Boluses can cause temporary apnea and/or bradycardia, and although this is extremely unlikely in painful patients at clinical doses, it is recommended that it is injected slowly if given via the intravenous (IV) route. Methadone has been used as an IV infusion at approximately 0.1-0.2 mg/kg/h, but this author recommends caution as commercially available methadone contains preservatives, so it is recommended to limit an infusion to a maximum of 12 hours.

- Morphine: morphine is not currently licensed in veterinary species. However, it is very hydrophilic compared to other full mu agonist opioids and is therefore still commonly given by epidural injection, where it remains in the epidural space, providing analgesia for up to 24 hours. If given IV or IM to pancreatitis patients, care should be taken as administration can lead to histamine release and occasional vomiting (with the first dose only), although this is less likely in already painful patients –see above.
- Fentanyl: fentanyl is a full mu agonist with an extremely rapid onset and short duration of action licensed in dogs in Europe and the USA for IV bolus or infusion. A fentanyl bolus can cause bradycardia or apnea, and for this reason, it is usually given as a constant rate infusion. Fentanyl transdermal patches (unlicensed) have been used in dogs and can provide analgesia for several days. The author will sometimes use an initial fentanyl CRI to offer immediate analgesia to pancreatitis cases, and when the pain is at an acceptable level, switch to methadone boluses as required, depending on pain scores.
- Pethidine: pethidine (meperidine) is a full mu agonist licensed in dogs in Europe. It is unique in that it is unlikely to cause bradycardia but must not be administered IV as it can cause histamine release, which would be detrimental in hypovolemic pancreatitis patients. Unfortunately, intramuscular injection of pethidine appears painful and has a short duration of action (around 90 minutes), therefore reducing its clinical usefulness. However, the author finds pethidine to be a very useful drug to use as a "test analgesic" to confirm that pain is present, and it appears to offer excellent abdominal analgesia at appropriate doses (author's dose range 3-5 mg/kg IM). Its use is contraindicated with other drugs which increase serotonin concentrations.
- Buprenorphine: buprenorphine is a partial mu agonist licensed in dogs and cats to treat mild to moderate pain. Its relatively weak analgesic properties, together with its slow onset, mean it is not recommended as the initial opioid in acute pancreatitis cases. It has a longer duration of action than most opioids (up to 6 hours in dogs). Buprenorphine has been administered to dogs via the oral transmucosal route at the same or higher doses as systemic injections (generally between 20 µg/kg and 120 µg/kg) and has been useful for owners to administer in the home environment.
- Butorphanol: butorphanol is a kappa agonist and a mu antagonist. Butorphanol is a good sedative but a poor analgesic, and it is unlikely to provide adequate analgesia in any pancreatitis case.

"Traditional" nonsteroidal anti-inflammatory drugs

Nonsteroidal anti-inflammatory drugs (NSAIDs) include many agents used to provide analgesia, decrease inflammation, and reduce temperature. Several licensed NSAIDs have an important role in both perioperative and long-term analgesia. The mechanism of action of most NSAIDs is via peripheral inhibition of the activity of cyclo-oxygenase enzyme (COX-1 and COX-2), reducing prostaglandin (PG) synthesis, which are peripheral proinflammatory mediators.

There is controversy surrounding the use of NSAIDs in acute pancreatitis, mainly around the potential side effects of these agents in clinically unwell patients. Many acute pancreatitis patients will have a combination of vomiting, diarrhea, and anorexia and often be hypovolemic. NSAIDs are contraindicated in hypovolemia, and therefore, the use of this class of drug should only be considered once the patient is cardiovascularly stable with normal renal, hepatic, and GI function.

Piprant class nonsteroidal anti-inflammatory drugs

Because of the potential for adverse events associated with the inhibition of COX enzymes, an EP4 prostaglandin receptor antagonist, grapiprant (Galliprant™), has been developed for use in dogs, which blocks the action of prostaglandin E2 (PGE2), one of the major proinflammatory prostaglandins. Grapiprant is a piprant class NSAID licensed for the treatment of mild to moderate osteoarthritis pain and inflammation in dogs in Europe and the U.S. There are currently no reports of the use of grapiprant for acute medical presentations, and the reader is urged to exercise the same caution and criteria as if using a traditional NSAID as discussed above. Adverse events reported include vomiting, diarrhea, decreased appetite, and tiredness, although these are often self-limiting.

Paracetamol

Paracetamol is not classed as an NSAID, and its major action is as a central analgesic and antipyretic agent. Despite widespread use, there is limited clinical data to support the use of paracetamol as an analgesic in dogs, but it is commonly used at a dose rate of 10 to 15 mg/kg by slow IV injection up to three times daily as part of a multimodal analgesic regime.

Although the use of paracetamol may be considered controversial in cases of acute pancreatitis because of the potential for concurrent hepatic disease, it is commonly used as an adjunct analgesic agent when there is no overt reduced liver function, and anecdotally it appears to add useful analgesia with minimal side effects.

Paracetamol can be combined with other agents, including NSAIDs and steroids. Paracetamol is also available as a licensed formulation for dogs in the UK only in combination with codeine (a weak opioid prodrug with limited efficacy), but it is only licensed for up to 5 days of use. However, the author uses paracetamol under the drug cascade for longer-term administration and control of low-grade, chronic pain, including that from recurrent pancreatitis. Paracetamol should never be administered to cats.

Local anesthetic agents

Local anesthetics are versatile and inexpensive agents that can be applied in a number of ways, including systemic, topical, regional, and intravenous routes.

In dogs, lidocaine can be administered as an intravenous infusion, where it has been shown to have analgesic properties. Unfortunately, there are no controlled veterinary trials looking at the use of lidocaine in pancreatitis cases as a sole agent, and it is very difficult to quantify its effect as part of a multimodal approach to pain control. In humans, current recommendations are "There is no evidence to support the use of parenterally administered local anesthetics (procaine) in the management of pain associated with acute pancreatitis".[14] Despite this, in severe, intractable pancreatic pain, the author does add in lidocaine as part of an infusion alongside opioids and ketamine (see below) as it is unlikely to have significant side effect and may contribute to the patient's comfort.

Ketamine

Ketamine is a very versatile licensed analgesic agent in dogs that acts via noncompetitive inhibition of the N-methyl-D-aspartate (NMDA) receptor. Ketamine can be useful as part of a multimodal approach to pancreatitis pain and may be an important agent in stopping the development of chronic, pathological pain via interaction with spinal cord receptors. A single bolus (0.25-1 mg/kg IV) lasts around 20 minutes, and it is therefore often administered as an infusion at 10 µg/kg-1 min-1. In the UK, ketamine is a controlled drug and should be stored and recorded accordingly.

Alpha-2 receptor agonists

Medetomidine, dexmedetomidine, and xylazine offer excellent "visceral" analgesia and can be used as an adjunct method of relieving pain. The analgesia after a single administration is short-lived (up to 40 minutes), and these drugs are thus administered as an intravenous infusion at doses around 1-2 µg/kg/h (dexmedetomidine/medetomidine). They are particularly useful in anxious patients who may also require mild sedation.

There are two areas of concern with the use of these agents in pancreatitis cases. The primary concern is that they cause profound peripheral vasoconstriction and resultant bradycardia and reduction in cardiac output, which could be extremely dangerous in patients with compromised fluid balance, and they should only be considered in cardiovascularly stable patients. Secondly, they possess potent anti-insulin effects, leading to glucosuria, polyuria, and increased blood glucose levels. As a significant number of pancreatitis patients present either with diabetes mellitus or with a reduced islet cell reserve (acute on chronic cases), the use of alpha-2 agonists as analgesic agents in this group of patients should be considered only if no alternatives exist.

Constant rate infusions

For severe and intractable pain, it is often useful to combine some of the agents listed above as a constant rate infusion. In hospitalized patients, this involves the use of morphine or methadone, lidocaine, and ketamine in a so-called "MLK" infusion. This combination should not be used in cats who are very sensitive to the toxic effects of local anesthetics, but the use of methadone/ketamine infusions is possible. There are several approaches to the infusion, but the author will add 50 mg ketamine, 50 mg morphine or methadone, and 500 mg of adrenaline-free lidocaine to 500 ml 0.9% saline and infuse at 1 ml/kg/h with a pump or syringe driver (range 0.5-2 ml/kg/h depending on the response). Dogs receiving this treatment are often sedated, and good monitoring is essential, but excellent analgesia is obtained.

Tramadol

Tramadol acts as a synthetic opioid drug via the M1 metabolite (O-desmethyl tramadol), which is the active component. Even though there is a formulation licensed for use in dogs in the UK and Europe, there is a growing body of evidence that the efficacy of tramadol in dogs is extremely limited, and this author does not recommend its use as a sole agent to control pain, with very few dogs being able to produce the active metabolite.

Gabapentin and pregabalin

These are unlicenced anticonvulsant drugs with analgesic effects, particularly for treating neuropathic pain. The exact mode of action is uncertain, and there are no controlled trials examining the efficacy in chronic pancreatitis. However, as part of a multimodal approach to pain therapy, their use should be considered alongside other analgesic agents where they may exhibit some benefit, using pain scales to guide effectiveness. The drugs are totally eliminated via the renal route, so care should be taken in patients with significant renal disease. A degree of sedation is likely when initially administering these drugs, and owners should be informed accordingly.

Amantadine and memantine

These human antiviral drugs have significant NMDA receptor antagonist effects similar to ketamine and are available in tablet and liquid (amantadine) form, but unlike ketamine, they are not controlled substances. The drugs appear to be synergistic with opioids and NSAIDs and have been successfully used as sole analgesic agents in various pain states, including neuropathic pain, although there are no reports of sole use to control pancreatic pain. They may cause sedation and occasionally vomiting, which may require symptomatic treatment and may be a concern in pancreatic disease patients.

Currently, the use of amantadine in animal medications is subject to an EU ban due to the discovery of resistance to its antiviral effects in human populations. The author now uses memantine as an alternative.

Amitriptyline

There is emerging evidence of the direct analgesic effects of amitriptyline, a tricyclic antidepressant, and it could be considered part of a multimodal approach in complex cases. The dose is between 0.25 mg/kg and 2 mg/kg once to twice a day in dogs, with lower doses reported to be more efficient in terms of analgesia in human medicine.

Miscellaneous analgesic agents

Maropitant

Maropitant is a neurokinin-1 receptor (NK-1) antagonist used to treat and prevent emesis by blocking NK-1 receptors in the chemoreceptor trigger zone in the CNS. Studies in mice and rabbits have demonstrated that NK-1 receptor antagonists consistently induce analgesia to visceral noxious stimulation, but this information should not be extrapolated to small animals as clinical analgesia does not seem to be relevant, and there is no clear evidence that maropitant should be relied upon as an analgesic in the clinical setting.[20]

Ondansetron

Ondansetron is a serotonin type 3 (5-HT3) receptor antagonist acting as an antiemetic and antinausea drug.[21] Although maropitant and ondansetron have no proven analgesic actions, they are still important components in the overall management of patients with pancreatitis, bearing in mind the autonomic components of visceral pain as outlined previously.

KEY POINTS

- Pain from acute or chronic pancreatitis is relentless, debilitating, and can contribute directly to morbidity and mortality. From both a welfare and a clinical point of view, aggressive and timely treatment is essential to improve the outcome.
  While no gold standard recommendations exist, by careful titration of drug combinations (guided by modes of action and side effects) and doses, plus responding to the outcome of the treatments (ideally using pain scales and recording the effects of the analgesics chosen), an individualized plan should be constructed for each case which will improve outcome and contribute to animal welfare.

References

1. Raja SN, Carr DB, Cohen M, Finnerup NB, et al. The revised International Association for the Study of Pain definition of pain: concepts, challenges, and compromises. *Pain* 161(9):1976-1982, 2020.
2. Monteiro BP, Lascelles BDX, Murrell J, Robertson SP, Steagall VM, Wright B. WSAVA guidelines for the recognition, assessment and treatment of pain. *J Small Anim Pract* 64:177- 254, 2022.
3. Self I, Grubb T. Physiology of pain. In Self, I (editor). BSAVA Guide to Pain Management in Small Animal Practice. UK, 2019, BSAVA.
4. Watson P. Pancreatitis in dogs and cats: definitions and pathophysiology. *J Small Anim Pract* 56(1):3-12, 2015.
5. Catanzaro A, Di Salvo A, Steagall PV, Zampini D, Angela Polisca A, della Rocca G. Preliminary study on attitudes, opinions and knowledge of Italian veterinarians with regard to abdominal visceral pain in dogs. *Vet Anaesth Analg* 43(4):361-370, 2016.
6. Peligrand L, Mora SS. Pain assessment methods. In Duke-Novakovski T, De Vries M, Seymour C (editors). BSAVA Manual of Canine and Feline Anaesthesia and Analgesia. Gloucester, 2015, BSAVA.
7. Kisielewicz C. Abdominal pain. In Self, I (editor) .BSAVA Guide to Pain Management in Small Animal Practice. UK, 2019, BSAVA.
8. Sharma GS, Kirsten Tillisch K. (). Visceral pain: mechanisms, syndromes, and treatment. In Pangarkar S, Pham QG, Eapen BC (editors). Pain Care Essentials and Innovations. Elsevier, 2021, pp 45-58.
9. Slingerland LI, Hazewinkel HAW, Meij BP, Picavet P, Voorhout G. Cross-sectional study of the prevalence and clinical features of osteoarthritis in 100 cats. *Vet J* 187(3):304-309, 2011.
10. Lascelles BDX, Hansen BD, Roe S, DePuy V, Thomson A, Pierce CC, Smith ES, Rowinski E. Evaluation of client-specific outcome measures and activity monitoring to measure pain relief in cats with osteoarthritis. *J Vet Intern Med* 21(3):410-416, 2007.
11. Vetmetrica HRQOL (health-related quality of life) system. Available from: http://www.newmetrica.com/
12. Good JM. Acute pancreatitis. In Silverstein DC, Hopper K (editors). Small Animal Critical Care Medicine 3rd edition. Elsevier, 2023.
13. Anekar AA, Hendrix JM, Cascella M. WHO Analgesic Ladder. [Updated 2023 Apr 23]. In StatPearls [Internet]. Treasure Island (FL), StatPearls Publishing, 2023. Available from: https://www.ncbi.nlm.nih.gov/books/NBK554435/
14. Leppäniemi A, Tolonen M, Tarasconi A, Segovia-Lohse H, Gamberini E, et al. WSES guidelines for the management of severe acute pancreatitis. *World J Emerg Surg* 14: 27, 2019.
15. Stigliano S, Sternby H, de Madariac E, Capursoa G, Petrov MS. Early management of acute pancreatitis: A review of the best evidence. *Dig Liver Dis* 49(6):585-594, 2017.
16. Gunduz OH, Kenis-Coskun O. Ganglion blocks as a treatment of pain: current perspectives. *J Pain Res* 10:2815-2826, 2017.
17. Bartholomew KJ, Ferreira TH. Ultrasound-guided erector spinae plane block as part of a multimodal analgesic approach in a dog with acute pancreatitis. *Vet Anaesth Analg* 48:629, 2021.
18. Lindley S. Physical methods used to alleviate pain. In Self, I (editor). BSAVA Guide to Pain Management in Small Animal Practice. UK, 2019, BSAVA.
19. Corletto F, Jolliffe C. Pharmacological treatment of pain. In Self, I (editor). BSAVA Guide to Pain Management in Small Animal Practice. UK, 2019, BSAVA.
20. Kinobe RT, Miyake Y. Evaluating the anti-inflammatory and analgesic properties of maropitant: A systematic review and meta-analysis. *Vet J* 259:105471, 2020.
21. Foth S, Meller S, Kenward H, Elliott J, Pelligand L, Volk HA. The use of ondansetron for the treatment of nausea in dogs with vestibular syndrome. *BMC Vet Res* 17(1):1-9, 2021.

Nonspecific laboratory tests in hepatobiliary disease

Cassia Hare
MA, VetMB, AFHEA, DACVP (Clin Path), DECVCP, MRCVS

Given the central role of the liver in the metabolism of lipids, carbohydrates and vitamins, the synthesis of proteins and the excretion of nitrogenous waste products, it is logical that hepatobiliary disease may result in abnormalities in laboratory parameters outside of commonly measured "hepatobiliary markers". In the patient with liver disease, such changes are most often encountered due to reduced hepatic functional capacity and as such, many are considered indirect indicators of hepatic function and of liver failure, in which there is significant loss of functional mass (<20% remaining). However, they are by their nature nonspecific and may also be affected by numerous extrahepatic diseases.

Nonspecific changes on biochemistry screens

Total protein

Total protein comprises albumin and globulins, with the latter including all nonalbumin proteins. Whilst albumin is produced solely by the liver, globulins may be produced either by the liver (most alpha and beta globulins) or by cells of the immune system (gamma globulins). Hypoproteinemia due to hypoalbuminemia is one of the most common abnormalities encountered in patients with liver disease. However, since changes in both albumin and globulins can have additive or opposing effects on total protein concentration, they are addressed separately.

Albumin

Hypoalbuminemia is a common finding in dogs with liver disease and is typically mild to moderate in severity (albumin usually >20 g/L, occasionally lower), with marked hypoalbuminemia due to isolated liver disease being uncommon except in end-stage disease. Decreased albumin is one of the few laboratory-derived negative prognostic indicators in dogs with hepatitis.[1,2] Although most often interpreted as a result of reduced hepatic synthetic capacity when there is overt liver failure, hypoalbuminemia in these patients is often multifactorial, and other contributory factors may include inflammation (albumin is a negative acute phase protein, decreased when production of positive acute phase proteins is increased)[3] and gastrointestinal malabsorption, maldigestion, or loss associated with secondary pathology such as gastroduodenal ulceration.[4] Decreased or inadequate dietary intake (nutritional risk), which may accompany numerous diseases, including liver disease, has been considered a cause of hypoalbuminemia in humans,[5] and is suggested to occur in dogs.[6] A diagnostic algorithm for hypoalbuminemia can be found in chapter 13.

Albumin is a significant contributor to plasma oncotic pressure, and so hypoalbuminemia is a potential contributory factor in effusion formation in patients with liver disease (see ascites section below), where it may compound the effects of portal hypertension in causing ascites. In addition, its role as a carrier for insoluble organic molecules (such as unconjugated bilirubin) and positively charged minerals (such as calcium, magnesium, and copper) means that reductions in albumin may result in altered distribution of these substances, for example, reduced total calcium concentration.

Increased albumin concentrations (hyperalbuminemia) have been reported in association with hepatocellular carcinoma[7] and in a subset of Scottish Terriers with progressive vacuolar hepatopathy.[8] However, in practice, hyperalbuminemia is uncommon in liver disease except as the result of volume contraction in dehydrated patients.

Globulins

Globulins represent a diverse range of proteins with a variety of functions. However, the globulin concentration available as part of routine biochemistry profiles is simply a calculated value, total protein minus albumin. More specific measurement of globulin fractions requires serum protein electrophoresis, which separates globulins into alpha, beta, and gamma fractions based on their size and charge. Decreases in calculated globulin are uncommon in patients with liver disease, and isolated reductions in the alpha and beta globulins produced by the liver are generally not considered clinically significant. However, hepatobiliary disease associated with inflammation may result in increases in globulins driven by acute phase proteins and immunoglobulins. Inflammation may be further perpetuated by the disruption of immunological function in the diseased liver, which in health is responsible for tolerance and clearance of antigens originating in the GI tract.[9] Beta-gamma bridging (a lack of separation between beta and gamma globulin fractions) on electrophoresis has been linked with chronic hepatitis in dogs and humans.[10] However, it is nonspecific and also found in dogs with infectious diseases.[11] Detectable increases in globulin on routine biochemistry are typically attributable to immunoglobulins, whilst specific measurement of major acute phase proteins, including C-reactive protein (CRP) and serum amyloid A (SAA), is available commercially in some laboratories, with increases sometimes seen in inflammatory liver disease.

Urea

Urea is produced in the liver from detoxification of ammonia, which is derived from the breakdown of amino acids from both dietary proteins and tissues.[12] Severely reduced hepatic function may, therefore, result in decreases in urea on biochemistry. In patients with congenital PSS (portosystemic shunt), reduced delivery of ammonia to the liver for use in the urea cycle may result in low urea and raised ammonia, and in chronic liver disease, acquired portosystemic shunting is an important contributor to this. Negative nitrogen balance associated with anorexia and feeding a low protein diet can contribute to low urea, as can fluid therapy. There are rare reports of dogs with inherited disorders of metabolism associated with deficiencies in urea cycle enzymes. Since such errors of metabolism result in an inability to convert ammonia to urea, ammonia accumulates, and clinical signs of encephalopathy may occur. As such, the clinical presentation of these dogs may mimic that of primary hepatic disease (e.g., PSS). However, other evidence of hepatic dysfunction is lacking.

Approximately 50% of renal medullary tonicity and the resultant concentration gradient required for water reabsorption is due to urea, and so reductions in urea may contribute to reduced renal concentrating ability and, therefore, polyuria and polydipsia (PU/PD), with reduced urine specific gravity (USG). However, the clinician is sometimes faced with a diagnostic conundrum since diuresis and PU/PD of many causes are also mechanisms by which decreases in urea may occur. This is highlighted in Algorithm 24.1.

Increases in urea are most often encountered in association with reduced glomerular filtration rate (GFR), which is associated with azotemia. In the context of liver disease, increases in urea may occur when there is concurrent dehydration (resulting in prerenal azotemia, including in patients receiving diuretic therapy) or renal injury, for example, in the context of leptospirosis. Increased breakdown of protein in the gastrointestinal tract associated with bleeding is also a cause of increased urea and may occur with gastroduodenal ulceration (see chapter 13 for a more detailed discussion of causes of increases in urea).

Algorithm 24.1 Note 1 Acquired nephrogenic diabetes insipidus (NDI) is associated with an inadequate renal tubular response to antidiuretic hormone (ADH, also known as vasopressin) via many mechanisms. Although renal disease is a common cause of nephrogenic diabetes insipidus, it is uncommon for intrinsic renal disease to cause reductions in urea, given the concurrent reduction in glomerular filtration rate (GFR) and associated azotemia. The mechanism by which many conditions cause NDI is incompletely understood. As well as the mechanisms occurring with hepatic disease outlined in the urinalysis section, causes include:

- Hypercalcemia: the finding of total hypercalcemia on biochemistry should ideally be followed by measurement of ionized calcium. Since idiopathic hypercalcemia does not occur in dogs (unlike cats), further investigations into the underlying cause are warranted if ionized hypercalcemia is confirmed. Differential diagnoses include primary hyperparathyroidism, hypoadrenocorticism, vitamin D toxicosis, osteolytic or granulomatous disease, and neoplasia (most commonly via production of PTHrP).
- Hypoadrenocorticism: other typical associated hematological and biochemical changes in hypoadrenocorticism include the lack of a stress leukogram with or without lymphocytosis and eosinophilia, hyponatremia and hyperkalemia, azotemia, and hypercalcemia.
- Hyperadrenocorticism: the mechanism of altered renal concentrating ability may involve inhibition of ADH secretion and/or impaired tubular response to ADH. Typical signs of hyperadrenocorticism are anticipated and may include PU/PD and polyphagia, a potbellied appearance, and dermatological changes. Typical laboratory findings include a stress leukogram, increases in ALP (often marked due to induction of the corticosteroid isoenzyme) with or without accompanying increases in other liver enzymes (if there is an associated hepatopathy), and increases in lipase, cholesterol, and triglyceride.
- Persistent, marked hypokalemia.
- Endotoxemia, especially with pyometra.

Algorithm 24.1 Note 2 Any type of water deprivation should only be considered once other causes of polyuria/polydipsia (including causes of secondary nephrogenic diabetes insipidus) have been excluded. This testing can be dangerous if not adequately monitored and result in worsening of renal compromise if present. A safer alternative is to assess the response to DDAVP (a synthetic ADH).

Algorithm 24.1 Note 3 See chapter 25 for further information regarding more specific hepatic function tests. A persistent increase in ALT (particularly in the absence of evidence of a reactive hepatopathy) is more likely to indicate ongoing hepatocellular damage and, therefore, warrants further investigation.

Lipids

The liver plays a key role in lipid metabolism, acting as a hub for fatty acid and lipoprotein synthesis. Lipoproteins are molecules that enable the transport of water-insoluble lipids throughout the body and are made up of varying proportions of cholesterol and triglycerides, which may be readily measured as part of routine biochemistry and so are the focus of this section.

Cholesterol

Cholesterol is a steroid and a precursor of bile acids, cholesterol esters, and steroid hormones, as well as a vital component of cell membranes alongside phospholipids. Bile is the primary route of cholesterol excretion and so both hepatic and posthepatic causes of cholestasis may result in hypercholesterolemia,[13] with or without an accompanying increase in triglycerides (refer to chapter 13 for further information on hypercholesterolemia and a diagnostic algorithm). However, increases in cholesterol may occur in the absence of other evidence of cholestasis, and many alternative mechanisms of hyperlipidemia have been proposed in dogs with chronic hepatitis.[14] Abnormal lipid metabolism, hypercholesterolemia, and increases in red blood cell (RBC) membrane cholesterol content are implicated in the formation of poikilocytes (abnormally shaped RBCs) such as acanthocytes, which may accompany liver disease (Fig. 24.1).

ALGORITHM 24.1

Diagnostic approach to patients with low urea concentrations.

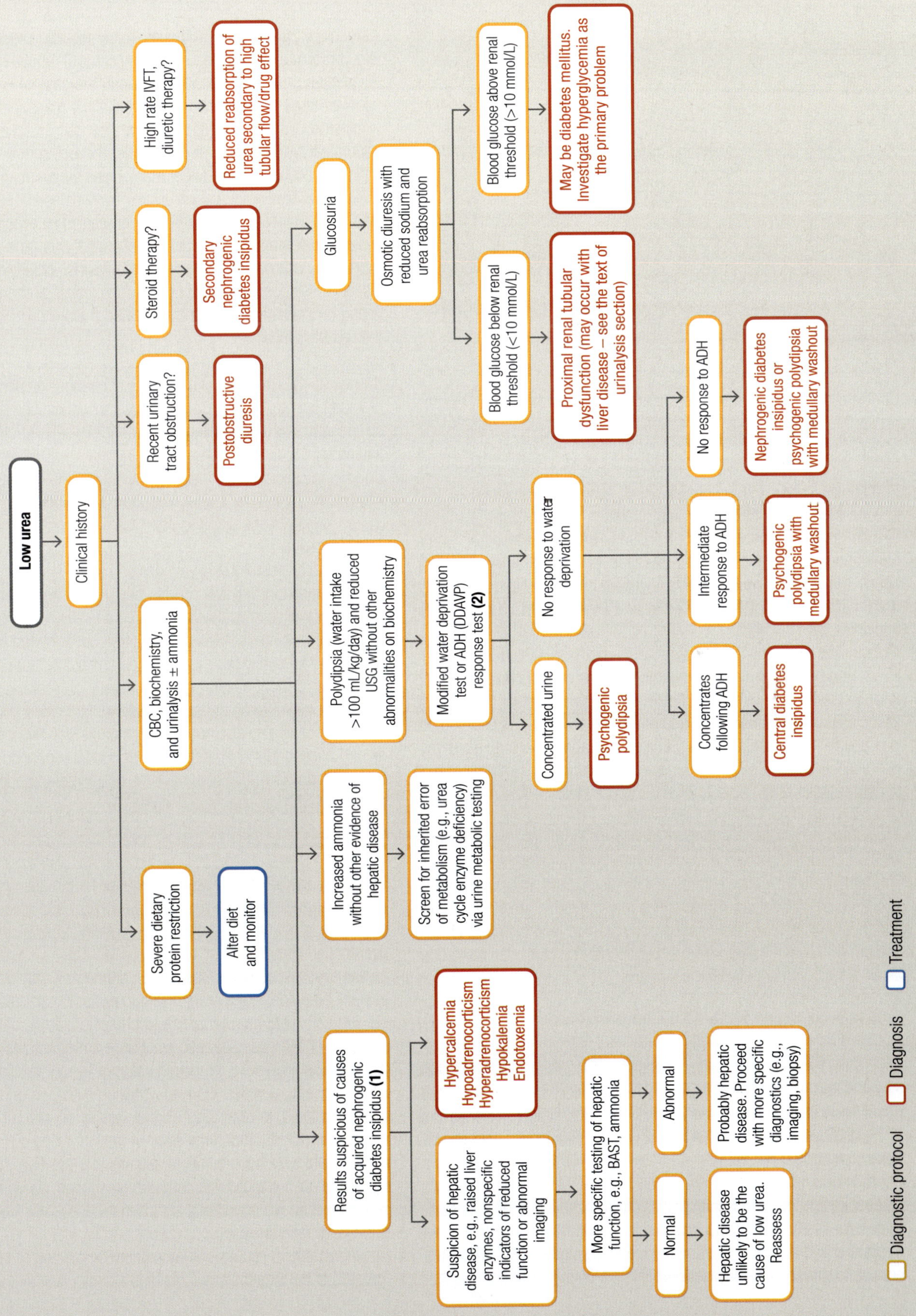

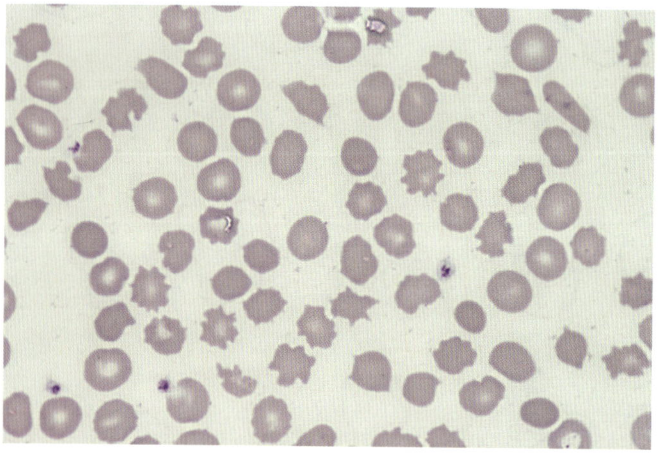

FIG. 24.1 Acanthocytes on the blood film of a dog, Wright's Giemsa, 100× objective view. Note the irregular projections of the RBC surface.

Cholesterol is derived from dietary sources or synthesized in tissues, primarily the liver, from acetyl-CoA. As such, hepatic disease associated with reduced function, particularly congenital or acquired portosystemic shunt (PSS), is a possible cause of hypocholesterolemia. Additionally, proposed mechanisms of hypocholesterolemia in PSS include hormonal alterations[15] and inhibition of cholesterol synthesis by bile acids.[16] Dogs with PSS frequently present with other typical hematological and biochemical changes discussed in this chapter, which may include microcytosis, hypoalbuminemia, and decreased urea, with or without hypoglycemia and increases in liver enzymes, bile acids, and bilirubin.

A diagnostic approach to hypocholesterolemia is presented in Algorithm 24.2. As well as liver disease, common causes of hypocholesterolemia in dogs include hypoadrenocorticism and gastrointestinal (GI) disease associated with malabsorption and maldigestion, especially when there is concurrent lymphangiectasia. Similarly, malabsorption and maldigestion associated with exocrine pancreatic insufficiency (EPI) may result in decreases in both cholesterol and triglycerides.

Algorithm 24.2 Note 1 Although, as with all laboratory tests, a single isolated change may be the result of individual variation, there are few differentials for hypocholesterolemia in dogs, and it is infrequently encountered incidentally, especially as many patients presented to veterinary practices have been inadequately starved, and therefore tend to present with hypercholesterolemia. Hypocholesterolemia can also occur as an artifact in markedly icteric samples.

Algorithm 24.2 Note 2 See algorithm 24.1 Note 1.

Algorithm 24.2 Note 3 Clinical evidence of GI disease could include weight loss, vomiting, and diarrhea. Further biochemical evidence of GI malabsorption/maldigestion typically includes hypoproteinemia due to hypoalbuminemia, often with concurrent hypoglobulinemia (or low normal globulin).

Algorithm 24.2 Note 4 Abnormalities on ultrasound that would support GI disease as a cause of hypocholesterolemia could include intestinal wall thickening and/or loss of layering or striations suggestive of lymphangiectasia. Identifying any mass lesions, lymphadenopathy, abnormalities of other organs, or presence of free fluid warrants sampling for cytological assessment if feasible and may guide the biopsy method and location.

Algorithm 24.2 Note 5 Although many disease processes implicated (e.g., chronic enteropathies, lymphangiectasia) require histopathology for diagnosis, cytology is often rewarding in the case of neoplastic disease such as large cell lymphoma, particularly if mass lesions are present within the GI tract or additional aspirates can be taken from enlarged abdominal lymph nodes. It should also be noted that hypocholesterolemia can occur in neoplasia of many types via an unknown mechanism (thought to involve increased uptake by neoplastic cells or changes in cytokines). Hypocholesterolemia, accompanied by hypoalbuminemia and hyperbilirubinemia, is a common biochemical change in hemophagocytic syndrome, which may accompany neoplasms, including lymphoma and histiocytic sarcoma amongst others. Also, consider the feasibility of FNA based on platelet count (contraindicated if platelets $<50 \times 10^9$/L due to the risk of hemorrhage).

Algorithm 24.2 Note 6 The absence of changes on ultrasound does not preclude primary GI disease and further investigations (e.g., biopsy) may still be warranted depending upon other clinical and clinicopathological findings.

Algorithm 24.2 Note 7 See Algorithm 24.1 Note 3.

Triglycerides

Similarly to cholesterol, triglycerides can either be obtained from the diet or synthesized in the liver, in this case, from nonesterified fatty acids (NEFA). However, low triglycerides are generally not considered diagnostically relevant, nor is this a change often encountered in disease states except in cases of severe malnutrition, including those associated with EPI. Hypertriglyceridemia may accompany cholestasis or dyslipidemia (similar to cholesterol) in hepatic disease. Increases in both cholesterol and triglyceride may also accompany increases in hepatobiliary enzymes as part of secondary hepatopathies induced by endocrine diseases such as hypothyroidism, diabetes mellitus, and hyperadrenocorticism, which are important rule-outs (see chapter 13).

Glucose

Glucose is the principal energy source for mammalian cells and may be derived from dietary sources, glycogenolysis, and gluconeogenesis. In dogs, the latter two are performed predominantly in the liver, so liver dysfunction may result in hypoglycemia. This is uncommon in most canine liver diseases, including PSS, although it may occur particularly in small breed dogs and is important to exclude, particularly in dogs presenting with seizures. As with hypocholesterolemia, other biochemical evidence of decreased hepatic function is anticipated when liver disease is the cause. However, the combination of hypoglycemia and acute hepatic necrosis, in which there may not be evidence of reduced hepatic function initially, is reported in xylitol toxicity, in which hypoglycemia is driven primarily by the stimulation of insulin secretion.[17] Hypoglycemia accompanied by hyperbilirubinemia is also seen in severe systemic inflammation (systemic inflammatory response syndrome; SIRS) and sepsis, and these conditions should not necessarily be confused with primary hepatic disease.

Hyperglycemia in excess of that induced by feeding or stress (e.g., >10 mmol/L) is not expected as a result of primary liver disease, but as with

ALGORITHM 24.2

Diagnostic approach to hypocholesterolemia.

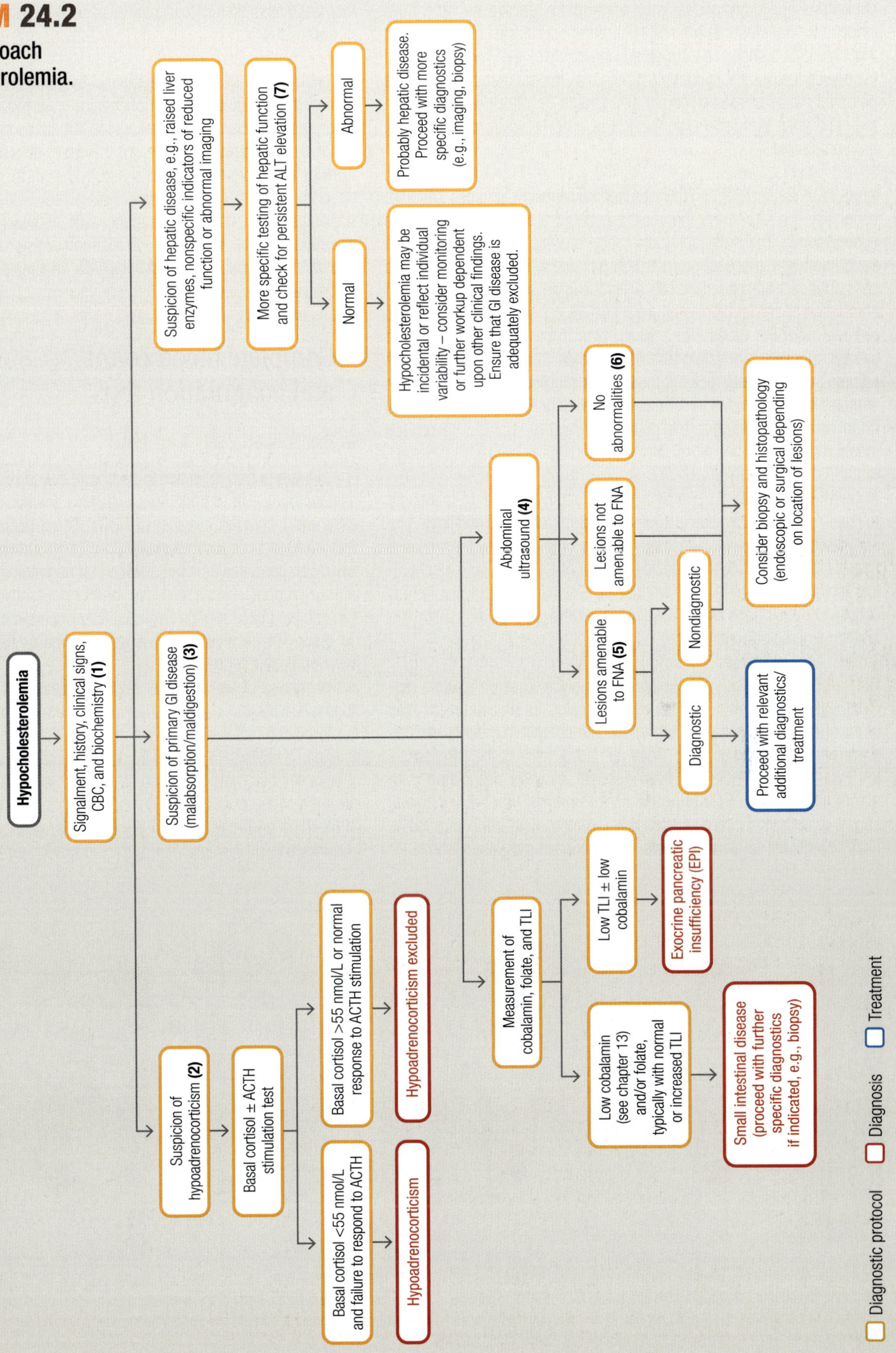

cholesterol and triglycerides, may accompany reactive hepatopathies induced by diabetes mellitus and hyperadrenocorticism.
Algorithm 24.3 shows a suggested approach to the investigation of hypoglycemia. As for hypocholesterolemia, hypoadrenocorticism is a potential cause of hypoglycemia and should be considered as a differential when the patient signalment or other laboratory parameters are compatible.

Algorithm 24.3 Note 1 When presented with low glucose reading, especially if unexpected, the clinician should first exclude artifactual hypoglycemia, the most common cause of which is delayed sample separation and processing, in which glucose is consumed by blood cells after sample collection. This artifact can be avoided by the prompt separation of serum or plasma from cellular constituents and, ideally, removal from gel tubes into a fresh, plain tube. The use of fluoride oxalate tubes is a possible alternative when facilities for immediate sample processing are lacking, though it is not recommended, as these samples cannot be used to measure other biochemical parameters and often result in hemolysis, the dilutional effect of which is to reduce measured glucose.

Algorithm 24.3 Note 2 Juvenile and toy breed hypoglycemia is thought to result from a combination of inadequate glycogen stores and limited fat and muscle mass.[18] The signalment of these patients may be similar to that of congenital PSS, and consideration of other clinical and biochemical factors is required for differentiation. Exertional hypoglycemia may occur in hunting dogs and is associated with excess glucose utilization and inadequate glycogen stores.

Algorithm 24.3 Note 3 Fructosamine is a glycated serum protein representing a longer-term glucose level indicator. Its measurement may be helpful when few other abnormalities are present in order to exclude a transient change in glucose. However, since many of the differentials for hypoglycemia (including liver disease) may be associated with chronicity, this is unlikely to be beneficial routinely when the initiating cause is already evident. Additionally, fructosamine concentration is highly correlated to albumin levels, so concurrent hypoalbuminemia (or increased albumin turnover) may be associated with a spurious decrease in fructosamine.

Algorithm 24.3 Note 4 In a patient with confirmed hypoglycemia at the time of testing (and a low fructosamine concentration supportive of a long-standing effect), insulin secretion should be suppressed (i.e., a low result is anticipated). If this is not the case, abnormal insulin secretion from an insulinoma is likely.

Algorithm 24.3 Note 5 Extrapancreatic neoplasia may induce hypoglycemia through increased glucose utilization or through secretion of insulin analogues. Examples include hepatocellular carcinoma and leiomyosarcoma.

Complete blood count and coagulation tests

Red blood cells and iron

Anemia is a common finding in dogs with liver disease and is frequently multifactorial, with contributors including anemia of inflammatory disease and increased turnover of RBCs. Of particular note in dogs with liver disease is microcytosis (RBCs with decreased size, reflected by low mean corpuscular volume [MCV] on hematology), which may occur with or without anemia and may be normochromic (normal mean cell hemoglobin concentration [MCHC]) or hypochromic (decreased MCHC). On blood film evaluation, RBCs appear smaller than normal and may have increased central pallor (Fig. 24.2).
In the context of liver disease, microcytosis is seen most frequently in dogs with PSS and is poorly characterized but is thought to be the result of altered iron metabolism (sequestration in the liver and other tissues resulting in functional iron deficiency),[19] a mechanism also associated with anemia of inflammatory disease. In contrast, absolute iron deficiency is a common cause of microcytic hypochromic anemia in dogs with chronic GI bleeding and may be seen in cases with gastroduodenal ulceration associated with liver disease, particularly with portal hypertension[4] or

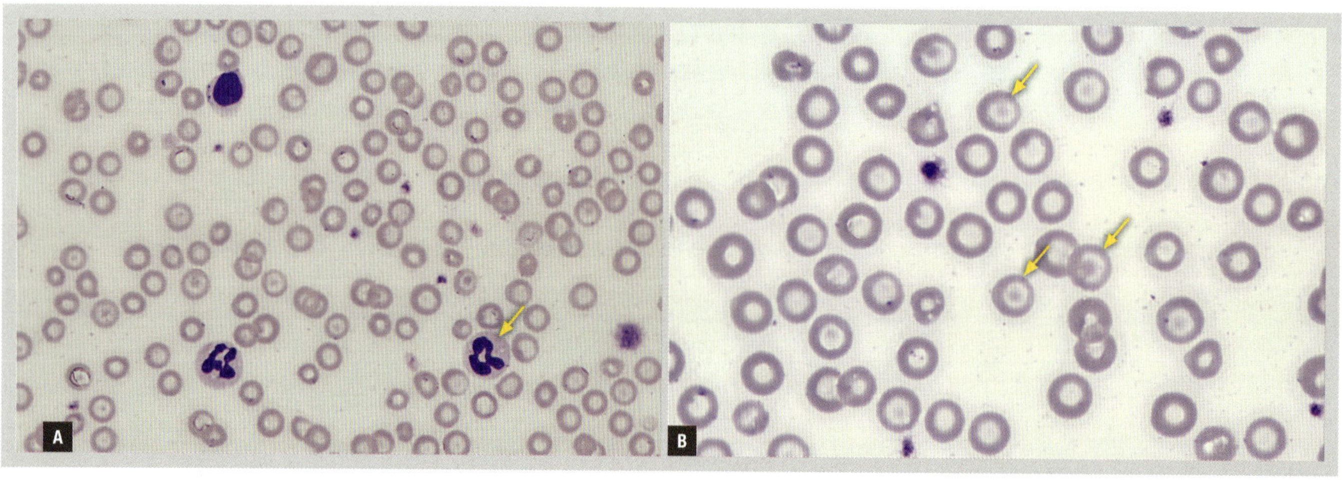

FIG. 24.2 Microcytic hypochromic RBCs in a dog, Wright's Giemsa, (A) 50× and (B) 100× objective views. (A) The RBCs are smaller than normal, as seen in comparison to the neutrophil (arrow) and confirmed by the automated MCV (57.9 fL, normal 60-77 fL). They have increased central pallor, with only a narrow rim of hemoglobin at their periphery, confirmed by a low MCHC (31.7 g/dL, normal 32-37 g/dL). This blood film is from a dog with a congenital intrahepatic portosystemic shunt, with a PCV of 27% (normal 37-55%). (B) Also pictured are moderate numbers of codocytes or "target cells" (arrows).

ALGORITHM 24.3

Diagnostic approach to hypoglycemia.

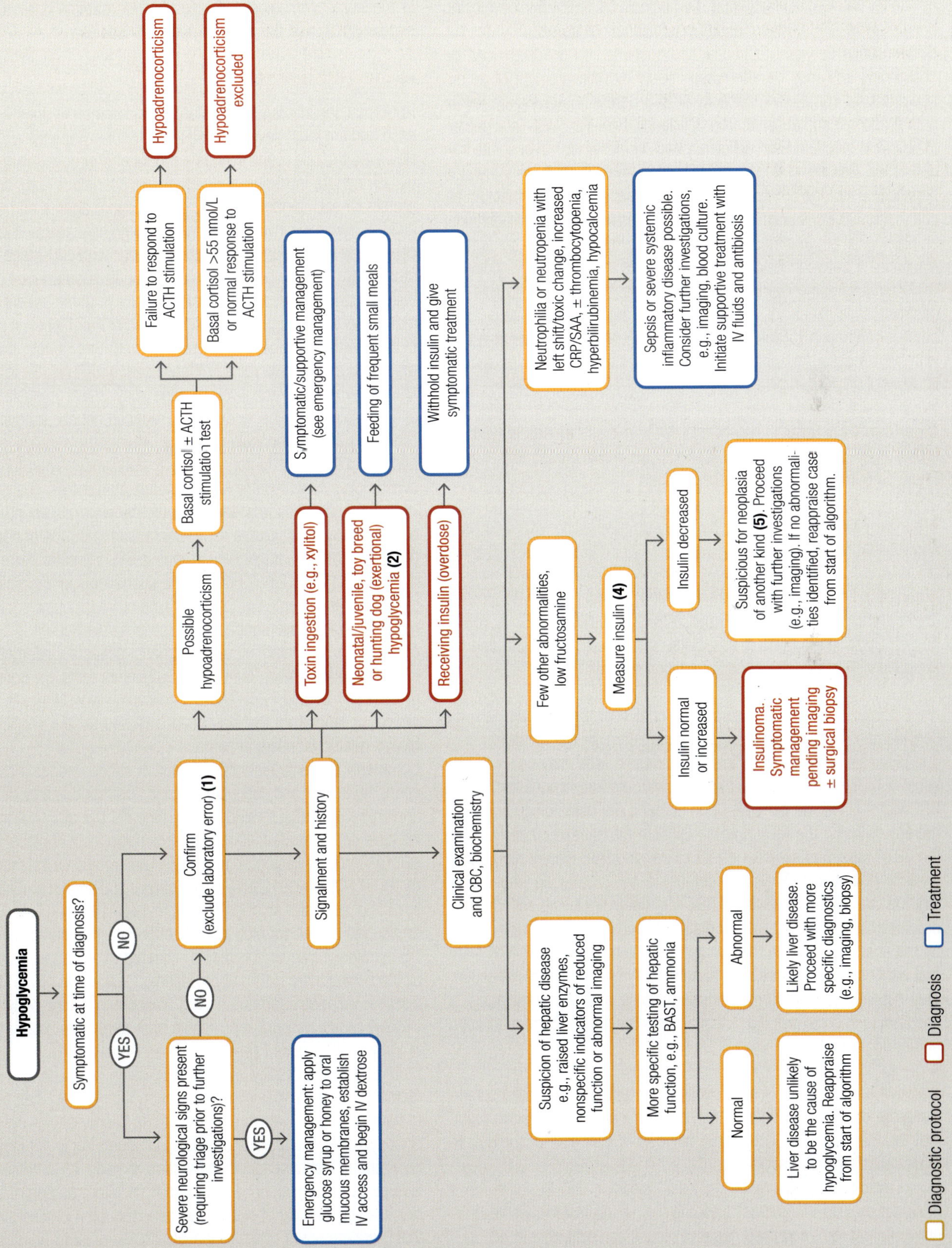

due to other causes. Hepatic dysfunction alone is typically associated with only mild or moderate anemia (if present, hematocrit [HCT] typically >26%). Therefore, the lower the HCT, the greater the concern should be for concurrent gastrointestinal blood loss. The microcytosis in iron deficiency is a result of inadequate hemoglobin content within developing bone marrow RBCs, which results in additional cell division.

Differentiation between functional and absolute iron deficiency can be challenging and may be attempted initially by measurement of serum iron and total iron binding capacity (TIBC). Serum iron levels are low in both functional and absolute iron deficiency. However, TIBC is expected to be low in functional iron deficiency and normal or high in absolute iron deficiency. Results in dogs with PSS are variable, although increased hepatic iron storage on histopathology is a consistent finding that can be confirmed with Perls stain. More recent studies have examined additional hematological parameters, including reticulocyte hemoglobin content, to discriminate between functional and absolute iron deficiency, although there remains some overlap between groups.[20] Attempting to rule out gastrointestinal bleeding, as detailed in the algorithm, may be a more practical approach to determining the cause of microcytosis in a dog with liver disease. An approach to the assessment of microcytic anemia is shown in Algorithm 24.4.

Algorithm 24.4 Note 1 The normal MCV in these breeds is typically in the region of 50-60 fL (microcytic). Other Asian breeds (e.g., Chow Chow, Shar Pei) may show similar changes.

Algorithm 24.4 Note 2 Young puppies can have a low MCV and have a lower HCT than adult dogs.

Algorithm 24.4 Note 3 A rare inherited disorder of erythropoiesis (dyserythropoietic anemia and myopathy syndrome; DAMS) in young English Springer Spaniels is associated with microcytosis and can be excluded via testing for a genetic mutation in EHBP1L1.

Algorithm 24.4 Note 4 Exclusion of analytical error should include consideration of other hematological parameters, biochemical changes, and blood film evaluation. A falsely decreased MCV may occur in patients with hypo-osmolal plasma (e.g., with marked hyponatremia), as RBC water is lost via osmosis upon entering the hematology analyzer, thereby reducing the MCV. Excess EDTA in the sample (underfilling of the EDTA tube) has a similar effect by causing RBC dehydration. Most in-clinic hematology analyzers determine MCV using an impedance method, and so the presence of RBC fragments (including with marked poikilocytosis), large platelets, or platelet clumps (which may be counted by the analyzer as small RBCs) can result in a falsely low MCV. Note that although spherocytes may appear small on blood film evaluation, they typically have a normal internal volume and so microcytosis is uncommon in dogs with IMHA (usually macrocytic due to regeneration and/or agglutination).

Algorithm 24.4 Note 5 A fecal occult blood test can be a useful screen alongside other clinical findings and biochemical data. A positive result may be the result of GI bleeding; however, it can also occur due to cross-reactivity with enzymes contained in some plants or with meat-based diets. A negative result makes GI bleeding unlikely, although it does not exclude intermittent bleeding (i.e., if the tested sample does not contain blood), and false-negative results can occasionally occur.

Algorithm 24.4 Note 6 MCHC is calculated from HCT (a function of RBC concentration and MCV) and hemoglobin concentration. Increases in MCHC are unphysiological and imply analytical error. This may either be due to a falsely low MCV (see Algorithm Note 4) or a false increase in measured hemoglobin. Causes include sample lipemia, hemolysis, excess EDTA, and the presence of Heinz bodies.

Coagulation status

Abnormalities in coagulation status are common in dogs with liver disease and are most severe in dogs with chronic hepatitis and cirrhosis.[21] However, the role of the liver as a producer of procoagulant (e.g., coagulation factors including fibrinogen), anticoagulant (e.g., antithrombin, protein C) and fibrinolytic (e.g., plasminogen) agents and the complex disease dynamics involved means that both hypocoagulable and hypercoagulable states can occur, although dogs with end-stage disease are more likely to be hypocoagulable. Although spontaneous pathological bleeding at the time of presentation is rare in these patients, it is common to perform coagulation testing ahead of liver biopsy. A small subset of dogs with liver disease may present with thrombosis, particularly of the portal and splenic veins.[22] Please see Algorithm 13.1 in chapter 13.

Mechanisms by which liver disease may affect coagulation include altered platelet number or function, reduced hepatic production of procoagulant and anticoagulant factors, impaired clearance of factor VIII and von Willebrand factor, vitamin K deficiency, hyperfibrinolysis and consumptive coagulopathy (disseminated intravascular coagulation; DIC). In a cohort of 102 dogs undergoing percutaneous ultrasound-guided liver biopsy, packed cell volume (PCV) decreased in 85.3% of dogs following the procedure, with major hemorrhage (a 6% or greater decrease in PCV) documented in 42.2%.[23] Fortunately, such bleeding is typically clinically silent, and the overall complication rate of liver biopsy is low. Although human studies have suggested some possible benefit in preoperative coagulation screening of asymptomatic patients undergoing elective surgery,[24] others have found that coagulation tests are poor predictors of clinical bleeding,[25] particularly following liver biopsy.[26] Indeed, no clinical or laboratory test has been validated for the prediction of liver biopsy-related bleeding in humans.

Commonly available tests of coagulation status in dogs include platelet count, fibrinogen and coagulation times, prothrombin time (PT or OSPT), and activated partial thromboplastin time (PTT or aPTT). Although studies have demonstrated altered patterns using tests of global hemostasis such as thromboelastography (TEG)[27,28] and rotational thromboelastometry (ROTEM),[29] these require rapid analysis and are not routinely available outside of specialist settings. Buccal mucosal bleeding time (BMBT) may be used to screen for high-risk patients (which generally have a BMBT >5 minutes); however, this test is of limited value and explicitly contraindicated when there is thrombocytopenia.[22] Exclusion of von Willebrand's disease via measurement of von Willebrand factor activity (with or without genetic testing) is advisable prior to elective biopsy, particularly in known predisposed breeds such as Dobermanns. Measurement of protein C (commercially available alongside measurement of specific factor activities in specialist coagulation laboratories) has been shown to have diagnostic value in differentiating microvascular dysplasia from portosystemic vascular abnormalities in dogs[30] but is not recommended as a routine test of coagulation function. In dogs, as in humans, there is little evidence to support a clear cutoff for interpretation of coagulation results in the context of planned surgery, though it is generally accepted that platelet counts of less than 50×10^9/L present an increased risk

ALGORITHM 24.4

Diagnostic approach to microcytosis.

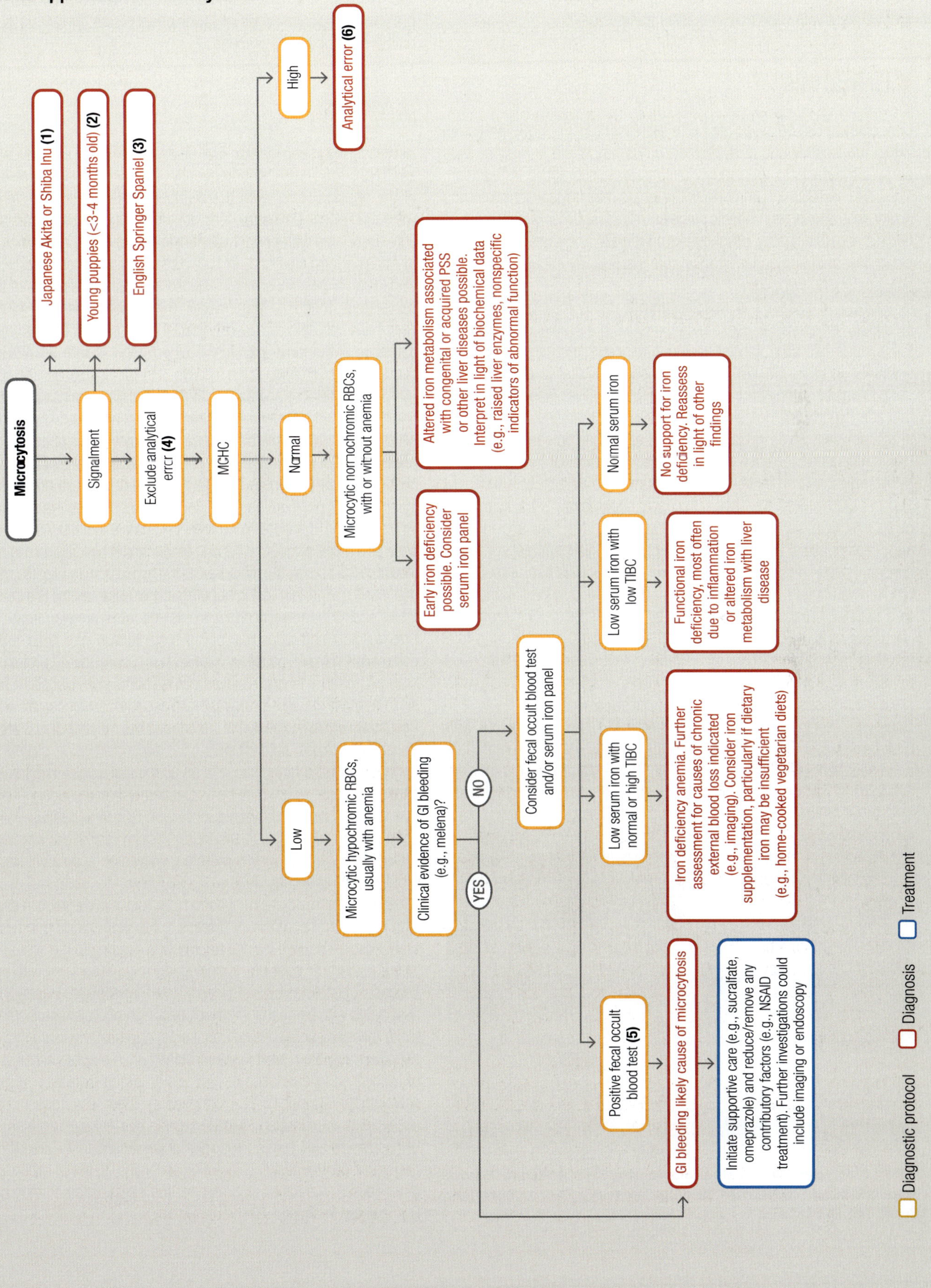

of bleeding. Prolongations in PT and aPTT should prompt the surgeon to take extra care with hemostasis and have blood products ready in case they are needed. There is currently no evidence to support routine pretreatment with vitamin K or plasma transfusion.[22]

Urinalysis

Liver disease can be associated with decreased USG (<1.030 and often within the isosthenuric or hyposthenuric range), which is likely at least partly attributable to urea reductions, as explained above. In addition, increased excretion of ammonia is thought to impair renal concentrating ability, resulting in nephrogenic diabetes insipidus. Other factors such as hepatic encephalopathy, psychogenic polydipsia, and alterations in renal blood flow and glomerular filtration rate (particularly in cases of PSS)[31] may compound the issue.

In addition to changes in specific gravity, there may be alterations in urinary biochemical constituents, including bilirubin and glucose. Bilirubinuria can be a normal finding in concentrated canine urine (for example, up to 2+ positive reaction on semiquantitative dipstick analysis). However, it may be increased in dogs with liver disease and may precede hyperbilirubinemia due to the low renal threshold for bilirubin in this species. Some dogs with liver disease may present with euglycemic glucosuria (positive glucose reaction on dipstick in the absence of hyperglycemia on biochemistry). This may be as part of a transient Fanconi-like syndrome in dogs with copper hepatopathy[32,33] or as a result of an infectious or toxic insult that affects both the liver and kidneys (e.g., leptospirosis, NSAID toxicity). Euglycemic glucosuria occurs as a consequence of reduced glucose reabsorption because of proximal renal tubular dysfunction, and so is typically accompanied by proteinuria (due to a failure of reabsorption reflected by an increased urine protein to creatinine ratio; UPC) and hyperchloremic metabolic acidosis (due to a failure to reabsorb bicarbonate). Increases in UPC associated with renal tubular dysfunction alone are typically mild to moderate (UPC <2), with greater increases suggestive of glomerular proteinuria.

Dogs with liver disease, particularly with PSS, may also present with urate urolithiasis and ammonium biurate crystals may be identified on urine sediment examination (Fig. 24.3). This is the result of inefficient transport of serum uric acid into hepatocytes, where it is normally degraded to allantoin for excretion. Once urolith formation has occurred, secondary changes associated with lower urinary tract inflammation, such as hematuria, pyuria, and proteinuria, may be seen, and dogs may present with clinical signs of lower urinary tract disease or sublumbar pain if nephroliths are present.

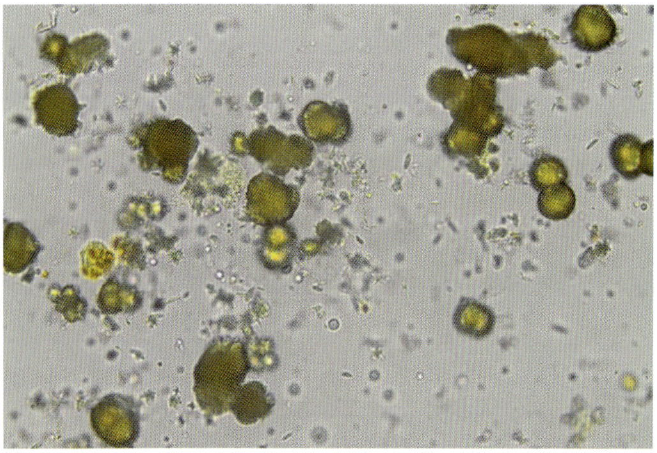

FIG 24.3 Ammonium biurate crystals in canine urine, 50× objective view. Note the typical golden-brown coloration and "thorn apple" appearance. Image courtesy of Holly Brown, DVM, PhD, DACVP.

Ascites

Ascites formed secondary to liver disease is typically a transudate, with a low TNCC ($<5\times10^9$/L and frequently $<1.5\times10^9$/L). The protein content of the effusion varies with the distribution and severity of the disease. Although hypoalbuminemia may contribute, increased hydrostatic pressure associated with portal hypertension is the largest contributory factor to effusion formation and, in liver disease, may be either presinusoidal, sinusoidal, or postsinusoidal (classified according to the area of the portal vasculature affected). The "overfill" hypothesis of ascites formation in portal vein hypertension describes splanchnic pooling of blood resulting in activation of the renin-angiotensin-aldosterone system (RAAS) with subsequent water retention in the kidneys, a further increase in the splanchnic hydrostatic pressure and ascites formation. This explains why aldosterone antagonists can be effective diuretics in dogs with portal hypertension. In severe cases, hypervolemic hyponatremia may occur due to nonosmotic release of ADH secondary to peripheral hypotension. This is a poor prognostic indicator in humans but has not been reported in dogs.[34,35]

In isolation, hypoalbuminemia is unlikely to cause ascites unless marked (and even then, there are likely other contributory factors). As hypoalbuminemia as a result of reduced hepatic production is typically mild to moderate (see proteins above), the more severe the hypoalbuminemia, the more likely that loss (e.g., protein-losing nephropathy or enteropathy) is a contributory factor and further investigations to exclude these are warranted.

Presinusoidal and sinusoidal portal hypertension (the latter being most common) typically cause a protein-poor transudate (protein content <25 g/L, often <10 g/L). Causes include portal vein hypoplasia and fibrosis from many causes, including those associated with chronic hepatitis.[34] Postsinusoidal hypertension is uncommon but may result in a protein-rich transudate (protein content >25 g/L), dependent upon plasma albumin levels. Another common cause of an abdominal protein-rich transudate is cardiac disease, which may be associated with a secondary hepatopathy due to congestion and hypoxia. Exclusion of severe cardiac disease (associated with congestive heart failure) through clinical examination with or without echocardiography is therefore warranted upon identification of a protein-rich transudate.

A less frequent mechanism of abdominal fluid accumulation in association with suspected hepatobiliary disease is bleeding resulting in hemoabdomen. Possible causes include trauma (e.g., trauma to the liver associated with a road traffic collision), coagulopathy (e.g., associated with defects of secondary hemostasis, as outlined above), or neoplasia. Hepatic neoplasia associated with hemoabdomen includes hepatocellular carcinoma (particularly massive hepatocellular carcinoma) and hemangiosarcoma. Hepatic neoplasia may also result in the formation of an exudate either as a result of associated inflammation or necrosis or due to exfoliation of neoplastic cells into the effusion (e.g., in lymphoma). Other less frequent causes of ascites with hepatobiliary disease include bile leakage resulting in sterile bile peritonitis and, rarely, septic peritonitis secondary to hepatic abscess, perforated gastrointestinal ulceration secondary to portal hypertension, or other causes. A detailed algorithm for the investigation of abdominal fluid is presented in chapter 10 (Algorithm 10.2).

KEY POINTS

- Nonspecific laboratory changes in liver disease reflect the wide-ranging role of the liver in synthesis, metabolism, and excretion.
- Reductions in cholesterol, urea, albumin, and glucose result from reduced hepatic synthesis.
- Increases in cholesterol and triglyceride may occur with cholestasis or dyslipidemia.
- Urinalysis changes include reduced USG and urate urolithiasis.
- Liver disease is often accompanied by inflammation, which may contribute to hyperglobulinemia (including increases in acute phase proteins) and anemia of inflammation.
- Microcytosis of RBCs occurs due to abnormal iron metabolism.
- Abnormal coagulation results are common and screening for high-risk patients prior to biopsy is advisable.
- Ascites occurs due to increases in hydrostatic pressure associated with portal hypertension and reductions in plasma oncotic pressure associated with hypoalbuminemia.

References

1. Strombeck DR, Miller LM, Harrold D. Effects of corticosteroid treatment on survival time in dogs with chronic hepatitis: 151 cases (1977-1985). *J Am Vet Med Assoc* 193(9):1109-1113, 1988.
2. Poldervaart JH, Favier RP, Penning LC, Van Den Ingh TSGAM, Rothuizen J. Primary hepatitis in dogs: A retrospective review (2002-2006). *J Vet Intern Med* 23(1):72-80, 2009.
3. Torrente C, Manzanilla EG, Bosch L, Fresno L, Rivera Del Alamo M, Andaluz A, et al. Plasma iron, C-reactive protein, albumin, and plasma fibrinogen concentrations in dogs with systemic inflammatory response syndrome. *J Vet Emerg Crit Care (San Antonio)* 25(5):611-619, 2015.
4. O'Kell AL, Gallagher AE, Cooke KL. Gastroduodenal ulceration in dogs with liver disease. *J Vet Intern Med* 36(3):986-992, 2022.
5. Eckart A, Struja T, Kutz A, Baumgartner A, Baumgartner T, Zurfluh S, et al. Relationship of nutritional status, inflammation, and serum albumin levels during acute illness: A prospective study. *Am J Med* 133(6):713-722.e7, 2020.
6. Watson P. Letter to the Editor. *J Vet Intern Med* 24(1):1-2, 2010.
7. Cooper ES, Wellman ML, Carsillo ME. Hyperalbuminemia associated with hepatocellular carcinoma in a dog. *Vet Clin Pathol* 38(4):516-520, 2009.
8. Cortright CC, Center SA, Randolph JF, McDonough SP, Fecteau KA, Warner KL, et al. Clinical features of progressive vacuolar hepatopathy in Scottish Terriers with and without hepatocellular carcinoma: 114 cases (1980-2013). *J Am Vet Med Assoc* 245(7):797-808, 2014.
9. Robinson MW, Harmon C, O'Farrelly C. Liver immunology and its role in inflammation and homeostasis. *Cell Mol Immunol* 13(3):267-276, 2016.
10. Gori E, Pierini A, Tulone F, Abramo F, Marchetti V. Serum protein electrophoresis in 26 dogs with chronic hepatitis. *J Vet Diagn Invest* 34(4):738-741, 2022.
11. Camus MS, Krimer PM, Leroy BE, Almy FS. Evaluation of the positive predictive value of serum protein electrophoresis beta-gamma bridging for hepatic disease in three domestic animal species. *Vet Pathol* 47(6):1064-1070, 2010.
12. Dimski DS. Ammonia metabolism and the urea cycle: function and clinical implications. *J Vet Intern Med* 8(2):73-78, 1994.
13. Center SA. Diseases of the gallbladder and biliary tree. *Vet Clin North Am Small Anim Pract* 39(3):543-598, 2009.
14. Assawarachan SN, Chuchalermporn P, Maneesaay P, Thengchaisri N. Changes in serum lipid profiles among canine patients suffering from chronic hepatitis. *Vet Sci* 8(10):221, 2021.
15. Francavilla A, Jones AF, Benichou J, Starzl TE. The effect of portacaval shunt upon hepatic cholesterol synthesis and cyclic AMP in dogs and baboons. *J Surg Res* 28(1):1-7, 1980.
16. Stockham SL, Scott MA. Lipids. In Stockham SL, Scott MA (editors). Fundamentals of Veterinary Clinical Pathology 2nd edition. Ames, Iowa, Blackwell Publishing, 2008, pp. 763-782.
17. Murphy LA, Dunayer EK. Xylitol Toxicosis in dogs: an update. *Vet Clin North Am Small Anim Pract* 48(6):985-990, 2018.
18. Idowu O, Heading K. Hypoglycemia in dogs: causes, management, and diagnosis. *Can Vet J* 59(6):642-649, 2018.
19. Laflamme DP, Mahaffey EA, Allen SW, Twedt DC, Prasse KW, Huber TL. Microcytosis and iron status in dogs with surgically induced portosystemic shunts. *J Vet Intern Med* 8(3):212-216, 1994.
20. Schaefer DMW, Stokol T. The utility of reticulocyte indices in distinguishing iron deficiency anemia from anemia of inflammatory disease, portosystemic shunting, and breed-associated microcytosis in dogs. *Vet Clin Pathol* 44(1):109-119, 2015.
21. Prins M, Schellens CJMM, van Leeuwen MW, Rothuizen J, Teske E. Coagulation disorders in dogs with hepatic disease. *Vet J* 185(2):163-168, 2010.
22. deLaforcade A, Bacek L, Blais MC, Boyd C, Brainard BM, Chan DL, et al. 2022 Update of the Consensus on the Rational Use of Antithrombotics and Thrombolytics in Veterinary Critical Care (CURATIVE) Domain 1- Defining populations at risk. *J Vet Emerg Crit Care (San Antonio)* 32(3):289-314, 2022.
23. Reece J, Pavlick M, Penninck DG, Webster CRL. Hemorrhage and complications associated with percutaneous ultrasound-guided liver biopsy in dogs. *J Vet Intern Med* 34(6):2398-2404, 2020.
24. Lim K, Satkunasivam R, Nipper C, Xu J, Hsu E, Slawin JR, et al. Association between isolated abnormal coagulation profile on transfusion following major surgery: A NSQIP analysis of individuals without bleeding disorders. *Transfusion (Paris)* 62(11):2223-2234, 2022.
25. Chee YL, Crawford JC, Watson HG, Greaves M. Guidelines on the assessment of bleeding risk prior to surgery or invasive procedures. British Committee for Standards in Haematology. *Br J Haematol* 140(5):496-504, 2008.
26. Bissonnette J, Riescher-Tuczkiewicz A, Gigante E, Bourdin C, Boudaoud L, Soliman H, et al. Predicting bleeding after liver biopsy using comprehensive clinical and laboratory investigations: A prospective analysis of 302 procedures. *J Thromb Haemost* 20(12):2786-2796, 2022.
27. Kelley D, Lester C, Shaw S, de Laforcade A, Webster CRL. Thromboelastographic evaluation of dogs with acute liver disease. *J Vet Intern Med* 29(4):1053-1062, 2015.

28. Fry W, Lester C, Etedali NM, Shaw S, DeLaforcade A, Webster CRL. Thromboelastography in dogs with chronic hepatopathies. *J Vet Intern Med* 31(2):419-426, 2017.
29. Enk NM, Kutter APN, Kuemmerle-Fraune C, Sigrist NE. Correlation of plasma coagulation tests and fibrinogen Clauss with rotational thromboelastometry parameters and prediction of bleeding in dogs. *J Vet Intern Med* 33(1):132-140, 2019.
30. Toulza O, Center SA, Brooks MB, Erb HN, Warner KL, Deal W. Evaluation of plasma protein C activity for detection of hepatobiliary disease and portosystemic shunting in dogs. *J Am Vet Med Assoc* 229(11):1761-1771, 2006.
31. Deppe TA, Center SA, Simpson KW, Erb HN, Randolph JF, Dykes NL, et al. Glomerular filtration rate and renal volume in dogs with congenital portosystemic vascular anomalies before and after surgical ligation. *J Vet Intern Med* 13(5):465-471, 1999.
32. Appleman EH, Cianciolo R, Mosenco AS, Bounds ME, Al-Ghazlat S. Transient acquired Fanconi syndrome associated with copper storage hepatopathy in 3 dogs. *J Vet Intern Med* 22(4):1038-1042, 2008.
33. Langlois DK, Smedley RC, Schall WD, Kruger JM. Acquired proximal renal tubular dysfunction in 9 Labrador Retrievers with copper-associated hepatitis (2006-2012). *J Vet Intern Med* 27(3):491-419, 2013.
34. Buob S, Johnston AN, Webster CRL. Portal hypertension: pathophysiology, diagnosis, and treatment. *J Vet Intern Med* 25(2):169-186, 2011.
35. DiBartola SP. Disorders of sodium and water: hypernatremia and hyponatremia. In DiBartola SP (editor). Fluid, Electrolyte, and Acid-Base Disorders in Small Animal Practice. Elsevier Inc., 2012, pp. 45-79.

CHAPTER 25

Laboratory tests more specific for hepatobiliary disease

Alice Tamborini
DVM, MRCVS,
DECVIM-CA (Internal Medicine), RCVS

In this chapter, we will discuss laboratory tests more specific for hepatobiliary disease, with a particular focus on liver enzyme activities, bilirubin, bile acids, ammonia, and other potential diagnostic tests.

Liver enzyme activities

Elevated serum liver enzyme activities are often encountered during routine biochemical testing and can represent the first recognizable sign of hepatobiliary disease or a nonspecific finding. For an enhanced assessment of liver enzyme aberrations, it is important to consider the possibility of extra hepatobiliary factors that might influence the liver enzyme activities, as well as the predominant pattern and the magnitude of the enzyme activity increases.[1,2] The hepatocellular enzymes are metabolic enzymes that have constant activity in normal hepatocytes and are increased with hepatocellular disease or stimulation, whereas the biliary enzymes are induced by disease or drugs. A mild increase is defined as an elevation up to five-fold the upper limit of the reference interval (RI), a moderate increase as an elevation of five to ten-fold the upper limit of the RI, while a marked increase as an elevation greater than ten-fold the upper limit of the RI.[2,3]

Hepatocellular enzymes

Alanine aminotransferase

Alanine aminotransferase (ALT) is found in high concentrations within the cytoplasm of canine hepatocytes. ALT is also present in lower enzyme activities in muscle (cardiac and skeletal), kidney, and red blood cells (RBCs).[2-5] Therefore, although ALT is considered to be relatively liver-specific, correlation with serum creatine kinase (CK) activity is often useful in differentiating ALT activity of muscle origin from that of hepatic origin.[2,3] Hemolysis has a minimal effect on ALT in dogs because there is a low RBC to plasma ALT ratio.[6] It is also important to consider the impact of drugs, such as anticonvulsants (phenobarbital, phenytoin, primidone) and corticosteroids, on the alanine aminotransferase activity. Phenobarbital can increase ALT activity up to four-fold normal, mostly secondary to hepatocellular necrosis rather than increased ALT synthesis. Corticosteroids (endogenous or exogenous) can increase ALT to approximately two- to three-fold normal due to altered hepatocyte permeability rather than increased ALT synthesis.[6] The increase may vary and can be higher in dogs with steroid hepatopathy where hepatocellular injury occurs.[2,3] Any drug (e.g., tetracycline, acetaminophen, etc.) can potentially cause hepatotoxicity and result in increased ALT activity; therefore, a thorough clinical history is essential.

As increased ALT activity is generally associated with reversible or irreversible damage to the hepatocellular membrane by inflammatory diseases, hypoxia, toxins, drugs, and neoplasia, this enzyme is considered to be a useful marker of hepatocellular injury in dogs and cats.[1-5] Although the degree of ALT elevation may be roughly proportional to the severity of liver disease, an underlying liver pathology cannot be ruled out on the basis of a normal ALT activity, which could result from a quantitative decrease in hepatocytes (e.g., advanced cirrhosis, portosystemic shunting with hepatocyte atrophy).[2,3]

Following hepatocellular injury, serum ALT levels increase within 12 hours and reach peak concentration in approximately 24-48 hours. Serum half-life is approximately 40-61 hours in dogs.[1-6]

Aspartate aminotransferase

Aspartate aminotransferase (AST) is found within the cytoplasm and mitochondria of canine and feline hepatocytes. Skeletal muscle contains the highest concentration of this enzyme, followed by liver, cardiac muscle, renal epithelial cells, RBCs, and brain tissue. Therefore, this enzyme is considered less liver-specific than ALT.[2,3,5] Intravascular or *in vitro* hemolysis may increase activity due to the AST being released from the RBCs because dogs have a high RBCs to plasma AST ratio.[3] In the case of increased AST activity, it is therefore useful to correlate with CK, ALT, and hematocrit in order to determine its origin.[2,3]

As increased AST activity can be associated with reversible or irreversible hepatocellular injury by inflammatory diseases, hypoxia, toxins, drugs, and neoplasia, this enzyme is considered to be a sensitive (although not specific) marker of hepatocellular injury in dogs and cats.[2-5]

The half-life of AST is approximately 12 hours in dogs.[1-5]

Glutamate dehydrogenase

Glutamate dehydrogenase (GLDH) is found within the mitochondria of canine and feline hepatocytes of the centrilobular areas of the liver. Although GLDH is found in other tissues of the body (kidney, intestine, muscle, and salivary gland), most of the serum GLDH originates from hepatocytes; therefore, GLDH is considered to be a specific marker of liver disease.[7]

An increase in GLDH activity is thought to reflect a centrilobular area injury (e.g., hypoxia) and leakage from severely damaged or necrotic hepatocytes. The half-life of GLDH is about 8 hours in the dog.[7]

Biliary enzymes

Alkaline phosphatase

Alkaline phosphatase (ALP) is found in the membranes of hepatocytes that line bile canaliculi and sinusoids, and therefore ALP is considered to be a sensitive marker for cholestasis (intrahepatic or extrahepatic). In dogs, several ALP isoenzymes have been identified, and its elevation may be due to extrahepatic sources (kidney, pancreas, brain, bone marrow, spleen, testes, lymph node, placenta, cardiac and skeletal muscle. The intestinal form has a very short half-life).[1-3] However, it should be noted that the magnitude of the increase resulting from extrahepatic sources is likely to be minimal.[1-3,5] The corticosteroid-induced isoenzyme of ALP is, however, important in dogs. It is not recognized in other species, such as cats and humans, and is due to hyperglycosylation of the intestinal isoenzyme, which increases its half-life.[1] Technically, it is possible to selectively measure the activity of glucocorticoid-induced ALP as a way to distinguish between increases due to corticosteroids versus cholestasis. Unfortunately, measuring glucocorticoid-induced ALP is not clinically useful because this enzyme can be increased in a variety of conditions, such as chronic cholestasis, diabetes mellitus, hypothyroidism, hyperadrenocorticism, and pancreatitis.[3]

Other than induction by drugs (such as anticonvulsants in addition to corticosteroids), an increased ALP activity can be associated with primary biliary tract disease (such as cholangitis, cholecystitis, cholelithiasis, neoplasia), extrahepatic biliary obstruction (such as by pancreatitis), parenchymal liver disease or systemic disease particularly associated with vacuolar hepatopathy (such as hyperadrenocorticism, diabetes mellitus, tick-borne disease, hyperparathyroidism, hypothyroidism, or right-sided heart failure). Elevated ALP can also be seen in growing dogs, particularly of large breeds, due to the bone isoenzyme (typically two- to three-fold normal) and in certain breeds (Siberian Huskies and Scottish Terriers).[1-3,8]

In other words, an increased ALP activity can indicate primary hepatobiliary disease (such as cholestasis, in which cases it is often markedly increased), canalicular cell necrosis, or increased hepatic synthesis induced by drugs.[1-3] Hemolysis is thought to decrease serum ALP activity. The increase of ALP following hepatic injury is delayed compared to ALT and AST. The reason for this is that it takes time for alkaline phosphatase to be synthesized and released into systemic circulation.[2] The serum half-life of hepatic ALP is approximately 66-70 hours in the dog.[1-5]

Gamma-glutamyl transferase

Gamma-glutamyl transferase (GGT) is found in the membranes of biliary epithelial cells and hepatocytes. GGT is also found in pancreatic, renal tubular, and mammary gland epithelial cells, where is involved in glutathione synthesis and degradation.[1-3]

Drugs (such as anticonvulsants and corticosteroids) may result in increased serum GGT activity; however, to a lesser extent than with ALP.[3] Therefore, an increased GGT activity can generally be attributed to cholestasis. In dogs, GGT can be considered more specific (87%) but less sensitive (50%) than ALP for the detection of hepatobiliary disease.[2,3,5]

Marked icterus and hemolysis can decrease serum GGT activity.

GGT has a half-life of approximately 72 hours in dogs.[1-5]

Please refer to Algorithm 25.1 for the approach to increased hepatocellular leakage of liver enzymes and biliary enzymes.

Algorithm 25.1 Note 1 Further workup is advised if hepatic enzyme activities are elevated (<five-fold the upper limit of the reference range) for 6-8 weeks with no obvious cause detected (such as hypoxia, hypothyroidism, diabetes mellitus, myositis, pancreatitis, hyperadrenocorticism, and enteritis). Please note that clinical signs in canine chronic hepatopathy might only appear at the onset of end-stage liver disease; therefore, an early diagnosis is warranted.

Algorithm 25.1 Note 2 Details and evidence of breed, sex, and age predispositions for liver diseases are discussed in chapters 33-38. It is strongly advised to review the patient's medical history, with particular attention to clinical signs, medications (e.g., phenobarbital, phenytoin, primidone, corticosteroids, nonsteroidal anti-inflammatory drugs), travel history, vaccination status, exposure to toxins.

Algorithm 25.1 Note 3 Depending on the epidemiology/travel history, testing for *Leptospira* spp., *Leishmania* spp., *Ehrlichia* spp., protozoa (*Neospora* spp., *Sarcocystis* spp., *Toxoplasma* spp.), Histoplasmosis infection might be recommended.[9]

Algorithm 25.1 Note 4 Other tests (such as specific pancreatic lipase) could be performed to identify possible pancreatitis (acute or chronic) as a cause of extrahepatic biliary obstruction.

Bilirubin

Bilirubin is formed during the degradation of hemoglobin of senescent RBCs through the mononuclear phagocyte system in the liver and spleen. Following transfer to the liver, bilirubin is transformed into a conjugated water-soluble form which is transported from the hepatocytes to the intestine as a component of the bile and then degraded into urobilinogen. About 10% of the urobilinogen is reabsorbed, and most (90%) is broken down into urobilin and stercobilin, which are both excreted in the feces. Of the resorbed urobilinogen, most is taken up by the liver and re-excreted into the bile, while a small amount is excreted into the urine.[2-4]

The causes of serum hyperbilirubinemia are prehepatic (hemolytic) disease, primary hepatic disease and posthepatic disease (see Table 8.1 for more detail). As concerns primary hepatic hyperbilirubinemia, this is often caused by conditions that lead to significant hepatocyte dysfunction (such as acute or chronic hepatitis, hepatic necrosis, neoplasia, cholangitis, and hepatic lipidosis in cats), and so decreased bilirubin uptake, conjugation, and excretion often combined with intrahepatic canalicular obstruction by hepatocyte swelling and fibrosis. Posthepatic hyperbilirubinemia is secondary to abnormal biliary excretion of bilirubin due to extrahepatic bile duct obstruction, which can frequently be observed in pancreatitis, pancreatic neoplasia, cholecystitis, biliary mucocele, and neoplasia. Biliary tract rupture also results in posthepatic hyperbilirubinemia. Extrahepatic biliary duct obstruction is often characterized by hypercholesterolemia and by a greater increase in cholestatic enzymes

ALGORITHM 25.1

Approach to increased hepatocellular leakage liver enzymes and biliary enzymes.

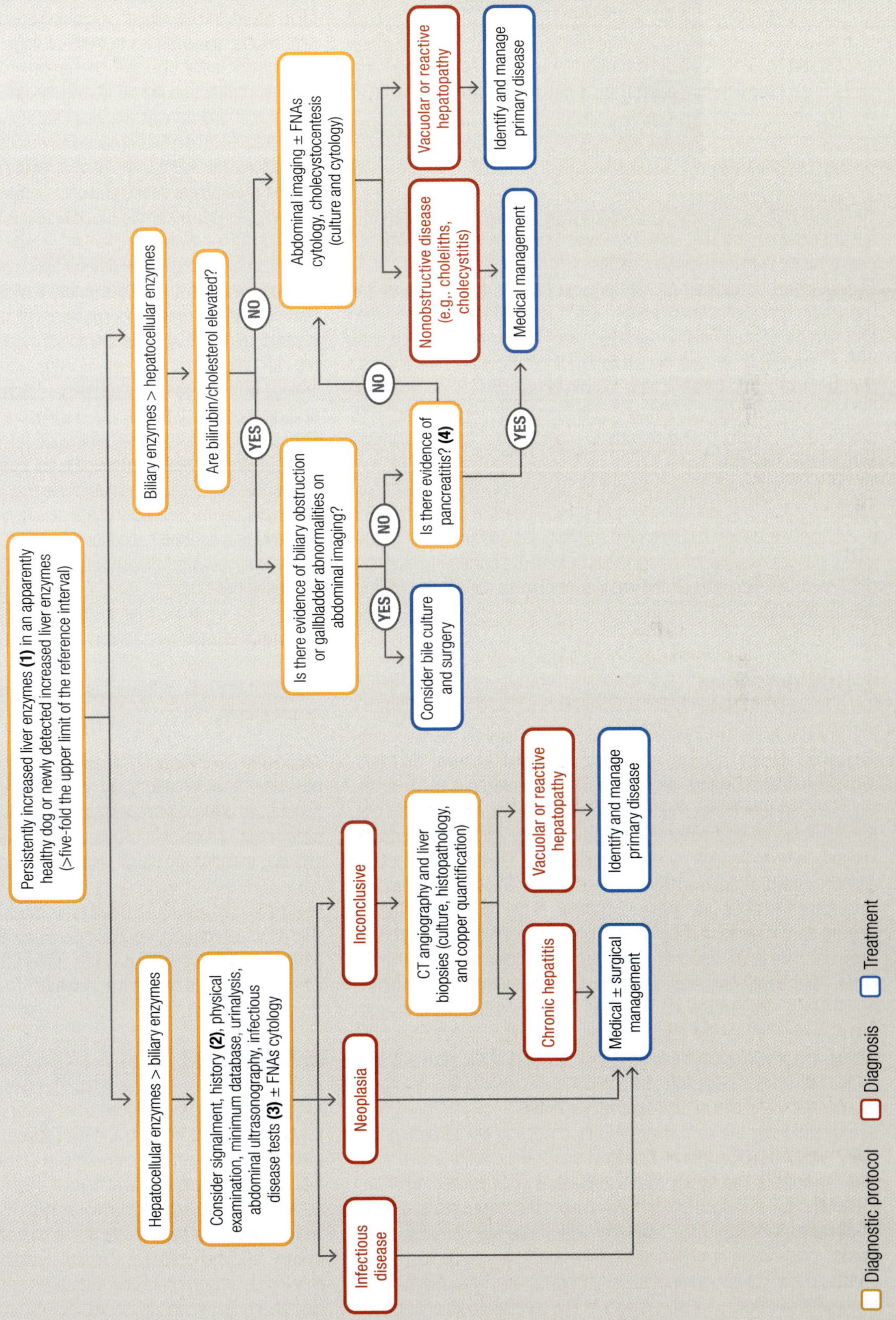

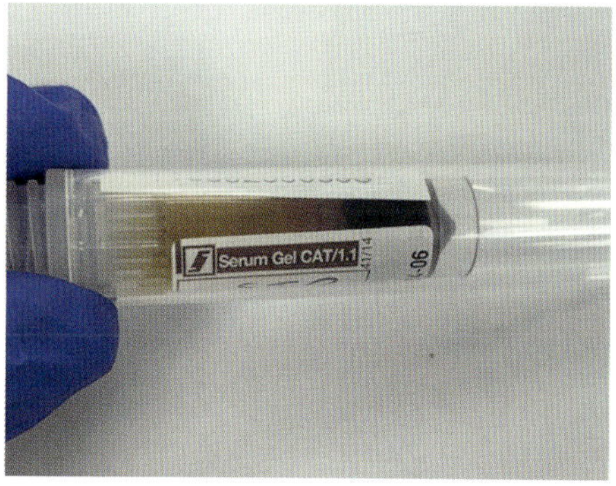

FIG. 25.1 Serum from a dog with clinical jaundice (Photo courtesy of Nikki Marshall, IDEXX).

compared with hepatocellular leakage enzymes.[2-4] When measured with some analyzers and reagents, hemolysis and lipemia (even mild) will cause falsely high total bilirubin values.

Clinical icterus is defined as high enough bilirubin to be seen by the naked eye on mucous membranes, and it is generally the case when total bilirubin concentrations exceed 50 µmol/L (3.0 mg/dL). This means that it is possible to have hyperbilirubinemia without visible icterus.[4] On the other hand, visibly icteric plasma or serum (Fig. 25.1) can be observed when total bilirubin concentrations are greater than 7-15 µmol/L (0.5-1 mg/dL).[4] Please refer to Algorithm 8.1 for the approach to hyperbilirubinemia.

As the liver enzyme activities cannot be used to assess the functional capacity of the liver, measurement of substances that are synthesized or excreted exclusively by the liver (e.g., bile acids and ammonia) can be useful in those cases where there is a suspicion of a portosystemic shunt (PSS) or to aid diagnosis of end-stage liver disease, before considering hepatic biopsies.

Bile acids

Primary bile acids are synthesized from cholesterol in the liver, conjugated to glycine, taurine, glucuronic acid and sulfates, and then excreted into the canaliculi as sodium salts. The presence of bile acids, salts, and sodium draws water by osmosis from the cells into the bile. Upon gallbladder contraction (after a meal), they are excreted into the intestine, where, through micelle formation, they facilitate the digestion and absorption of fats and liposoluble vitamins. Once in the intestine, conjugated bile acids are mainly reabsorbed in the ileum, while 10% or less are deconjugated or dehydroxylated by intestinal bacteria to produce secondary bile acids, which are absorbed in the colon or excreted in the feces. After absorption, conjugated or unconjugated bile acids enter the portal blood, where they are extracted by the hepatocytes and again excreted into the bile. Bile acids are typically recycled several times after a meal. In a physiological state, very small amounts of bile acids are seen in blood samples of dogs and cats due to the efficiency of ileal resorption and hepatic extraction of the recycled bile acids.[2-5]

Serum bile acids are best measured by collecting paired preprandial (after withholding food for 8-12 hours) and 2-hour postprandial samples. As lipemia can falsely increase the bile acids concentration, an extremely fat-dense food should be avoided.[2-4] Increases in fasting and/or postprandial serum bile acids concentrations are consistent with hepatic dysfunction or abnormal portal blood flow (i.e., portosystemic shunts, either congenital or acquired or portal vein hypoplasia) in patients without evidence of cholestasis.[2-5] The measurement of bile acids would not be useful in patients with cholestasis and increased serum hyperbilirubinemia since bile acids are excreted in the bile. They will be elevated due to cholestasis; therefore, the test could not be relied upon to give any information on the liver functional capacity.[3-5] In these cases, the measurement of ammonia would be preferable.

Most animals have higher postprandial than preprandial bile acid concentrations; however, up to 20% of dogs may have higher preprandial than postprandial bile acid concentrations due to a recent meal, gallbladder contraction during fasting, or delayed gastric emptying. In this scenario, if both results are less than 25 µmol/L, hepatobiliary disease is unlikely.[2-5] When interpreting the results, the higher of the two concentrations should be taken versus relying on the postprandial to always exceed preprandial concentrations. Serum bile acid concentrations are the most sensitive hepatic function test for PSS and end-stage chronic hepatitis (CH); however, not for early-stage CH.[10] Although the magnitude of elevation does not allow differentiation of the category of the disease, marked elevation (>75-100 µmol/L) of pre- and/or postprandial bile acids should increase the suspicion of congenital or acquired PSS.[4] A more recent study has identified overlap between bile acids, both pre- and postprandial values, in dogs with or without liver disease and in dogs with different liver diseases, potentially limiting the utility of bile acid measurement as a test to diagnose and differentiate between liver diseases.[12] Please note that prolonged fasting, intestinal malabsorption, rapid gastrointestinal transit, delayed gastric emptying, or ineffective gallbladder contraction and hemolysis may lower bile acid concentrations and decrease the sensitivity of bile acid testing for hepatobiliary diseases, therefore it is advised to cautiously interpret the test results if any of the above is suspected.[4] Please refer to Algorithm 25.2 for the approach to increased bile acids.

Algorithm 25.2 Note 1 Please be aware that measurement of bile acids would not be useful in patients with cholestasis and increased serum hyperbilirubinemia. In these cases, the measurement of ammonia would be preferable.

Algorithm 25.2 Note 2 Measurement of bile acids in Maltese dogs may have questionable utility, based on a study that found this breed might have artifactually elevated serum bile acids caused by a reacting substance;[11] however, it is believed that many of these dogs might have clinically insignificant portal vein hypoplasia.

Algorithm 25.2 Note 3 Other tests (such as abdominal imaging, specific pancreatic lipase, low dose dexamethasone suppression test) could be performed to identify possible pancreatitis or hyperadrenocorticism as a cause of mild cholestatic disorder.

Ammonia

Ammonia is mostly produced from dietary amino acids by bacteria in the gastrointestinal system and then absorbed into the portal circulation, taken up by the liver, and converted, via the urea cycle, into urea. Urea is then excreted via the urine and, as it freely crosses membranes, is also secreted into the gastrointestinal system.[2-5]

Ammonia plays a central role in the pathogenesis of hepatic encephalopathy, and therefore it is a useful marker for this condition. Note that only increased ammonia concentrations are diagnostically useful, as the plasma ammonia concentrations of patients with hepatic encephalopathy

ALGORITHM 25.2

Approach to the patient with increased bile acids.

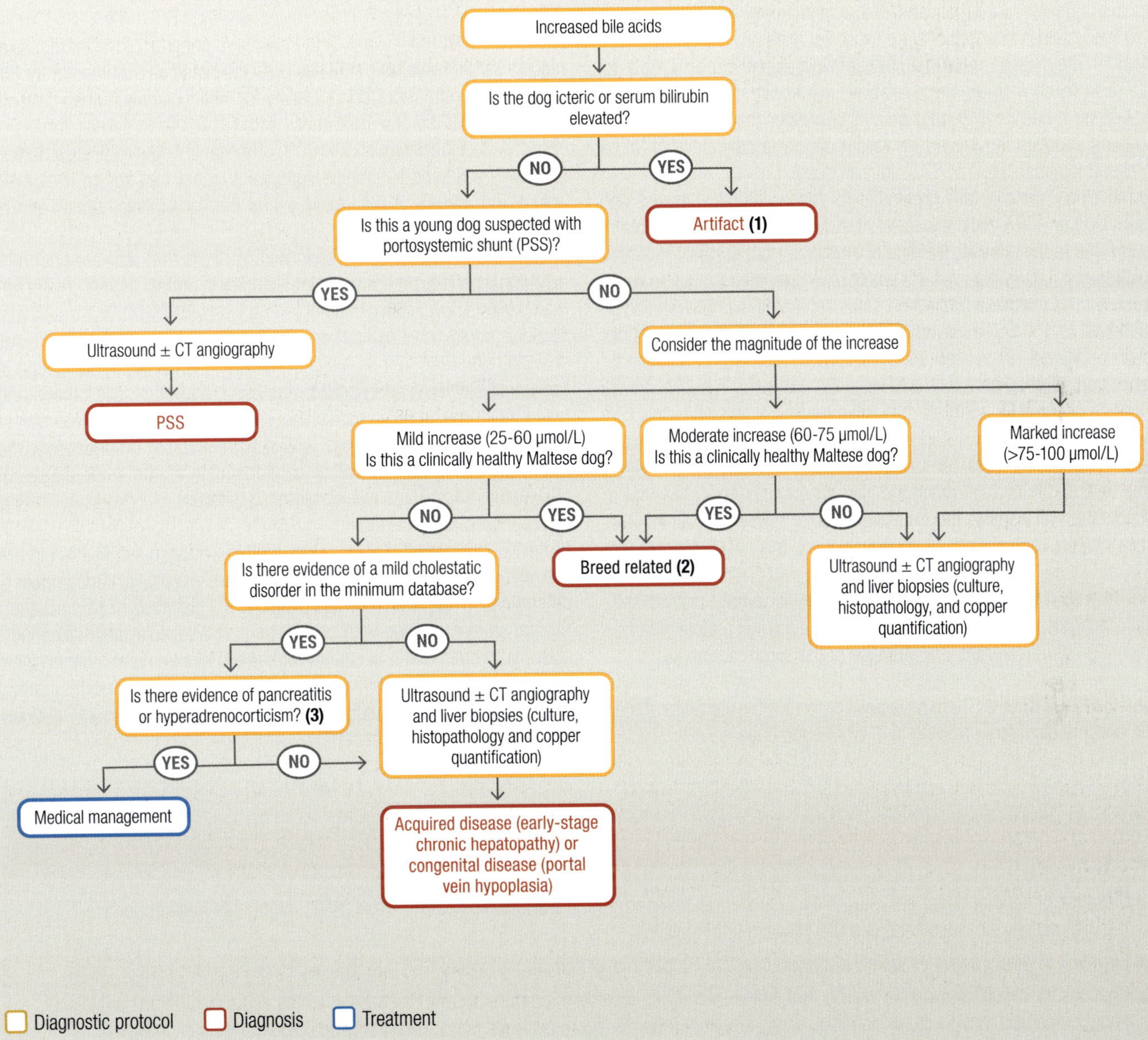

are often normal.[2] Other causes of hyperammonemia include high-protein meals, strenuous exercise/seizures (causing ammonia liberation from the muscle), inherited disorders of the urea cycle (described in Irish Wolfhounds), and use of drugs (i.e., narcotics, diuretics) that can lead to alkalosis. Congenital cobalamin deficiency in dogs has been reported to cause hyperammonemic hepatic encephalopathy. The mechanism appears to be increased methylmalonic acid indirectly inhibiting the urea cycle.[13] Bile acid concentrations are expected to be normal in these conditions.[2-5] The measurement of ammonia levels can be a specific (it is not influenced by cholestasis) but a relatively insensitive marker for hepatic function as it has been suggested that a greater than 70% reduction of hepatic function is required for serum ammonia concentration to be increased (optimal cutoff of 57 µmol/L in dogs).[14]

Arterial blood samples are preferable to venous blood samples, and heparinized or EDTA-anticoagulated plasma samples are preferable to serum. Due to the possible leakage of ammonia from erythrocytes (that could result in falsely high values), whole blood samples should be separated within 15 minutes of collection. Once separated, samples should be maintained at 4°C until assayed (stable for a maximum of 3 hours under these conditions). Separated samples can also be frozen and stored frozen (and shipped as such) until analysis. However, result accuracy cannot be assured for samples that arrive thawed at the laboratory.[2-5,13]

Please refer to Algorithm 25.3 for the approach to hyperammonemia.

Ammonia tolerance tests can be performed to increase the sensitivity of the test, and it involves giving the animal ammonia as a challenge to see how the liver handles the excess ammonia.[2-5] However, as this test can precipitate clinical signs of encephalopathy, it is not recommended.

Algorithm 25.3 Note 1 Please consider hemolytic sample, delayed separation/analysis, strenuous exercise, alkalosis, and high protein meals as reasons for spurious/artifactual increase of the serum ammonia.

Algorithm 25.3 Note 2 There have been reports in the literature of urea cycle enzyme disorders involving Irish Wolfhound dogs.[13]

Algorithm 25.3 Note 3 The breeds most reported with congenital cobalamin deficiency include Giant Schnauzers, Border Collies, Chinese Shar Peis, Beagle dogs, and Australian Shepherd dogs.[15]

Other potential diagnostic tests

Hyaluronic acid (HA) is one of the main components of the extracellular matrix. Serum hyaluronic acid has been evaluated as a biomarker for hepatic fibrosis with reported sensitivity for distinguishing human patients with no to mild fibrosis from those with moderate to severe fibrosis of 75-87% and specificity of 80-100%.[3] Preliminary studies using a human HA assay validated for canine samples suggest that serum hyaluronic acid might also be a potentially useful marker of liver fibrosis and/or cirrhosis in dogs.[16-18]

MicroRNAs are small non-protein-coding RNAs that regulate posttranscriptional gene expression. Various studies in animal models and in human patients have shown hepatocyte-derived microRNAs as a stable and sensitive noninvasive biomarker of hepatocellular injury.[3] Recent studies showed microRNA-122 as a highly sensitive marker for the detection of hepatocellular injury in Labrador Retrievers and other dog breeds and could be a promising biomarker that may be used for early detection of subclinical liver injury in dogs with normal ALT.[19-21] Unfortunately, the specificity of this test seems to be inadequate as the same degree of elevation of microRNAs was observed in different liver diseases, limiting its diagnostic utility in dogs.[21]

Protein C is a vitamin K-dependent protein zymogen synthesized in the liver with an important role in coagulation. In humans, plasma protein C determination has been reported to help in the diagnosis of liver disease.[3] Clinical studies in dogs with congenital portal vascular anomalies indicate that protein C is a biomarker of hepatic function and a noninvasive measure of portal blood flow with a role in distinguishing portosystemic shunting from microvascular dysplasia although this is not routinely measured in clinical practice.[22]

KEY POINTS

- Elevation of hepatocellular enzymes (alanine aminotransferase [ALT], aspartate aminotransferase [AST], glutamate dehydrogenase [GLDH]) usually indicates hepatocellular disease or stimulation.
- Elevation of biliary enzymes (alkaline phosphatase [ALP], gamma-glutamyltransferase [GGT]) is typically induced by disease or drugs.
- Reasons for hyperbilirubinemia include prehepatic (hemolytic) disorders, primary hepatic diseases (such as acute or chronic hepatitis, hepatic necrosis, neoplasia, cholangitis), or posthepatic diseases (such as cholecystitis, biliary mucocele or extrahepatic biliary obstruction due to pancreatitis or neoplasia).
- A mild to moderate increase in bile acids can be observed in cholestatic disorders, portal vein hypoplasia, and in some Maltese dogs, while a marked elevation (>75-100 µmol/L) in bile acids is typically seen in PSS and end-stage chronic liver disease.
- The measurement of serum ammonia, in order to assess for portosystemic shunting or the functional capacity of the liver, is preferable in cases of hyperbilirubinemia. However, it has been suggested that a greater than 70% reduction of hepatic function is required for serum ammonia concentration to be increased.
- A spurious increase of ammonia can be observed in the case of hemolytic samples, delayed separation/analysis, strenuous exercise, alkalosis, and high-protein meals.
- Other potential diagnostic tests include hyaluronic acid (a biomarker of liver fibrosis and/or cirrhosis in dogs), microRNAs (biomarker for early detection of subclinical hepatitis in dogs with normal ALT) and protein C (biomarker of hepatic function and a noninvasive measure of portal blood flow in dogs).

ALGORITHM 25.3

Approach to the patient with hyperammonemia.

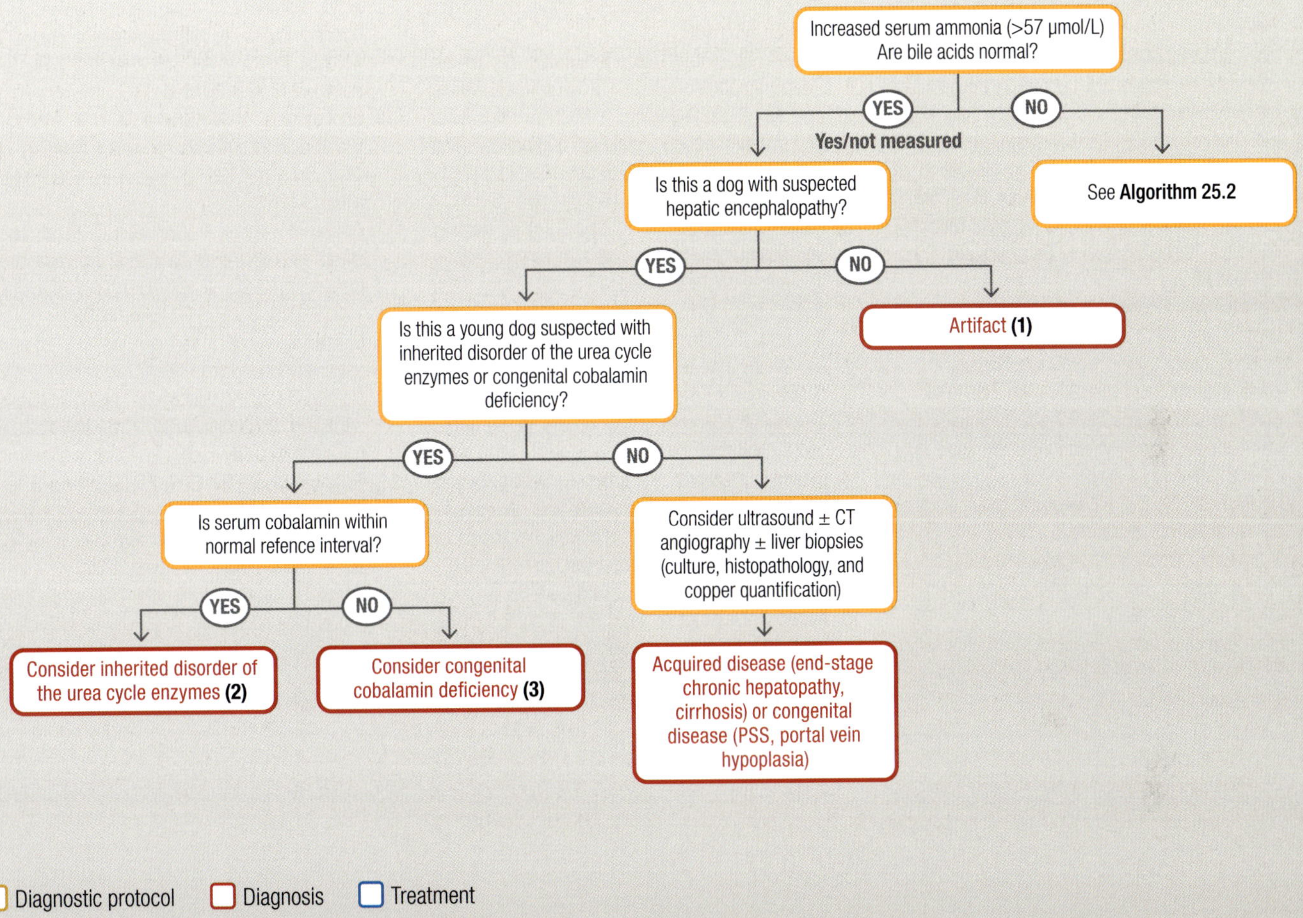

References

1. Center SA. Interpretation of liver enzymes. *Vet Clin North Am Small Anim Pract* 37(2):297-333, 2007. doi:10.1016/j.cvsm.2006.11.009
2. Chapman SE, Hostutler RA. A laboratory diagnostic approach to hepatobiliary disease in small animals. *Vet Clin North Am Small Anim Pract* 43(6):1209-1225, 2013. doi:10.1016/j.cvsm.2013.07.005
3. Lawrence YA, Steiner JM. Laboratory evaluation of the liver. *Vet Clin North Am Small Anim Pract* 47(3), 2017. doi:539-553 10.1016/j.cvsm.2016.11.005
4. Cocker S, Ritcher K. Diagnostic evaluation of the liver. In Ettinger SJ, Feldman EC, Côté E (editors). Textbook of Veterinary Internal Medicine 8th edition. St Louis, Elsevier Saunders, 2017, pp. 1613-1617.
5. Webster CRL, Cooper JC. Diagnostic approach to hepatobiliary disease. In Bonagura JD, Twedt DC (editors). Kirk's Current Veterinary Therapy XV. St Louis, Elsevier Saunders, 2014, pp. 569-573.
6. eClinPath.com. https://eclinpath.com/chemistry/liver/liver-injury/alanine-aminotransferase/ [Accessed 11th August 2023]
7. Hoffman WE, Solter PF. Diagnostic enzymology of domestic animals. In Kaneko JJ, Harvey JW, Bruss M (editors). Clinical Biochemistry of Domestic Animals 6th edition. Cambridge MA, Academic Press, 2008, pp. 351-378.
8. eClinPath.com https://eclinpath.com/chemistry/liver/cholestasis/alkaline-phosphatase/ [Accessed 11th August 2023]
9. Webster CRL, Center SA, Cullen JM, et al. ACVIM consensus statement on the diagnosis and treatment of chronic hepatitis in dogs. *J Vet Intern Med* 33(3):1173-1200, 2019. doi: 10.1111/jvim.15467
10. Center SA. Serum bile acids in companion animal medicine. *Vet Clin North Am Small Anim Pract* 23:625-657, 1993.
11. Tisdall PL, Hunt GB, Tsoukalas G, et al. Post-prandial serum bile acid concentrations and ammonia tolerance in Maltese dogs with and without hepatic vascular anomalies. *Aust Vet J* 72(4):121-126, 1995. doi: 10.1111/j.1751-0813.1995.tb15029.x
12. Pena-Ramos J, Barker L, Saiz R, et al. Resting and postprandial serum bile acid concentrations in dogs with liver disease. *J Vet Intern Med* 35(3):1333-1341, 2021. doi: 10.1111/jvim.16134
13. Battersby IA, Giger U, Hall EJ. Hyperammonaemic encephalopathy secondary to selective cobalamin deficiency in a juvenile Border collie. *J Small Anim Pract* 46(7):339-344, 2005. doi: 10.1111/j.1748-5827.2005.tb00330.x
14. Ruland K, Fischer A, Hartmann K. Sensitivity and specificity of fasting ammonia and serum bile acids in the diagnosis of portosystemic shunts in dogs and cats. *Vet Clin Pathol* 39(1):57-64, 2010. doi: 10.1111/j.1939-165X.2009.00178.x
15. Kather S, Grützner N, Kook PH, Dengler F, Heilmann RM. Review of cobalamin status and disorders of cobalamin metabolism in dogs. *J Vet Intern Med* 34(1):13-28, 2020. doi: 10.1111/jvim.15638
16. Ceplecha V, Rehakova K, Lendon C, et al. Hyaluronic acid and TGF-β1 in dogs with hepatobiliary diseases. *Acta Veterinaria Brno* 87:231-240, 2018. doi:10.2754/avb201887030231
17. Glin'ska-Suchocka K, Orłowska A, Spuz'ak J, et al. Suitability of using serum hyaluronic acid concentrations in the diagnosis of canine liver fibrosis. *Polish J Vet Sci* 18(4):873-878, 2015. doi:10.1515/pjvs-2015-0113
18. Kanemoto H, Ohno K, Sakai M, et al. Blood hyaluronic acid as a marker for canine cirrhosis. *J Vet Med Sci* 71(9):1251-1254, 2009. doi:10.1292/jvms.71.1251
19. Dirksen K, Verzijl T, Grinwis GC, et al. Use of serum microRNAs as biomarker for hepatobiliary diseases in dogs. *J Vet Intern Med* 30(6):1816-1823, 2016. doi:10.1111/jvim.14602
20. Dirksen K, Verzijl T, van den Ingh TS, et al. Hepatocyte-derived microRNAs as sensitive serum biomarkers of hepatocellular injury in Labrador retrievers. *Vet J* 211:75-81, 2016. doi: 10.1016/j.tvjl.2016.01.010
21. Oosthuyzen W, Ten Berg PWL, Francis B, et al. Sensitivity and specificity of microRNA-122 for liver disease in dogs. *J Vet Intern Med* 32(5):1637-1644, 2018. doi:10.1111/jvim.15250
22. Toulza O, Center SA, Brooks MB, et al. Evaluation of plasma protein C activity for detection of hepatobiliary disease and portosystemic shunting in dogs. *J Am Vet Med Assoc* 229(11):1761-71, 2006. doi:10.2460/javma.229.11.1761

CHAPTER 26

Imaging the liver, biliary system, and portal vasculature

Abby Caine
MA, VetMB, CertVDI, DECVDI, FRCVS

The liver may be imaged for many reasons: there may be a clinical suspicion of hepatic disease, or it may be imaged as part of a more global assessment of the patient, e.g., to look for evidence of metastasis in patients with neoplasia elsewhere. For all indications of hepatic imaging, the process is the same:

- Ask a question: i.e., is there a structural abnormality in the liver to explain why my patient has elevated liver enzymes? Imaging without a question may make interpreting the significance of any findings difficult.
- Choose the right imaging modality. The mainstay of liver and biliary imaging in dogs is ultrasound, with radiographs usually employed as an initial screening test to look for any abnormalities in animals with nonspecific clinical signs such as vomiting. If ultrasound is not sufficient to identify a specific liver pathology, either an advanced imaging modality may be chosen. For example, computed tomography (CT) is frequently used to assess the liver, particularly for vascular abnormalities, with contrast-enhanced ultrasound (CEUS), magnetic resonance imaging (MRI), and scintigraphy described in research but not often employed in clinics. Frequently, the next step following ultrasound is a biopsy, as few pathognomic imaging findings can achieve a definitive diagnosis without a biopsy.
- Acquire the images carefully, and then interpret the images thoroughly –use the six Roentgen signs to assess for differences from normal: changes to size, shape, margination (smooth or irregular outline), location (displacement –such as in a diaphragmatic rupture or torsion of a lobe), number (there should only be one liver. However, the gallbladder may be duplicated or congenitally absent) and opacity on radiographs (is it soft tissue opacity or is there any abnormal mineral/fat/gas opacity in the liver) or echogenicity for ultrasound (is the echogenicity uniform, and appropriate compared to other organs).

Once the images have been thoroughly assessed, any abnormalities identified can be given a list of potential differential diagnoses and integrated back into the case to see if the clinical question is answered or if further tests are indicated.

eFigure

eFigures gallery.

We will consider the imaging modalities used to assess the liver, biliary tract, and portal vasculature in turn.

Imaging the liver parenchyma

Radiographic imaging of the liver parenchyma

Normal anatomy and imaging appearance

The liver should be of uniform soft tissue opacity. It is located within the costal arch, with only a tiny portion extending caudal to the last rib and associated costal cartilage. It has a triangular shape, with the caudal border not rounded. A full assessment of the liver involves at least one lateral view, where the margin of the liver is observed as it is highlighted by the diaphragm cranially, gastric gas caudodorsally, and fat in the falciform fat pad caudoventrally; and a ventrodorsal view that allows any lateralized liver masses to be observed.

Assessing for abnormalities

Markers for abnormality are change of size, change of shape, and change of opacity.

To help assess for change of size, look for alterations in the gastric axis, an imagined line placed from the fundus to the body of the stomach, which in most dogs is parallel to the most caudal rib (Fig. 26.1). In normal deep-chested dogs, the gastric axis is perpendicular to the spine (**eFig. 26.1**).

Change in size

If the liver is enlarged, it displaces the body of the stomach caudally, so the gastric axis rotates anticlockwise (Fig. 26.2). Conversely, if the liver is small, the gastric axis may rotate clockwise (**eFig. 26.2**). Enlargement of the liver is a nonspecific feature associated with benign vacuolar hepatopathy, neoplasia, and sometimes hepatitis. It is often accompanied by a change of shape and rounding of the caudal border of the liver as it swells, and a large mass may cause a visible focal bulge. Microhepatica (a small liver) is uncommon. It may be seen with congenital portosystemic shunts and rarely in end-stage fibrotic/cirrhotic liver disease.

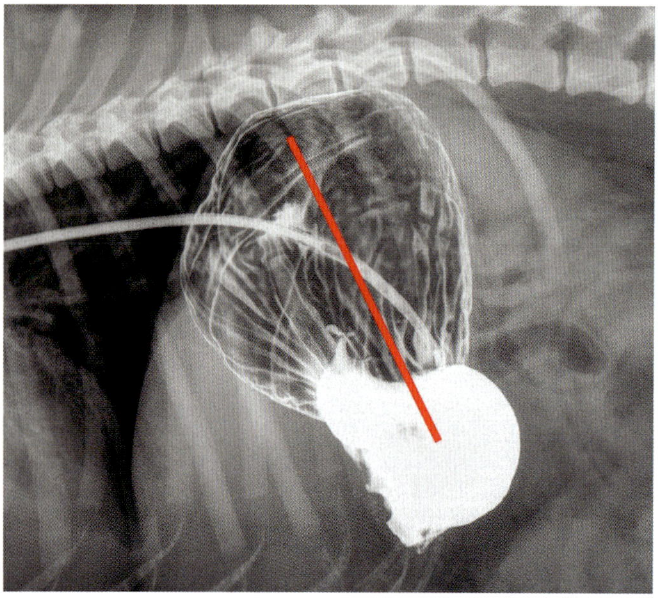

FIG. 26.1 The normal radiographic size of the liver. A normal dog has the liver just peeping out from the costal arch and a gastric axis (red line) parallel to the last rib.

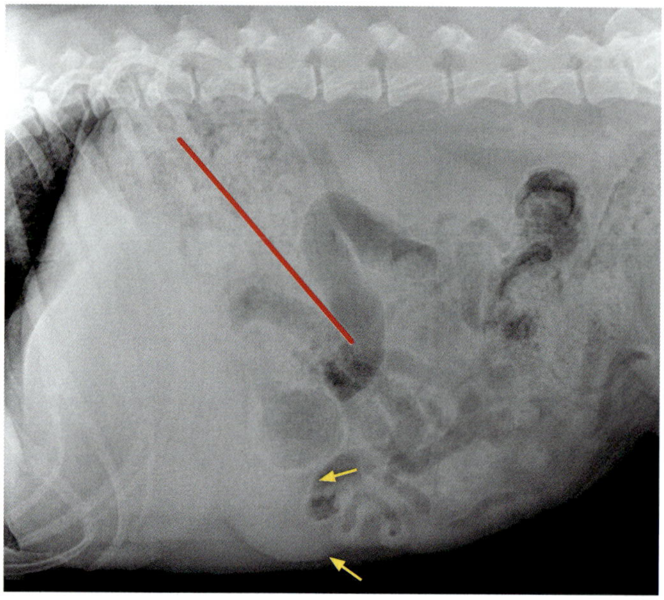

FIG. 26.2 Hepatomegaly leads to the liver extending further into the abdomen (arrows), rotating the gastric axis (red line) anticlockwise, usually with a rounded caudal border (arrows).

Change of opacity

The liver may have dystrophic mineralization if a mass is present. However, mineralization superimposed on the liver is most commonly within the biliary system (see the section later). It may be due to mineralization of the intrahepatic bile ducts (**eFig. 26.3A**) or to choleliths in the gallbladder (**eFig. 26.3B** and **eFig. 26.3C**).

Very rarely, gas may be seen in the liver (**eFig. 26.4**). It is usually difficult from a radiograph to be sure if the gas is in the liver parenchyma, biliary system, or the portal vasculature, and either ultrasound or computed tomography may be used to determine the location of hepatic gas, which would help determine its origin and significance.

Ultrasound imaging of the liver parenchyma

Normal anatomy and imaging appearance

An understanding of the anatomy is critical to be able to understand the appearance on ultrasound and is detailed in chapter 30 and Fig. 30.1 and Fig. 30.2. On ultrasound, it is usually not possible to see the divisions between the lobes unless there is a peritoneal effusion dissecting between them, although they may slide slightly against each other with breathing. A few other anatomic landmarks may be helpful in identifying individual lobes: the caudate lobe is the most caudodorsal part of the liver on the right, where the right kidney lies against the liver in the renal fossa. In addition, the gallbladder lies slightly to the right of the midline between the right medial and quadrate lobes. With experience in ultrasound, sometimes the portal veins can be followed from the porta hepatis into the lobes so an individual lobe can be confidently identified.

On ultrasound, the liver should be homogenous with a "coarse" echotexture due to multiple small nonspecular echoes making small, short linear speckles uniformly distributed through the liver (**eFig. 26.5**). The liver has an echogenic margin due to the capsule, and this should be smooth and each lobe coming to a sharp edge without rounding –often described as looking like a shark's fin (Fig. 26.3). The liver contains many anechoic tubular structures that are either the hepatic veins or the portal veins. The portal veins tend to have more echogenic walls than hepatic veins. Hepatic arteries also pass through the liver that can generally only be identified with Doppler. Bile ducts are only seen when they are enlarged when they appear as anechoic tubes parallel with the portal veins without a Doppler signal.

How to image

The entire liver should be scanned, sweeping through each part in two planes (laterolateral sweeping in a plane parallel to the long axis of the liver, and craniocaudal sweeping in a transverse plane). This involves placing the probe in several locations as the dorsal liver cannot be accessed from ventrally in most dogs. In fat patients, the falciform fat pad can cause problems when scanning from ventrally –fat is hyperechoic and semistructured and can be mistaken for the abnormal liver. It can also attenuate the beam, making an examination of the liver in large

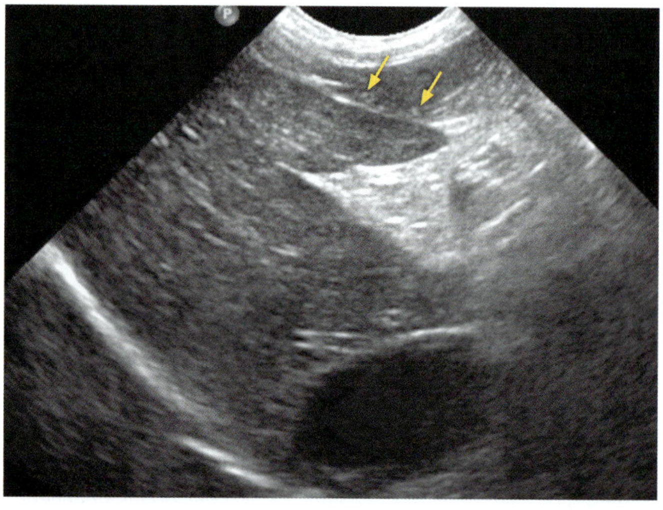

FIG. 26.3 Ultrasound of a normal liver. Note the smooth echogenic capsule and caudal margin with a "shark's fin" appearance (arrows).

fat dogs challenging, and may necessitate a lower frequency setting or low-frequency probe compared to the remainder of the abdomen.

When selecting settings, ensure the depth is sufficient that the diaphragm can be seen on the image as a highly echogenic curved interface, which may yield a mirror image artifact (where it appears as if the liver is mirrored on the other side of the diaphragm). The focal zone should be set in the far half to a third of the screen, and the frame rate and frequency should be adjusted to optimize the image.

Assessing for abnormalities

Liver size

There is no definitive assessment of hepatic size, although a liver that extends caudal to the stomach or caudal to the right kidney is considered enlarged. Subjective signs of enlargement are if the probe is positioned reasonably caudal to the costal arch and yet the liver remains visible and if the liver capsule loses its shark's fin shape (Fig. 26.3) and becomes rounded.

Margination and shape

An undulating or irregular capsule may indicate a diffuse abnormality. A mass may be seen, or a single lobe may be abnormal.

Echotexture

The overall echotexture should be examined for any areas where it is altered focally. The overall echogenicity should be compared to adjacent organs (e.g., the liver should be very slightly hypoechoic to the spleen and slightly hyperechoic or isoechoic to the renal cortex). Both organs should be on the same image during comparison since moving the probe and particularly altering machine settings between views makes the comparison worthless.

Focal vs. diffuse hepatic parenchymal imaging abnormalities

Ultrasound is very good at identifying focal changes such as nodules (eFig. 26.6), although it is not so good at concluding the cause of the change. It is moderately good at identifying diffuse changes in echogenicity. However, it tends to be better if there is also concurrent size and shape change, and in almost all circumstances, findings should be backed up by cytology/histopathology to confirm the cause of the abnormalities.

Differentials for nodular/focal liver abnormalities where liver appearance between nodules is normal

Nodules may be single or multiple and have very similar differentials. Any nodule (or mass) may be neoplasia (primary hepatic, metastatic), hematoma, inflammatory nodule (abscess, granuloma), benign (nodular hyperplasia, extramedullary hematopoiesis, or a "nodule" with more normal tissue between areas of fibrosis).

A nodule with an anechoic (fluid-filled) core may be a cyst (thin-walled) or due to fluid/necrosis within the center of an abscess, granuloma, or neoplasia if the wall is thicker, causing a cavitary mass (Fig. 26.4). Both benign and malignant nodules have the potential to be hypoechoic, isoechoic, or hyperechoic to the surrounding liver.

Multiple nodules are most commonly benign associated with normal aging and a variety of age-related diseases, with endocrine disease (hyperadrenocorticism, diabetes mellitus) or some drugs such as phenobarbitone, although metastatic neoplasia may also lead to multiple nodules. It is not possible to distinguish benign from malignant nodules with B-mode ultrasound, underlining the importance of cytological or histological examination of tissue before diagnosing malignancy.

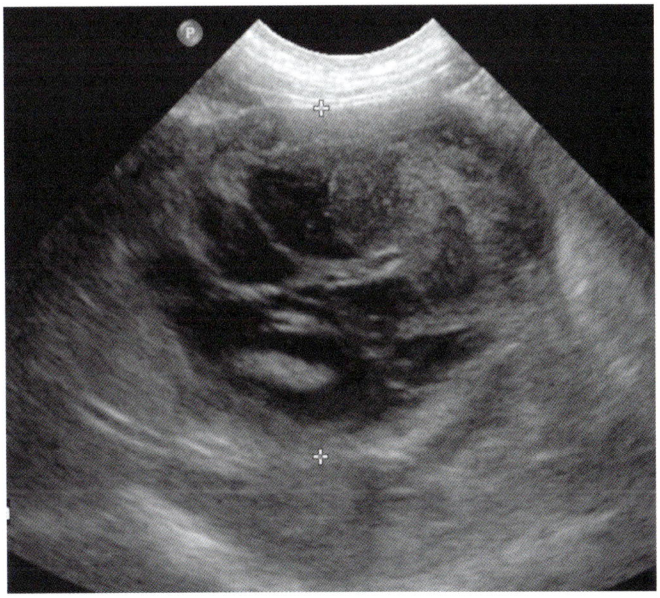

FIG. 26.4 Ultrasound appearance of a cavitary hepatic mass due to hemangiosarcoma.

Specific differentials for liver nodules with different ultrasound appearances are shown in Table 26.1.

One feature associated with neoplasia is the target lesion (Fig. 26.5), where a nodule looks like an archery target with an inner core of relative hyperechogenicity and an outer rim of hypoechogenicity. In a study of a small number of dogs, a target lesion has a 74% positive predictive value for malignancy, although target lesions may be benign.[1] A separate study identified that the presence of a larger mass (over 3 cm) and peritoneal effusion were the only two features that helped differentiate neoplastic lesions from benign lesions on ultrasound, although target lesions were not evaluated.[2] Ultimately, cytology or histology is required to diagnose neoplasia. Identifying enlarged hepatic lymph nodes (found on either side of the portal vein just caudal to the porta hepatis) may suggest hepatic neoplasia with metastasis, although enlarged lymph nodes also occur with benign conditions. Therefore, identifying enlarged lymph nodes is concerning but not definitive for malignancy. If a very large mass is found, its position in relation to the caudal vena cava and portal vein should be evaluated (eFig. 26.7) to assess if the mass is amenable to surgical resection.

A liver lobe torsion can mimic a hypoechoic, round-to-ovoid "mass", affecting an entire liver lobe.[3] This is an uncommon presentation, typically in medium to large breed dogs. It is more often a left-sided lobe; however, the lobe may be displaced to the midline after torsing, and the lobe is typically hypoechoic or heterogenous, enlarged, and slightly rounded, and therefore may mimic a neoplastic mass. Reduced or absent Doppler signal in the vessels supports the diagnosis of a lobar torsion (eFig. 26.8).

Differentials for disease affecting the entire liver diffusely

Diffuse abnormality is harder to recognize than a nodule. There could be diffuse hyperechogenicity or hypoechogenicity (compared to the kidney or spleen) or diffuse alteration of the echoarchitecture of the liver, such as in cirrhosis/fibrosis. Multiple nodules affecting a large percentage of the liver may also have the appearance of diffuse hepatic abnormality. Diffuse hypoechoic changes may make the normal portal vascular structures stand out from the hypoechoic parenchyma to a greater extent;

TABLE 26.1 Differential diagnoses for alterations in hepatic echogenicity, nodules, and diffuse alterations in hepatic parenchymal echogenicity.

	Nodular	Diffuse
Anechoic	■ Cyst, cystic tumor, necrosis, abscess, hematoma	■ N/A
Hypoechoic	■ Nodular hyperplasia/ hematopoesis ■ Neoplasia (lymphoma, metastasis, primary) ■ Abscess ■ Necrosis ■ Hematoma ■ Complex cyst ■ Torsion (entire lobe)	■ Passive venous congestion ■ Acute hepatitis (e.g., leptospirosis) ■ Neoplasia (round cell neoplasia: e.g., lymphoma, leukemia, and histiocytic) ■ Amyloidosis (has a familial association in the Shar Pei; may also be slightly heterogeneous in appearance)
Hyperechoic	■ Hyperplasia ■ Neoplasia (primary, metastasis) ■ Mineralization ■ Abscess ■ Granuloma ■ Gas (hepatic emphysema)	■ Steroid hepatopathy (iatrogenic and hyperadrenocorticism) ■ Chronic hepatitis ■ Neoplasia (e.g., lymphoma and mast cell tumor metastasis) ■ Fatty liver (uncommon; e.g., with diabetes mellitus, hypothyroidism, or rarely in young toy breed dogs) ■ Mixed/disordered architecture (some overlap with multifocal)
Mixed echogenicity	■ Hyperplasia ■ Neoplasia (primary, metastasis) ■ Abscess ■ Hematoma	■ Cirrhosis, fibrosis, chronic hepatitis ■ Neoplasia (lymphoma, hepatocellular carcinoma, metastasis) ■ Hepatocutaneous syndrome (a classic honeycomb pattern seen) ■ Multiple processes, e.g., steroid hepatopathy and nodular hyperplasia

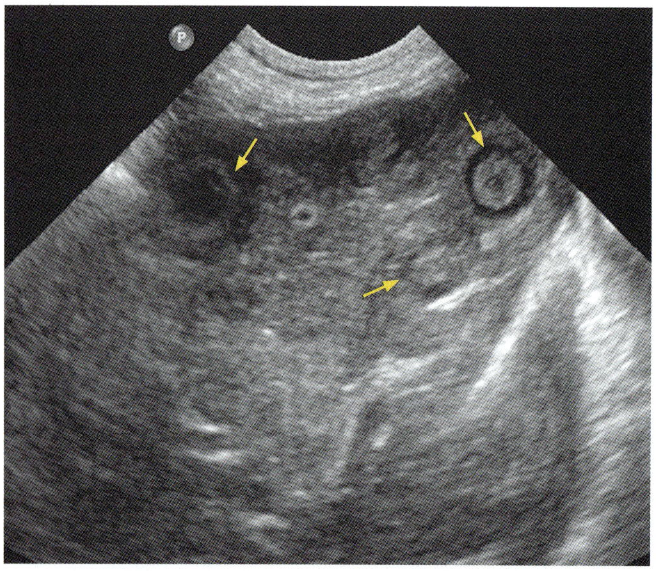

FIG. 26.5 Ultrasound appearance of multiple hepatic target lesions in a patient with metastatic gastrointestinal stromal cell tumor (arrows).

hyperechoic changes render the liver more echogenic than the kidney, and it becomes similar to the spleen, and the portal vascular structures are less visible than typically expected (**eFig. 26.9**).

Patterns of ultrasound findings associated with common diffuse hepatic diseases

The main categories of diffuse disease are benign liver disease, inflammatory liver disease, and neoplasia (Table 26.1). It is important to note that each disease category can show multiple different echogenicities –i.e., ultrasound is nonspecific for benign, inflammatory, or neoplastic liver disease. Both neoplasia and chronic hepatitis may have a range of ultrasound appearances from normal to diffusely abnormal parenchyma and irregular capsular margins due to multiple nodules and/or fibrosis. Some ultrasound features may help prioritize neoplasia vs. hepatitis. Neoplasia usually leads to a liver that is normal-sized to enlarged, while chronic hepatitis usually leads to a liver that is normal-sized to shrunken. Neoplasia may also have enlargement of the local hepatic lymph nodes, which would not usually be seen with (sterile) chronic hepatitis. Chronic hepatitis is frequently associated with portal hypertension and sometimes acquired shunts, which are not so consistently identified in neoplasia. Finally, on close inspection of the parenchyma, chronic hepatitis often has an impression of echogenic thickened and sometimes irregular periportal regions that dissect between more normal or nodular hepatic parenchyma, with the periportal changes less consistent with neoplasia. A biopsy is needed for a definitive diagnosis of diffuse liver disease, but some features may help to prioritize a diagnosis pending a biopsy, as summarized below:

- Acute hepatitis, for example, an infectious process such as leptospirosis, has little structural change and tends to lead to a uniform reduction in echogenicity; for leptospirosis, remember other organs are likely to be affected, such as the kidney where the renal cortex becomes more hyperechoic, so there is a bigger discrepancy in echogenicity when the right kidney is compared to the liver.[4]
- Chronic hepatitis usually leads to disruption of the liver architecture as there is fibrosis with regions of nodular regeneration, and there is generally an overall increase in echogenicity (Fig. 26.6 and **eFig. 26.10**),[5] although the liver may appear ultrasonographically normal in some cases.
- Diffuse infiltration with round cell neoplasia may have a variety of appearances ranging from normal to uniform alteration of echogenicity (may increase or decrease) and the presence of diffuse nodular change. When performing a metastasis check for round cell neoplasia, the liver may have lymphoma or mast cell tumor infiltration and yet remain ultrasonographically normal. A fine-needle aspirate would be necessary for diagnosis.[6]

Differentials for the presence of gas or mineralization in the liver

Gas may be identified within the hepatic vessels, intrahepatic bile ducts, or parenchyma. Gas will usually be echogenic and may cast a dirty acoustic shadow (**eFig. 26.11**), and if in the vessels may appear as small shadowing bubbles. It may be due to sepsis, gastrointestinal disease, trauma, neoplasia, or it may be iatrogenic. It is important to distinguish if the gas is confined to the portal vasculature within the liver or is located within the parenchyma itself, as there is a significant difference between mortality reported, 90% if the gas is in the parenchyma, and 22% if in the vessels, where the gas was in some cases transient and not identified on follow-up.[7]

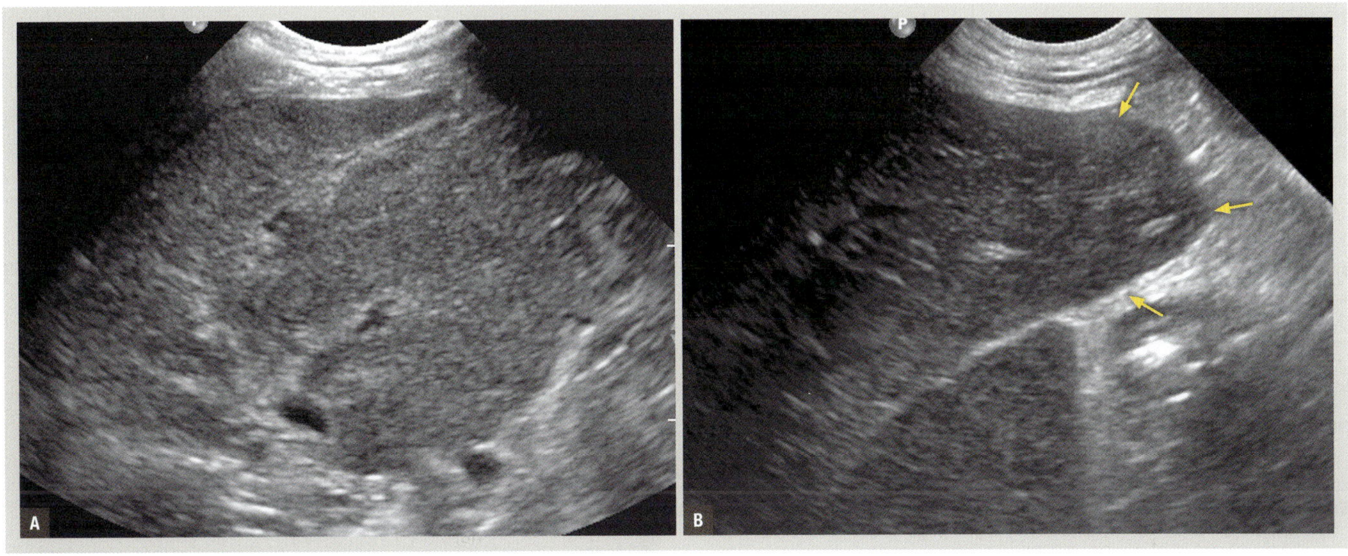

FIG. 26.6 (A) Ultrasound image showing mixed hepatic architecture in a dog with chronic hepatitis, showing irregular hyperechoic periportal regions and a diffusely heterogeneous background. (B) Mixed hepatic architecture in the same dog with chronic hepatitis, showing that the lobar margin may also be rounded and have an undulating capsule (arrows).

Hepatic mineralization appears as an echogenic interface, often with a strong acoustic shadow. As in radiographs, it may be due to mineralization of the bile ducts, which can be an incidental finding, the presence of choleliths in the intrahepatic bile ducts, or due to dystrophic mineralization of a hepatic mass or abnormality. The presence of linear branching mineralization following the bile ducts may not necessarily be associated with clinically significant disease. Cavalier King Charles Spaniels may be overrepresented.[8] More focal pinpoint or larger choleliths within the intrahepatic bile ducts often lack clinical or ultrasound evidence of further biliary abnormality such as cholestasis.[9]

Mineralization of hepatic masses or cysts is uncommon, with mineralization of hepatic cystic lesions described with parasites such as liver fluke.

Use of advanced imaging techniques to image the liver parenchyma

Advanced ultrasound: contrast-enhanced ultrasound and elastography

Advanced ultrasound techniques are available on certain high-specification ultrasound machines. They include contrast-enhanced ultrasound, elastography, and microvascular assessment of lesions.

Contrast-enhanced ultrasound (CEUS) uses very tiny bubbles (called microbubbles), which are in a liquid suspension and are injected into the patient intravenously. The contrast agent remains circulating within the vasculature for a few minutes. Its use is described in the veterinary literature, particularly for assessing hepatic masses based on their perfusion. The unique perfusion of the liver gives it three distinct phases following contrast administration: the arterial phase (starts approximately 7-10 seconds after IV injection and lasts for 10-15 seconds), the portal phase starting at 30-45 seconds postinjection, and lasting up to 2 minutes), and the later delayed or parenchymal phase (when contrast is seen enhancing the hepatic sinusoids until it is cleared from circulation). At the portal and parenchymal phase, many benign lesions are isoechoic to hyperechoic to the surrounding tissues since they have a similar vascularization to normal liver and, therefore, a uniform enhancement (**eFig. 26.12A**). Malignant lesions tend to have a greater proportion of vascularization from the hepatic artery. Consequently, they tend to be strongly enhanced in the arterial phase but poorly enhanced (compared to the surrounding tissues) in the portal and parenchymal phases (early wash and early wash-out pattern (**eFig. 26.12B**).[10] The technique is particularly useful in cases where metastasis checks are being carried out in urgent cases (e.g., ruptured hemangiosarcoma), where a cytologist might not be available to guide decision-making or if a patient is not suitable for fine-needle aspiration (e.g., has a coagulopathy).

Elastography

Elastography is another advanced ultrasound technique that is under evaluation for its applicability to veterinary patients. It is a method using the physical properties of the ultrasound beam moving through soft tissues to assess differences in the stiffness of the tissue, with potential clinical application in assessing the alteration of tissue stiffness associated with a variety of pathologies. Normal values of one method for elastography have been published for the liver, spleen, and kidneys in dogs.[11] Elastography has shown that there is increased stiffness in the liver of brachycephalic dogs, indicating that canine patients may have hepatic effects of hypoxia or inflammatory status similar to that seen in human patients who suffer from obstructive sleep apnea.[12]

Transient elastography (a cut-down consulting-room-based elastography method, which does not have an equivalent B-mode image for planning the plane for image acquisition) is used in humans with chronic hepatic disease as a method of staging the degree of hepatic fibrosis and has been described in a small number of dogs experimentally infected with viral hepatitis.[13] However, there are no robust publications demonstrating the reproducible clinical utility of elastography in veterinary patients yet. There are additional challenges in our species compared to human patients –the shape of some dogs with deep chests will challenge the ability to place the probe appropriately, and a breath hold is usually required, which is not possible for our patients (unless anesthetized, which makes the process more invasive).

Computed tomography

Computed tomography (CT) is commonly used for further investigation of a known or suspected focal liver lesion such as a mass or lobar torsion, usually with a view to surgical planning, and in patients with neoplasia looking for disease spread –for example, a metastasis check (Fig. 26.7). CT is best at identifying focal lesions such as nodules and masses. However, as with ultrasound, it cannot definitively distinguish between benign and malignant masses, although one paper identified that the overall transverse width of the mass (being over 4.5 cm) and being heterogenous in the delayed phase postcontrast were features associated with malignancy.[14] Generally, benign liver masses are hyper- to isoattenuating and homogenously enhancing on the delayed phase postcontrast.[15] CT is generally poor in identifying diffuse liver diseases, with little literature describing its appearance, so it would not usually be the imaging technique of choice in suspected hepatitis, although it may help identify consequences of acute and chronic hepatitis such as acquired shunts and portal thrombi.[16]

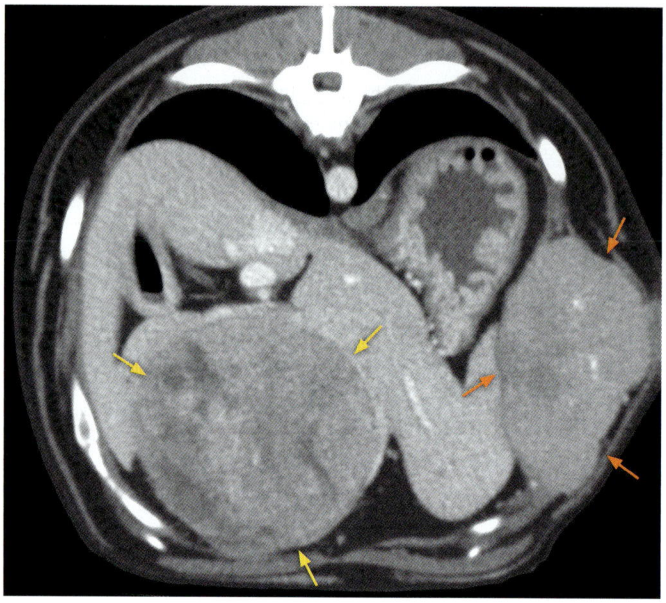

FIG. 26.7 A transverse CT image showing a large heterogeneously enhancing liver mass (yellow arrows), which is a metastatic lesion from the body wall sarcoma (orange arrows).

Magnetic resonance imaging

Magnetic resonance imaging (MRI) is also not currently used in veterinary medicine for investigation of liver disease, although it is used in humans to identify active inflammation in acute liver disease (abnormal enhancement) and can identify fat accumulation and fibrosis in more chronic inflammation, in addition to a host of advanced MRI sequences for specific diseases.

Ultrasound-guided biopsy and fine-needle aspiration of the liver parenchyma

Options for liver sampling include fine-needle aspiration (FNA), tissue core biopsy under ultrasound guidance, or laparoscopic or open wedge biopsies. Several considerations are necessary when deciding which technique to select. First, it needs to be understood what can be diagnosed with the sample type and size likely acquired. An FNA provides a reasonable chance in terms of diagnosing the cause of a hepatic nodule (see chapter 28 for more details on interpreting liver cytology). However, an FNA provides too small a sample size to distinguish causes of diffuse hepatic disease other than neoplastic infiltration (e.g., lymphoma, mast cell tumor). For the diagnosis of diffuse diseases such as chronic hepatitis and ductal plate malformation, a tissue biopsy is required as pathologists need a number of portal triads to generate an accurate diagnosis (12-15 portal triads are recommended).[5] This can be achieved with ultrasound tissue core biopsies but usually necessitates obtaining several (four are recommended) biopsy samples, with the risk of hemorrhage increasing with the number of samples taken. For this reason, if available, wedge biopsies taken at laparoscopy or laparotomy are preferred for the investigation of diffuse liver disease as they are larger and more representative.[5]

Potential complications and risks

In terms of anticipated complications, the most common complication to consider is hemorrhage. The risk of hemorrhage is higher with a tissue core than an FNA. However, since the liver is very vascular and dogs with diffuse liver disease such as chronic hepatitis have the potential for coagulopathy and may also have chronic anemia, there is a risk of potentially fatal hemorrhage following even an FNA technique. All dogs with suspected chronic hepatitis where a needle aspirate or biopsy is planned are therefore recommended by the ACVIM consensus statement to have a hematocrit, platelet count, clotting times, and fibrinogen measurement, and dogs at risk of von Willebrand's factor deficiency should additionally have buccal mucosal bleeding time and von Willebrand factor tests.[5] Any dog with abnormalities on these tests may have correction of these abnormalities on a case-by-case basis, although the consensus statement did not find evidence for routine prophylaxis, and blood component treatment should be available during and after the biopsy. Laparoscopic biopsies are preferred in these cases if a tissue biopsy is needed.

Other potential complications of ultrasound-guided biopsies include perforation of a hollow viscous and infection. Very rare, theoretical complications may include seeding of a carcinoma along a needle tract or induction of fatal vagotonia when using a fully automated tissue core biopsy. This is a theoretical risk in dogs but has been described in cats.

Fine-needle aspiration

For FNAs, a needle is first chosen –the author prefers a 22-gauge, 1.5-inch needle, which is then inserted through clipped and aseptically prepared skin into the liver with ultrasound guidance. Sedation is usually necessary since the patient must not move during sampling. Ultrasound is used to avoid passing through big intrahepatic vessels and allows the selection of a path for the needle while avoiding both the gallbladder cone within the liver and other organs. The needle is "stabbed" three to four times, avoiding redirection between stabs. The tip of the needle must remain in the ultrasound field of view during the stabbing to prevent damage to deeper organs. No aspiration is performed unless there is little yield. The sample is sprayed gently onto a slide and then smeared gently. Overenthusiastic spraying and smearing can damage cells, rendering the sample nondiagnostic. Usually, 2-3 samples from each lesion are taken, depending on the yield.

Ultrasound-guided tissue core biopsy

This procedure requires heavy sedation, often general anesthesia. If a tissue core biopsy is elected, the largest tissue core biopsy needle that can be safely used is ideal since the more intact portal triads obtained, the more accurate a diagnosis is. Ideally, a liver biopsy should be performed with a 14 gauge Trucut needle and 2 cm length since needles smaller than this will reduce the diagnostic yield and necessitate a greater number of biopsies. If it is not considered safe to obtain an adequate sample this way, another biopsy technique, such as laparoscopy or exploratory laparotomy, should be performed instead to obtain the biopsy. Again, ultrasound is used to guide the needle through a safe path to the liver, avoiding other organs and large vessels. The tissue core sample is submitted in formalin, and observing that the sample sinks in the pot helps to confirm that an inadvertent falciform fat sample has not been acquired (fat would float).

Imaging the biliary system

The biliary system can be divided into the intrahepatic portion (progressively larger intrahepatic bile ducts take bile from the portal triads to the extrahepatic biliary system) and the extrahepatic biliary system, which comprises the gallbladder and a duct that runs from the gallbladder neck to the major duodenal papilla. This duct is called the cystic duct at the level that arises from the gallbladder neck, and several intrahepatic bile ducts join it. It changes its name to the common bile duct after the last intrahepatic duct joins it.

Radiographic imaging of the biliary system

Radiographs are not a useful method to evaluate the gallbladder and biliary tree. They will only show abnormalities if the intrahepatic bile ducts become mineralized or mineral opacity choleliths are seen in the gallbladder or extrahepatic bile duct. Even more rarely, gas may be seen in the gallbladder in cases of emphysematous cystitis.

Ultrasound imaging of the biliary system

Normal anatomy and imaging appearance

The gallbladder lies in the right ventral part of the liver and should have a smooth echogenic wall (Fig. 26.8A), which usually appears as a pencil-thin echogenic line, with an upper measurement of thickness for fasted dogs <40 kg being 1.3 mm.[17] Note that there may be differences in gallbladder wall thickness with feeding, and with some sedatives such as dexmedetomidine. The neck of the gallbladder is usually found at the most dorsal part and tapers to a nondistended (usually less than 3 mm) cystic duct, which may be traced with ultrasound to the major duodenal papilla in some dogs, although not all. The cystic/common bile duct is easier to follow if it becomes distended. As described above, the intrahepatic bile ducts should only be seen if distended.

How to image

The gallbladder should be examined by a sweep from base to apex in both short and long axes. Special attention is paid to the neck of the gallbladder to ensure it tapers down to being empty or near empty –any visibility of more than a few mm diameter of fluid in the neck suggests bile duct distension. If possible, the extrahepatic biliary duct should be followed from the gallbladder neck (close to the midline of the patient) dorsally and to the right, where it enters the duodenal papilla near the proximal duodenal flexure.

Assessing for abnormalities

Size

Assess the gallbladder and bile duct walls for any thickening and gallbladder size and identify any distension of the intra- or extrahepatic bile ducts. Note that the gallbladder empties postprandially, and there is a wide physiologic range in gallbladder volume, which is associated with body weight. Standard measures for the gallbladder are estimated on 2D ultrasound by measuring the height, width, and length of the gallbladder and using the formula to estimate the volume of an ellipsoid (H×W×L×0.53). It may be an option for the ultrasound machine to calculate this). As standard, "normal" values are therefore given for fasted animals. This method calculates 80-90% of normal fasted dogs with a volume of less than 1 mL/kg.[18]

Echogenicity

Look for any abnormal gallbladder material (whether it is gravity-dependent) in the extrahepatic and intrahepatic bile ducts or gas or mineralization in the biliary tract.

Number

Various congenital abnormalities may be recognized (see chapter 37), including dilation of multiple intra- and/or extra-hepatic bile ducts (Caroli's disease), with or without atresia of the gallbladder.[19] Occasionally, a very empty gallbladder may be overlooked on ultrasound and appear missing.

Location

The gallbladder may pass into the thorax in the case of congenital or traumatic diaphragmatic hernias/ruptures.

Patterns of ultrasound findings associated with common biliary diseases

Appearance of chronic inflammatory disease

Gallbladder wall abnormalities may be seen in chronic inflammatory disease. These include thickening or loss of the normal smooth-walled appearance (Fig. 26.8B). Thickening is often irregular; however, it may be diffuse and uniform, leading to a "double wall" sign where there is a hypoechoic layer sandwiched between the two outer hyperechoic layers (**eFig. 26.13**). This double wall sign is thought to show gallbladder edema, which may be due to edematous gallbladder inflammation/cholecystitis, but is more frequently seen with anaphylaxis, portal hypertension, and infrequently with hypoalbuminemia.[20] A survey of 54 dogs with confirmed cholangiohepatitis showed ultrasound abnormalities in 84%. A spectrum of changes was seen in the liver itself and the biliary tract. Abnormalities included gallbladder wall thickening (sometimes with a double rim, sometimes with irregular thickening of the wall), gallbladder and/or extrahepatic bile duct distension, and varying degrees of echogenic content.[21] Sometimes cholecystitis may become polypoid or emphysematous (more common in diabetic patients, **eFig. 26.14**). Emphysematous cholecystitis may show gas, either tracking through the wall or within the lumen. A differential for echogenic shadowing foci noted within the wall would be adenomyomatosis (**eFig. 26.15**), a poorly described pathology uncommonly encountered, thought to be due to cholesterol crystals becoming trapped in the wall, and of unclear clinical significance.

Presence of echogenic material in the gallbladder

- Sludge: many aging dogs have some echogenic gallbladder content that moves dependently within the gallbladder and that we regard as

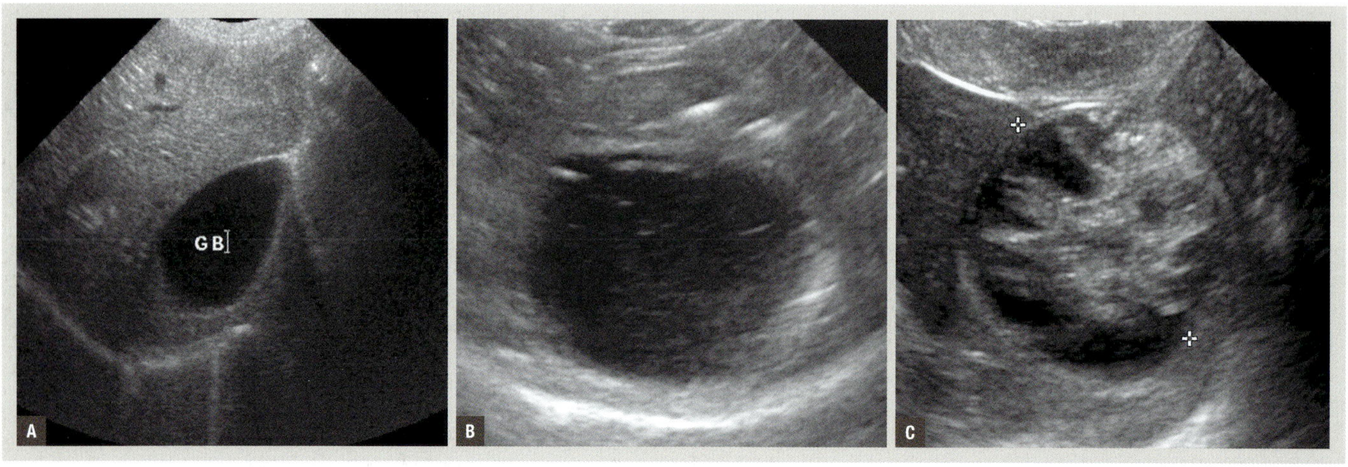

FIG. 26.8 (A) Normal ultrasound appearance of the gallbladder –anechoic lumen and a pencil-thin echogenic wall. (B) Ultrasound image of gallbladder irregular wall thickening due to cholangitis. (C) A stellate/kiwi pattern of gallbladder content on ultrasound, consistent with a mucocele.

incidental "sludge" in most cases[22] unless there are other indications of cholestasis (Video 26.1).

- Mucocele: a mucocele is an abnormal accumulation of mucinous content within the gallbladder in association with mucosal hypertrophy. Gallbladder mucocele is a common diagnosis in dogs, with extensive literature on the imaging appearance. Ultrasound is the most commonly employed imaging modality for diagnosis,[23] with a "classic" mucocele having a stellate appearance of echogenic content fixed within the otherwise anechoic gallbladder contents. However, there are a variety of gallbladder mucocele appearances on ultrasound, ranging from a streak of fixed echogenic content to the more classic "cut kiwi fruit" or stellate appearance described by Choi in 2013 (Fig. 26.8C).[24] Six different subtypes are described: 1: echogenic immobile bile occupying the gallbladder; 2: incomplete stellate pattern; 3: classic stellate pattern; 4: combined stellate and kiwi fruit pattern; 5: kiwi fruit pattern; 6: kiwi fruit pattern without central echogenic bile. Types 1, 2, 4, and 5 were most common, and type of mucocoele may be associated with likelihood of having clinical signs.[25] The key feature of all subtypes of mucocele is the lack of change of location within the gallbladder despite the different recumbency of the patient. Additional findings may include other abnormalities within the extrahepatic biliary tract (dilation of the common bile duct, thickening of the gallbladder wall and the remaining extrahepatic biliary tract), and potentially local mesenteric reaction or bile peritonitis if the gallbladder ruptures, with the mucocele sometimes identified in the abdomen outside the gallbladder. One study showed that the identification of nondependent biliary sludge was a risk factor for the future development of gallbladder mucocele, warranting imaging monitoring.[26]
- Choleliths: gallbladder choleliths are seen with reasonable frequency, in some cases without clinical signs (although monitoring should always be advised). They can, of course, be associated with obstruction or cholelithiasis.

Video 26.1

Video showing that echogenic particles of sludge can be seen to slowly reposition dependently in the gall bladder.

Gallbladder masses

Focal thickenings of the gallbladder may be a gallbladder polyp, a carcinoid, or neoplasia (eFig. 26.16). Neoplasia of the biliary tract is rare. In a case series of 14 patients with gallbladder neoplasia, all showed a sessile vascularized gallbladder mass.[27]

Extrahepatic bile duct abnormalities

Ultrasound abnormalities of the extrahepatic bile duct include dilation of the duct, or having abnormal thickening of the wall, or abnormal content. Dilation of the duct is seen with infection or obstruction or in a subset of currently healthy cats if previous duct dilation is now resolved.

Infection or sterile inflammation is usually seen as part of a wider picture of cholangitis, or cholangiohepatitis (eFig. 26.17). These patients often have generalized thickening of the bile duct wall and may have abnormal sludge or cholelith content within the biliary tract, which may not be causing obstruction. The duodenal papilla may be enlarged, with a normal papilla size of 15 mm by 6 mm by 4 mm.[28] Obstruction may be caused by a luminal lesion (e.g., sludge or a cholelith lying within the lumen) or a mural lesion (e.g., fibrosis, inflammation or neoplasia of the bile duct wall itself) or rarely, a duodenal wall mass or foreign body at the level of the papilla. However, most commonly, it is due to compression from an adjacent structure with an inflamed pancreas due to pancreatitis being the commonest cause of extrahepatic biliary obstruction (see chapter 15 for details of pancreas imaging). All forms of obstruction will cause the extrahepatic bile duct to distend proximal to the obstruction, so identification of a distended bile duct should prompt a search for obstruction. Ultrasound is a helpful clinical tool in identifying biliary obstruction and its cause. It is often easiest to look for the bile duct at the neck of the gallbladder, and if a dilated duct is found, it should be followed towards the papilla to attempt to identify the source of the obstruction.

Intrahepatic bile duct distension

Intrahepatic bile duct distension is described as giving the liver a "too many tubes" appearance, as additional anechoic "vessels" are seen in the liver parallel with the intrahepatic portal veins. These intrahepatic bile ducts lack a Doppler signal as opposed to the signal obtained from hepatic and portal veins (**eFig. 26.18**). Intrahepatic bile ducts become visible around 5-7 days after extrahepatic biliary obstruction. Therefore, dilation may be seen in cases of obstruction. However, it may also be seen in cases of cholangitis. Intrahepatic biliary mineralization or choleliths may occasionally be seen as echogenic, sometimes shadowing lines/foci that are along the path of the biliary system.

Ultrasound-guided gallbladder aspiration

Bile aspiration from the gallbladder (cholecystocentesis) may be beneficial to distinguish infectious from sterile cholangitis. The primary complications with potentially severe clinical consequences are rupture of the gallbladder leading to bile peritonitis and cardiopulmonary arrest during the procedure (associated either with sedation or general anesthesia or with vasovagal reflex (biliary cardiac reflex). There are few publications to guide risk-benefit analysis –one publication of 300 cholecystocentesis procedures reported eight cases of severe complications, including two gallbladder ruptures, three cardiopulmonary arrests, and one each of acute kidney injury, hypotension, and SIRS (7/8 patients died).[29] This suggests a low rate of complications, although those complications were potentially very severe. There are no specific guidelines associating gallbladder ultrasound appearance with the risk of complications. Indeed, in that study, the patients with complications did not necessarily have the most severely abnormal gallbladder appearance. Speculatively, risk factors to consider may include an obstructed gallbladder or a severely abnormal gallbladder wall in case there is necrosis/friability that could increase the risk of rupture following sampling. A mature mucocele would, therefore, not usually be considered a candidate for cholecystocentesis due to the likelihood of mucocele-associated wall necrosis. In addition, the usual considerations of risk factors in ultrasound-guided sampling discussed in the previous section remain applicable to cholecystocentesis.

Use of advanced imaging techniques to image the biliary tract

Advanced ultrasound techniques –contrast-enhanced ultrasound

Contrast-enhanced ultrasound (CEUS) has a role in identifying gallbladder rupture. B-mode ultrasound has difficulty distinguishing between an intact and a ruptured gallbladder in many conditions (e.g., gallbladder necrosis following gallbladder mucocele or due to cholangitis or obstruction). A paper by Bargellini in 2018 introduced additional information that CEUS can offer in gallbladder conditions, particularly for assessing the wall for enhancement that might discriminate between wall edema/cystic mucosal hyperplasia and necrosis.[30] CEUS also helped determine if echogenic structures adjacent to the wall were polypoid nodules/masses or sediment/content lying alongside the wall. CEUS was found to be 100% sensitive and specific for identifying wall necrosis (determined at surgery), while B-mode ultrasound was 75% sensitive and 81% specific.[31]

Computed tomography

Some data on normal biliary and gallbladder anatomy on CT in dogs have been published.[32,33] The clinical application of CT in biliary tract disease is currently limited. It has been used to understand abnormal biliary anatomy in a dog with Caroli's syndrome.[34] The CT of common biliary pathologies have been retrospectively reported[35] including attenuation values of the gallbladder content in gallbladder mucocele,[36] showing hyperattenuating contents centrally in the gallbladder (not dependently). This provides useful data for clinicians who identify an abnormal appearance of the gallbladder on CT of the abdomen performed for other reasons, and in centers where ultrasound is not available as frequently as CT, may provide an option for evaluation of mucoceles.

Magnetic resonance imaging

Magnetic resonance cholangiopancreatography is routinely used to evaluate the gallbladder and biliary tree in humans. However, it is not widely used in veterinary medicine at the current time.

Scintigraphy

Scintigraphy can be used to assess for obstruction of the biliary tract by administering a scintigraphic agent that is excreted well into bile and observing if it reaches the small intestines. While an effective technique, this is little used because other modern imaging techniques are generally sufficient to identify biliary obstruction and its causes, and there is a lack of availability of scintigraphy in veterinary medicine.[37]

Imaging the portal vasculature

The portal vein is the third largest abdominal vessel and the vessel most commonly examined with imaging, primarily to identify a congenital abnormality (congenital portosystemic shunt or arterioportal malformation) and, at times, to obtain evidence of acquired vascular abnormality such as acquired portosystemic shunting or portal vein thrombosis. The portal vein drains venous blood from the gastrointestinal tract, pancreas, and spleen into the liver. Its origin can be identified as the cranial mesenteric vein in the mid-abdomen amongst the mesentery. It becomes the portal vein when the caudal mesenteric vein joins the cranial mesenteric vein. Two further tributaries join (the splenic vein from the left and the gastroduodenal vein from the right) before the portal vein enters the liver and divides into left, central, and right branches within the liver to supply the liver parenchyma.

Radiographic imaging of abnormalities of the portal vasculature

Radiographs are of limited use in imaging portal vasculature. Historically, radiographs acquired following a contrast portovenogram (injection of iodinated contrast media into a mesenteric vein via a mini-laparotomy) were used to diagnose a portosystemic shunt. However, this has now been superseded by less invasive ultrasound or CT evaluation. Fluoroscopic contrast portovenograms may still be acquired by some surgeons at the time of shunt ligation surgery.

The main feature of congenital portosystemic shunting on a plain radiograph is a small liver (microhepatica) and, in some cases, enlarged kidneys. Uroliths may be identified in the bladder or kidneys, although the ammonium urate uroliths associated with portosystemic shunts are often radiolucent and can, therefore, be overlooked on plain radiographs unless they are mixed with struvite as a result of secondary infection. Dogs with acquired portosystemic shunts are also likely to have ascites due to portal hypertension, further limiting radiographic detail.

Ultrasound imaging of abnormalities of the portal vasculature

Normal anatomy and imaging appearance

A detailed discussion of ultrasound of the portal vasculature is beyond the scope of this book but can be found in D'Anjou and Penninck's reference textbook "Atlas of Small Animal Ultrasonography 2nd edition", 2015.

How to image

A thorough examination of the entire portal tributary system is necessary to identify the origin of an extrahepatic PSS, of the intrahepatic portal divisions to identify an intrahepatic PSS origin, and of the caudal vena cava and azygous veins for the termination of the anomalous vessel. An understanding of locations for commonly encountered shunt anatomy may help to find the majority of shunt types.[38] Doppler may be used to confirm that blood in the main portal vein as it enters the liver at the porta hepatis is hepatopetal (**eFig. 26.19**).

Differential diagnoses for specific imaging abnormalities

Congenital portosystemic shunts

The most common portal anomaly seen is a portosystemic shunt. These are often congenital, where they may have an anomalous vessel connecting the portal to systemic circulation either within or outside the hepatic parenchyma. The types of portosystemic shunts can be divided into intrahepatic and extrahepatic (see chapter 36). Small breed dogs more commonly have extrahepatic shunts; however, it is possible to get any type of shunt in any dog, so a thorough examination of the entire portal system is necessary. The most common termination vessel is the caudal vena cava, with the anomalous vessel most frequently entering the CVC between the renal and hepatic veins if extrahepatic.[39] It is possible for a portosystemic shunt to enter the caudal vena cava elsewhere (including in its intrathoracic portion) or into another systemic vein –most commonly the azygous vein, although other vessels, including the internal thoracic, colic, external iliac veins, etc. are described. Additional features such as microhepatica, renomegaly, and the presence of renal or bladder uroliths may be suggestive of a shunt, although identifying the shunt via imaging is required for diagnosis.[40]

Congenital extrahepatic portosystemic shunts

These arise from the tributaries of the portal vein and exit the portal vein caudal to the porta hepatis, most commonly in the splenic vein (left-sided shunts) and the gastroduodenal vein (right-sided shunts). They enter the caudal vena cava most commonly and the azygous vein second most commonly. They are often looping, tortuous vessels that run dorsally from close to the portal vein up to a systemic vein. The portal vein cranial to the shunt exit is reduced in diameter compared to the portal vein caudal to the shunt exit, as blood preferentially passes up the shunt.

Congenital intrahepatic portosystemic shunts

These arise from the intrahepatic branches, where the portal vein divides into left, right, and central branches (cranial to the porta hepatis, where the portal vein enters the liver). These usually form a wide, short shunt with a swirling Doppler signal, connecting a dilated intrahepatic vessel to the caudal vena cava via the hepatic veins.

Acquired portosystemic shunts

Acquired portosystemic shunts occur secondary to portal hypertension, which may be prehepatic (portal vein compression/hypoplasia, tumor, or thrombus), hepatic (end stage of many liver diseases including chronic hepatitis, neoplasia, nodular regeneration, arteriovenous malformations) or posthepatic (e.g., caudal vena cava obstruction, pericarditis restricting the right heart). Acquired shunts lead to the opening up of multiple small vessels from the mesentery to the systemic circulation, which most commonly drain via the left renal and left gonadal veins (**eFig. 26.20**), so the shunt may be identified by looking for a plexus of abnormal small vessels close to the left kidney, although several other locations of varices of collateral circulation may be identified. Reduced portal blood flow may be identified with spectral Doppler (mean less than 10 cm/s, normal range 18 ± 7 cm/s) in the dog.[41] Ascites is a common consequence of portal hypertension, so identifying some free fluid in the abdomen supports the diagnosis. Hepatic parenchymal anomalies may also be seen if it is secondary to chronic hepatitis.

Portal vein thrombosis

Portal vein thrombosis is a rare complication, seen associated with any hypercoagulable state and often with hepatic disease or neoplasia.[42] It may be asymptomatic or may lead to signs associated with portal hypertension, such as acquired shunting and ascites. A thrombus appears on ultrasound as a slightly echogenic structure filling the portal vein (**eFig. 26.21**), with a lack of Doppler signal.

Arterioportal malformation

Rarely, an arterioportal malformation is identified in a young patient, leading to portal hypertension (as the arterial pressure blood communicates with the portal system), and the communication may be recognized since there are many tortuous vessels within a portion of the liver.

Use of advanced imaging techniques to image the portal vasculature

Computed tomography

Contrast CT vascular studies are widely used in the diagnosis of portal vascular abnormalities.[43] CT has the advantages of being noninvasive compared to portovenography and can image the vessels at different time points postinjection, timing the acquisition so the contrast may be seen most strongly in the arteries and/or in the portal veins, with a more delayed scan 1-2 minutes postinjection where contrast uptake should be mostly in the hepatic parenchyma. As with ultrasound, congenital portosystemic shunts are the most common vascular anomaly diagnosed. However, an arterioportal malformation is a rare congenital vascular anomaly that may be diagnosed with a triple-phase (arterial, portal, then delayed phase) CT contrast study, with arterial phase contrast noted in the hepatic portal veins due to the arterioportal communication,[44] and the consequences of the secondary portal hypertension seen such as ascites. CT is very helpful for identifying shunts, as there is no concern regarding being able to access the vessels for assessment as with ultrasound (it may be difficult to find the portal vasculature in large dogs on ultrasound or those with a lot of bowel gas). It also allows the whole abdomen to be examined to minimize the risk of missing an unusual shunt variant or double shunting vessel, and it allows for surgical planning or shunt measurements to be taken in patients going for interventional management of intrahepatic shunts (**eFig. 26.22** and **eFig. 16.23**).[45] Ultrasound may be the initial approach as it is noninvasive and can be performed with light sedation (particularly useful if the patient is being evaluated while presenting with neurological signs). Ultrasound by an experienced operator may be sufficient for a definitive diagnosis if an extrahepatic shunt is found. However, if ultrasound is nondiagnostic or equivocal, or if an intrahepatic shunt is suspected/found, and if surgical/interventional management is planned, then a CT is usually warranted once the patient has been stabilized.

CT may be useful in identifying signs of portal hypertension (acquired shunts[46] and ascites); however, it cannot obtain an actual measurement to confirm portal hypertension. It readily identifies a portal vein thrombus,[47] although this should be confirmed in the delayed phases as earlier phases may have a "streaming" effect as blood with different concentrations of contrast agent mix, which can mimic a thrombus.

Magnetic resonance imaging

MRI of portosystemic shunts is described and avoids the use of iodine contrast administration if an animal has a known reaction to this. However, MRI is not used for shunt diagnosis on the clinic floor, where ultrasound and CT are more widely available.

Scintigraphy

Scintigraphy is very accurate for diagnosing the presence of portosystemic shunting[48] but gives no anatomic information, so it is not routinely used clinically.

KEY POINTS

- Many imaging modalities may be used to evaluate the liver. Radiography is helpful for an overview; however, ultrasound and computed tomography are the main methods of detailed hepatic imaging.
- Ultrasound of the liver encompasses a thorough examination of the hepatic parenchyma, the intra- and extrahepatic biliary tracts, and the portal vasculature.
- Abnormalities affecting the hepatic parenchyma may be nodular or diffuse, and there is a great deal of overlap in imaging appearance between different hepatic diseases. Therefore, a liver biopsy or fine-needle aspirate sample is needed for a definitive diagnosis.
- The most common portal vascular abnormality is a portosystemic shunt. Both ultrasound and computed tomography are commonly used to image the portal vascular system to identify and characterize portosystemic shunts.

References

1. Cuccovillo A, Lamb CR. Cellular features of sonographic target lesions of the liver and spleen in 21 dogs and a cat. Vet Radiol Ultrasound 43(3):275-278, 2002.
2. Murakami T, Feeney DA, Bahr KL. Analysis of clinical and ultrasonographic data by use of logistic regression models for prediction of malignant versus benign causes of ultrasonographically detected focal liver lesions in dogs. *Am J Vet Res* 73(6):821-829, 2012.
3. Schwartz SG, Mitchell SL, Keating JH, Chan DL. Liver lobe torsion in dogs: 13 cases (1995-2004). *J Am Vet Med Assoc* 228(2):242-247, 2006.
4. Sonet J, Barthélemy A, Goy-Thollot I, Pouzot-Nevoret C. Prospective evaluation of abdominal ultrasonographic findings in 35 dogs with leptospirosis. *Vet Radiol Ultrasound* 59(1):98-106, 2018.
5. Webster CRL, Center SA, Cullen JM, Penninck DG, Richter KP, Twedt DC, Watson PJ. ACVIM consensus statement on the diagnosis and treatment of chronic hepatitis in dogs. *J Vet Intern Med* 33(3):1173-1200, 2019.
6. Book AP, Fidel J, Wills T, Bryan J, Sellon R, Mattoon J. Correlation of ultrasound findings, liver and spleen cytology, and prognosis in the clinical staging of high metastatic risk canine mast cell tumours. *Vet Radiol Ultrasound* 52(5):548-554, 2011.
7. Manfredi S, Fabbi M, Bonazzi M, Leonardi F, Miduri F, Parroccini I, Daga E, Gnudi G, Volta A. Ultrasonographic differentiation between portal venous and parenchymal gas may be important for the prognosis of canine and feline hepatic emphysema: 37 cases. *Vet Radiol Ultrasound* 60(6):734-744, 2019.
8. Genain MA, Barbosa A, Herrtage M, Watson P. Clinical relevance of radiographic linear branching mineral opacities in the canine liver. *J Small Anim Pract* 59(7):432-437, 2018.
9. Leoni FP, Puccinelli C, Pelligra T, Gori E, Marchetti V, Diana A, Linta N, Citi S. Ultrasonographic appearance and possible clinical relevance of hyperechoic foci of mineralization in the canine intrahepatic biliary tree. *Open Vet J* 13(5):541-549, 2023.
10. O'Brien RT, Iani M, Matheson J, Delaney F, Young K. Contrast harmonic ultrasound of spontaneous liver nodules in 32 dogs. *Vet Radiol Ultrasound* 45(6):547-453, 2004.
11. Holdsworth A, Bradley K, Birch S, Browne WJ, Barberet V. Elastography of the normal canine liver, spleen and kidneys. *Vet Radiol Ultrasound* 55(6):620-627, 2014.
12. Facin AC, Uscategui RAR, Maronezi MC, Pavan L, Menezes MP, Montanhim GL, Camacho AA, Feliciano MAR, Moraes PC. Liver and spleen elastography of dogs affected by brachycephalic obstructive airway syndrome and its correlation with clinical biomarkers. *Sci Rep* 10(1):16156, 2020.
13. Rivero-Juárez A, Morgaz J, Camacho A, Muñoz-Rascón P, Dominguez JM, Sánchez-Céspedes R, Torre-Cisneros J, Rivero A. Liver stiffness using transient elastography is applicable to canines for hepatic disease models. *PLoS One* 7(7):e41557, 2012.
14. Leela-Arporn R, Ohta H, Shimbo G, Hanazono K, Osuga T, Morishita K, Sasaki N, Takiguchi M. Computed tomographic features for differentiating benign from malignant liver lesions in dogs. *J Vet Med Sci* 81(12):1697-1704, 2019.
15. Kutara K, Seki M, Ishikawa C, Sakai M, Kagawa Y, Iida G, Ishigaki K, Teshima K, Edamura K, Nakayama T, Asano K. Triple-phase helical computed tomography in dogs with hepatic masses. *Vet Radiol Ultrasound* 55(1):7-15, 2014.
16. Dröes FC, Suchodolski JS, Steiner JM, Lidbury JA. Prevalence of portal vein and splanchnic venous thrombosis in dogs with chronic hepatitis. *J Small Anim Pract* 64(6):375-383, 2023.

17. Martinez C, Davies D, Hoey S, Shiel RE, O'Neill EJ. Ultrasonographic measurement of gallbladder wall thickness in fasted dogs without signs of hepatobiliary disease. *J Vet Intern Med* 37(5):1766-1771, 2023.
18. Ramstedt KL, Center SA, Randolph JF, Yeager AE, Erb HN, Warner KL. Changes in gallbladder volume in healthy dogs after food was withheld for 12 hours followed by ingestion of a meal or a meal containing erythromycin. *Am J Vet Res* 69(5):647-51, 2008.
19. Pillai S, Center SA, McDonough SP, Demarco J, Pintar J, Henderson AK, Cooper J, Bolton T, Sharpe K, Hill S, Benedict AG, Haviland R. Ductal plate malformation in the liver of Boxer dogs: clinical and histological features. *Vet Pathol* 53(3):602-613, 2016.
20. Murakami M, Heng HG, Steinbach S, Sola M. Ultrasonographic features of gallbladder wall thickening in dogs with hypoalbuminemia. *Vet Quart* 43(1):1-7, 2023.
21. Harrison JL, Turek BJ, Brown DC, Bradley C, Callahan Clark J. Cholangitis and cholangiohepatitis in dogs: A descriptive study of 54 cases based on histopathologic diagnosis (2004-2014). *J Vet Intern Med* 32(1):172-180, 2018.
22. DeMonaco SM, Grant DC, Larson MM, Panciera DL, Leib MS. Spontaneous course of biliary sludge over 12 months in dogs with ultrasonographically identified biliary sludge. *J Vet Intern Med* 30(3):771-778, 2016.
23. Besso JG, Wrigley RH, Gliatto JM, Webster CR. Ultrasonographic appearance and clinical findings in 14 dogs with gallbladder mucocele. *Vet Radiol Ultrasound* 41(3):261-271, 2000.
24. Choi J, Kim A, Keh S, Oh J, Kim H, Yoon J. Comparison between ultrasonographic and clinical findings in 43 dogs with gallbladder mucoceles. *Vet Radiol Ultrasound* 55(2):202-207, 2014.
25. Jaffey JA, Kreisler R, Shumway K, Lee YJ, Lin CH, Durocher-Babek LL, Seo KW, Choi H, Nakashima K, Harada H, Kanemoto H, Lin LS. Ultrasonographic patterns, clinical findings, and prognostic variables in dogs from Asia with gallbladder mucocele. *J Vet Intern Med* 36(2):565-575, 2022.
26. Butler T, Bexfield N, Dor C, Fantaconi N, Heinsoo I, Kelly D, Kent A, Pack M, Spence SJ, Ward PM, Watson P, McCallum KE. A multicenter retrospective study assessing progression of biliary sludge in dogs using ultrasonography. *J Vet Intern Med.* 36(3):976-985, 2022.
27. MacLeod AN, Reichle JK, Szabo D, Cohen EB, Artiles C, Fulkerson CV, Kurihara M, Mattoon J. Ultrasonographic appearance of gallbladder neoplasia in 14 dogs and 1 cat. *Vet Radiol Ultrasound* 64(3):537-545, 2023.
28. Mortier JR, Maddox TW, White GM, Blundell RJ, Monné JM, Lillis SM. Ultrasonographic appearance of the major duodenal papilla in dogs without evidence of hepatobiliary, pancreatic, or gastrointestinal tract disease. *Am J Vet Res* 77(6):597-603, 2016.
29. Schiborra F, McConnell JF, Maddox TW. Percutaneous ultrasound-guided cholecystocentesis: complications and association of ultrasonographic findings with bile culture results. *J Small Anim Pract* 58(7):389-394, 2017 58:389-394.
30. Bargellini P, Orlandi R, Paloni C, Rubini G, Fonti P, Righi C, Peterson ME, Rishniw M, Boiti C. Contrast-enhanced ultrasound complements two-dimensional ultrasonography in diagnosing gallbladder diseases in dogs. *Vet Radiol Ultrasound* 59(3):345-356, 2018.
31. Bargellini P, Orlani R, Paloni C, Rubini G, Fonti P, Peterson M, Rishniw M, Boiti C. Evaluation of contrast-enhanced ultrasonography as a method for detecting gallbladder necrosis or rupture in dogs. *Vet Radiol Ultrasound* 57:6:611-620, 2016.
32. Mattolini M, Citi S, Gianni B, Carozzi G, Caleri E, Puccinelli C, Rossi F. CT features of divisional bile ducts in healthy Labrador Retrievers. *Vet Radiol Ultrasound* 64(3):448-454, 2023.
33. Park HY, Cho YG, Lee YW, Choi HJ. Evaluation of gallbladder and common bile duct size and appearance by computed tomography in dogs. *J Vet Sci* 19(5):653-659, 2018.
34. Serrano G, Mortier F, Bosseler L, Taylor O, and Paepe D. Diagnosis of Caroli syndrome in a crossbreed dog. *Vet Rec Case Rep* 6:2:e000576, 2018.
35. Brand EM, Lim CK, Heng HG, Grosso FV, Hanlon J, Jones-Hall Y. Computed tomographic features of confirmed gallbladder pathology in 34 dogs. *Vet Radiol Ultrasound* 61(6):667-679, 2020.
36. Fuerst JA, Hostnik ET. CT attenuation values and mineral distribution can be used to differentiate dogs with and without gallbladder mucoceles. *Vet Radiol Ultrasound* 60(6):689-695, 2019.
37. Head LL, Daniel GB. Correlation between hepatobiliary scintigraphy and surgery or postmortem examination findings in dogs and cats with extrahepatic biliary obstruction, partial obstruction, or patency of the biliary system: 18 cases (1995-2004). *J Am Vet Med Assoc* 227(10):1618-1624, 2005.
38. White RN, Shales C, Parry AT. New perspectives on the development of extrahepatic portosystemic shunts. *J Small Anim Pract* 58(12):669-677, 2017.
39. Lamb CR. Ultrasonography of portosystemic shunts in dogs and cats. *Vet Clin North Am Small Anim Pract* 28(4):725-753, 1998.
40. d'Anjou MA, Penninck D, Cornejo L, Pibarot P. Ultrasonographic diagnosis of portosystemic shunting in dogs and cats. *Vet Radiol Ultrasound* 45(5):424-437, 2004.
41. Nyland T and Fisher P. Evaluation of experimentally induced canine hepatic cirrhosis using duplex Doppler ultrasound. *Vet Radiol Ultrasound* 31:4:189-194, 1990.
42. Respess M, O'Toole TE, Taeymans O, Rogers CL, Johnston A, Webster CR. Portal vein thrombosis in 33 dogs: 1998-2011. *J Vet Intern Med* 26(2):230-237, 2012.
43. Zwingenberger A. CT diagnosis of portosystemic shunts. *Vet Clin North Am Small Anim Pract* 39(4):783-792, 2009.
44. Specchi S, Rossi F, Weisse C, Morabito S, Petrovitch NP, Drees R, Thierry F, Ricciardi M, Penchome R, Armenise A, Pey P, Paek M, Panopoulos I, Nicoli S, Schwarz T. Canine and feline abdominal arterioportal communications can be classified based on branching patterns in computed tomographic angiography. *Vet Radiol Ultrasound* 59(6):687-696, 2018.
45. Plested MJ, Zwingenberger AL, Brockman DJ, Hecht S, Secrest S, Culp WTN, Drees R. Canine intrahepatic portosystemic shunt insertion into the systemic circulation is commonly through primary hepatic veins as assessed with CT angiography. *Vet Radiol Ultrasound* 61(5):519-530, 2020.
46. Specchi S, d'Anjou MA. Diagnostic imaging for the assessment of acquired abdominal vascular diseases in small animals: A pictorial review. *Vet Radiol Ultrasound* 60(6):613-632, 2019.
47. Sato K, Sakamoto Y, Sakai M, Ishikawa C, Nakazawa M, Cheng CJ, Watari T, Nakayama T. Diagnostic utility of computed tomographic angiography in dogs with portal vein thrombosis. *J Vet Med Sci* 82(10):1421-1427, 2020.
48. Daniel GB. Scintigraphic diagnosis of portosystemic shunts. *Vet Clin North Am Small Anim Pract* 39(4):793-810, 2009.

CHAPTER 27

Liver biopsy

Laura J. Owen
BVSc, AFHEA, DECVS, MRCVS

Indications for biopsy and preoperative assessment

Hepatic biopsy in dogs is indicated for investigation of persistent elevations in liver enzymes, characterization of lesions identified on diagnostic imaging, and the staging of neoplastic disease in order to guide treatment and inform prognosis.

Ultrasound-guided fine-needle aspiration and core needle biopsies are the least invasive methods of biopsy but may not yield an accurate diagnosis due to the lack of complete portal triads available for examination.[1] A prospective study comparing needle and surgical wedge biopsies in 124 dogs and cats showed discordance in histological diagnosis for paired samples in 53% of dogs.[1] A minimum of 12 intact portal triads is recommended to obtain an accurate histological diagnosis, and this requires a larger sample size obtained via either open surgical or laparoscopic biopsy.[2]

A PCV and standard coagulation profile, including platelet count, one-stage prothrombin time (OSPT), activated partial thromboplastin time (aPPT), and plasma fibrinogen concentrations, are recommended prior to liver biopsy to assess the risk of hemorrhage in an individual patient. In hepatobiliary disease, either the production of coagulation factors or absorption of vitamin K necessary for their activation may be affected, resulting in the prolongation of clotting. Animals may also be hypercoagulable due to reduced production of anticoagulant factors in the liver. Knowledge of any abnormalities prior to biopsy can impact the technique chosen and minimize complications. Blood products should be available in dogs with pre-existing anemia/thrombocytopenia or an increased risk of bleeding.

Video 27.1

Laparoscopic liver biopsy with ascites. Video demonstrating suction of ascitic fluid prior to examination of the liver and biopsy. Note the grossly abnormal appearance of this liver.

Surgical anatomy of the liver

The liver has six lobes, the parenchyma of which merge at the hilus (see chapter 30). These lobes are grouped into three "divisions" according to their portal vein supply:

- Right division: caudate lobe and right lateral lobe.
- Central division: right medial lobe and quadrate lobe.
- Left division: left medial lobe and left lateral lobe.

The gallbladder lies between, and is closely adherent to, the right medial and quadrate lobes.

The hepatic artery is a branch of the celiac artery and is responsible for supplying the liver with 50-75% of its oxygen demands but represents only 20% of hepatic blood flow. The remainder of the liver's blood flow is derived from the portal vein, on which it is dependent for essential nutrients, hormones, and growth factors. The hepatic veins drain directly into the caudal vena cava.

Bile is channeled out of each of the liver lobes via the hepatic ducts, which join with the cystic duct of the gallbladder. Bile passes along the cystic duct towards the gallbladder, which acts as a reservoir for bile. Bile also passes in the opposite direction along the cystic duct to enter the common bile duct, which empties into the duodenum at the major duodenal papilla, approximately 3-6 cm distal to the pylorus.

Open vs. laparoscopic approach

Liver biopsy can be performed via a ventral midline celiotomy, mini-laparotomy, or laparoscopy as described for pancreatic biopsy (see chapter 16). In patients with ascites, suction of the abdominal fluid is required to improve visibility and reduce hemorrhage (Video 27.1). Regardless of the approach or biopsy method used, multiple liver lobes should be sampled, even if grossly uniform in appearance, and adequate-sized samples should be obtained to improve the likelihood of an accurate diagnosis.[3]

Biopsy technique

Open surgical biopsy

The entire liver is visually inspected and gently palpated to identify gross abnormalities, e.g., change in color, texture, rounding of lobar edges, presence of nodules, etc. If the liver is diffusely uniform in appearance, biopsies are taken from the most accessible edges of multiple lobes. If specific lesions are identified, more targeted samples may be required.

Several methods of open liver biopsy have been reported in dogs. Traditionally, the crush, guillotine/suture fracture, and punch biopsy techniques have been used. These techniques have been shown to yield adequately sized samples with a low complication rate.[1,4,5] More recently, the use of a pretied ligature loop and ultrasonically activated (harmonic) scalpel have been described and may have some advantages in higher-risk patients.[4,6]

Crush technique

The crush biopsy technique is most applicable to dogs with normal coagulation and minimal gross abnormalities of their liver (Fig. 27.1). A "pointed" section of the edge of a liver lobe is selected, and a mosquito artery forceps is applied across it. The separated tissue is excised with a number 11 blade, manipulating it gently to avoid crush artifact. The mosquito forceps remain in place for 2-3 minutes, after which they are removed, and the cut edge is checked for hemorrhage. A hemostatic sponge or diathermy can be used to provide additional hemostasis if required, although this is rarely necessary.

Suture fracture/guillotine technique

These techniques utilize ligatures to provide hemostasis and thus may be a preferred option for dogs with prolonged clotting times or ascites. They are also more applicable for biopsy of rounded liver edges or friable liver tissue.

If a "pointed" edge of liver lobe can be identified, a single ligature can be placed around this section and tightened to secure the biopsy site (guillotine technique) (Fig. 27.2). A number 11 blade or Metzenbaum scissors and Debakey forceps are used to excise the liver tissue distal to the ligature. A 5 mm stump of the liver should remain to ensure the ligature does not become dislodged. The same technique can also be performed using a pretied ligature loop.[6]

If the liver lobes are more rounded, two divergent sutures can be placed to isolate a triangular tissue area at the edge of the liver parenchyma. A wedge biopsy is cut from this triangular zone with a number 11 blade, leaving a small cuff of tissue adjacent to each suture to prevent dislodgement and taking care not to cut either suture during the procedure (suture fracture technique).

Punch biopsy technique

The use of a 6-8 mm punch biopsy instrument is an effective method for biopsy of central areas of the liver, although this method is associated with a mild increased risk of hemorrhage.[4] The punch biopsy is

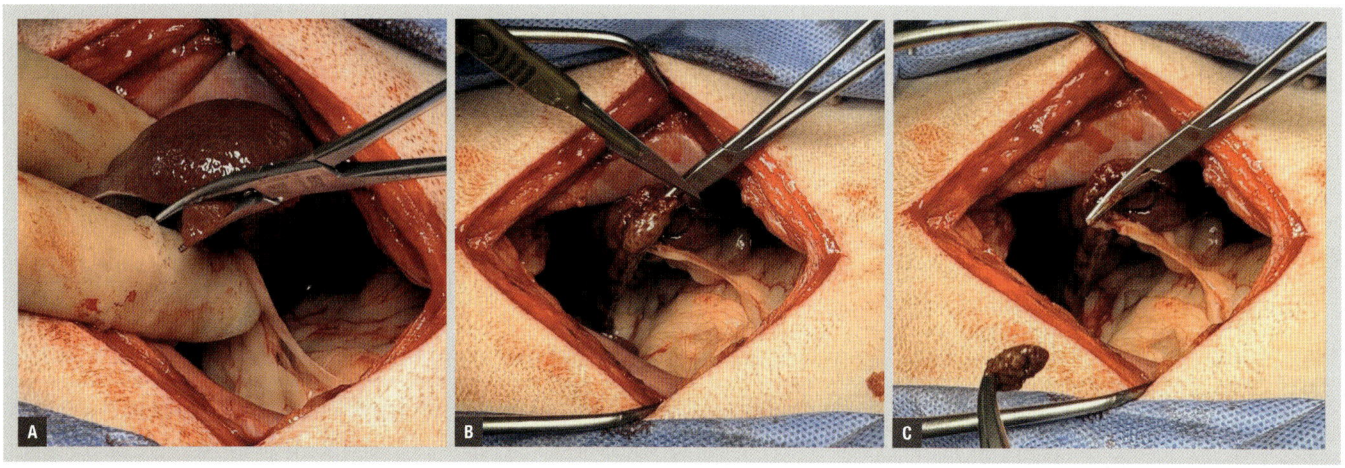

FIG. 27.1 Crush liver biopsy technique. (A) Application of forceps to the edge of the liver to be biopsied. (B) Use of a number 11 scalpel to excise the biopsy sample. (C) Excised biopsy specimen.

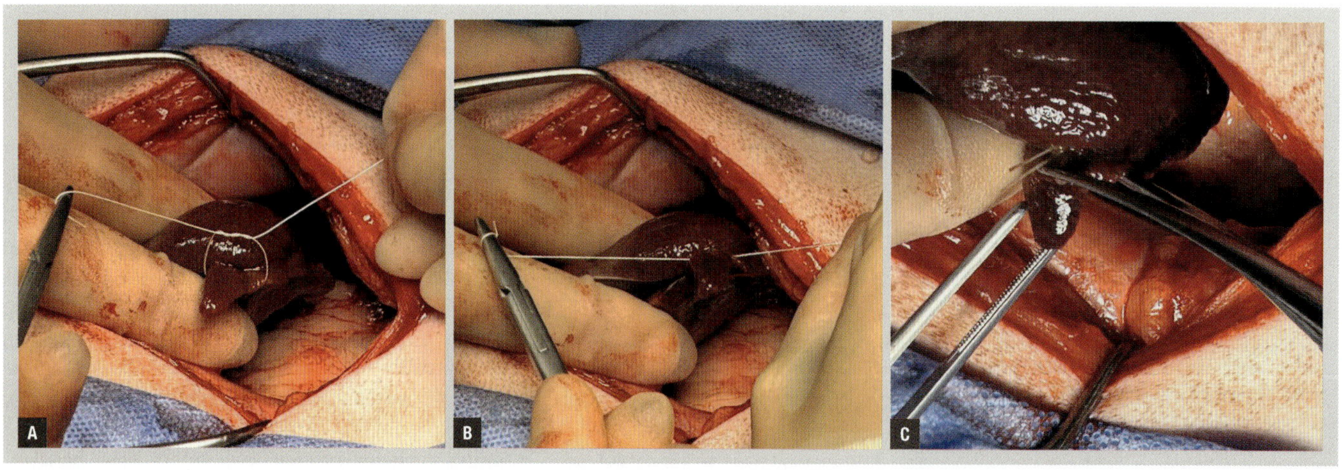

FIG. 27.2 Guillotine suture technique. (A) Placement of the guillotine suture. (B) Tightening of the guillotine suture. (C) Biopsy excision using Metzenbaum scissors.

pressed into the liver parenchyma to its full depth, gently twisted, and then removed. The biopsy is manipulated with Debakey forceps and excised using a number 11 blade or Metzenbaum scissors. A lug of a hemostatic sponge or gel is placed into/over the resultant defect to achieve hemostasis.

Laparoscopic biopsy

Laparoscopic liver biopsy is most commonly performed as a two-port technique, with a subumbilical camera port (see chapter 16) and a 6 mm instrument cannula placed in a paramedian position in the left or right cranial abdominal quadrant. In smaller patients, care should be taken not to place these cannulas too cranially, as this will reduce working space. Exploration of the liver is performed using the blunt probe (maneuvering around the falciform fat as necessary), and any gross lesions/abnormalities are recorded. Biopsies are performed according to the preferred technique of the surgeon and/or individual patient status. All sites are assessed for ongoing hemorrhage before closure. Hemostasis can be assisted by applying pressure to the site with a blunt probe or hemostatic sponge. Conversions to laparotomy are rare (3/80 dogs and 2/106 dogs, respectively, in two retrospective studies[7,8]); this can become necessary as a result of injury to other organs, e.g., the spleen, during laparoscopic entry or following identification of a lesion requiring partial/total liver lobectomy or as a result of an unexpected complication, e.g., pneumothorax (due to an undiagnosed diaphragmatic defect), but is unlikely to be directly related to the liver biopsy procedure.[7,8]

Cup biopsy technique

The simplest laparoscopic biopsy technique uses 5 mm laparoscopic cup forceps to grasp liver tissue along the free edges of the lobes. The lobe should be partially elevated during the application of the forceps to ensure no aberrant tissue is grasped. The forceps are held closed for 30 seconds to achieve hemostasis, followed by the removal of the instrument to obtain the biopsy (Video 27.2). Pull, twist, and cannula separation methods are all reported. A 360° unidirectional twisting motion has been demonstrated to achieve reduced tearing of the liver and fewer histological artifacts compared to the pull method, but these differences were minor, and thus, either of these can be recommended.[9] The cannula separation method was inferior in this study.[9] The technique is repeated to obtain 4-6 biopsy samples from multiple lobes.

Pretied ligature loop

A pretied ligature loop (PLL) can be used for laparoscopic liver biopsies, as described for pancreatic biopsy (see chapter 16). The technique is more challenging in patients with friable liver tissue and rounded edges, making it difficult to grasp the liver tissue and slide the suture loop over the lobe respectively. The advantages of the PLL over the cup biopsy method are a much larger sample size (>3×), a greater number of portal triads (median 69 vs. 19), reduced crush and fragmentation artifacts, and reduced hemorrhage.[10] The disadvantages are the requirement for an additional instrument cannula, a more skilled laparoscopic surgeon and a surgical assistant, increased time taken to complete the biopsy, and acquisition of a sample originating from just one lobe rather than multiple lobes.[10]

Video 27.2

Laparoscopic liver biopsy. Video demonstrating examination of the liver with a blunt probe and liver biopsy using cup forceps. Note the absence of a gallbladder in this dog.

Harmonic scalpel and vessel-sealing devices

See pancreatic biopsy (chapter 16) for the advantages and disadvantages of these techniques. The use of a harmonic scalpel to obtain hepatic biopsies (both peripheral and central) via laparoscopy in normal dogs has been reported to result in reduced hemorrhage and may be a safer alternative in patients with coagulation abnormalities.[4,11] As for the pancreas, a larger sample size should be obtained (compared to the cup biopsy) to account for increased artifact as a result of collateral thermal injury to the tissue.[11]

Bile sampling

Aspiration of the gallbladder to obtain samples of bile for cytology and culture is performed in most dogs undergoing liver biopsy. Cytology samples are placed in EDTA tubes to preserve cell morphology, whilst samples for culture are placed in a plain sterile pot or applied to a charcoal transport swab.

At open surgery, sampling is performed with a 23G needle and a 10-20 mL syringe. Bile should be aspirated until the gallbladder is flaccid to reduce the risk of postoperative leakage. If there is concern about the integrity of the gallbladder wall, the aspiration can be performed through adjacent liver tissue to reduce this risk further.

During laparoscopy, a 22G, 3-inch spinal needle is used to allow for greater depth penetration. The abdominal clip should be extended over the caudal thorax to allow for optimal needle placement. The external body wall is palpated firmly until an optimal location for needle entry is observed via the laparoscope (depression of the body wall immediately above or lateral to the gallbladder on the right side). The needle is passed through the body wall and into the gallbladder to aspirate bile. A reduction in insufflation is helpful during this procedure to reduce the distance between these two surfaces. Aspiration until the gallbladder is flaccid and aspiration through adjacent liver tissue are considered as for open surgery. A small amount of bile leakage may be observed following the procedure, but this does not require intervention.

Processing of biopsy samples

Liver biopsies are routinely submitted for histopathology and bacterial culture and/or copper analysis. A recent international consensus statement recommended a minimum of five laparoscopic or surgical biopsy specimens be attained from at least two different liver lobes: three for histopathology, one for culture, and one for copper analysis.[2] Any additional samples can be placed in formalin or frozen and stored in the event additional testing is required, e.g., fluorescent *in situ* hybridization (FISH) or molecular techniques (e.g., PCR).[2]

Postoperative care

Analgesia, IV fluid therapy, nutritional support, and exercise restriction are performed as for pancreatic biopsy (see chapter 16).

Complications of liver biopsy

Although rare, hemorrhage is a potentially life-threatening complication of liver biopsy. This risk is greater in dogs with coagulation abnormalities and severe liver pathology or ascites, but the overall risk remains low in all patients provided the biopsy sites are thoroughly examined at the end of surgery and action is taken if persistent bleeding is noted. Dogs should be monitored for at least 6 hours postoperatively to enable hemorrhage to be identified and treated if required.

Most dogs undergoing liver biopsy do not encounter significant complications, and 95% of dogs are reported as surviving to discharge.[7,8] In these studies, the rare causes of death were stated as requested euthanasia in dogs with a poor prognosis or deteriorating clinical signs and cardiopulmonary arrest in dogs with end-stage liver pathology.[7,8]

KEY POINTS

- Surgical or laparoscopic liver biopsy provides the most accurate antemortem histopathological diagnosis of liver disease in the dog.
- A coagulation profile should be performed prior to the procedure to determine the optimal method of biopsy and reduce the risk of complications.
- In dogs with ascites, abdominal fluid should be suctioned prior to biopsy to improve visualization and assist with clotting.
- Suture guillotine or fracture methods (or use of harmonic scalpel/vessel sealing device) are advised in dogs with prolonged coagulation.
- Direct pressure or application of hemostatic sponge/gel is used to control hemorrhage at liver biopsy sites when necessary.
- A minimum of five biopsy specimens should be obtained: three for histology, one for culture, and one for copper analysis. Biopsies should be taken from multiple lobes to improve the accuracy of diagnosis.
- Dogs should be monitored in the initial postoperative period in case of postoperative hemorrhage. However, liver biopsy is a safe procedure in the majority of dogs, with approximately 95% survival to discharge and rare complications attributed directly to the biopsy procedure rather than the underlying disease.

References

1. Cole TL, Center SA, Flood SN, et al. Diagnostic comparison of needle and wedge biopsy specimens of the liver in dogs and cats. *J Am Vet Med Assoc* 220(10):1483-1490, 2002.
2. Webster CRL, Center SA, Cullen JM, et al. ACVIM consensus statement on the diagnosis and treatment of chronic hepatitis in dogs. *J Vet Intern Med* 33:1173-1200, 2019.
3. Kemp SD, Zimmerman KL, Panciera DL, et al. Histopathologic variation between liver lobes in dogs. *J Vet Intern Med* 29:58-62, 2015.
4. Vasanjee SC, Bubenik LJ, Hosgood G, et al. Evaluation of haemorrhage, sample size, and collateral damage for five hepatic biopsy methods in dogs. *Vet Surg* 35(1):86-93, 2006.
5. Kemp SD, Zimmerman KL, Panciera DL, et al. A comparison of liver sampling techniques in dogs. *J Vet Intern Med* 29:51-57, 2015a.
6. Cuddy LC, Risselada M, Ellison GW. Clinical evaluation of a pre-tied ligating loop for liver biopsy and liver lobectomy. *J Small Anim Pract* 54:61-66, 2013.
7. Petre SL, McClaran JK, Bergman, PJ, et al. Safety and efficacy of laparoscopic hepatic biopsy in dogs: 80 cases (2004-2009). *J Am Vet Med Assoc* 240:181-185, 2012.
8. McDevitt HL, Mayhew PD, Giuffrida MA, et al. Short-term clinical outcome of laparoscopic liver biopsy in dogs: 106 cases (2003-2013). *J Am Vet Med Assoc* 248:83-90, 2016.
9. Buote NJ, Loftus JP, Miller AD. Laparoscopic twist technique has the best overall artifact profile when comparing three laparoscopic hepatic cup biopsy techniques for dogs. *Am J Vet Res* 83(12):ajvr.22.08.0127, 2022.
10. Fernandez N, Del-Pozo J, Shaw D et al. Comparison of two minimally invasive techniques for liver biopsy collection in dogs. *J Small Anim Pract* 58:555-561, 2017.
11. Barnes RF, Greenfield CL, Schaeffer DJ, et al. Comparison of biopsy samples obtained using standard endoscopic instruments and the harmonic scalpel during laparoscopic and laparoscopic-assisted surgery in normal dogs. *Vet Surg* 35:243-251, 2006.

CHAPTER 28

Interpretation of cytological examination of the liver

Carlo Masserdotti
DVM, DECVCP

Cytological examination of the liver is a reliable method for recognizing many hepatic diseases, but diagnostic accuracy is generally variable and related to the type of hepatic lesion and the sampling method used. Concordance of cytological examination, obtained with fine-needle aspiration (FNA), and histological diagnosis was complete in 16 and partial in 7 samples from 25 dogs;[1] in another study in cytological samples obtained with ultrasonographic guided FNA concordance was 30,3%,[2] and in another, diagnostic sensitivity was 52% in cytological samples of focal nodular lesions.[3]

Although cytological examination allows a final diagnosis in some selected lesions, it is necessary to remember that in other instances, cytology is able to recognize some changes that need clinical correlation or histological evaluation to address a diagnosis; moreover, nonspecific cytological changes are found in many of the inflammatory diseases of the liver, that are not useful for diagnostic purposes without histological examination.

To date, FNCS (fine-needle capillary sampling) is the preferred technique to sample the liver; this technique is based on the principle of capillarity and can be performed just by putting, under ultrasonographic guidance, a needle into the liver, without aspiration with a syringe.[4] This technique has diagnostic sensitivity similar to FNA, with the advantage of reducing blood contamination when sampling the highly vascular tissue of the liver.

Differences in the values of concordance between cytological and histological examination are the consequence of some factors that are always to be taken into account when approaching a hepatic disease by FNCS:

- The tip of the needle samples areas affected by nonspecific changes that are located around other sites where primary alteration occurs; for example, sampling the areas that surround a portal tract, where a biliary disease occurs, may collect hepatocytes with reversible nonspecific changes, sometimes with evidence of extracytoplasmic cholestasis, although specific cytological features that help in recognition of the primary disease are generally lacking.
- Cytology is not able to evaluate vascular disorders or ductal plate abnormalities; portosystemic disturbances or centrilobular congestion need imaging evaluation or, in many instances, histological confirmation for final diagnosis.
- Although morphological features may help in suspecting them, the final diagnosis of most biliary diseases is not evaluable by cytology.
- Some changes, although easily observed and evaluated by cytology, need to be correctly addressed by histology; for example, fibrosis, although evident in a cytological sample, needs histological examination for a correct diagnosis of a fibrotic process, like chronic hepatitis or lobular dissecting hepatitis.

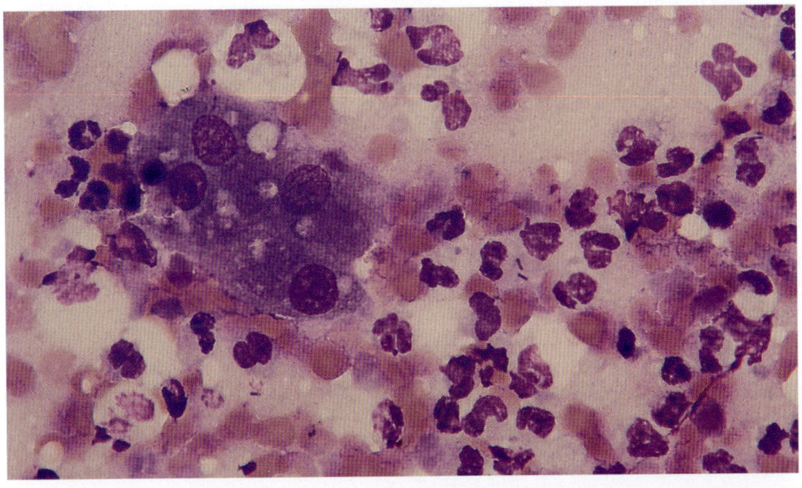

FIG. 28.1 Dog, septic suppurative hepatitis; FNCS: degenerate neutrophils surround a small cluster of hepatocytes; notice the phagocytosis of rod bacteria (MGG – May-Grünwald Giemsa, 100×).

From this point of view, cytology is useful only if properly correlated with all the clinical and historical information, with hematological and biochemical data, and with ultrasonographic results.

Cytological examination provides morphological information that leads to different types of diagnosis. In cases where cytology provides a definitive diagnosis, cytological examination may provide a definitive diagnosis that does not need histological confirmation or further evaluation unless there is another underlying or concurrent disease process that may need later identification. This diagnosis can be achieved in:

- Septic suppurative hepatitis or septic suppurative cholecystitis: these may be diagnosed on aspirates of liver

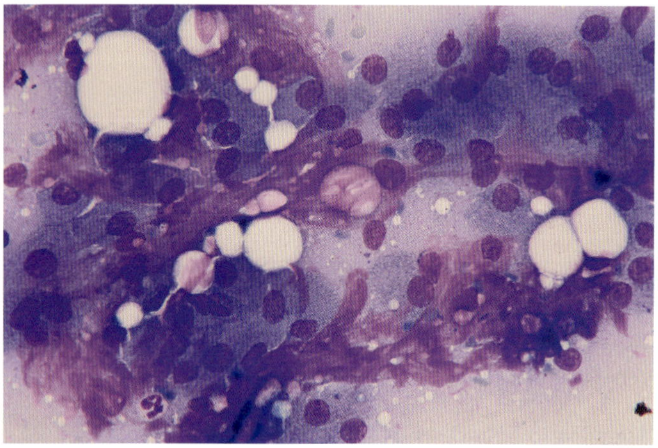

FIG. 28.2 Dog, hepatic amyloidosis; FNCS: dense, wispy tufts of eosinophilic material surround clusters of hepatocytes (MGG, 100×).

or gallbladder bile by the presence of a high number of degenerate neutrophils, sometimes with phagocytosis of bacteria (Fig. 28.1) that surround sheets of hepatocytes or scattered on the bile background.

- Amyloidosis: although rare in dogs and described mostly in some breeds, like Shar Pei and Chow Chow, this pathological condition is characterized by the presence of pink, dense material in tufts that surround the hepatocytes (Fig. 28.2).[4]
- Neoplasia: a definitive diagnosis by cytology of nodular hyperplasia, hepatocellular adenoma, and well-differentiated hepatocellular carcinoma should be difficult since the three conditions share many morphological features; in all these lesions, grossly represented by hepatic masses, apparently normal hepatocytes are generally observed, although in well-differentiated hepatocellular carcinoma a high number of naked nuclei (Fig. 28.3A) crowded around sheets of hepatocytes may represent a reliable differential cytological feature.[5] Nevertheless, always consider that differential diagnosis of these lesions is challenging with histology too, if performed on small fragments of tissue, where peripherical infiltrative behavior, frequently the only diagnostic feature between benign and malign lesions, is not evaluable. When properly addressed by clinical and historical data, cytological features of many other neoplasms, like cholangioma, cholangiocarcinoma (Fig. 28.3B), large cell hepatic lymphoma (Fig. 28.3C), histiocytic neoplasms (Fig. 28.3D) or involvement of hepatic parenchyma in metastasis, when properly compared with primary lesions, are generally mandatory for diagnosis. Cytological features of the main types of hepatic neoplasia have been described elsewhere.[6]

In some cases, cytology gives useful information, but the definitive diagnosis may not be reached. Cytological examination provides useful information in identifying hepatic diseases, but a definitive diagnosis cannot be reached without a complete clinical, historical, hematochemical, ultrasonographic examination and, sometimes, without histological examination. Some of these cytological diagnoses are represented by:

- **Extracytoplasmic cholestasis.** Cholestasis is easy to recognize by cytology, represented by linear or branched casts of green to bluish or black material among the cytoplasmic borders of the hepatocytes (Fig. 28.4); sometimes by cytology, this change is recognizable much more easily than with histological examination, mostly when focal and minimal. Nevertheless, cholestasis may be the consequence of many prehepatic (acute massive hemolysis), hepatic (acute and chronic hepatitis), and posthepatic (biliary obstruction) diseases for which further diagnostic investigation is necessary.
- **Liver fibrosis.** The presence of bundles of spindle cells embedded in pink fibrillary material that cross or interconnect the hepatocyte clusters (Fig. 28.5) is indicative of a fibrotic process.[7] Although fibrosis is easy to detect cytologically, histology is necessary to stage and grade the extent and severity of the fibrosis and to correlate it with some specific diagnoses, such as chronic hepatitis.

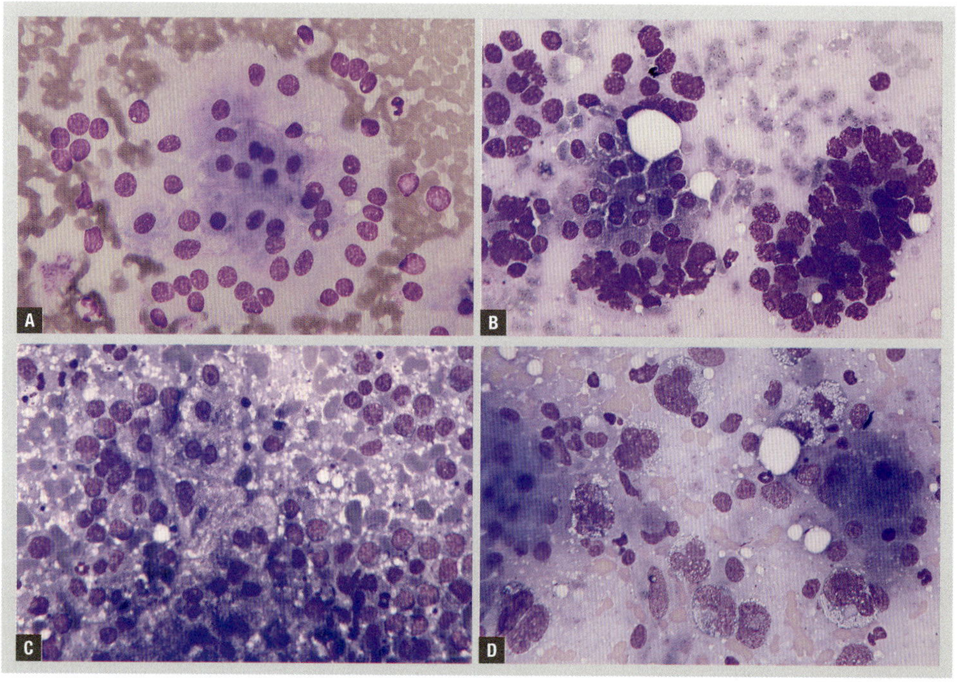

FIG. 28.3 (A) Dog, hepatic mass; FNCS; well-differentiated hepatocellular carcinoma; notice the high number of naked nuclei surrounding a small cluster of intact, apparently normal hepatocytes (MGG, 100×). (B) Dog, multiple hepatic masses; FNCS: cholangiocarcinoma; there are a lot of epithelial cells with indistinct cytoplasm and large round to ovoid nuclei around a small group of hepatocytes; notice the presence of microacinar structures (MGG, 100×). (C) Dog, hepatic enlargement: large cell lymphoma; a lot of round, atypical lymphoid cells surround a small cluster of hepatocytes (MGG, 100×). (D) Dog, multiple hepatic masses: histiocytic sarcoma; large round cells with lobulated nuclei scattered around small clusters of hepatocytes (MGG; 100×).

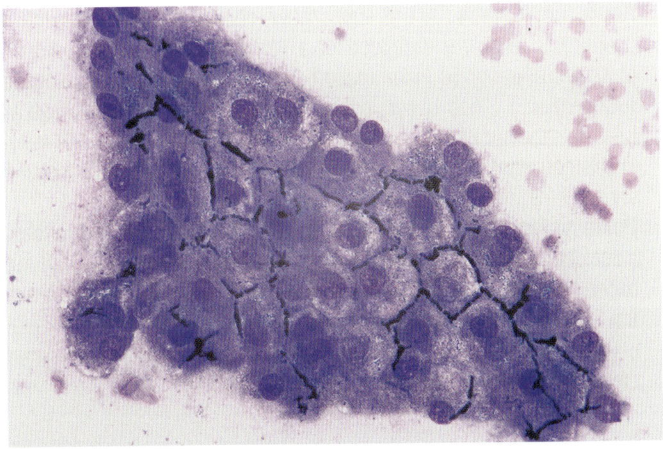

FIG. 28.4 Dog, cholestasis; FNCS: presence of branched casts of bluish, dense material accumulated among hepatocyte borders (MGG, 100×).

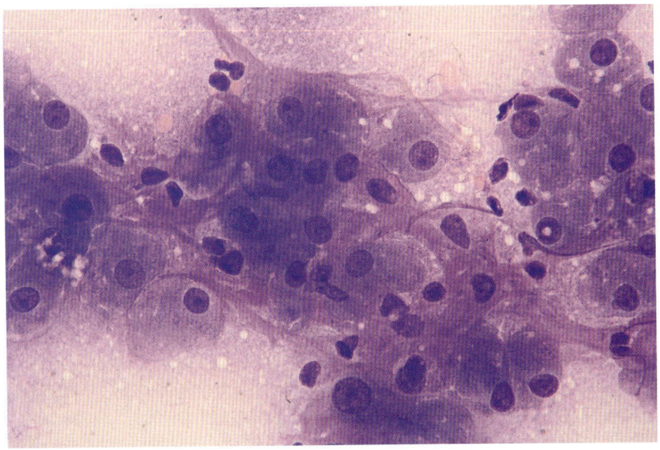

FIG. 28.5 Dog, fibrosis; FNCS: presence of bundles of collagen surround and cross the hepatocytes (MGG, 100×).

- **Glycogen accumulation.** This change is represented by the enlargement of cytoplasm because of the accumulation of achromatic material (Fig. 28.6A); although traditionally associated with the so-called "steroid-induced hepatopathy", many primary diseases, both hepatic and extrahepatic, induced by disease-related physiologic stress, may lead to this nonspecific injury.[8]
- **Lipid accumulation.** This change is represented by round, achromatic globules of different sizes that accumulate inside the cytoplasm and sometimes displace the nucleus (Fig. 28.6B); their presence is generally a consequence of metabolic disturbance, such as diabetes mellitus, hypothyroidism, or hypertriglyceridemia, that lead to an accumulation of fat into the hepatocytes. Other causes are represented by alteration of the energetic pathways of the hepatocytes, like mitochondrial injury, mostly induced by drugs or toxins, or damage to microtubules for intracytoplasmic lipoprotein transport.[9]
- **Cytoplasmic copper accumulation.** The presence of copper inside the cytoplasm of hepatocytes is represented by very small, indistinct, blurred, teal-colored granules, which may be detected by Romanowsky stains (Fig. 28.6C), although rhodanine or rubeanic acid stains provide much more reliable results.[10] This should be considered a nonspecific finding and insufficient for a final diagnosis of copper toxicosis. Nevertheless, the cytological accumulation of copper should represent the starting point of a diagnostic workup when copper-associated hepatopathy is suspected and should be properly addressed with histological examination.
- **Chronic cholangitis.** Although the presence of large sheets of cholangiocytes, sometimes associated with inflammatory cells, frequently allows a suspicion of chronic biliary diseases (Fig. 28.6D),[10] histological examination is necessary to correct and recognize the primary pathological process.

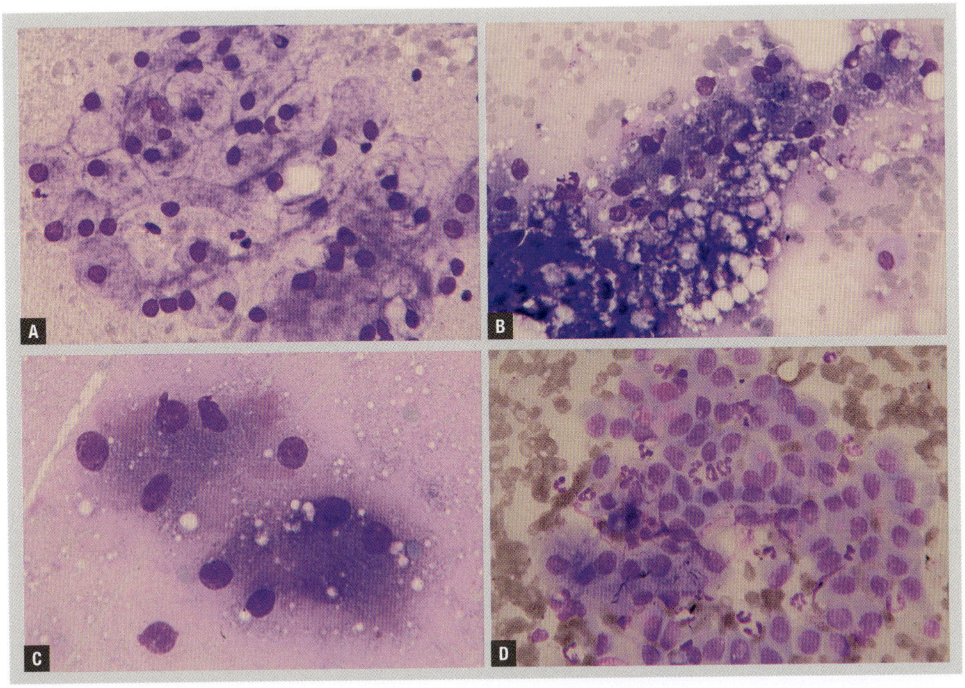

FIG. 28.6 (A) Dog, glycogen cytoplasmic accumulation; FNCS: cytoplasm is enlarged by the accumulation of achromatic material (MGG, 100×). (B) Dog, lipid cytoplasmic accumulation; FNCS: presence of sharply demarcated, round, achromatic globules that sometimes displace the nucleus (MGG, 100×). (C) Dog, copper accumulation; FNCS: notice the presence of very small, refractile, teal-colored granules that accumulate into the cytoplasm (MGG, 100×). (D) Dog, chronic suppurative cholangitis; FNCS: a large sheet of cholangiocytes surrounded by neutrophilic granulocytes (MGG, 100×).

In some other cases, cytology shows nonspecific pathological processes and does not give a diagnosis. Sometimes, cytological examination provides insufficient morphological changes to allow recognition of the pathological process despite a complete clinical and hematological evaluation, and only histological examination can help in definitive diagnosis.

- **Inflammation.** With the exception of severe suppurative hepatitis, inflammatory processes are generally difficult to address by cytology correctly. The first obstacle in this diagnosis is to properly differentiate true inflammation from leukocyte presence secondary to blood contamination. In cases of reactive nonspecific hepatitis, subacute or mild chronic hepatitis, all of which are very frequent in clinical practice, finding the presence of rare inflammatory cells among the hepatocytes on cytology is not useful; in these cases, histologic examination is necessary for a definitive diagnosis.[12]
- **Acute cholangitis.** Acute suppurative cholangitis and destructive cholangitis, with the exception of a variable degree of nonspecific or septic neutrophilic inflammation, are not evaluable by cytological examination.[11] Since a cytological diagnosis of a biliary disease is based on the number of cholangiocytes present on a smear, generally, in this condition, no biliary cells exfoliate, and a diagnostic suspicion cannot be formulated.
- **Portosystemic shunt and ductal plate abnormalities.** Portal vascular disturbances are generally not detectable by cytology, with the exception of a mild, nonspecific, sometimes detectable reduced size of the hepatocytes. Ductal plate abnormalities and other developmental disturbances of intrahepatic bile ducts may be correctly investigated only with imaging and histology.

KEY POINTS

- Cytological examination of the liver should be selected by clinicians when a hepatic disease is suspected based on historical and clinical data, hematological and biochemical changes, or abnormalities detected by imaging investigation.
- Cytological examination may provide suitable results for a final diagnosis, although many changes need to be addressed by histological examination.

References

1. Roth L. Comparison of liver cytology and biopsy diagnoses in dogs and cats: 56 cases. *Vet Clin Pathol* 30(1):35-38, 2001.
2. Wang KY, Panciera DL, Al-Rukibat RK, Radi ZA. Accuracy of ultrasound-guided fine-needle aspiration of the liver and cytologic findings in dogs and cats: 97 cases (1990-2000). *J Am Vet Med Assoc* 224(1):75-78, 2004.
3. Bahr KL, Sharkey LC, Murakami T, Feeney DA. Accuracy of US-guided FNA of focal liver lesions in dogs: 140 cases (2005-2008). *J Am Anim Hosp Assoc* 49(3):190-196, 2013.
4. Mair S, Dunbar F, Becker PJ, Du Plessis W. Fine needle cytology – Is aspiration suction necessary? A study of 100 masses in various sites. *Acta Cytol* 33(6):809-813, 1989.
5. Masserdotti C. Nonneoplastic disorders of the liver. In Sharkey LC, Radin MJ, Seelig D (editors). Veterinary Cytology. Hoboken, Wiley Blackwell, 2021, pp 413-431.
6. Masserdotti C, Drigo M. Retrospective study of cytologic features of well-differentiated hepatocellular carcinoma in dogs. *Vet Clin Pathol* 41(3):382-390, 2012.
7. Wiedmeyer CE, Bryan J. Hepatobiliary neoplasia and cancer staging. In Sharkey LC, Radin MJ, Seelig D (editors). Veterinary Cytology. Hoboken, Wiley Blackwell, 2021, pp 432-444.
8. Masserdotti C, Bertazzolo W. Cytologic features of hepatic fibrosis in dogs: a retrospective study on 22 cases. *Vet Clin Pathol* 45(2):361-367, 2016.
9. Sepesy LM, Center SA, Randolph JF, Warner KL, Erb HN. Vacuolar hepatopathy in dogs: 336 cases (1993-2005). *J Am Vet Med Assoc* 229(2):246-252, 2006.
10. Cullen JM, Van den Ingh TSGAM, Van Winkle T, Charles JA, Desmet VJ. Morphological classification of parenchymal disorders of the canine and feline liver. In WSAVA Liver Standardization Group. Standard for Clinical and Histological Diagnosis of Canine and Feline Liver Disease. St. Louis, Saunders, 2006, pp 80-82.
11. Moore AR, Coffey E, Hamar D. Diagnostic accuracy of Wright-Giemsa and rhodanine stain protocols for detection and semi-quantitative grading of copper in canine liver aspirates. *Vet Clin Pathol* 45(4):689-697, 2016.
12. Masserdotti C. The cytologic features of biliary diseases: A retrospective study. *Vet Clin Pathol* 49(3):440-450, 2020.
13. Wang KY, Panciera DL, Al-Rukibat RK, et al. Accuracy of ultrasound-guided fine-needle aspiration of the liver and cytologic findings in dogs and cats: 97 cases (1990-2000). *J Am Vet Med Assoc* 224:75-78, 2004.

CHAPTER 29

Interpretation of liver biopsy reports

Sean McDonough
DVM, PhD, DACVP

eFigure

eFigures gallery.

The liver biopsy remains the most reliable way to diagnose diffuse hepatic disease and hepatic nodules. When submitting the biopsy, the clinician should indicate if the biopsy is unfocused (suspect diffuse liver disease) or focused (suspect focal liver disease, such as a liver mass), the type of biopsy (needle, wedge, punch or laparoscopic cup), the location, and the number of specimens obtained.[1] Matching the number and type of biopsies received with those indicated on the accession form is critical for laboratory quality control and ensures that all specimens submitted have been processed and examined. A typical liver biopsy report includes a morphologic diagnosis, which summarizes the major histologic pattern(s), a comment, and a histologic description of the tissue section(s).

The morphologic diagnosis summarizes the major histologic pattern(s) of injury present in the biopsy. Like other organs, the liver has a limited repertoire of responses to a wide array of injurious agents. The features that make up a pattern of liver response to a specific injury often overlap with other injuries. Further, multiple patterns often coexist in a liver biopsy. Thus, while the morphologic diagnosis may indicate a specific disease, it will more likely reflect a pattern of disease rather than a specific entity.

In the comment, the pathologist will discuss likely differential diagnoses and explain why other differential diagnoses are or are not excluded. To write a clinically relevant comment, the clinician must provide the pathologist with appropriate clinical information, including history, physical exam findings, laboratory data, results of relevant imaging studies, drug history, gross appearance of the liver (if available), and differential diagnoses under consideration. Many clinicians justify not providing a history since they "do not want to bias the pathologist". This is illogical since the hepatopathologist will first assess the biopsy without knowledge of the clinical information and will then determine the reasonableness of their interpretation based on the clinical features. Do not send a copy of the complete medical record. The busy pathologist will not have time to evaluate the record critically, and the reason for obtaining the liver biopsy may be overlooked. The clinical information need not be extensive; several well-thought-out sentences are usually sufficient.

The pathologist should include a comment on the adequacy of the biopsy so the clinician can assess the likelihood that the results accurately reflect the patient's condition. Biopsies that are too small, severely fragmented, have excess crush artifact or are poorly fixed may obscure important diagnostic features leading to a misdiagnosis (Fig. 29.1). In some cases, poor-quality liver biopsies are due to operator error. In other cases, the nature of the liver (fibrosis, vacuolar change) may result in collection artifacts even with excellent operator technique.

A biopsy report includes the histologic description: the bulk of the liver biopsy will consist of a description of the tissue sections. While hematoxylin-eosin-stained sections are the mainstay of liver biopsy evaluation, the accuracy and diagnostic yield of liver biopsies are improved by the evaluation of a panel of histochemical stains (Table 29.1 and **eFig. 29.1**). Many terms used in liver pathology are specific to the discipline and may not be familiar to the clinician. Finding definitions can be a challenge since authoritative sources for definitions are sparse. The meaning of a specific term can "drift" since different pathologists may use the same term slightly differently. Finally, regionally distinct usage of terms often reflects training provided by a single influential hepatopathologist.

Definition of common terms used in liver pathology

Lobule vs. acinus

Multiple concepts of the functional unit of the liver have been proposed beginning as early as the 17th century, but the lobule of Kiernan and the acinus of Rappaport are the most widely accepted models.[2] The lobule is divided into periportal, midzonal, and central lobular regions, which correspond to zone 1, zone 2, and zone 3, respectively, in the acinus (**eFig. 29.2**).

Hepatocyte necrosis

Regardless of the mechanism of cell death, dead hepatocytes have a similar histologic appearance. If they occur as single dead cells, they are referred to as either acidophil bodies or Councilman bodies. Individual necrotic

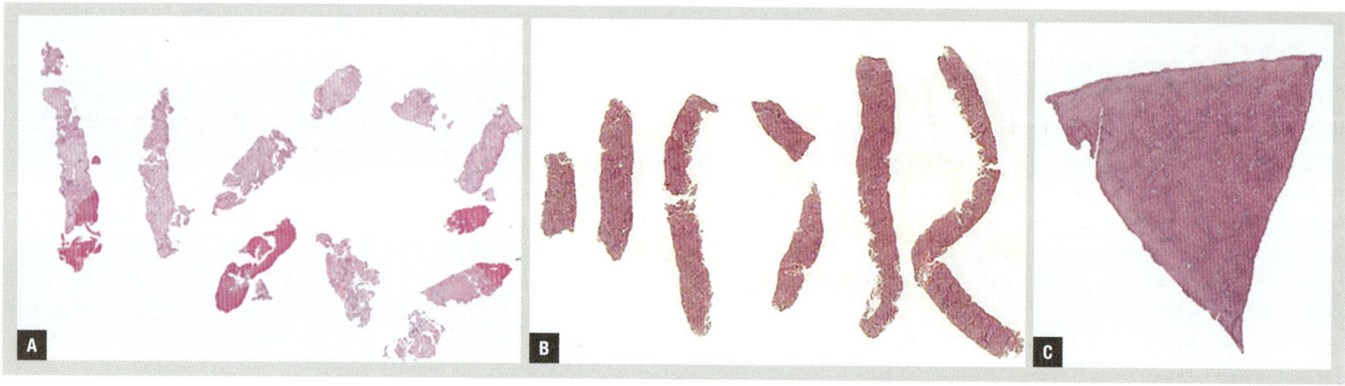

FIG. 29.1 (A) An example of a poor-quality needle biopsy of the liver. The sections are severely fragmented, and 40% of the tissue is skeletal muscle. This may reflect poor biopsy technique, indicating a need for practice. Dull biopsy instruments or excessive force used to retrieve the biopsy may lead to significant crush artifact and torsional distortion. In some cases, fibrosis or severe vacuolar change, which increases hepatocyte membrane fragility, may lead to excessive fragmentation. Hematoxylin and eosin stain. (B) An example of an excellent quality needle biopsy. The samples have minimal fragmentation and crush artifact. At least 12 to 15 portal tracts are available for inspection, which allows for the assessment of lobular architecture. Hematoxylin and eosin stain. (C) An example of an excellent quality wedge biopsy that has minimal collection artifact and a sufficient number of portal tracts to allow for assessment of lobular architecture. When obtaining focused biopsies, avoid the quadrate lobe whenever possible since changes in the gallbladder may alter the adjacent hepatic architecture. If portal vein hypoperfusion is suspected (e.g., congenital portosystemic shunt), avoid the caudate liver lobe since this is supplied by the first branch of the portal vein, and typical changes may not be evident. Hematoxylin and eosin stain.

TABLE 29.1 Histochemical stains used routinely in diagnostic hepatopathology.

Stain	Diagnostic utility
Reticulin	■ Facilitates assessment of hepatic architecture. ■ Demonstrates parenchymal collapse. ■ Widened hepatic plates with a reduction in the reticulin substructure indicate hepatocyte proliferation.
Masson's trichrome	■ Highlights portal tracts and central veins, facilitating assessment of architecture. ■ Demonstrates fibrosis. ■ Accentuates necrotic hepatocytes. ■ Can impart a blue-green tint to bile aiding recognition of cholestasis.
Picrosirius red	■ Enhances natural birefringence of collagen under polarized light. ■ Demonstrates delicate collagen fibers in the space of Disse not visible with Masson's trichrome.
Perls Prussian blue	■ Demonstrates the presence, extent, and site of iron accumulation. ■ Helps identify pattern of hepatitis due to distribution of hemosiderin-laden macrophages.
Rhodanine	■ Demonstrates the presence, extent, and site of copper accumulation.
PAS (with diastase)	■ Helps distinguish glycogen accumulation from other causes of vacuolar hepatopathy.
Oil red O ("wet" tissue only)	■ Demonstrates the presence of fat in nonfixed tissue.

hepatocytes are often called apoptotic bodies, but this should be avoided since the molecular mechanism of cell death cannot be reliably identified based solely on histologic features. Spotty necrosis (eFig. 29.3) refers to individual acidophil bodies scattered about the lobule. Piecemeal necrosis is an archaic term and should be avoided. Focal necrosis may be indicated by the aggregation of lymphocytes ("tombstone"; eFig. 29.4) or lipogranulomas (eFig. 29.5), which are thought to represent a "clean-up" reaction. The term microgranuloma for small aggregates of hemosiderin and lipid-laden macrophages should be avoided to avoid giving the false impression of infectious hepatitis.

Confluent necrosis of multiple adjacent hepatocytes can be either coagulative or lytic. Severe acute hypoxia and indirect-acting hepatotoxins can cause zonal necrosis, primarily affecting centrilobular (zone 3) regions (eFig. 29.6). Submassive necrosis affects 26% to 75% of a lobule, whereas massive (panacinar) necrosis affects >75% of the lobule.

Parenchymal extinction (eFig. 29.7), typically occurring in the subcapsular regions, is devoid of hepatocytes and has scattered remnants and proliferative bile ducts. The bile ducts are embedded in variable amounts of fibrosis with arterial neovascularization and congestion. Lymphocytes, plasma cells, hemosiderin-laden macrophages, and fewer neutrophils are scattered randomly between the remnant bile ducts. An estimation of the proportion of the biopsy occupied by extinct parenchyma should be reported.

Vacuolar change

Hepatocytes can become distended due to hydropic degeneration (reversible cell injury resulting in cellular swelling with small clear vacuoles that represent distended and pinched-off segments of the endoplasmic reticulum due to water accumulation), the accumulation of glycogen or the accumulation of lipids. In glycogen-type vacuolar hepatopathy, hepatocytes are distended with multiple, clear, rough-bordered vacuoles separated by thin wisps of cytoplasm that extend from the cell membrane to the nucleus (**eFig. 29.8**). A PAS stain with and without diastase digestion can confirm the presence of glycogen, if necessary. Ballooning degeneration (balloon cell change) refers to hepatocytes that are at least 50% larger than normal and may occur singly, in clusters, or rarely have a zonal distribution (**eFig. 29.9**). Degenerative vacuolar hepatopathy has been arbitrarily defined as groups of ten or more hepatocytes with severe ballooning degeneration. Degenerative vacuolar hepatopathy can lead to multifocal fibrous partitions. Degenerative vacuolar hepatopathy must be distinguished from hepatocutaneous syndrome (see chapter 38) and progressive vacuolar hepatopathy with dysplastic foci due to abnormal adrenal sex steroid hormone synthesis.

Hepatic lipidosis (steatosis) is another histological manifestation of reversible degeneration. With macrovesicular lipidosis, a single large vacuole displaces the nucleus to the periphery of the cell as a thin, hyperchromatic crescent. In cases of microvesicular lipidosis, multiple small lipid vacuoles accumulate without displacement of the nucleus (**eFig. 29.10**). Phospholipidosis is a lysosomal storage disorder that imparts a foamy appearance to hepatocytes (**eFig. 29.11**). In people, phospholipidosis is most often an adverse reaction to over 50 different drugs that inhibit lysosomal phospholipases. The cause in veterinary medicine is largely unknown but is also suspected to represent an adverse drug reaction.

Ductular reaction

A wide variety of liver injuries induce the proliferation of reactive bile ducts, and the extent of the ductular reaction reflects the extent of liver damage. Typical bile duct reaction (bile duct hyperplasia) arises from the proliferation of pre-existing bile ductular cells that form ducts with well-defined lumens and are confined to the portal tracts (**eFig. 29.12A**). Atypical ductular reaction consists of "transitional cells" that form anastomosing cords with no or only poorly defined lumens and extend to the periphery of the portal tract (**eFig. 29.12B**). In oval cell hyperplasia, bipotential progenitor cells in the canals of Hering proliferate as disorganized clusters of cells with bland oval nuclei and cytoplasm reminiscent of cholangiocytes (**eFig. 29.12C**).

Cholestasis

Cholestasis refers to the abnormal accumulation of bile in the liver. Bile may accumulate in bile ducts (**eFig. 29.13A**), canaliculi (**eFig. 29.13B**), or more rarely in hepatocytes. Accumulation of bile in hepatocytes is referred to as "feathery" degeneration or cholate stasis. Cholate stasis is seen primarily in periportal regions, where maximum bile transport occurs. Affected hepatocytes are swollen with rounded, distinct cell borders and web-like membranous and perinuclear granular material (**eFig. 29.13C**). Affected hepatocytes may contain copper; cholestasis-induced copper accumulation is common in cats but rare in dogs. Occasionally, cholestasis can lead to hepatocellular death and accumulation of extracellular lakes of bile (**eFig. 29.13D**).

Fibrosis

Subcapsular hepatic biopsies, such as laparoscopic cup biopsies and shallow punch biopsies, often lead to an overestimation of the degree of hepatic fibrosis. This author recommends taking both a wedge biopsy and a needle biopsy of deeper hepatic tissue whenever possible if hepatic fibrosis is suspected.

Different patterns of hepatic fibrosis are recognized. Portal tract sclerosis is a common age-associated change of no significance (**eFig. 29.14A**). Ischemic cholangiopathy is associated with hepatic arteriole thrombosis (**eFig. 29.14B**). Hepatic stellate cells in the space of Disse, between the sinusoidal endothelium and the hepatocyte, store vitamin A in lipid droplets (**eFig. 29.14C**). In chronic liver injury, stellate cells differentiate into myofibroblast-like cells with high fibrogenic capacity. Dissecting fibrosis (chicken wire fibrosis; archaic term), due to the transformation of the hepatic stellate cells into a myofibroblast phenotype, has pericellular fibrosis with strands of collagen extending along the space of Disse (**eFig. 29.14D**). Progressive dissecting fibrosis, especially in zone 3 (centrilobular regions), can cause sinusoidal obstruction syndrome (veno-occlusive disease) with encroachment on the diameter of the efferent hepatic venules, causing hepatic congestion that can mimic occlusion of the large hepatic veins (**eFig. 29.14E**).

Incomplete bridging has small, sharp-pointed trabeculae that end blindly in the parenchyma (**eFig. 29.14F**). Bands of connective tissue that span between lobular elements are termed bridging fibrosis. Bridging fibrosis has bands of collagen that may extend portal-to-portal, portal-to-central, or central-to-central (**eFig. 29.14G**).

Basic patterns of liver injury

Near-normal

Biopsies are usually taken when serum biochemistry detects elevated liver enzymes and/or the clinical signs (jaundice, ascites, encephalopathy) suggest liver disease. The near-normal biopsy is a diagnostic challenge since subtle histologic findings may be overlooked, leading to a misdiagnosis.[3] When confronted with a liver biopsy that has minimal changes (Fig. 29.2), the hepatopathologist will first determine if the biopsy is adequate, if all lobular elements are present with normal morphology, and attempt to correlate the biopsies with clinical features. Possible explanations for a near-normal liver biopsy include a biopsy that missed a focal lesion, portal vein hypoperfusion, such as what occurs with portosystemic shunts, end-stage destructive cholangitis, amyloidosis, alpha-1 antitrypsin storage disease, ischemic cholangiopathy, resolved cirrhosis, and nonspecific reactive (secondary) hepatitis.

Nonspecific reactive (secondary) hepatitis

Nonspecific reactive (secondary) hepatitis (Fig. 29.3) is the most common histological change to occur in the dog liver and is by far the most common cause of elevated liver enzymes.[4] A small number (10-25) of mixed inflammatory cells accumulate singly without forming aggregates in the portal tracts, do not target bile ducts, do not breach the limiting plate, and are not accompanied by fibrosis. Similarly, small numbers of individual mixed inflammatory cells are confined to the adventitia around central veins. Variable activation of Kupffer cells, occasional multifocal random to periportal hepatocellular necrosis, and scattered lipogranulomas, thought to reflect a "clean-up reaction" of individual

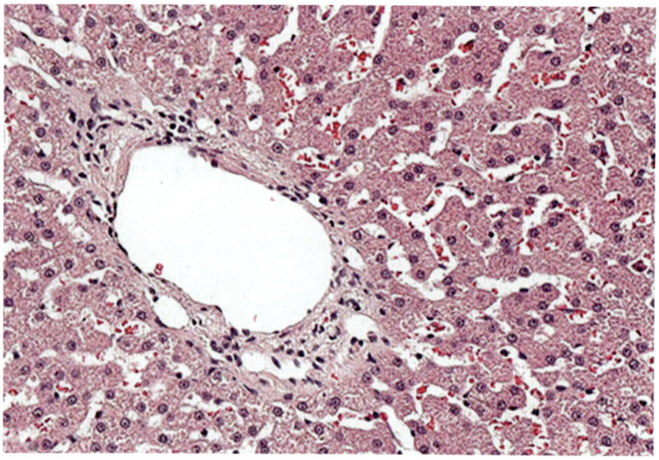

FIG. 29.2 A near-normal liver biopsy in a young toy breed dog with a congenital portosystemic shunt. Hematoxylin and eosin stain.

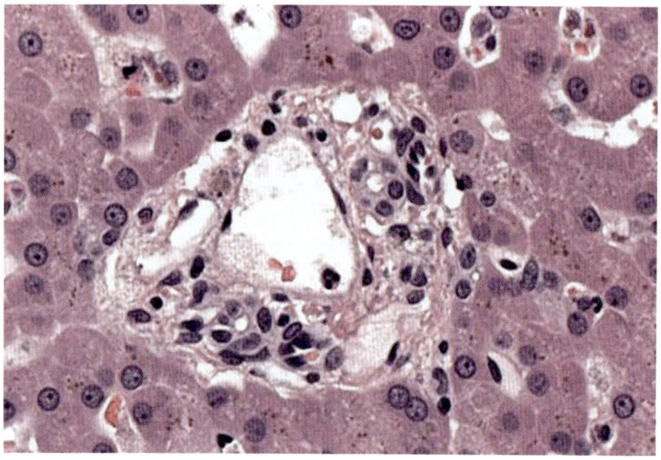

FIG. 29.3 Nonspecific reactive (secondary hepatitis) often presents a near-normal histologic picture. The portal tracts are infiltrated with small numbers of mixed inflammatory cells that do not target bile ducts and do not cross the limiting plate, which is the row of hepatocytes immediately adjacent to the portal tract. Hematoxylin and eosin stain.

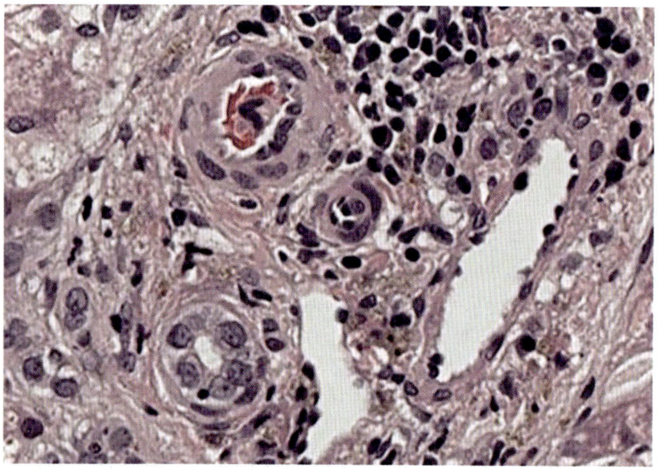

FIG. 29.4 Mild lymphocytic portal hepatitis in a dog. Note the lymphocytes form a vague nodular aggregate compared to the randomly dispersed lymphocytes in nonspecific (reactive) hepatitis (Fig. 29.3). Hematoxylin and eosin stain.

necrotic hepatocytes, are found in the parenchyma. Nonspecific reactive (secondary) hepatitis occurs most often in response to inflammatory bowel disease. Other conditions that can induce nonspecific reactive (secondary) hepatitis include pancreatitis, neoplasia, renal disease, autoimmune disease, dermatologic disorders, dental disease, heart failure, and pulmonary disease.

Portal cellular infiltrates

Portal hepatitis

Inflammatory cells are largely confined to the portal tracts with little interface (periportal) or lobular involvement (Fig. 29.4). No other abnormalities, such as cholangitis, are present. The primary rule-out is nonspecific reactive (secondary) hepatitis. Lymphocytic leukemia and lymphoma in dogs preferentially infiltrate the portal tracts. Mild portal infiltrates are often found adjacent to primary or metastatic tumors. If an attempt was made to biopsy a tumor and only portal hepatitis was found, the biopsy likely missed the mass. Viral hepatitis in people (e.g., hepatitis B virus) and in horses (e.g., equine parvovirus, equine hepacivirus) are associated with portal hepatitis, but to date, no viral cause of portal hepatitis has been recognized in dogs.

Cholangitis/cholangiohepatitis

Bile duct pathology is broadly classified as cholangitis (neutrophilic, lymphocytic to lymphoplasmacytic, destructive, associated with liver flukes), sclerosing, and extrahepatic bile duct obstruction.[5] In all cases, evidence of bile duct injury must be demonstrated, but it can be subtle, especially in cases of mild lymphocytic to lymphoplasmacytic cholangitis. Morphologic manifestations of bile duct injury may include a ductular reaction, hydropic degeneration or lipidosis, loss of nuclear polarity, nuclear pleomorphism, and nuclear hyperchromasia (Fig. 29.5A). Inflammatory targeting of the bile duct basement membrane is frequent, but inflammatory cell exocytosis and exudate accumulation in bile duct lumens are uncommon. Biliary epithelial cell necrosis may be accompanied by sloughed epithelial cells in the bile duct lumen, stratification of nuclei, and an uneven luminal profile with atrophied biliary epithelial cells interspersed with hypertrophied cells. Cholestasis is variable (**eFig. 29.13A**). Changes can be highly variable between lobes, within a single lobe, or even within a single biopsy. Thus, at least three separate lobes should be sampled. Extrahepatic bile duct obstruction or obstruction of large intrahepatic bile ducts will typically have mixed inflammatory infiltrates, often with neutrophils, accompanied by edema and periductal fibrosis, especially if chronic (Fig. 29.5B).

Portal venous hypoperfusion

Portal vein hypoperfusion (PVH) summarizes a constellation of histopathologic changes associated with decreased portal vein blood flow due to a variety of congenital and acquired vascular changes.[6] All causes of PVH result in stereotypic histopathologic changes that cannot be distinguished by histopathology. Low-power inspection of uncomplicated cases reveals a quiescent parenchyma with close spacing of portal tracts and unapparent central veins (Fig. 29.6A). The reticulin stain confirms the lack of parenchymal collapse compatible with lobular atrophy. Multifocal random lipogranulomas are a prominent feature in many cases of PVH. These lipogranulomas may or may not contain abundant hemosiderin. A paucity of central veins and/or obstruction of central veins by lipogranulomas may preclude complete shunt ligation. An increased number of

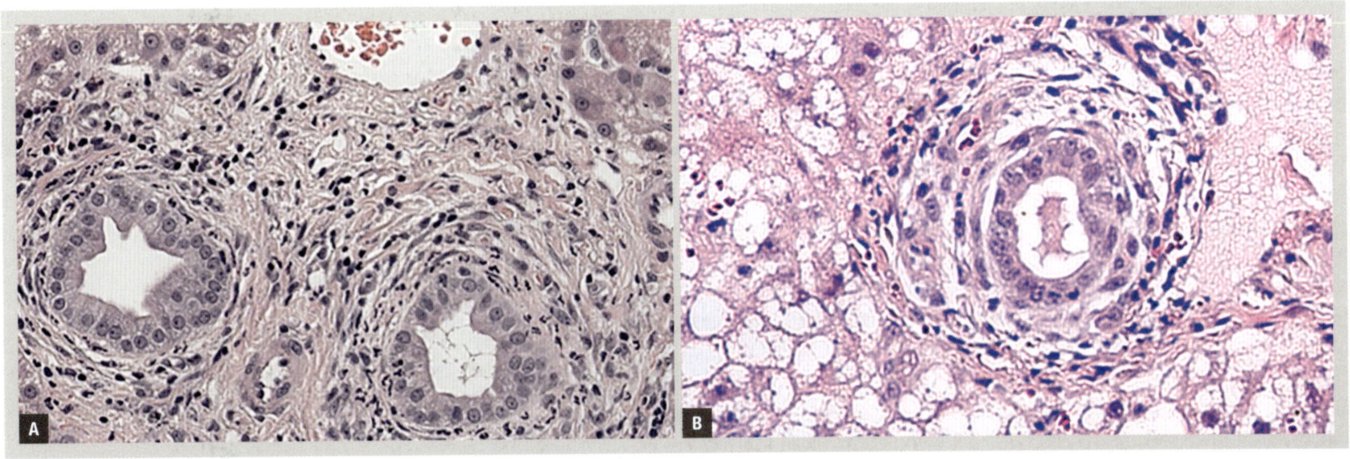

FIG. 29.5 (A) Neutrophilic cholangitis with stratification of nuclei, irregular luminal profiles, and mild peribiliary fibrosis. Note the lack of transmigrating leukocytes across the biliary epithelium or the accumulation of luminal exudate. Hematoxylin and eosin stain. (B) Mild edematous peribiliary fibrosis with mucus accumulation in the bile duct lumen in a dog with acute extrahepatic bile duct obstruction due to a duodenal foreign body. Hematoxylin and eosin stain.

monads and dyads ("miniaturized" portal tracts; "bonsai" portal tracts) are often accompanied by abnormal arterioles in the parenchyma ("orphan" arterioles). Monads consist of a portal tract with only a bile duct, while dyads contain a bile duct and a hepatic arteriole. Hepatic arteriolar reduplication of varying severity (Fig. 29.6B) reflects increased tortuosity due to increased arteriolar blood flow (hepatic arteriolar buffer response) as well as proliferation. Tributaries of the portal vein are variably absent, but large portal veins with irregular contours can be found in medium and large-sized portal tracts, sometimes opening directly into the sinusoids.

Chronic hepatitis

Chronic hepatitis is characterized by the presence of individual hepatocyte necrosis and a variable mononuclear or mixed inflammatory cell infiltrate that usually originates or is most severe in portal regions with spillover into the hepatic lobule.[7] With time, nodular regeneration and fibrosis may develop (advanced liver disease with fibrotic remodeling; cirrhosis) (**eFig. 29.14G**). Chronic hepatitis supplants older terminology of persistent hepatitis, chronic active hepatitis, and lobular hepatitis since these designations have no diagnostic or prognostic value. Interface hepatitis is dominated by lymphocytes and fewer plasma cells that breach the limiting plate and obscure the boundaries of the portal tract (**eFig. 29.15A**). Individual dead hepatocytes in the limiting plate may be noted as well. Inflammation and hepatocellular necrosis cause disruption of the lobular sinusoidal architecture, leading to lobular disarray (**eFig. 29.15B**). Known causes of chronic hepatitis are numerous, but in most cases, the etiology of chronic hepatitis remains unknown (see chapter 34 for more details). Immune-mediated hepatitis may be true autoimmune hepatitis (reaction to normal self-antigens) or a reaction to neoantigens as a result of a free radical-induced alteration of macromolecules leading to a breakdown in tolerance. Features strongly suggestive of immune-mediated hepatitis include interface activity and lymphocytic satellitosis around individual necrotic hepatocytes.

Copper hepatopathy is an extremely common cause of chronic canine hepatitis (see chapter 33). The degree of copper accumulation should be graded on a semiquantitative scale (Table 29.2). The report should

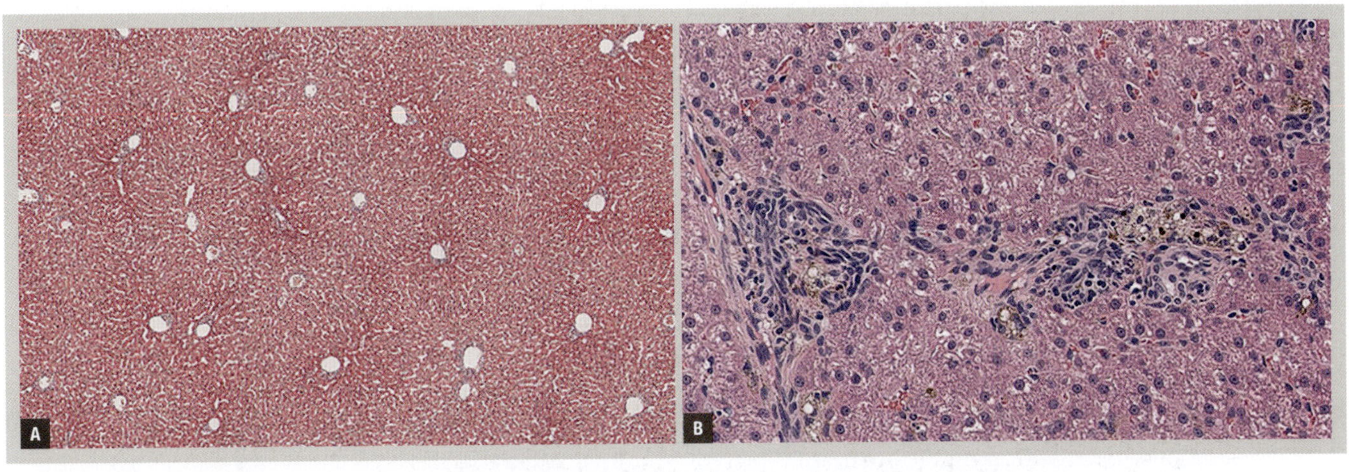

FIG. 29.6 (A) Liver biopsy from a young Yorkshire Terrier with a congenital portosystemic shunt.Low-power inspection reveals a quiescent biopsy with abnormally close spacing of portal tracts and a relative paucity of central veins. (B) Higher magnification of the same liver biopsy as in (A). Hepatic arteriolar reduplication forms a plexiform pattern as it wraps around mildly hyperplastic bile ducts. Note the hemosiderin-laden lipogranulomas in the portal tracts. Hematoxylin and eosin stain.

specify the distribution of the copper and whether it maps to areas of hepatocellular degeneration, necrosis, inflammation, parenchymal collapse, or fibrosis. Whenever possible, an additional fresh liver sample should be frozen and submitted for quantitative copper analysis if indicated by the biopsy results. If no fresh liver sample is available, the amount of copper can be determined using a digitized image of a rhodanine-stained section (Cornell University).

Granulomatous to pyogranulomatous hepatitis is an uncommon necroinflammatory chronic hepatitis that may reflect infection, immune-mediated disease, an immunoregulatory disorder, or a proliferative/neoplastic histiocytic syndrome. Meticulous exclusion of an infectious etiology, including both aerobic and anaerobic bacterial culture, PCR for mycobacteria, and/or fluorescent in situ hybridization (FISH), is recommended. Systemic fungal infection (i.e., histoplasmosis, blastomycosis, coccidioidomycosis, pythiosis) should be ruled out with priority given to those systemic fungal infections more likely to be encountered in the dog's geographic region or based on the travel history. A variety of bacterial agents have been isolated from cases of pyogranulomatous hepatitis in dogs, including *Brucella* spp., *Nocardia* spp., *Propionibacterium acne*, *Pantoea septicum*, mycobacteria, *Leptospira* spp., *Burkholderia* spp., and *Bartonella* spp. Baermann's technique to detect fluke eggs (e.g., schistosomiasis) might also be prudent but is often negative since the eggs are trapped in areas of hepatic fibrosis.

The biopsy report for cases of chronic hepatitis should have an indication of the grade and stage. Grade refers to the amount of necroinflammatory activity and indicates the rate of disease progression. Stage refers to the amount of fibrosis in the biopsy and indicates how far the disease has progressed. The biopsy will typically have a range of severity from field to field, but the most severe area will generally be reported in the morphologic diagnosis. While liver fibrosis is a consequence of necroinflammatory activity, the two processes should be assessed separately since they may not progress in parallel. Multiple grading and staging schemes have been proposed, but no formal grading and staging schemes have gained widespread acceptance in veterinary medicine. Table 29.3 outlines the staging scheme used by the author.

Ductal plate malformation

Ductal plate malformation refers to improper or arrested modeling of the ductal plate during embryogenesis[8] (see chapter 37). Depending on the level of the biliary tree affected, ductal plate malformation includes von Meyenburg complexes (biliary microhamartomas) (**eFig. 29.16A**), polycystic liver disease (**eFig. 29.16B** and **eFig. 29.16C**), small duct proliferative-like (**eFig. 29.16D**) and Caroli's disease (**eFig. 29.16E**). Caroli's syndrome is Caroli's disease in combination with another subtype of ductal plate malformation. Ductal plate malformation can be associated with a number of other congenital defects, including gallbladder hypoplasia/aplasia, choledochal cysts, left-sided liver lobe hypoplasia/aplasia, and diaphragmatic hernias.

Liver nodules

The liver is a frequent site of metastasis, and a diligent search for a primary tumor elsewhere should always be conducted. A variety of tumors can arise in the liver, but tumors of the biliary tree and those derived from hepatocytes are most frequent. See chapter 39 for more details.

Tumors of the biliary tree include biliary adenomas, biliary cystadenoma, and cholangiocellular carcinoma (**eFig. 29.17** and **eFig. 29.18**). Cholangiocellular carcinoma may be difficult or impossible to distinguish from a metastatic adenocarcinoma since bile pigment is rarely detectable. No immunohistochemical markers are currently available to make this distinction.

Nodular proliferations of hepatocytes can represent regenerative nodules, nodular hyperplasia, dysplastic foci, hepatocellular adenomas and hepatocellular carcinomas. Hepatoma has been used to designate both benign and malignant hepatocyte tumors. Because of this ambiguity, the term should be abandoned in favor of more specific designations. A needle biopsy through the center of a hepatic nodule without adjacent hepatic parenchyma for comparison may be impossible to categorize accurately.

Nodular hyperplasia is a common, age-related liver mass in dogs, beginning at 6 to 7 years of age and present in all dogs older than 14 years.[9] On histologic examination, the masses are mildly compressive but nonencapsulated and composed of variably sized and shaped lobules (**eFig. 29.19**). Normal hepatic parenchyma surrounds the nodules. Hepatocytes are arranged in somewhat disorganized cords one to two cells wide, accompanied by a reduction in the reticular meshwork. Hepatocytes have variable degrees of vacuolar change (hydropic, glycogen, lipid), and lipogranulomas are common.

Nodular regeneration arises from a background of hepatocellular degeneration, necrosis, and inflammation. Regenerative nodules are expansile and compress the adjacent parenchyma. Hepatocytes will

TABLE 29.2 Semiquantitative grading scheme for copper accumulation.

Grade	Comments
0	No visible copper
1	Only rare individual to <10% of centrilobular hepatocytes positive for copper
2	>10% to ≤25% of centrilobular hepatocytes positive
3	25% to 50% of centrilobular hepatocytes positive. A few mid-zonal hepatocytes may be positive and may have rare copper granulomas
4	>50% to 100% of centrilobular hepatocytes positive with variable numbers in mid-zonal regions. Copper granulomas may be numerous.
5	Panlobular copper accumulation in hepatocytes with frequent copper granulomas

TABLE 29.3 Staging scheme for the assessment of hepatic fibrosis.

Grade	Comments
0	No fibrosis
1	Fibrous expansion of <50% of portal tracts with no fibrous septa
2	Fibrous expansion of >50% of portal tracts with no fibrous septa
3	Fibrous expansion of >50% of portal tracts with fibrous septa
4	Fibrous expansion of >50% of portal tracts with <50% bridging septa
5	Fibrous expansion of >50% of portal tracts with >50% bridging septa
6	Cirrhosis (advanced liver disease with fibrous remodeling and nodular regeneration)

have an increased volume of slightly granular basophilic cytoplasm due to an increased amount of rough endoplasmic reticulum. Nuclei are often displaced toward the sinusoids and have an increased amount of euchromatin with a prominent nucleolus. With time, the nodules will become invested by a peripheral layer of connective tissue (**eFig. 29.20**). Hepatocytes are arranged in somewhat disorganized single to double-wide cords with a reduction in the reticulin substructure.

Dysplastic foci are nonencapsulated, nonexpansile, and noncompressive foci of proliferative hepatocytes with an irregular margin with the adjacent parenchyma (**eFig. 29.21**).[10] The hepatocytes are smaller than normal, resulting in a crowded appearance. The hepatocytes have hyperintense cytoplasm, and dysplastic foci stand out in stark relief to the adjacent nondysplastic parenchyma. The hepatocytes are arranged in single to double-wide cords, but the cords can occasionally be wider. Mega-canaliculi may be present where hepatocytes palisade around a clear central lumen. Sinusoids are often irregular, with dead-ends, hairpin turns, and meandering pathways. The reticulin stain demonstrates a decrease in the reticulin meshwork. Dysplastic foci are thought to have premalignant potential.

Hepatocellular adenomas are well-demarcated but usually encapsulated hepatocellular tumors devoid of portal tracts and bile ducts. Hepatocytes are cytologically bland and form variably wide trabeculae that can be separated by dilated sinusoids and cystic blood-filled spaces. Nuclei resemble normal hepatocytes, and mitotic figures are rare. The cytoplasm often displays "clear cell change" due to the accumulation of glycogen or lipids.

Hepatocellular carcinomas (HCC) are uncommon in dogs. Numerous histologic subtypes are recognized, but the most common are trabecular, solid, and telangiectatic. Low-grade, well-differentiated trabecular-type hepatocellular carcinomas are difficult to distinguish from hepatocellular adenomas. Careful inspection reveals an infiltrative rather than expansile growth pattern (**eFig. 29.22A**). Cytologic atypia, when observed, helps distinguish hepatocellular carcinoma from hepatocellular adenoma but is not often evident (**eFig. 29.22B**).

KEY POINTS

- A liver biopsy can provide valuable information for the management of liver disease.
- A brief summary of the history, physical exam findings, laboratory data, results of relevant imaging studies, drug history, the gross appearance of the lesion, whether the biopsy is focused (suspect focal liver disease) or unfocused (suspect diffuse liver disease) and the number, type and location of biopsies obtained should be reported to the pathologist to aid in diagnosis and ensure all specimens have been processed and examined.
- The morphologic diagnosis will typically summarize the major histologic pattern or injury patterns present in the biopsy but seldom provides a specific etiologic diagnosis.
- Hepatopathology uses many terms specific to the discipline and may not be familiar to the clinician. Authoritative sources for definitions are sparse and difficult to find. A few of the more commonly misinterpreted terms are defined, and the major patterns of hepatocellular injury are briefly described in this chapter. The chapter is not exhaustive, and many pathologic entities are not considered. Should the biopsy report cause confusion, call the pathologist for clarification.

References

1. Kemp SD, Zimmerman KL, Panciera DL, Monroe WE, Leib MS, Lanz OI. A comparison of liver sampling techniques in dogs. *J Vet Intern Med* 29(1):51-57, 2015.
2. Crawford, James M., Burt, Alistair D. Microanatomy of the liver. In Burt AD, Ferrell LD, Hübscher SG (editors). MacSween's Pathology of the Liver 6th edition. New York, Churchill Livingstone Elsevier, 2012, pp. 7-12.
3. Ettel MG, Appelman HD. Approach to the liver biopsy in the patient with chronic low-level aminotransferase elevations. *Arch Pathol Lab Med* 142(10):1186-1190, 2018.
4. Neumann S, Danner W. Reactive hepatitis in dogs. In 2012 [cited 2023 Nov 22]. Available from: https://www.semanticscholar.org/paper/Reactive-Hepatitis-in-Dogs-Neumann-Danner/eabfb72e649fde7299b7c00dee5adfeb01faffd5
5. Harrison JL, Turek BJ, Brown DC, Bradley C, Callahan Clark J. Cholangitis and cholangiohepatitis in dogs: A descriptive study of 54 cases based on histopathologic diagnosis (2004-2014). *J Vet Intern Med* 32(1):172-180, 2018.
6. Bertolini G. Anomalies of the portal venous system in dogs and cats as seen on multidetector-row computed tomography: an overview and systematization proposal. *Vet Sci* 6(1):10, 2019.
7. Webster CRL, Center SA, Cullen JM, Penninck DG, Richter KP, Twedt DC, et al. ACVIM consensus statement on the diagnosis and treatment of chronic hepatitis in dogs. *J Vet Intern Med* 33(3):1173-1200, 2019.
8. Pillai S, Center SA, McDonough SP, Demarco J, Pintar J, Henderson AK, et al. Ductal plate malformation in the liver of Boxer dogs: clinical and histological features. *Vet Pathol* 53(3):602-613, 2016.
9. Meyer, Denny J. Hepatic Pathology. In Strombeck DR, Guilford WG (editors). Small Animal Gastroenterology 3rd edition. Philadelphia, Saunders, 1996, pp. 649-650.
10. Cortright CC, Center SA, Randolph JF, McDonough SP, Fecteau KA, Warner KL, et al. Clinical features of progressive vacuolar hepatopathy in Scottish Terriers with and without hepatocellular carcinoma: 114 cases (1980-2013). *J Am Vet Med Assoc* 245(7):797-808, 2014.

Introduction to the liver anatomy and physiology

Francesco Lotti
DVM, MSc, DECVIM-CA
(Internal Medicine)

The liver is a highly vascular organ located in the cranial abdomen, immediately caudal to the diaphragm. It has a central importance in body homeostasis and is responsible for many different functions that support metabolism, blood volume regulation, hematopoiesis, immunity, digestion, detoxification, vitamin storage, and coagulation. This chapter will explore the basic anatomy and the major physiologic functions of the liver.

Liver anatomy: gross anatomy and anatomic relationships

The liver is a reddish brown, wedge-shaped organ representing approximately 3.4% of the body weight of an adult dog.[1] It is located in the most cranial region of the abdominal cavity immediately caudal to the diaphragm and within the confines of the rib cage.

The liver has two distinct surfaces, as shown in Fig. 30.1 and Fig. 30.2. A convex, diaphragmatic surface lies adjacent to the diaphragm, and the concave, visceral surface lies in contact with adjacent abdominal organs. The visceral surface contains impressions of the stomach, pancreas, duodenum, and right kidney in respective adjacent liver lobes.

The liver is grossly divided into six major lobes (right medial and lateral, left medial and lateral, quadrate and caudate lobes). The caudate lobe also contains a papillary process that projects into the vestibule of the omental bursa. The quadrate lobe is located between the right and the left medial lobes on the midline. The lateral aspect of the quadrate lobe, along with the right medial lobe, defines the gallbladder fossa. The gallbladder is attached to the quadrate lobe.

Blood supply

The liver has a unique circulation in that it is perfused by a dual blood supply: the hepatic artery and the portal vein. Both enter the liver at the level of porta hepatis (Fig. 30.1). The hepatic artery provides well-oxygenated blood (approximately 20% of the total afferent blood volume).[2,3] It arises from the celiac artery and merges into branches that perfuse individual liver lobes. The portal venous system carries the remaining 80% of the blood.[2,3] The portal vein is formed by the confluence of the cranial and caudal mesenteric veins, draining blood from the stomach, pancreas, spleen, and intestines. Portal blood is poorly oxygenated but rich in nutrients, hormones, metabolic substrates, and trophic factors, as well as noxious substances, particularly from the gut, that are removed by the liver.

The arterial and portal blood merge in the portal triad of the liver lobule and flow into the sinusoids, a specialized capillary system of the liver. Once passing through the sinusoids, blood enters the collecting branches of the central vein and leaves the liver via the hepatic veins. Six to eight hepatic veins usually drain venous blood from the canine liver, flowing into the caudal vena cava.[3]

The biliary system

Bile is produced within the hepatocytes and secreted into hepatic canaliculi. Canalicular bile first flows through the canals of Hering, an interconnected branching system of minute ductules, converging into interlobular bile ducts.[4] The interlobular ducts eventually fuse into hepatic ducts and unite to form the common bile duct, which enters the duodenum through the major duodenal papilla. Approximately 50% of all bile produced is temporarily stored, concentrated, and modified in the gallbladder. Bile enters the gallbladder through the cystic duct. The common bile duct starts where the first hepatic duct joins the cystic duct.[4] Bile flow into the duodenum through the common bile duct is regulated by the sphincter of Oddi, a muscular valve within the papilla.

Microscopic structure of the liver

Liver cells are organized around the microscopic structural unit of the liver —the liver lobule, as shown in (Fig. 30.3). The hepatic lobule is roughly hexagonal in shape and receives vascular blood flow at the portal triads. Each triad is composed of branches of the

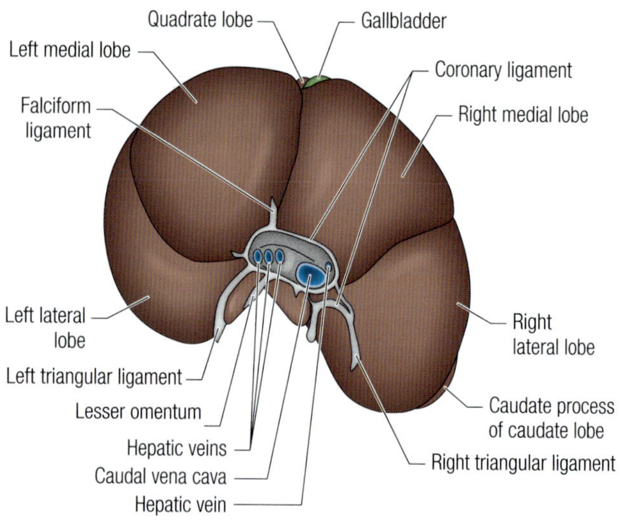

FIG. 30.1 Diaphragmatic surface of the liver.

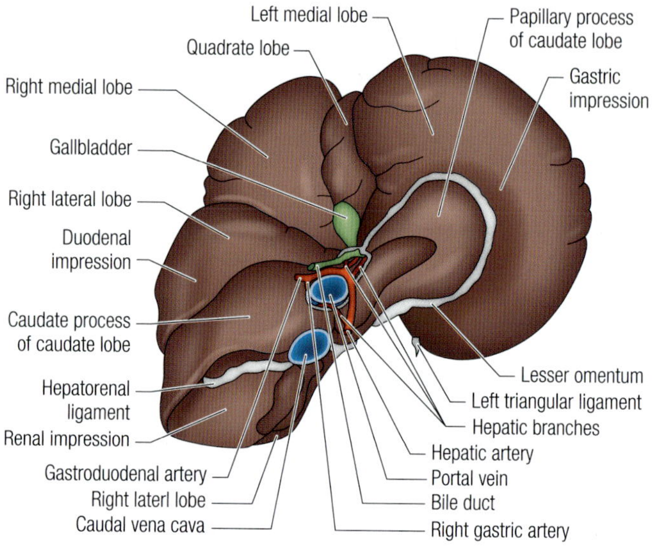

FIG. 30.2 Visceral surface of the liver.

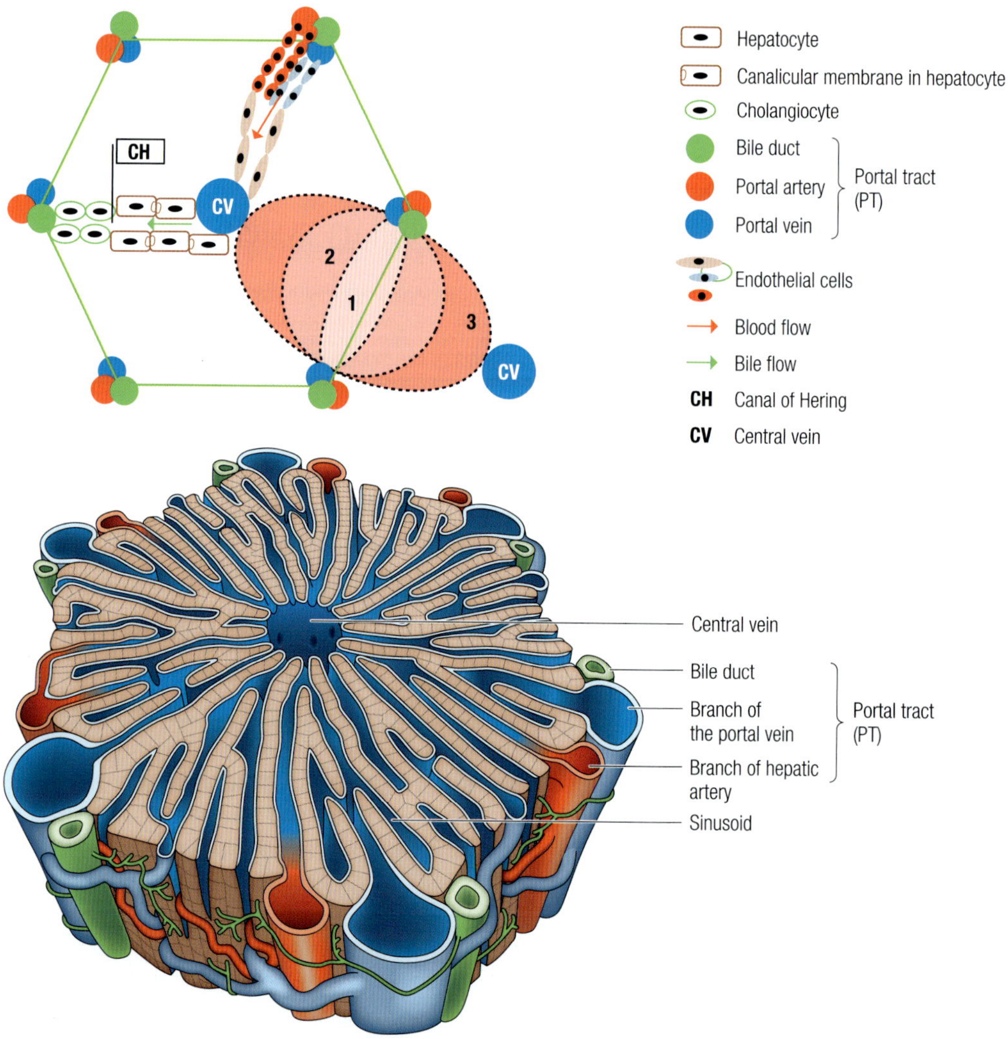

FIG. 30.3 Representation of liver microanatomy. The hepatic lobule is roughly hexagonal in shape. Its vertices are the portal triads, composed of branches of the hepatic artery, portal vein, bile ducts, and lymphatics. Blood flows from the portal triad into the hepatic sinusoids before merging into the central vein. Bile flows in the opposite direction, through the bile canaliculi and canals of Hering away from the central vein, toward the triad. Based on their function, parenchymal hepatocytes are divided into three zones, as depicted in the diagram at the top.

hepatic artery, portal vein, bile ducts, and lymphatics. Within the lobule, radiated chords of hepatocytes converge from the periphery of the "hexagon", extending toward the center and the central hepatic vein. Blood flows from the portal triad into the hepatic sinusoids before emptying into the central vein. The central vein joins the hepatic veins, carrying blood out of the liver. Secreted bile flows through small ductules in the opposite direction to blood flow, going from the central vein toward the portal triad.

The functional unit of the liver is the acinus. The functional acinus is described by both blood flow and metabolic functions of hepatocytes. The portal triad is the center of the acinus, and blood flows circumferentially through sinusoids toward terminal hepatic veins located in the periphery. Within the acinus, parenchymal hepatocytes are divided into three zones, as represented in Fig. 30.3. Zone 1 is located in the periportal region of hepatocytes. Due to its high perfusion and proximity to oxygenated blood and nutrients, zone 1 plays a large role in oxidative metabolisms such as beta-oxidation, gluconeogenesis, bile formation, cholesterol formation, and amino acid catabolism.[5] Zone 2 is a transitional zone and sits between zones 1 and 3. Zone 3 has the lowest perfusion and receives less oxygen due to its distance from the portal triad. It plays the largest role in detoxification, drug metabolism, ketogenesis, glycolysis, lipogenesis, glycogen synthesis, and glutamine formation.[5] New hepatocytes arise in zone 3 and move toward zone 1 as they age.

Physiology of the liver

Table 30.1 summarizes the major functions of the liver.

Biliary system and enterohepatic circulation of bile acids

One important function is the production of bile. Bile contains cholesterol, bilirubin, electrolytes, water, and bile acids (BAs), with the latter being the predominant component. BAs synthesis and enterohepatic circulation are illustrated in Fig. 30.4. The primary bile acids are cholic acid (CA) and chenodeoxycholic acid (CDCA). They are synthesized from cholesterol within the hepatocytes. The water solubility of primary BAs is increased by conjugation primarily to taurine or glycine. BAs conjugation prevents passive intestinal absorption, enabling their intraluminal involvement in digestion. Primary BAs are secreted into bile and stored in the gallbladder.[6] The presence of food (particularly fat) in the duodenum stimulates the release of cholecystokinin from duodenal I cells, which in turn stimulates gallbladder contraction as well as sphincter of Oddi relaxation.[7] In the intestine, BAs emulsify fat to enhance the digestion of dietary cholesterol, triglycerides, and fat-soluble vitamins by the formation of micelles. BAs then move distally and are efficiently (i.e., >95%) reabsorbed in the distal ileum and transported back to the liver.[7] Bile acid reabsorption occurs via the sodium-dependent bile transporter present in the apical membrane of the intestinal enterocyte. A small fraction of unabsorbed BAs enters the colon and undergoes deconjugation or 7α-hydroxylation to the secondary BAs by the resident gut microbiota. CA is converted to deoxycholic acid (DCA), and CDCA is converted to lithocholic acid (LCA). Almost all secondary BAs undergo passive colonic reabsorption and enter the enterohepatic circulation, with only 5% of BAs lost in feces daily.[7]

TABLE 30.1 Summary of the major functions of the liver.

Liver function	Examples
Digestive functions	■ Bile acid synthesis ■ Facilitating lipid digestion in the GI tract

Detoxification and excretion	■ Bilirubin
	  ■ Conjugation (UDP-glucuronyl-transferase)
	■ Ammonia
	  ■ Conversion to urea through Krebs-Henseleit urea cycle
	■ Hormones
	  ■ Steroids
	  ■ Thyroid hormones
	■ Drugs and toxin
	  ■ Phase I (oxidation, reduction, hydrolysis)
	  ■ Phase II (conjugation/cytochrome P450 system)

Hemostasis	■ Synthesis of coagulation factors
	  ■ Factors II, VII, IX, XI, XII and XIII
	  ■ Also, factor VIII in sinusoidal endothelium
	■ Synthesis of fibrinogen
	■ Site of vitamin-K-dependent carboxylation of prothrombin, and factors VII, IX, and X, protein C, and protein S
	■ Anticoagulant factors synthesis
	  ■ Antithrombin, protein S, tissue factor pathway inhibitor
	■ Control of fibrinolysis
	  ■ Synthesis of plasminogen, plasminogen activator inhibitor-1, thrombin activatable fibrinolysis inhibitor and alpha-2-antiplasmin

Nutrient metabolism	■ Carbohydrate metabolism
	  ■ Glucose homeostasis
	  ■ Glycogen metabolism and storage
	■ Lipid metabolism
	  ■ Fatty acid synthesis, mobilization, and degradation
	  ■ Triglyceride synthesis
	  ■ Secretion of lipoproteins
	■ Protein metabolism
	  ■ Albumin synthesis and turnover
	  ■ Amino acid regulation

Vitamin metabolism	■ Vitamin A metabolism and storage ■ Gamma-carboxylation of vitamin K-dependent coagulation factors ■ Vitamin D_3 conversion into 25-OH-vitamin D_3 ■ Vitamin E storage ■ Activation of water-soluble vitamin C and B complex

Bilirubin metabolism

The liver plays a significant role in bilirubin metabolism and excretion. Bilirubin is the major pigment in bile.[8] It originates from hemoprotein catabolism, primarily from hemoglobin. Unconjugated bilirubin enters the plasma and binds to albumin, which carries the lipid-soluble unconjugated bilirubin to the liver. As unconjugated bilirubin enters the hepatocyte, it is taken up and transported by anionic binding proteins (ligandin or Y protein) for hepatic conjugation to render bilirubin water-soluble. Conjugation occurs through the binding of bilirubin to glucuronide. This process is catalyzed by the UDP-glucuronyl-transferase. Conjugated bilirubin then moves through the canalicular membrane and enters the bile. In the intestine, conjugated bilirubin is either excreted through the feces

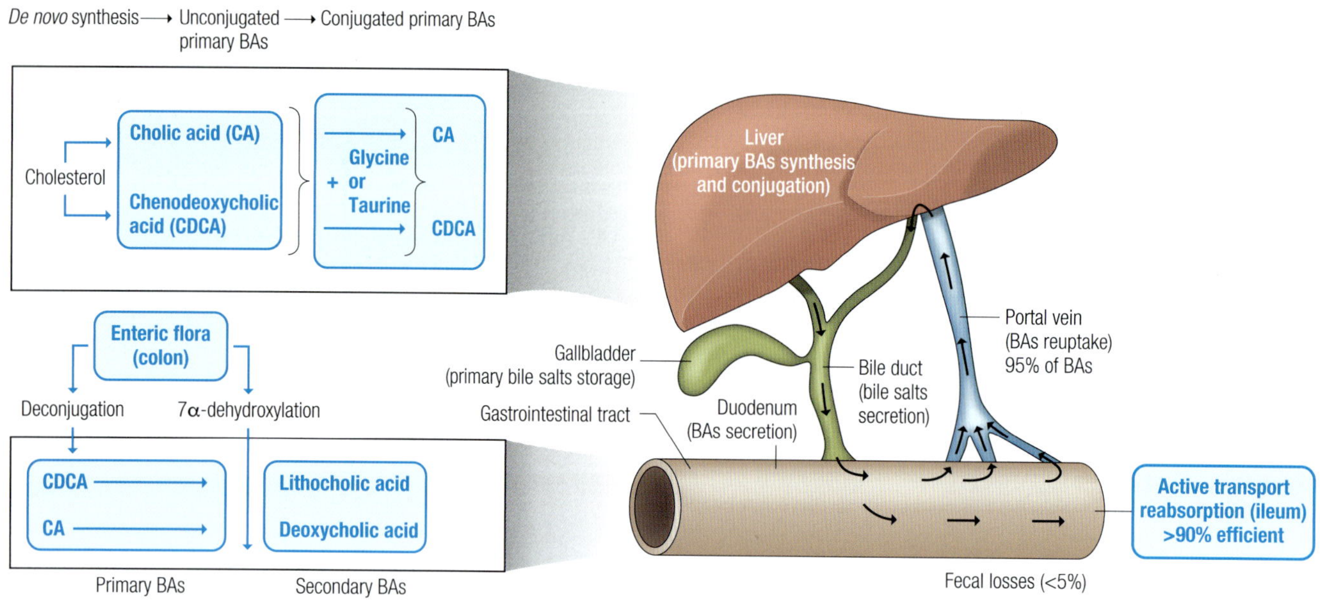

FIG. 30.4 Enterohepatic circulation and bile acid metabolism.

or deconjugated by colonic microbiota to other products (urobilinogens and stercobilinogens). Approximately half of urobilinogen is reabsorbed in the large intestine, enters the portal circulation, and is removed by the liver to be re-excreted back into bile, completing an enterohepatic pathway.[8] A small fraction of urobilinogen bypasses the liver and is eliminated in urine. Urobilinogen is a colorless pigment but is oxidized to yellow urobilin when exposed to air, which gives urine its color. Unabsorbed intestinal urobilinogen undergoes oxidation to urobilins and stercobilins, substances responsible for the normal brown fecal pigmentation.[8]

Nutrients and vitamin metabolism

The liver is of central importance for protein, lipid, and carbohydrate metabolism. It is also the primary site of synthesis for most plasma proteins, including albumin and alpha and beta globulins. Through plasma protein production, the liver is actively involved in the regulation of tissue inflammation, oncotic pressure, iron metabolism, hemostasis, enzyme production, and binding functions.[9]

The liver also plays a major role in determining the metabolic fate of lipids absorbed from the intestine or released from adipose tissue. Generally, lipid metabolism in hepatocytes can be summarized by three processes: 1) uptake of lipids and fatty acids and fatty acid synthesis (*de novo* lipogenesis); 2) lipid storage, including triglyceride synthesis; and 3) lipid consumption, including fatty acid degradation (lipolysis), β-oxidation, and the secretion of lipoproteins.[10]

The normal liver is actively involved in carbohydrate metabolism by providing energy substrates. In particular, it becomes critical in the fasted state due to its role in maintaining euglycemia. In conjunction with insulin and glucagon, the liver prevents excessive fluctuations in blood glucose concentration by stimulating glycogen synthesis, gluconeogenesis, or glycolysis.[9]

Liver function is important in the metabolism, utilization, storage, and degradation of many vitamins. Examples include the liver's role in vitamin A metabolism and storage, gamma-carboxylation of vitamin K-dependent coagulation factors (II, VII, IX, X, protein C, and protein S), vitamin D_3 conversion into 25-OH-vitamin D_3, vitamin E storage and activation of water-soluble vitamin C and B complex.[9]

Coagulation

The liver is crucial in all aspects of coagulation homeostasis. Most factors that regulate procoagulation, anticoagulation, and fibrinolysis are produced and/or activated in the liver.[11] The liver produces thrombopoietin, a hormone that regulates bone marrow production of platelets. Fibrinogen, prothrombin, factors V, VII, IX, X, XI, XII, and XIII are all synthesized at least to some extent in the liver.[11] It used to be believed that the liver did not make factor VIII, but it is now recognized that hepatic sinusoidal endothelial cells are the main source of this coagulation factor.[12] Hepatocytes are also the site of vitamin K-dependent carboxylation of prothrombin, FVII, FIX, FX, protein C, and protein S. Many anticoagulant proteins, including antithrombin, protein S, and tissue factor pathway inhibitors, are synthesized in the liver. The liver also synthesizes factors that control fibrinolysis, including plasminogen, plasminogen activator inhibitor-1, thrombin activatable fibrinolysis inhibitor, and alpha-2-antiplasmin.[11]

Drug and toxin metabolism

A critical function of the liver is metabolism and/or detoxification of xenobiotics. It has central importance because of its strategic position between the digestive tract and the systemic circulation, which permits immediate access to substances absorbed from the intestines.[9,13] The liver functions to transform xenobiotics mainly by converting lipophilic forms to hydrophilic forms through two metabolic reactions: phase I and phase II.[13] These reactions mainly take place in the smooth endoplasmic reticulum of hepatocytes. Phase I reactions create a more hydrophilic solute via oxidation, reduction, and hydrolysis using primarily the cytochrome P450 (CYP450) family of enzymes. The product of phase I has an oxygen species that reacts better with enzymes involved with phase II reactions.[9,13] Phase II reactions conjugate the metabolites created in phase I, making them more hydrophilic for secretion into the blood or bile. There are three main avenues for conjugation performed in phase II reactions: conjugation to glucuronate, glutathione, or sulfate.[13]

Ammonia metabolism

Ammonia is a catabolic product of amino acid and nitrogen compound metabolism. About half of the ammonia in the portal vein originates from small intestinal enterocyte catabolism of glutamine as an energy source, with some also originating from dietary proteins and bacterial metabolism of nitrogenous products to ammonia, particularly in the large intestine.[14,15] Production of ammonia in the GI tract is increased by the ingestion of a protein-rich meal (with some evidence that meats produce more ammonia than dairy or vegetable protein),[15] GI hemorrhage, and constipation. The rate of intestinal absorption depends on the ionization state of the ammonia molecule. The nonionized form NH_3 is lipid soluble and readily crosses cell membranes, while the ammonium ion NH_4^+ is favored by a low pH (pH <6) and is poorly absorbed across the enterocyte membrane. Ammonia is then delivered to the liver through the portal vein circulation. Under normal conditions, almost all the ammonia delivered to the liver is effectively converted to urea through the Krebs-Henseleit urea cycle.[14] About 25% of the urea produced in the liver diffuses back into the GI tract, where it undergoes conversion to ammonia by bacterial ureases.[9] The remainder of the urea is removed through the kidneys.[15] Pathological increases in serum ammonia concentrations are usually associated with abnormal hepatic function or portosystemic shunting of blood bypassing the liver. Excess ammonia is one of the factors responsible for hepatic encephalopathy.[15]

KEY POINTS

- The liver is a highly vascular gland located in the anterior abdominal cavity, caudal to the diaphragm.
- It is composed of two surfaces and six major lobes.
- The liver is perfused by a dual blood supply: the hepatic artery and the portal vein. Arterial and portal blood merge and flow into the sinusoids. The blood then enters the collecting branches of the central vein and leaves the liver via hepatic veins.
- The biliary system includes hepatic canaliculi, canals of Hering, bile ductules, interlobular bile ducts, hepatic ducts, common bile duct, cystic duct, and the gallbladder.
- Liver cells are organized around the microscopic structural unit of the liver —the hepatic lobule. The hepatic lobule is roughly hexagonal in shape and receives vascular blood flow at the portal triads. Each triad is composed of branches of the hepatic artery, portal vein, bile ducts, and lymphatics.
- The liver plays a major role in body homeostasis, being responsible for many different functions that help support metabolism, blood volume regulation, hematopoiesis, immunity, digestion, detoxification, vitamin storage, and coagulation.

References

1. Hermanson JW, De Lahunta A, Evans HE. Liver. The digestive apparatus and abdomen. In Hermanson JW, De Lahunta A, Evans HE (editors). Miller and Evans' Anatomy of the Dog. 5th edition. St. Louis, Elsevier Health Sciences, 2020, pp. 767-780.
2. Kan Z, Madoff DC. Liver anatomy: microcirculation of the liver. *Semin Intervent Radiol* 25(2):77-85, 2008.
3. Mari L, Acocella F. Vascular anatomy of canine hepatic venous system: a basis for liver surgery. *Anatomia, histologia, embryologia* 44(3):212-224, 2015.
4. Jaffey JA. Canine hepatobiliary anatomy, physiology and congenital disorders. *J Small Anim Pract* 63(2):95-103, 2022.
5. Sasse D, Spornitz UM, Piotr Maly I. Liver architecture. *Enzyme* 46(1-3):8-32, 1992.
6. Scott RB, Eidt PB, Shaffer EA. Regulation of fasting canine duodenal bile acid delivery by sphincter of Oddi and gallbladder. *Am J Physiol* 249:622-633, 1985.
7. Scott RB, Strasberg SM, El-Sharkawy TY, et al. Regulation of the fasting enterohepatic circulation of bile acids by the migrating myoelectric complex in dogs. *J Clin Invest* 71:644-654, 1983.
8. Rothuizen J, Van Den Brom WE. Bilirubin metabolism in canine hepatobiliary and haemolytic disease. *Vet Quart* 9(3):235-240, 1987.
9. Center SA. Pathophysiology of liver disease: normal and abnormal function. In Guilford WG (editor). Strombeck's Small Animal Gastroenterology 3rd edition. Philadelphia, W.B. Saunders, 1996, pp. 563-632.
10. Nguyen P, Leray V, Diez M et al. Liver lipid metabolism. *J Anim Physiol Anim Nutrition* 92(3):272-283, 2008.
11. Prins M, Schellens CJ, Van Leeuwen MW. Coagulation disorders in dogs with hepatic disease. *Vet J* 185(2):163-168, 2010.
12. Pradhan-Sundd T, Gudapati S, Kaminski TW, et al. Exploring the complex role of coagulation factor VIII in chronic liver disease. *Cell Mol Gastroenterol Hepatol* 12(3):1061-1072, 2021.
13. Apte U, Krishnamurthy P. Detoxification functions of the liver. In Cagle PT (editor). Molecular Pathology of Liver Diseases. Springer, 2011, 147-163.
14. Huizenga JR, Gips CH, Tangerman A. The contribution of various organs to ammonia formation: a review of factors determining the arterial ammonia concentration. *Annals Clin Biochem* 33(1):23-30, 1996.
15. Wright G, Noiret L, Olde Damink SW, et al. Interorgan ammonia metabolism in liver failure: the basis of current and future therapies. *Liver Intl* 31(2):163-175, 2011.

CHAPTER 31

Acute toxic hepatopathy

Karyn Bischoff
DVM, DABVT

Introduction to hepatic detoxification and toxicity

A major function of the liver is to protect the animal body from chemical injury. A large proportion of cardiac output (25% in humans) goes through the liver. The liver receives blood from the gastrointestinal tract via the portal circulation, which contains absorbed endotoxins, ammonia, and other compounds that can potentially cause cell injury. Some toxicants absorbed by the liver and eliminated through the bile can be reabsorbed into the portal circulation, termed enterohepatic cycling.

Blood percolates through the liver, starting at the portal vein, which branches to form multiple portal triads, including the hepatic artery and bile ducts. Blood from the hepatic artery is oxygenated and also flows through the sinusoids toward the central vein. Cords of hepatocytes radiate from the central vein to the portal triads, forming hexagonal hepatic lobules, and sinusoids are formed between those cords. The sinusoids are lined by microvilli on the hepatocyte membranes on each side, separated from fenestrated endothelial cells by the space of Disse. The large surface area of the hepatocyte membrane, in direct contact with the circulating plasma, allows the transport of nutrients, hormones, steroids, and xenobiotics into the cell by various mechanisms, whereupon they can be metabolized by phase I and phase II enzymes for elimination in the bile or the urine.

The purpose of the phase I and II enzyme systems is to increase the water solubility of lipophilic compounds in order to promote biliary or renal excretion. Most phase I enzymes (microsomal enzymes) are found in hepatocellular microsomes. Often, these enzymes are termed cytochrome P450s (abbreviated as P450s or CYPs) for the wavelength at which they absorb light (450 nm). CYPs are numerous, but all act by the addition of a functional group to the substrate through oxidation, reduction, or hydrolysis, producing reactive electrophilic metabolites.

Phase II enzymes are involved in conjugation reactions, adding a polar group to the reactive phase I metabolite and further enhancing water solubility. Molecules used in these conjugation reactions include glucuronic acid, sulfate, acetate, glutathione peroxidase, methyl groups, and amino acids. A mismatch between phase I and phase II enzymes can lead to the accumulation of toxic phase I metabolites. This mismatch occurs in paracetamol toxicosis. Paracetamol, or acetaminophen, is metabolized by phase I enzymes to N-acetyl-p-benzoquinone imine (NAPQI). NAPQI undergoes phase II conjugation to glutathione, but limited phase II substrate availability leads to NAPQI accumulation, resulting in toxicosis in the overdose situation.[1] There are species differences in phase II enzymes, such as the deficiency in uridine 5'-diphosphate-glucuronosyltransferase in cats and N-acetyltransferase in both cats and dogs, which can impair their ability to detoxify certain xenobiotics.[2] Deficient glucuronosyltransferase in cats diminishes their ability to conjugate NAPQI and other metabolites of paracetamol, which is the reason cats are so exquisitely sensitive to paracetamol toxicosis.

Also important are the phase III enzymes, which are transporters involved in eliminating chemicals. An example is the p-glycoprotein, involved in transport into bile canaliculi, which is defective in many dogs due to a base pair deletion in the ABCB1 gene. This genetic defect is likely to impact the elimination and toxic dose of p-glycoprotein substrates.

The hepatic lobule can be subdivided in two ways to describe liver injury. Zones 1 and 3 are approximately equivalent to periportal and centrilobular zones, respectively, with zone 2 hepatocytes equivalent to midzonal hepatocytes. The distribution of lesions is often described as zonal, bridging, or panlobular. The centrilobular zone is the most common distribution of hepatocellular necrosis in toxicoses. This area is relatively hypoxic compared to the portal zone because of arteriolar blood flow from the portal triads. This, and the higher density of phase I enzymes within centrilobular hepatocytes, predispose to centrilobular necrosis. Grossly, centrilobular necrosis presents with a reticulated pattern, with dark red centrilobular zones separated by the brown-to-yellow portal zone. When panlobular necrosis occurs (Fig. 31.1), the liver is grossly swollen and friable, necrosis extends through all three zones, and lobular architecture is completely lost on histology.

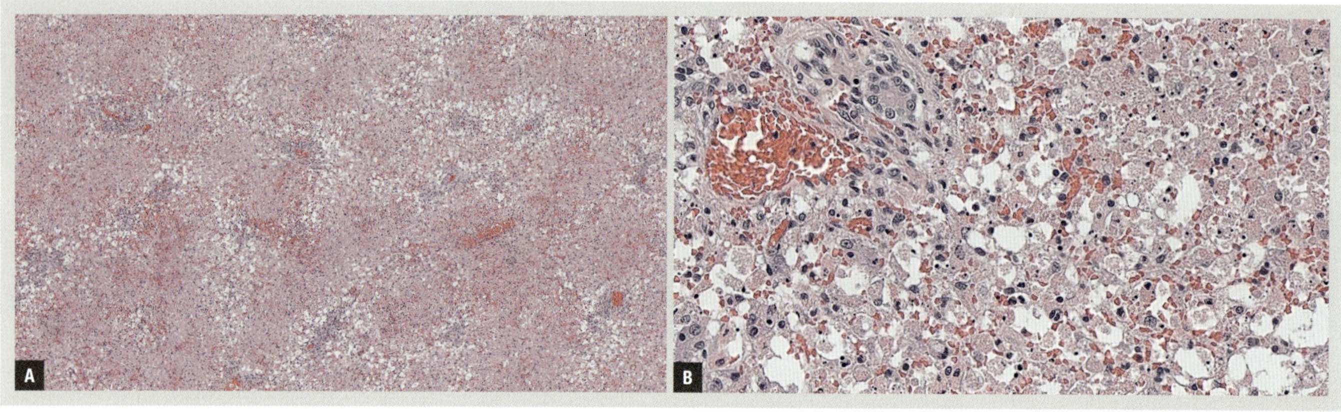

FIG. 31.1 (A) Histological section of liver from a dog showing panlobular hepatic necrosis with collapse of the lobular architecture due to ingestion of microcystins. (B) Close-up of a portal area in (A). Note the loss of hepatic cords and sinuses with extravascular erythrocytes, necrosis of hepatocytes as illustrated by nuclear pyknosis and fragmentation, cytoplasmic vacuolation, and loss of cellular integrity. Hematoxylin and eosin stain—photo courtesy of Dr. Ana Alcaraz.

Pathophysiology of acute toxic hepatitis

Rapid onset hepatopathy can be classified as acute liver injury (ALI) or acute liver failure (ALF). ALF occurs after loss of more than 70% of hepatic function and presents with a rapid onset of severe clinical signs, including icterus, coagulopathy, and hepatic encephalopathy. Coagulopathy is associated with both the decreased synthesis of vitamin K-dependent coagulation factors and reduced hepatic thrombopoietin production, resulting in thrombocytopenia. There are numerous agents that can cause acute hepatocellular degeneration and necrosis, several of which are listed in Table 31.1. These agents cause predictable, dose-dependent lesions, often with a latent period. The latent period is related to the time needed for absorption, distribution, and often bioactivation, plus the time it takes to meet the threshold of liver damage beyond which dysfunction becomes clinically evident. Therefore, despite the acute onset of severe clinical signs, hepatic lesions take time to develop.

Some pharmaceuticals can cause sporadic acute hepatocellular necrosis, termed idiosyncratic hepatotoxicosis. This occurs when the animal has been previously exposed to a drug and forms adducts of reactive drug metabolites that interact with cellular proteins to form neoantigens. Neoantigens are processed by antigen-presenting cells, such as Kupffer cells, leading to cellular and antibody-mediated immune responses.[18] Upon re-exposure to the drug, acute hepatic necrosis ensues, and the effect is not dose-dependent. Some drugs associated with idiosyncratic hepatotoxicity are listed in Table 31.2.

Overview of clinical and clinicopathological signs of acute toxic hepatopathy

There is often a latent period between xenobiotic exposure and clinical signs of hepatopathy, in some cases preceded by clinical signs of gastrointestinal dysfunction. The gastrointestinal epithelium is usually exposed to xenobiotics first. Thus, intestinal villus epithelium may be impacted. Rapid regeneration of crypt cells leads to villus repair and resolution of signs. Meanwhile, the absorbed toxicant causes hepatocellular necrosis, and hepatocytes are slower to regenerate than gastrointestinal mucosal epithelium. Once a threshold of up to 70% cell loss occurs, clinical liver failure is observed. Signs associated with acute liver failure can include a rapid onset of lethargy, vomiting, diarrhea, hematochezia or melena, icterus, coagulopathy, and ascites. Aside from idiosyncratic reactions, the severity of organ damage and clinical signs are dose-dependent.

Baseline serum chemistry at the start of hospitalization, with repeated monitoring of glucose (every 2-4 hours), electrolytes, and liver enzymes (every 12-24 hours) is warranted, and should continue for at least 3 days.[19] Ammonia is a specific and sensitive indicator of liver function, with hyperammonemia leading to hepatic encephalopathy, but serum analysis for ammonia must take place almost immediately after serum collection and thus is not always practical (see chapter 25 for more details on ammonia measurement). Bile acids are not helpful as tests of liver function in acute toxic hepatopathy if there is concurrent jaundice as they are elevated in cholestasis (see chapter 25).

Common serum chemistry findings associated with hepatotoxic events are related to hepatocyte membrane leakage, cholestasis, or liver function deficits. Enzyme leakage from hepatocytes is associated with changes in cell membrane permeability and cell death. The major enzymes associated with hepatocellular leakage include alanine aminotransferase (ALT) and aspartate aminotransferase (AST). ALT has high activity in canine hepatocytes and increases within 12 hours of hepatocyte injury, then peaks within 2 days, with a half-life of up to 60 hours. AST increases rapidly after liver injury but is found in lower concentrations in other tissues, such as muscle. AST has a much shorter half-life than ALT, around 12 hours, so while it also increases rapidly after liver injury, AST is less specific and returns to baseline more quickly than ALT. Additionally, since these enzymes are hepatocyte products, they can be relatively low in end-stage liver failure, as reported in aflatoxicosis.[3]

The production of certain membrane enzymes can be induced in biliary epithelium by cholestasis, including alkaline phosphatase (ALP) and gamma-glutamyl transferase (GGT). ALP is produced in different isoforms by multiple tissues in dogs, including bone ALP (B-ALP), while liver (L-ALP) and corticosteroid-induced (C-ALP) both produced in the liver. C-ALP predominates with anticonvulsant as well as with corticosteroid therapy. More details on the measurement of liver enzymes are found in chapter 25.

TABLE 31.1 Toxic agents causing acute hepatic necrosis in small animals.

Toxic agent	Source and toxicity	Toxicity	Proposed mechanism of action
Aflatoxins*	Produced by mold fungi, especially *Aspergillus* spp.	Food containing >60 ppb aflatoxins has been associated with aflatoxicosis in dogs	Activated by P450 enzymes to an epoxide that causes oxidative damage and binds macromolecules, especially DNA[3]
Amatoxins*	Fungal toxins from mushrooms of several genera, including *Amanita phalloides*, *A. ocreata*, and some *Lepiota* spp. and *Galerina* spp.	The LD_{50} for methyl-ϒ-amanitin is 0.5 mg/kg, and mushrooms can contain >2 mg amatoxins/g[4]	Cyclic octapeptide amatoxins inhibit RNA polymerase II, ceasing translation and protein production, causing death in cells with a high metabolic rate[4]
Azathioprine	Immunosuppressive prescription drug	A dose of 1.9 mg/kg every other day + and 1.3 mg/kg glucocorticoid	Not understood, but potentially related to polymorphisms in the thiopurine methyltransferase pathway and glutathione depletion[5]
Chondroitin and glucosamine joint supplements	Over-the-counter pharmaceutical products	A dose of 86 mg of Mn/kg was fatal in a dog[6]	Likely caused by manganese
Cycasin, methylazoxy-methanol (MAM)*	Palm trees of the genus *Cycas* or *Zamia* (e.g., "sago palms", Fig. 31.2), especially the seeds	Variable concentrations of cycasin based on plant species and tissues	Cycasin is a glucoside of MAM. Converted to the aglycone by intestinal microflora, MAM is activated by P450 enzymes to an electrophile, which intercalates DNA[7]
Iron	Supplements, hand warmers	Ingestion of 20-60 mg/kg elemental iron is associated with mild clinical signs. Ingestion of >100 mg/kg is potentially lethal[8]	Oxidative injury
Microcystins and nodularins*	Cyanobacterial toxins from genera including *Microcystis*, *Nodularis*, *Aphanizomenon*, and *Cylindrospermum*	The oral lethal dose of microcystin RR in mice was 10.9 mg/kg[9]	Cyclic peptides that inhibit protein phosphatases 1 and 2A, involved with cytoskeletal function, leading to cytoskeletal collapse, disruption of hepatic architecture, hemorrhage, and potential hypovolemic shock
Oak (*Quercus* spp.)	Ingestion of acorns reported in a dog	Toxic dose expected to be variable based on *Quercus* species and conditions, but toxicosis in a 23.4 kg dog was associated with ≥10 cracked acorns[10]	Not understood but may be related to tannin metabolism to gallic acid and pyrogallol causing oxidative damage to hepatocytes
Oxibendazole and mebendazole	Prescription anthelmintic, historically used in dogs, oxibendazole often combined with diethylcarbamazine	Therapeutic dose of 5 mg oxibendazole/kg/day for 10 days and 22 mg mebendazole/kg/day for 3+ days was associated with hepatotoxic effects in some dogs[11,12]	May impact cytoskeletal assembly[11]
Paracetamol (acetaminophen)*	Over-the-counter pain relievers, cold and flu products, etc.	A dose >150 mg/kg can be associated with toxicosis in dogs[13] There is no safe dose for cats[14]	Activated by P450 enzymes to the electrophile NAPQI, which binds cellular proteins, disrupting cell signaling and leading to mitochondrial dysfunction, oxidative stress, and cell death
Phenytoin, primidone, phenobarbital	Prescription use in combination to treat epilepsy	Increased ALT and ALP are commonly seen with phenobarbital in the absence of significant hepatic pathology.[15] Prolonged use in combination with phenytoin >30 mg/kg/day has been associated with hepatocellular degeneration and cholestasis	Potentially, metabolic activation to an epoxide intermediate, which causes oxidative damage[16]
Xylitol*	Sugar alcohol, used in dietetic and dental products	Hypoglycemia is reported in dogs ingesting >100 mg/kg Hepatic necrosis is reported at >500 mg/kg[17]	Unknown mechanism Preceded by hypoglycemia

* For more details on clinical and clinicopathological presentation of these toxins, see below.

TABLE 31.2 Drugs associated with idiosyncratic hepatotoxicity in dogs.

Drug	Breed affected
Carprofen	Labrador Retrievers may be predisposed[18,19]
Lomustine	Various breeds[19]
Sulfonamides	Various breeds, Doberman may be predisposed[19]
Zonisamide	Reported in a Boston Terrier and a Rottweiler[18,19]

The liver has important functions in synthesizing cholesterol and proteins, including coagulation factors. As liver function declines below 70% in acute toxic hepatopathies, coagulopathy becomes evident and is measured by increased activated partial thromboplastin time (aPTT) and prothrombin time (PT). Thromboelastography can be used to diagnose a hypocoagulable state. Other biomarkers for hepatic synthetic function useful in acute toxic hepatopathies include protein C and antithrombin.[3]

Summary of some important hepatotoxins

Aflatoxins[3]

Aflatoxin-producing fungi, often of the genus *Aspergillus*, can grow on a number of high-nutrient crops and seeds. Aflatoxicosis is thus often associated with pre- or postproduction contamination of pet foods but can be associated with other moldy material, as can occur in garbage or compost ingestion. The patient can present with acute signs up to 3 weeks after dietary exposure.[20] Vomiting, melena, depression, icterus, and ascites are commonly reported. ALT and AST elevation can be relatively mild. Hypocholesterolemia and decreased protein C are often seen as evidence of loss of hepatic function.

Amatoxins[19]

Toxicity associated with mushrooms including *Amanita phalloides*, *A. ocreata*, and some *Lepiota* spp. and *Galerina* spp. The toxic peptides are temperature- and time-stable, so dried, stored, and cooked mushrooms remain toxic. Dogs typically present with vomiting, diarrhea, abdominal pain, and hematochezia in the first 6-24 hours due to necrosis of villus epithelium, which is followed by apparent recovery. Hepatic necrosis occurs over time, leading to fulminant liver failure 36-84 hours postingestion, beginning with hypoglycemia and progressing to coagulopathy, encephalopathy, and renal failure.

Cycasin[19]

Cycas spp. and *Zamia* spp. are ancient plants found in warm climates and can grow into large trees, but they are also sold as potted plants to be kept in the home (Fig. 31.2). Vomiting and diarrhea are seen within the first 24 hours of exposure due to damage to the intestinal mucosa, followed by apparent recovery. Acute liver failure occurs 48-72 hours after ingestion.

Microcystins and nodularin[19]

Microcystins are peptides produced by naturally occurring freshwater cyanobacterial (blue-green algal) blooms. Nodularin is a similar peptide associated with the cyanobacterium *Nodularia spumigena* in brackish water. Cyanobacteria are microscopic organisms, and those that produce microcystins include *Microcystis* spp. (Fig. 31.3), *Planktothrix* spp., *Nostic* spp., and *Dolichispermum* spp. Blooms can be blue-green to brown or inapparent.[21] Access is usually by drinking contaminated water or ingesting bloom material during grooming or scavenging activity, although cyanobacteria-containing supplements can be purchased and are occasionally reported to cause hepatic injury due to the presence of microcystins. A rapid onset of vomiting, abdominal pain, and diarrhea with blood can be seen soon after ingestion, followed by a rapid progression to icterus, hypoglycemia, hyperammonemia, coagulopathy, and hepatic encephalopathy. Death after very high dose exposure can occur within hours from collapse of hepatic architecture and subsequent hemorrhage into the liver, causing hypovolemic shock. ALT and AST elevations range from mild to marked.

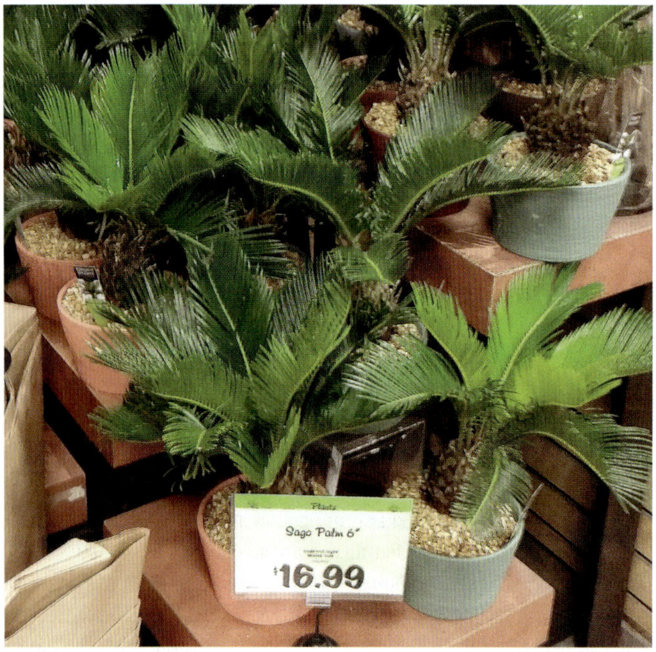

FIG. 31.2 Potted sago palms (*Cycad revoluta*) for sale at a grocery store.

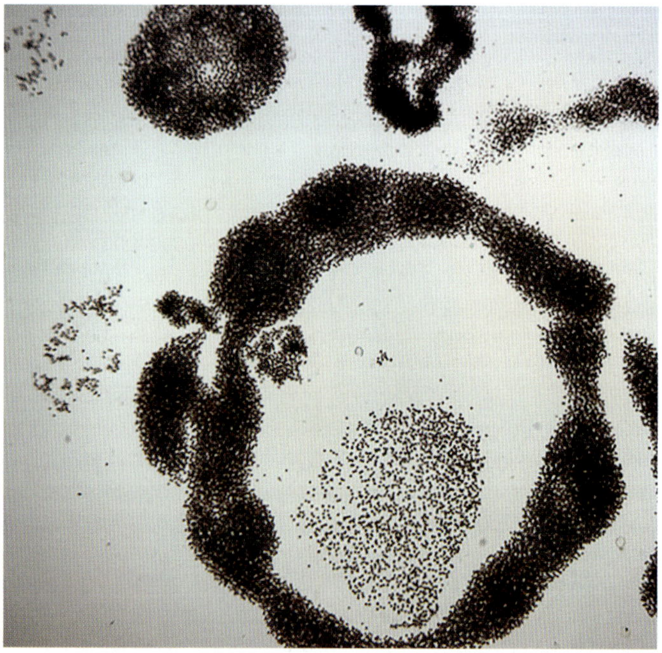

FIG. 31.3 Microscopic colonies of *Microcystin* spp. cyanobacteria. Courtesy of Dr. Gregory Boyer.

Paracetamol[19,22]

Cats are exquisitely sensitive to paracetamol toxicosis, but toxicosis is also reported in dogs and ferrets. Paracetamol is used in dogs as an analgesic and antipyretic despite a lack of documentation of efficacy. An oral product licensed for use in dogs is available in the UK. Overdose or use of paracetamol in patients with hepatic insufficiency can lead to acute liver failure.

Liver injury occurs 24-26 hours after ingestion due to formation of the phase I metabolite NAPQI and depletion of glucuronide needed for phase II metabolism. Methemoglobinemia, facial swelling, and paw swelling are seen early and are often the primary toxicosis in dogs, ferrets, and especially cats. The metabolite p-aminophenol causes methemoglobinemia.

Xylitol[19]

Hypoglycemia is seen 0.5-12 hours after ingestion, presenting as weakness, ataxia, collapse, and potentially seizures. Liver damage has been reported 12-72 hours after high-dose exposures. There is a self-limiting increase in AST. Acute hepatic necrosis and coagulopathy have been reported, but liver damage is often relatively mild.

Diagnostic approach to a suspected case of acute toxic hepatopathy

The investigation of a suspected case will start with a careful history and investigation of potential exposures, mindful of seasonal entities such as mushrooms, cyanobacteria, and acorns. Acorns, mushrooms, xylitol-containing gum, or other potentially toxic material may be evident in vomitus or stomach contents. Emergency real-time plant and mushroom identification is available at https://www.facebook.com/groups/144798092849300. The medical history should include a careful dietary and supplement history. A history of dietary indiscretions may indicate a behavior pattern predisposing to toxin ingestion. Treatment with pharmaceuticals may indicate toxic or idiosyncratic liver damage.

Remember that because the liver can continue to function even after significant loss of hepatocytes, clinical signs can be delayed for 24 to 72 hours and can include organomegaly, abdominal pain, ascites, icterus, hepatic encephalopathy, coagulopathy, hematochezia, or melena. The presence of extrahepatic clinical signs can help in the tentative diagnosis. For example, gastrointestinal signs are seen early with amatoxins, cycasin, and iron, whereas early hypoglycemia is recognized with xylitol ingestion. Cyanosis, methemoglobinemia, Heinz body anemia, and swelling of the paws and face may be seen with paracetamol exposure. Other criteria that can be used to support the diagnosis of a specific hepatotoxin include gastrointestinal metal densities on imaging secondary to ingestion of mineral supplements containing iron, microscopic observation of hepatotoxic cyanobacteria in water (Fig. 31.3), identification of foreign material such as pills, plant material, or mushroom fragments in vomitus or gastric lavage fluid, and aflatoxin screening of the food source.

Testing for specific toxins

Veterinary diagnostic laboratories have targeted analyses for some specific hepatotoxins, such as acetaminophen, amatoxins, and microcystins, which can be run on samples that may include urine, plasma, liver, kidney, stomach contents or vomitus, or suspected source of the toxicant (such as mushroom fragments or water with cyanobacteria). Contact your diagnostic laboratory for information on proper sample submission. Most analytical chemistries require technical skill, time, and financial resources, and results usually take too long to be of use for immediate clinical decision-making. There are, however, a few point-of-care diagnostic tests for some hepatotoxins:

- The lateral flow immunoassay AMATOXtest is available and can be used to test urine or mushroom samples for amatoxins.[23] Amatoxins are detectable in the urine before clinical signs become apparent and can remain in the urine for up to 72 hours.[4]
- There are also commercially available enzyme-linked immunosorbent assay (ELISA) kits for the detection of microcystin in water.

Treatment of hepatotoxicosis

Specific treatments that have been recommended for specific hepatotoxins, when available, are listed in Table 31.3.

Ending exposure to the toxicant is the most important step in treatment and can include changing the diet (as in aflatoxicosis), removing access to cyanobacterial blooms, and thorough surface decontamination through rinsing the haircoat and gastrointestinal decontamination after significant toxicant ingestion.

Gastrointestinal decontamination procedures are best used when there are no contraindications (such as ingestion of caustic or oily chemicals, evidence of central nervous system dysfunction which will increase the risk of aspiration, or animals presenting with vomiting) and can include emesis induction within one hour of exposure in the asymptomatic patient, using a species-specific emetic. In dogs, emesis can be induced using apomorphine: a 6.25 mg tablet whole or crushed is given in the conjunctival sac, flush the conjunctiva with saline after emesis; alternately 0.01-0.04 mg/kg of the injectable form can be given IV, SC, or IM. An injectable apomorphine preparation licensed for use in dogs is available in the EU and UK but not the USA.[15] Alternatively, ropinirole, licensed for use in dogs in the USA (but not in the EU and UK), can be used as a liquid formulation given intraocularly at 2.7-5.4 mg/m^3.[15] See package instructions for mg/kg dose estimates. Retrieved gastric contents should be checked for the suspected source of intoxication and saved for toxicology testing.

If emesis is not successful and no contraindicates apply, gastric lavage can be undertaken under anesthetic within an hour of ingestion of a lethal dose. Gastric lavage may be safer than emesis in brachycephalic breeds.

Depending on the toxicant involved, consideration should be given to the administration of a sequestrant. This should be used after inducing emesis or gastric lavage. Cholestyramine, a bile acid sequestrant, has been given to interrupt the enterohepatic cycling of xenobiotics eliminated in the bile, including cycasin, microcystins, amatoxins, and manganese.[24] Enterohepatic cycling can prevent the elimination of toxicants over time, and cholestyramine can be given at a dose of 1-3 g PO in water 2-3 times per day for 2 to 5 days, depending on the elimination half-life.[15] Activated charcoal, a nonspecific sequestrant, can be given within 6 hours of exposure. An initial dose of activated charcoal of 1-2 mg/kg, up to 5 g/kg, is given PO.[15] Subsequent doses can be given can be given by mouth, or can be given PO 0.5-2 g/kg every 4-8 hours for up to 48 hours to prevent portal-hepatic cycling. The first dose can include sorbitol as a cathartic, but subsequent doses should not. Monitoring for serum sodium is critical if sorbitol is used.

TABLE 31.3 Treatment recommendations for some specific hepatotoxins.

Toxicant	Treatment
Acetaminophen	N-acetylcysteine (see dosing below)
Amatoxins	IV silibinin has been effective in people and dogs but is not available for veterinary use at this time Silybin (see dosing below) for 3-4 days Penicillin G given IV 100 mg/kg within 5 hours can reduce amatoxin uptake
Iron	Deferoxamine is used to chelate until serum iron is below 300 µg/dL or anecdotally until the urine is clear and no longer red: ■ 15 mg/kg/hour intravenous CRI ■ Alternately, 40 mg/kg IM every 4 to 8 hours[15]
Manganese	Allopurinol treatment was used in a dog, 11.5 mg/kg PO every 12 hours[24] Calcium-EDTA can be given cautiously as a chelator ■ Dogs can be dosed at 25 mg/kg, diluted in 5% dextrose to 10 mg/mL, SC every 6 hours for 5 days, not to exceed 2 g/day[15]

Supportive care includes fluid and electrolyte support, ideally avoiding lactate due to reduced hepatic function, and maintaining normoglycemia. Volume loss can occur with dehydration and electrolyte abnormalities, but hypoproteinemia secondary to synthetic liver failure increases the risk of ascites or pulmonary edema with fluid therapy. Coagulopathy may require supportive care ranging from vitamin K_1 (phytonadione) supplementation to replacement of clotting factors. Plasma is recommended only in the presence of active bleeding or if invasive procedures, such as biopsies or feeding tube placement, are required.[25] The recommended vitamin K_1 doses in dogs are 2.5 mg/kg PO twice daily with a fatty meal or 2.5 mg/kg SC twice daily.[15] Gastrointestinal absorption of vitamin K_1 is almost equivalent to parenteral; thus, oral dosing is favored. PT and aPTT should be checked every 12-24 hours, and PT should normalize within 48 hours.[15]

Supportive care for the liver often includes use of one or more of the following hepatoprotectants:

- N-acetylcysteine is a thiol donor for glutathione synthesis that can be given extra-label either intravenously or orally and is often preferred when the patient cannot be dosed orally.[19] An initial dose of 140-180 mg/kg is given IV, diluted to 5%, and given through a 0.2-micron filter over 20 minutes or 280 mg/kg PO via gastric tube if the patient is not vomiting.[15] Subsequent doses of 70 mg/kg are given PO or IV every 6 hours for 48 hours or up to 4.5 days.[15]
- S-adenosylmethionine (SAMe) can be given to enhance glutathione production[19] at a dose of 20 mg/kg/day PO an hour before feeding.[15]
- Silybin can be given orally at a higher-than-labeled dose. Dogs can be given 20-40 mg/kg/day[15], and silybin can be a combined product with SAMe.
- Ursodeoxycholic acid, or ursodiol, is a bile acid that can be given with food and might be helpful in some hepatotoxicoses. Its use was reported in one case report of microcystin poisoning in a dog.[26] Dogs can be given 10-15 mg/kg PO every 24 hours or 5-7.5 mg/kg every 12 hours.[10]
- Vitamin E can be given orally as a lipophilic antioxidant to stabilize cell membranes. Depending on body weight, a dog can be given 50-400 IU PO per day.[15]

Animals with severe liver injury often have gastrointestinal ulceration and hemorrhage. Gastroprotectants such as pantoprazole (0.7-1 mg/kg IV every 12 hours for dogs) or omeprazole (1 mg/kg for dogs, given PO every 12 hours) can be given to reduce acid secretion, and sucralfate (250-1000 mg per dog every 6-12 hours) acts as a physical barrier to protect the mucosa.[15]

Prognosis for dogs with acute toxic hepatopathy

Generally, the prognosis for acute liver failure is poor. However, prognosis can vary greatly based on the toxicant, dose, time elapsed between exposure and treatment, and individual susceptibility, which may be breed-related in some cases. Although many hepatotoxin exposures, such as aflatoxins, amatoxins, and microcystins, carry a poor to grave prognosis, animals that do survive are likely to recover completely.[26] Acetaminophen poisoning has a good prognosis with early and intensive treatment.

KEY POINTS

- A variety of common toxicants cause hepatic injury, which can present acutely despite 24 to 72 hours or more between exposure and clinical signs.
- Clinical hepatotoxicosis may be preceded by other organ system impacts:
  - Transient gastrointestinal signs are seen with cycasin and amatoxins.
  - Hypoglycemia is seen soon after xylitol ingestion.
  - Methemoglobinemia and peripheral edema can also be seen early with paracetamol.
- Specific treatments are recommended for a few toxicants.
- Mainstays of therapy are decontamination, supportive care including hepatoprotectants and vitamin K_1 supplementation, and symptomatic care.
- Prognosis is often guarded, but it depends on the toxicant, dose, and promptness of therapy.

References

1. Court MH, Greenblatt DJ. Molecular basis for deficient acetaminophen glucuronidation in cats: An interspecies comparison of enzyme kinetics in liver microsomes. *Biochem Pharmacol* 53:1041-1047, 1997.
2. Tibbitts J. Issues related to the use of canines in toxicologic pathology—issues with pharmacokinetics and metabolism. *Toxicol Pathol* 31:17-24, 2003.
3. Dereszynski DM, Center SA, Randolph JF, Brooks MB, Hadden AG, Palyada KS, et al. Clinical and clinicopathologic features of dogs that consumed foodborne hepatotoxic aflatoxins: 72 cases (2005-2006). *J Am Vet Med Assoc* 232:1329-1337, 2008.
4. Puschner B, Wegenast C. Mushroom poisoning cases in dogs and cats: diagnosis and treatment of hepatotoxic, neurotoxic, gastroenterotoxic, nephrotoxic, and muscarinic mushrooms. *Vet Clin North Am Small Anim Pract* 48:1053-1067, 2018.
5. Eberhardy AC, Heinrich NA, McFadden RA, Reiter LV. Prevalence of hepatotoxicity and myelosuppression with alternate day use of azathioprine and glucocorticoids for treatment of dermatological conditions in dogs. *Vet Dermatol* 33:503-508, 2022.
6. Borchers A, Epstein SE, Gindiciosi B, Cartoceti A, Puschner B. Acute enteral manganese intoxication with hepatic failure due to ingestion of a joint supplement overdose. *J Vet Diagn Invest* 26:658-663, 2014.
7. Burrows GE, Tyrl RJ. Toxic Plants of North America 2nd edition. Ames, Iowa, John Wiley & Sons, 2013.
8. Albretsen J. The toxicity of iron, an essential element. *Vet Med* 101(2):82-90, 2006.
9. Roegner AF, Brena B, González-Sapienza G, Puschner B. Microcystins in potable surface waters: toxic effects and removal strategies. *J Appl Toxicol* JAT 34:441-457, 2014.
10. Camacho F, Stewart S, Tinson E. Successful management of suspected acorn (*Quercus petraea*) toxicity in a dog. *Can Vet J* 62:581-585, 2021.
11. Hardy RM, O'Brien T, Adams LG, Polzin DJ, Reidarson T. Periportal hepatitis associated with the use of a heartworm-hookworm preventive (diethylcarbamazine-oxibendazole) in 13 dogs. *J Am Anim Hosp Assoc* 25:419-429, 1989.
12. Polzin DJ, Stowe CM, O'Leary TP, Stevens JB, Hardy RM. Acute hepatic necrosis associated with the administration of mebendazole to dogs. *J Am Vet Med Assoc* 179:1013-1016, 1981.
13. Schlesinger DP. Methemoglobinemia and anemia in a dog with acetaminophen toxicity. *Can Vet J* 36:515-517, 1995.
14. Vulcano LAD, Confalonieri O, Franci R, Tapia MO, Soraci AL. Efficacy of free glutathione and niosomal glutathione in the treatment of acetaminophen induced hepatotoxicity in cats. *Open Vet J* 3:56-63, 2013.
15. Plumb's™ n.d. https://app.plumbs.com/ (accessed October 30, 2023).
16. Bunch SE, Conway MB, Center SA, Castleman WL, Baldwin BH, Hornbuckle WE, et al. Toxic hepatopathy and intrahepatic cholestasis associated with phenytoin administration in combination with other anticonvulsant drugs in three dogs. *J Am Vet Med Assoc* 190:194-198, 1987.
17. Schmid RD, Hovda LR. Acute hepatic failure in a dog after xylitol ingestion. *J Med Toxicol* 12:201-205, 2016.
18. Trepanier LA. Idiosyncratic drug toxicity affecting the liver, skin, and bone marrow in dogs and cats. *Vet Clin North Am Small Anim Pract* 43:1055-1066, 2013.
19. Weingarten MA, Sande AA. Acute liver failure in dogs and cats. *J Vet Emerg Crit Care* 25:455-473, 2015.
20. Bischoff K, Rumbeiha WK. Pet food recalls and pet food contaminants in small animals: An update. *Vet Clin North Am Small Anim Pract* 48:917-931, 2018.
21. Freshwater harmful algal blooms. Cornell Univ Coll Vet Med 2021. https://www.vet.cornell.edu/animal-health-diagnostic-center/laboratories/toxicology/fhab (accessed September 1, 2023).
22. Court MH. Feline drug metabolism and disposition: pharmacokinetic evidence for species differences and molecular mechanisms. *Vet Clin North Am Small Anim Pract* 43:1039-1054, 2013.
23. AMATOXtest – A rapid, sensitive and simple test for amanitin – As simple as a pregnancy test n.d. https://amatoxtest.com/ (accessed August 0, 2023).
24. Wolf J, Hoffman L, Southern C. Successful management of severe manganese toxicosis in two dogs. *J Am Anim Hosp Assoc* 59:152-157, 2023.
25. DeVries SE, Galey FD, Namikoshi M, Woo JC. Clinical and pathologic findings of blue-green algae (*Microcystis aeruginosa*) intoxication in a dog. *J Vet Diagn Invest* 5:403-408, 1993.
26. Bautista AC, Moore CE, Lin Y, Cline MG, Benitah N, Puschner B. Hepatopathy following consumption of a commercially available blue-green algae dietary supplement in a dog. *BMC Vet Res* 11:136, 2015.

CHAPTER 32

Acute infectious liver disease and hepatic abscess

Katie Elizabeth McCallum
BVM&S, PGCertSAM, FHEA, DECVIM-CA, MRCVS

Introduction and sequelae of acute infectious liver disease

Hepatobiliary infections can occur via hematogenous spread as part of a systemic infection, ascending infection via the biliary tract, or bacterial translocation from the portal circulation.[1,2] Gallbladder and biliary tract infections are discussed in chapter 35. In parenchymal infections, the liver may be the target organ (e.g., infectious canine hepatitis [ICH], leptospirosis), or it may be a multisystemic disorder with secondary hepatic involvement (e.g., sepsis, *Toxoplasma gondii*, parvovirus).[3] One of the challenges in diagnosing infectious causes of acute liver disease (ALD) is the overlap in clinical presentations with different etiologies, which means that the clinician has to consider specific tests to reach a diagnosis; otherwise, the primary infectious agent may not be identified.[4] Although a multitude of infectious diseases have been associated with acute hepatitis, determining causality can be challenging. In a study that extensively PCR screened the livers of dogs with acute and chronic hepatitis for infectious disease, only two dogs with acute hepatitis were positive for parvovirus, which was deemed a secondary reactive hepatitis.[5] Table 32.1 lists infectious diseases commonly associated with necroinflammatory parenchymal ALD, but please note that this list is not exhaustive; it may reflect multisystemic infections with secondary hepatic involvement, and there will inevitably be a degree of overlap with infectious causes of chronic and/or granulomatous hepatitis, particularly since the characterization of the chronicity of hepatitis relies on a combination of duration of clinical signs and histology.[6,7] Granulomatous hepatitis is discussed separately in chapter 34, but it is important to note that some of these dogs will present acutely.

A proportion of dogs with infectious ALD will develop acute liver failure (ALF) and multiorgan dysfunction. ALF has been defined as the development of acute clinical signs in patients without pre-existing liver disease with concurrent hyperbilirubinemia and coagulopathy (defined as PT>1.5× upper limit of reference interval) with or without hepatic encephalopathy (HE).[8,9] In a retrospective study of 49 dogs with ALF, only 8% of cases were attributed to an infectious etiology, which may reflect the large reserve capacity of the liver.[8] However, severe acute hepatic necrosis (e.g., in cases of ICH) can rapidly lead to ALF.[7]

Clinical features

History taking should involve a careful review of dietary history (paying particular attention to raw diet feeding), access to drugs and toxins, travel history, geographic location, exposure to other animals, and vaccination status. Pets with ALD can present with asymptomatic

TABLE 32.1 Infectious causes of acute liver disease in dogs.

Bacterial	■ *Leptospira* spp.[3,4,17,28,38,39] ■ *Helicobacter* spp.[4,47,48] ■ Gram-positive cocci, e.g., *Staphylococcus* spp., *Streptococcus* spp. ■ Gram-negatives, e.g., *Escherichia coli, Klebsiella pneumoniae, Enterobacter* spp., *Salmonella* spp., *Pseudomonas aeruginosa*[1,35,36,37] ■ Anaerobic infections, e.g., *Clostridium* spp.[3,4,49]
Fungal	■ *Histoplasma capsulatum*[3] ■ *Coccidiodes immitis*[3] ■ *Blastomyces dermatitidis*[3]
Viral	■ Canine adenovirus-1[2,3,4,5,51,52,53] ■ Canine herpesvirus[54,55] ■ Canine acidophil cell hepatitis[3,4,56,57]
Protozoal	■ *Sarcocystis* spp.[20,55,56] ■ *Hammondia* spp.[22,24] ■ *Toxoplasma gondii*[3,4,28] ■ *Babesia* spp.[3] ■ *Hepatozoon canis*[3,4] ■ *Neospora caninum*[4,24,58] ■ *Leishmania infantum*[3]
Rickettsial	■ *Ehrlichia canis*[3,50] ■ *Rickettsia rickettsiae*[3] ■ *Borrelia burgdorferi*[4]
Parasitic	■ Visceral larval migrans[3,23] ■ Liver flukes[3] ■ *Dirofilaria immitis*[3] ■ *Heterobilharzia americana*[3]

increases in liver enzymes. Clinical presentations can be vague and include an acute history of vomiting, diarrhea, polydipsia/polyuria (PU/PD), anorexia, lethargy, abdominal pain, and/or jaundice. There may be evidence of bleeding diathesis (petechiation, hematemesis, melena).[7,9] Signs of HE are uncommon with infectious etiologies but may manifest as behavioral changes, dull mentation, circling, head pressing, seizures, ataxia, and coma.[8,7,10]

Physical examination may be unremarkable, liver-specific (e.g., jaundice, cranial abdominal pain, alterations in liver size and/or ascites on abdominal palpation), or develop due to the systemic effects of the infectious etiology (e.g., pyrexia, dehydration, cardiovascular shock due to systemic inflammatory response syndrome [SIRS], uremic oral ulceration due to AKI, tachypnea/dyspnea due to respiratory involvement).[7] Concurrent acute kidney injury (AKI) can occur due to disseminated intravascular coagulation (DIC), sepsis, dehydration, hypovolemia, or direct nephrotoxicity (leptospirosis, CAV-1). Concurrent respiratory involvement can develop with leptospiral pulmonary hemorrhage syndrome, acute respiratory distress syndrome (ARDS), pulmonary thromboembolism (PTE), or aspiration pneumonia as a result of HE.[7] A baseline neurological examination is worth assessing for subtle mentation changes suggestive of HE. Patients with ALF can develop cerebral edema and intracranial hypertension (IH) with clinical signs such as mydriasis, altered mental state, altered respiratory pattern, or development of a Cushing reflex (concurrent acute arterial hypertension and bradycardia).[9]

Clinicopathological findings

Complete blood count

Anemia may develop as a result of inflammatory disease, acute hemorrhage (gastrointestinal, pulmonary), or DIC. Leukocytosis (due to neutrophilia and/or left shift, monocytosis) or leukopenia may occur with infectious disease; the latter is more likely with ICH and sepsis. Thrombocytopenia may be due to impaired thrombopoietin production by the liver, decreased platelet survival (e.g., increased platelet clearance due to SIRS), immune-mediated destruction, consumption due to DIC, splenic sequestration or a direct result of the causative agent (e.g., leptospirosis).[7,9,11]

Biochemistry

Biochemistry typically demonstrates marked increases in the hepatocellular leakage enzymes ALT and AST with variable increases in the inducible enzymes ALP and GGT. ALT is a liver-specific cytosolic enzyme that is released with hepatocyte damage or increased membrane permeability, increasing 100-fold within 12-24 hours of injury.[9,12] AST is found within both the hepatocellular cytosol and mitochondria, with activities generally paralleling ALT after hepatocellular injury.[9] Magnitude of increases roughly parallel the severity or extent of the hepatic injury but are affected by hepatocyte mass (which can be decreased in acute hepatic necrosis); therefore, a single ALT measurement is not prognostic.[3,7,9,12] ALP and GGT increases occur as a result of extrahepatic and intrahepatic cholestasis and/or drug induction. ALP usually increases 2-5-fold following acute severe hepatic necrosis and then gradually declines. Increases can be delayed in ALD due to the time taken to synthesize and release these enzymes.[9]

Dogs with ALD may show biochemical evidence of hepatic dysfunction, e.g., low blood urea nitrogen, cholesterol, and albumin. Hyperbilirubinemia in ALD is due to a combination of hepatocyte dysfunction and intrahepatic cholestasis.[7] Hypoglycemia can be seen with both hepatic dysfunction and sepsis, particularly in small breed/young dogs. A bile acid stimulation test can be performed to assess liver function in nonicteric animals. Ammonia is a relatively insensitive marker of liver function, and it can be normal even in patients with HE.[12] Electrolyte and acid-base derangements include hypokalemia, hyperphosphatemia, hypophosphatemia, hypernatremia, hyponatremia, and metabolic acidosis.[9] Increases in creatinine may be prerenal (dehydration or hypovolemia) or reflect concurrent AKI.

Urinalysis

Decreased urine specific gravity (due to PU/PD or concurrent AKI) is common. Icteric pets may have bilirubinuria, although this can be a normal finding, particularly in male dogs. Proximal renal tubular and glomerular damage (seen with leptospirosis and ICH, respectively) may manifest as glucosuria (acquired Fanconi's syndrome), granular casts, and proteinuria.[7] Ammonium biurate crystals may be documented with ALF.

Coagulation testing and thromboelastography

Most clotting factors are synthesized in the liver, as are anticoagulant proteins (antithrombin, protein C, protein S) and fibrinolytic proteins.[11] Vitamin K is responsible for carboxylation of factors II, VII, IX, and X, proteins C and S, and the liver is the site for activation. Deficiency (due to cholestasis, anorexia, antibiotic treatment) can lead to factor dysfunction and depletion.[9,11] The liver is also responsible for the clearance of activated pro- and anticoagulants, fibrin degradation products (FDPs), and D-dimers.[11]

People and dogs with ALF usually have balanced proportional deficiencies in procoagulant and anticoagulant clotting factors. This can shift to bleeding tendencies or hypercoagulability.[13,14] Factors impairing hemostasis include thrombocytopenia, thrombocytopathia, vitamin K and clotting factor deficiencies, hypofibrinogenemia, and hyperfibrinolysis. Factors that promote hypercoagulability include increased factor VIII and von Willebrand factor, SIRS-related endothelial dysfunction, and a decrease in anticoagulant factors (proteins C and S, antithrombin).[9,11,13,15] Prolongation in conventional prothrombin times (PT) and activated partial thromboplastin times (aPTT) are common. In fact, PT prolongation is included in the definition of ALF.[8] However, these tests do not reliably predict the risk of bleeding in people or dogs with ALF.[8,11,14] Evidence of spontaneous hemorrhage was only reported in 51% of dogs with ALF despite most of these dogs demonstrating prolonged coagulation times. In this same study, 8% of dogs had evidence of thrombosis, suggesting hypercoagulability can also occur.[8] Thromboelastography (TEG) provides information about the global coagulation status, including speed of clot formation, clot strength, and clot lysis. Conventional coagulation testing may overestimate hypocoagulability/bleeding risk compared to TEG in dogs with early ALD and sustained hepatic function. However, as ALF develops, both conventional coagulation times and TEG trend towards hypocoagulability.[15]

Diagnostic imaging findings

Thoracic radiographs may document pleural effusion or an alveolar pattern due to ARDS, aspiration pneumonia, atelectasis, hemorrhage, or PTE. Abdominal radiographs allow a rough assessment of liver size but are of limited value. Abdominal ultrasound (US) has poor accuracy in diagnosing diffuse hepatic parenchymal disease in dogs and can even be normal in ALD.[8,16] US abnormalities, when present, include decreased liver volume, hepatomegaly, variable diffuse echogenicity changes, and ascites.[6,7,8,9] Other findings include gallbladder wall thickening and common bile duct distension (if concurrent cholecystitis/cholangitis – see chapter 35), GI ulceration, evidence of thrombosis, and renal changes (increased renal cortical echogenicity, renomegaly, renal pelvic dilation, perirenal fluid).[1,8,17]

Prebiopsy considerations

FNAs of the liver are generally considered safe, but the true complication rate remains unknown.[3,18,19] The author routinely performs platelet counts and coagulation tests in ALD patients prior to FNAs as part of the general diagnostic approach. The risk of bleeding with a liver biopsy is higher, with 42.5% of dogs in one study experiencing asymptomatic hemorrhage, so coagulation profiles are strongly recommended prior to these procedures.[20] Risk factors for bleeding after percutaneous ultrasound-guided needle organ biopsy reported in one study include thrombocytopenia and increased PT in dogs; however, these risk factors were not identified in a recent study assessing risk factors after percutaneous ultrasound-guided liver biopsy in 102 dogs with liver disease (including acute hepatitis).[20,21] Fresh frozen plasma (FFP) (5-15 mL/kg) is a preferred first-line treatment for coagulopathies if there is active hemorrhage and should also be available to treat hemorrhage if there is a planned invasive procedure, e.g., liver biopsy. Criteria for ensuring blood product availability (whole blood/FFP) in high-risk cases prior to biopsy include the presence of thrombocytopenia (whole blood), prolonged coagulation times, or a hypocoagulable TEG (FFP). Prophylactic vitamin K_1 0.5-1.5 mg/kg IM/SC q12h for 3 days should be considered in all patients with evidence of cholestasis or prolonged coagulation times.[11] Treatment should be aimed at the resolution of bleeding and not at reversing abnormal coagulation times, which are unlikely to provide an accurate assessment of ongoing bleeding risk.[11]

Liver cytology

FNA cytology of the liver in infectious ALD can aid in the diagnosis of inflammation, hepatic abscesses, and directly visualize infectious agents.[22,23,24,25] One study documented high sensitivity and specificity to detect suppurative inflammation,[25] but other studies showed lower agreement with the cytological diagnosis of inflammatory liver disease when compared to histology.[26,27] Cytology does not provide information on parenchymal architecture, and hemodilution may hinder the interpretation of inflammatory hepatitis.[3,25,26,27]

Liver biopsy

Indications for a liver biopsy include establishing cause, severity, reversibility (acute versus chronic), and prognosis.[3] Acute hepatitis is characterized by hepatocellular necrosis or apoptosis, variable inflammation, which may be neutrophilic or mixed, and variable evidence of regeneration.[2,28] Histopathological changes in infectious acute hepatitis include centrilobular necrosis with typical nuclear inclusions in CAV-1 and random multifocal necrosis in herpesvirus and bacterial etiologies with hematogenous spread. Focal lesions may explain why ALF is uncommon in infectious hepatitis, as the damage to the hepatic parenchyma is not severe enough to lead to systemic clinical signs.[2] Protozoal etiologies may demonstrate cysts or protozoal organisms.[24,28] In most cases of ALD, liver biopsy does not confirm a specific cause[6,8] due to sampling variation (and histopathological heterogeneity) in concert with a nonspecific histological picture, e.g., cholestasis and necrosis, which does not identify the etiological agent.[29] The author's preference is to obtain a liver biopsy via laparoscopy or laparotomy (see chapter 27) due to the larger sample sizes yielded and the ability to control hemorrhage. A cholecystocentesis sample for bile cytology and culture can be obtained at the same time.

Bacterial causes of acute liver disease and hepatic abscesses

Liver defense mechanisms against bacterial infection

The liver has a dual blood supply and sinusoidal network, which increases susceptibility to both hepatic and systemic infections via hematogenous spread and drainage of bacterial organisms from the splanchnic circulation via the portal vein.[4] Furthermore, the healthy canine liver harbors bacteria and, therefore, any condition that leads to hypoxia, e.g., hepatic necrosis, neoplasia, trauma, can lead to overgrowth of anaerobic bacteria and bacterial hepatitis/hepatic abscessation.[3,30,31] The liver has several defense mechanisms to protect against infections, including Kupffer cells (liver macrophages) that efficiently extract bacteria drained by the splanchnic circulation; tight junctions between hepatocytes prevent bacterial translocation; antegrade bile flow; the mechanical barrier provided by the sphincter of Oddi; bacteriostatic effects of bile, and local biliary IgA.[1,32]

Etiology of hepatic parenchymal bacterial infections

Bacterial infections are associated with acute and chronic hepatitis, hepatic abscessation, granulomatous hepatitis, and cholangiohepatitis.[33] Potential routes of infection include ascending biliary infection; hematogenous infection via hepatic artery (systemic bacteremia), portal vein translocation or umbilical vein (omphalophlebitis); direct extension (e.g., cholecystitis); trauma (e.g., penetrating wound, blunt trauma) and iatrogenic (liver biopsy).[1,3,34] Conditions such as ischemia, inflammatory liver disease, cholestasis, portosystemic shunting, endotoxemia, gastrointestinal disease (e.g., inflammatory bowel disease (IBD), pancreatitis and neoplasia), and host factors such as immunosuppression (e.g., diabetes mellitus, hyperadrenocorticism) can predispose to bacterial infection.[1,4]

Diagnosis of bacterial infections

Bacterial hepatitis/cholangiohepatitis can be diagnosed by liver (aspirate or tissue) and bile (percutaneous ultrasound-guided cholecystocentesis) culture and liver histopathology. PCR and fluorescence *in situ* hybridization (FISH) can be performed on histological sections. Studies suggest that bile cultures are more often positive than liver culture (30% compared to 5%). Combining cultures (e.g., bile, liver) has been suggested to improve diagnostic sensitivity.[1,35] Bile is generally considered sterile; however, healthy dogs can harbor transient bactibilia, so results should be carefully interpreted as part of the whole clinical picture. Cytological abnormalities of bile include the presence of increased numbers of degenerate neutrophils, mononuclear cells, and bacteria.[1] Enteric *E.*

coli spp., *Enterococcus* spp., *Bacteroides* spp., and *Clostridium* spp. are most commonly isolated in association with hepatobiliary infections, and approximately 50% of infections are polymicrobial.[1,35,36] Following the advent of FISH, a culture-independent means of bacterial identification, the association of hepatitis with difficult-to-culture bacteria, including *Salmonella* spp. and leptospirosis infections, has been more frequently reported. FISH has also been able to confirm bacterial colocalization with inflammation (neutrophilic, pyogranulomatous, lymphoplasmacytic) in dogs.[33,37,38]

Specific bacterial causes

Leptospirosis

Leptospirosis, caused by the spirochete bacteria belonging to the genus *Leptospira*, is a systemic zoonotic disease characterized by renal and hepatic dysfunction, pulmonary hemorrhage, and abortion. Serovars are maintained in nature by subclinically affected wild and domestic mammalian reservoir hosts that serve as potential sources of infection for incidental animal hosts.[17] Dogs are infected directly via mucous membranes following contact with infected urine, venereal/placental transmission, ingestion of infected tissues, bite wounds, or indirectly from urine-contaminated water, soil, and mud.[17] Leptospires spread hematogenously during a bacteremic phase, then localize in the proximal renal tubules with subsequent renal excretion. While AKI is the most common manifestation of leptospirosis, the liver is also a target organ, and ALD may occur with or without concurrent renal involvement.[3] Other clinical manifestations include vasculitis and bleeding diathesis.[39]

The presence of concurrent acute cholestatic liver disease, AKI, thrombocytopenia, and evidence of proximal tubular damage (glucosuria) warrants further testing, regardless of vaccination status, due to lack of complete vaccinal cross-protection and epidemiological shifts in serovars. Leptospirosis is diagnosed using microscopic agglutination testing (MAT) serology, which provides an estimate of the antibody titer against different *Leptospira* serovars present in the blood. In acute cases, a fourfold increase in paired sera over 2-4 weeks is consistent with recent or active infection and differentiates the titer from previous exposure, vaccination, or chronic infection; however, antibiotic treatment can blunt seroconversion.[3,17] A single titer >1:800 raises the suspicion of leptospirosis but does not confirm the diagnosis, especially in vaccinated dogs,[17] as vaccinal titers of 1:6400 can be observed but do not usually persist for more than 3 months.[39] It is often assumed that the highest titer reflects the causative serovar; however, high titers to a noninfecting serovar within the same serogroup occur due to cross-reactivity, rendering definitive identification of the causative challenging serovar.[17] Serovars *icterohaemorrhagiae* and *pomona* have been reported to induce the most severe hepatic involvement. However, no definitive correlation has been made between the infecting serovar and clinical manifestation.[3,4,17] PCR can detect leptospiral DNA in blood and urine and can be used to diagnose vaccinated animals, although PCR does not identify the infecting serovar and is affected by antibiotic treatment. Culture is impractical for early diagnosis because leptospires are slow-growing and require 3-6 months of incubation.[17] In patients with acute hepatic manifestations of leptospirosis, histopathology may document diffuse mild hepatic necrosis, dissociation of liver cell plates, neutrophilic periportal reactive hepatitis, and intrahepatic cholestasis (Fig. 32.1).[28,39] Profound hepatic dysfunction may occur without significant histologic changes due to bacterial toxin-induced subclinical damage, endothelial damage, and DIC.[3,4]

Antibiotics are the mainstay of treatment for leptospirosis to both treat leptospiremia and eliminate renal excretion. Parenteral potentiated amoxicillin is recommended during initial hospitalization, followed by a 2-week course of 10 mg/kg PO q24h doxycycline to prevent a long-term carrier state. Survival rates of >80% have been reported but are poorer if there is respiratory involvement.[17] The risk of leptospirosis can be reduced with regular vaccinations, but these only provide serogroup-specific immunity.[17]

It should be noted that *Leptospira* can also cause chronic granulomatous hepatitis without obvious renal involvement[38] (see chapter 34).

Hepatic abscesses

This condition is relatively rare, and Table 32.2 summarizes case series detailing this condition. In puppies, abscessation is thought to occur secondary to omphalophlebitis, whereas in adults, it is thought to occur secondary to extrahepatic infections, ascending biliary tract infections, or due to regional hepatic parenchymal damage.[3,40] Although a proportion of cases remain idiopathic, hepatic abscesses have been reported in association with the following predisposing factors: neoplasia, endocrine disease (diabetes mellitus, hyperadrenocorticism, hypothyroidism), pancreatitis, liver fluke infection, trauma, liver lobe torsion, hepatobiliary disease, systemic infections (e.g., endocarditis, pyometra), and chronic phenobarbital or glucocorticoid administration.[1,3,31,34,40,41,42,43,44,45] Lethargy, vomiting and anorexia are the most common symptoms, in concert with elevated hepatobiliary parameters.[31]

Diagnosis is usually made by a combination of abdominal imaging and ultrasound-guided aspiration cytology and culture.[31] Abdominal radiographs can be normal or demonstrate hepatomegaly, a hepatic mass effect, poor abdominal serosal detail, and occasionally pneumoperitoneum if abscess rupture has occurred.[1] On abdominal ultrasound, abscesses usually appear as single to multiple hypoechoic to anechoic masses, with irregular hyperechoic margins and gas shadowing within the abscess. Other findings include abdominal effusion, regional lymphadenopathy, and echogenic perihepatic fat.[1,40,46] Cytology reveals large numbers of degenerate neutrophils and visible bacteria (Fig. 32.2). Culture and sensitivity of liver abscess aspirates, abdominal fluid, and/or blood should be performed.[1,3] The most common bacteria isolated is *E. coli*; other bacteria include *Clostridium*, *Staphylococcus*, *Streptococcus*, and *Klebsiella* species.

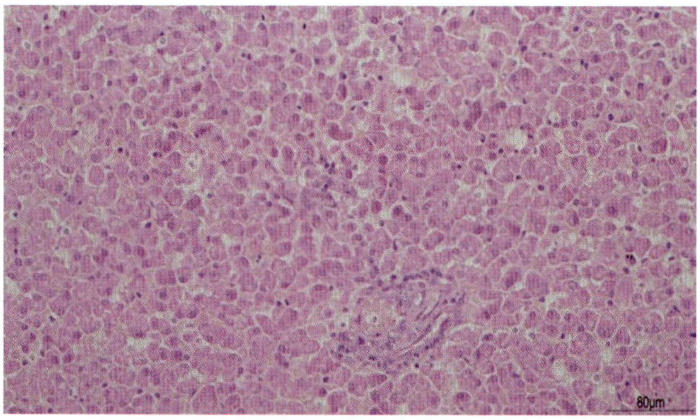

FIG. 32.1 Histological section of liver from a dog with acute leptospirosis showing dissociation of hepatocytes which is a common but nonspecific finding in canine leptospirosis (hematoxylin and eosin stain). Image courtesy of Dr. Fernando Constantino-Casas, Department of Veterinary Medicine, University of Cambridge.

TABLE 32.2 Summary of case series on hepatic abscesses.

Study	Grooters, et al.[40]	Farrar, et al.[34]	Schwartz, et al.[41]	Zatelli, et al.[46]	Dickinson, et al.[31]
Number of subjects	2	14	13	5	38
Mean age (range)	10 years (10)	10.6 years (8-15)	11.5 years (4-16)	8.4 years (3-15)	Median 11 years (0.2-15.9)
Sex (FN = female neutered, MN = male neutered)	■ FN (n = 2)	■ Male (n = 6) ■ MN (n = 3) ■ FN (n = 4) ■ Female (n = 1)	■ Male (n = 3) ■ MN (n = 3) ■ FN (n = 7)	■ Male (n = 2) ■ Female (n = 2) ■ FN (n = 1)	■ Male (n = 1) ■ MN (n = 18) ■ FN (n = 19)
Clinical presentation					
Anorexia/hyporexia	1	14	7	5	21
Vomiting	–	11	9	1	23
Diarrhea	–	6	5	–	5
Lethargy	1	14	13	–	28
Others	■ Weakness (n = 1) ■ Weight loss (n = 2) ■ PU/PD (n = 2)	–	■ PU/PD (n = 2) ■ Trembling (n = 4)	–	■ Weakness (n = 7) ■ Labored breathing (n = 3) ■ Inappropriate urination (n = 3) ■ PU/PD (n = 2)
Clinical examination findings					
Hepatomegaly	1	6	2	–	4
Dehydration	1	9	5	–	14
Pyrexia	2	12	11	3	12
Abdominal pain	1	8	10	4	20
Bleeding diathesis	–	5	2		2
Others	■ Tachypnea (n = 1) ■ Pendulous abdomen (n = 2)		■ Abdominal mass (n = 1) ■ Ascites (n = 1) ■ Tachypnea (n = 2) ■ Tachycardia (n = 7)	■ Ascites (n = 1)	■ Abdominal distension (n = 11) ■ Dyspnea (n = 9) ■ Depressed mentation (n = 14) ■ Pallor (n = 6)
Diagnostic tests: selected hematological variables					
Leukocytosis	2 of 2	11 of 14	9 of 12	5 of 5	16 of 34
Neutrophilia	2 of 2	11 of 14	10 of 12	–	19 of 34
Monocytosis	2 of 2	2 of 14	5 of 12	–	–
Lymphopenia	1 of 2	5 of 14	–	–	–
Anemia	2 of 2	8 of 14	6 of 12	–	13 of 36
Thrombocytopenia	–	7 of 14	11 of 12	–	20 of 33
Diagnostic tests: selected biochemical variables					
Increased ALT	1 of 2	11 of 14	10 of 13	5 of 5	24 of 34
Increased AST	N/A	2 of 3	8 of 13	5 of 5	–
Increased ALP	2 of 2	14 of 14	13 of 13	–	32 of 34
Hyperbilirubinemia	1 of 2	5 of 14	5 of 13	–	5 of 34
Hypoalbuminemia	2 of 2	11 of 14	–	–	8 of 34
Diagnostic tests: blood culture		3 of 3 positive (*Clostridium* spp. n = 1, *Staphylococcus intermedius* n = 2)			

continued

TABLE 32.2 Summary of case series on hepatic abscesses.

Study	Grooters, et al.[40]	Farrar, et al.[34]	Schwartz, et al.[41]	Zatelli, et al.[46]	Dickinson, et al.[31]
Diagnostic tests: liver histopathology	■ Chronic suppurative hepatitis (n = 2), with marked fibrosis in one dog	■ Hepatic abscessation (n = 13)	Performed in 8/13: ■ Hepatic adenoma (n = 3) ■ Hepatic abscess (n = 3) with suppurative hepatitis (n=2) and multifocal hepatic and cystic hyperplasia with gallbladder rupture (n=1) ■ Vacuolar hepatopathy (n = 1)		■ Abscessation (n = 36) ■ Hepatic adenoma (n = 7) ■ Hepatocellular carcinoma (n = 3) ■ Metastatic carcinoma (n = 1) ■ Liver lobe torsion (n = 1)
Medical treatment		■ 2 months antibiotics (n = 1)	■ Antibiotics alone (n = 4) ■ Antibiotics + ultrasound-guided percutaneous drainage (n = 4)	■ 1 month antibiotic treatment + percutaneous drainage and alcoholization (n = 5)	
Surgical treatment	■ Antibiotics + liver lobectomy (n = 2)	■ Antibiotics + full/partial liver lobectomy (n = 4) ■ Lobectomy + cholecystectomy (n = 1) ■ Abscess resection (n = 1)	■ Antibiotics + hepatic resection, including 1 dog that underwent percutaneous drainage) (n = 6)		■ Full/partial liver lobectomy (n = 27) + concurrent omentalization (n = 3) ■ Abscess omentalization (n = 6) ■ Debridement (n = 1)
Died/euthanized with no definitive treatment	0 of 2	7 of 14	All defined as treated but 3 of 13 died or euthanized within 4 days of diagnosis	0 of 5	2 perioperatively
Recurrence	N/A	■ Adhesion/abscess recurrence at 28 days (n = 1) ■ Splenic abscess (n = 1) responded to antibiotic change	■ 2 dogs with percutaneous drainage were drained on 2 occasions.	No recurrence	Suspected in one dog
Outcome in treated dogs	Good (9-19 month follow-up)	Successful outcome in 6 of 14 dogs at 12-month follow-up	10 of 13 alive at 4-12 months follow-up	Good in 5 of 5 dogs at 4 months	30 of 36 survived to discharge with median survival time of 638 days.

Medical management options include broad-spectrum antibiotics alone (4-6 weeks based on culture and sensitivity) or in combination with percutaneous drainage and alcoholization (ethanol instillation to sterilize the abscess).[34,41,46] Risks involved with percutaneous drainage include hemorrhage, rupture, and associated septic peritonitis. Treatment success is affected by depth, location, and number of abscesses, with surgery reserved for cases that have failed drainage, patients with septic peritonitis, or patients with multiabscessation.[31] Surgical management consists of antibiotics and debridement alone or in combination with omentalization, or liver lobectomy.[31,34] Although mortality rates reaching 50% were reported in earlier studies,[34] less invasive treatment options have reportedly excellent outcomes, particularly when solitary abscesses are present.[46]

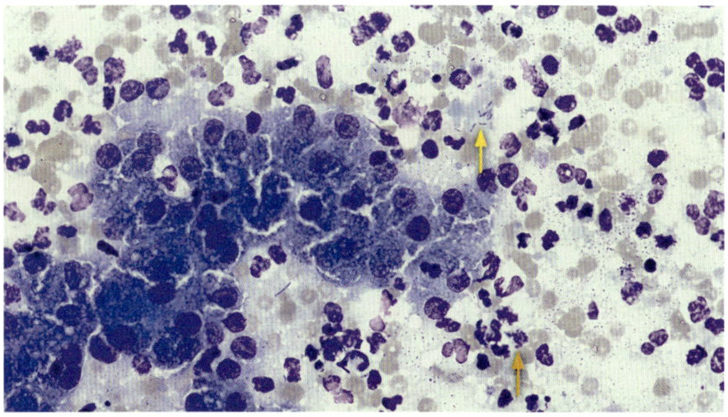

FIG. 32.2 Fine-needle aspiration cytology of liver from a 5-year-old female neutered Beagle presenting with diabetes mellitus and hepatic abscessation, documenting clusters of hepatocytes with degenerate neutrophils (orange arrow) and rod-shaped bacteria (yellow arrow). Wright-Giemsa stain (50× objective [500× magnification]). Image courtesy of Dr Cassia Hare, Queen's Veterinary School Hospital, University of Cambridge.

Helicobacter species

Helicobacter canis has been isolated from the liver of a puppy with hepatitis. Histopathology was consistent with multifocal necroinflammatory hepatitis with characteristic spiral bacteria seen following Warthin-Starry staining adjacent to necrotic lesions predominantly located within the bile duct system, suggesting an ascending infection. *Helicobacter* organisms are difficult to culture, so diagnosis can be achieved by PCR or FISH of the liver tissue.[4,47] A recent study detected *Helicobacter* spp. from the hepatobiliary tract in 21.2% of dogs with hepatic lesions, suggestive of an association with liver disease.[48]

Clostridium piliforme (Tyzzer's disease)

Tyzzer's disease is a spore-forming Gram-negative bacterial infection opportunistically infecting young and/or immunocompromised animals. Coinfections are common, e.g., with canine distemper virus or parvovirus. Histopathology documents multifocal neutrophilic necroinflammatory hepatitis. Filamentous bacteria can be visualized with silver staining; PCR testing of liver tissue can also be performed for diagnosis. Death rapidly ensues following hepatic infection.[3,4,49]

Extrahepatic biliary infections

The liver can be affected as part of systemic septicemia/endotoxemia or associated with extrahepatic bacterial septic foci, perhaps playing an "innocent bystander" role. These dogs can develop functional cholestasis with hyperbilirubinemia predominating over liver enzyme derangements. Liver histopathology may document intrahepatic cholestasis, mild periportal lymphocytic infiltrate, foci of macrophages/neutrophils, and necrosis. These dogs rarely develop ALF, and prognosis is dependent on the underlying disease.[3]

Rickettsial causes of acute liver disease

Ehrlichia canis and *Rickettsia rickettsiae* are systemic infections, although the liver is not usually the target organ for infection. However, *E. canis* has been associated with acute mixed inflammatory portal hepatitis in a dog. The diagnosis was achieved by cytology, serology, PCR, and immunohistochemistry (IHC) and confirmed with response to doxycycline therapy.[50]

Viral causes of acute liver disease

Infectious canine hepatitis (CAV-1)

Canine adenovirus type 1 (CAV-1) is a significant cause of fatal ALD in unvaccinated dog populations. The presence of neutralizing antibodies in unvaccinated dogs suggests natural exposure to the virus is common.[3,51] The prevalence of disease has decreased with widespread vaccination (with modified live CAV-2). However, re-emergence in vaccinated dogs leading to outbreaks in Europe have led to concerns regarding puppy trading in Eastern Europe, maternally-derived antibody (MDA) vaccinal interference in puppies, re-emergence of new strains and spillover from asymptomatic wild carnivore reservoirs, e.g., red foxes.[51,52] The disease usually affects mainly young and/or unvaccinated dogs and is both endotheliotropic and hepatotropic. Direct oronasal transmission occurs via saliva, feces and urine or indirectly via fomites.[51] Viral replication initiates in the tonsils, followed by lymphatic and hematogenous spread, the latter occurring 4-8 days postinfection, accompanied by leukopenia.[2,51] Response to infection is dependent on the production of a sufficient antibody response: susceptible dogs can develop fatal ALF or even peracute disease with sudden death, whereas dogs with adequate immunity can be asymptomatic or develop mild febrile illness.[2,3,51]

Acute clinical signs include neurological signs (due to encephalitis or HE), subcutaneous edema of the head, neck, and trunk, tonsillitis, bronchopneumonia, and lymphadenopathy.[3,51] Complications in those recovering include self-limiting corneal edema and anterior uveitis ("blue eye"), occurring in approximately 20% of infected dogs, and interstitial nephritis and glomerulonephritis due to immune complex deposition and viral persistence in the kidneys, however, chronic kidney disease has not been described.[51]

Liver histology demonstrates centri- to panlobular hepatic necrosis, neutrophilic and mononuclear cell infiltrates with large basophilic intranuclear inclusion bodies within hepatocytes and Kupffer cells (Fig. 32.3).[2,3,51] IHC, viral isolation, and PCR can be performed on histological sections. PCR techniques can also be utilized on conjunctival swabs, blood, feces, and urine.[51] Serological testing is also available; however, it can be challenging to interpret due to cross-reactivity with CAV-2 vaccination.[51] Seroconversion in acute cases requires the demonstration of a fourfold increase in titer over 2-3 weeks in an unvaccinated dog.[51]

There is no specific treatment for CAV-1, so treatment is supportive only with a reported mortality rate of 10-30%.[51] Prognosis depends on the severity of necrosis and complicating factors, e.g., DIC. Hepatic regeneration and clinical recovery are possible unless there is severe coagulation necrosis of entire hepatic lobules.[2,3] Progressive liver injury does not appear to be a feature of acute disease, even though chronic hepatitis has been experimentally reproduced in partially immunized dogs challenged with the virus.[2] Those that survive may go on to develop chronic hepatitis, likely secondary to viral damage-induced hepatitis rather than chronic infection, given that studies utilizing PCR, FISH, and IHC methods have not consistently detected CAV-1 in dogs with chronic hepatitis.[2,3,4,5,51,53] Prevention of disease is by vaccination from 6 weeks of age, with the last vaccination given no earlier than 16 weeks of age, to avoid interference with MDAs. Studies have shown that dogs are immune for at least 3 years after an initial vaccination course.[51]

Herpesvirus

Herpesvirus infection is a rapidly fatal disease that occurs more commonly in young puppies (particularly neonates) and immunocompromised adults, and causes disseminated multifocal hemorrhagic necrosis in parenchymal organs, including the liver, with the presence of intranuclear inclusion bodies.[2,3,54,55] It has been reported in one immunocompetent dog.[54] Oronasal transmission occurs through contact with respiratory, ocular, or genital tract secretions from an infected dog. Neonatal transmission can occur in utero or following contact with secretions from an infected bitch or littermate. Clinical presentation in adult dogs can be asymptomatic to mild, self-limiting respiratory and genital symptoms. Previously healthy puppies develop mucous membrane vesicles, seizures, abdominal pain, loss of interest in nursing, and depression. Definitive diagnosis has been made by viral isolation, PCR, immunohistochemistry, and FISH of liver and conjunctival samples. Treatment is generally unsuccessful, and the disease is rapidly fatal. Vaccination is available but not routinely performed due to low incidence of disease.[3,4,54,55]

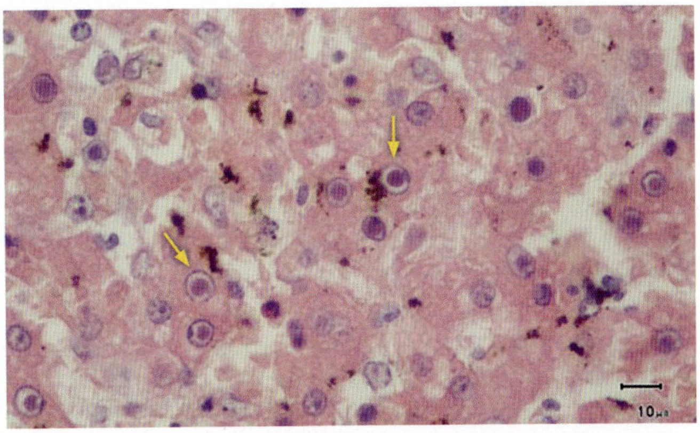

FIG. 32.3 Histological section of liver from a dog with infectious canine hepatitis (adenovirus type 1) showing hepatocytes with characteristic basophilic intranuclear inclusions (arrows). Hematoxylin-eosin stain. Image courtesy of Dr. Fernando Constantino-Casas, Department of Veterinary Medicine, University of Cambridge.

Canine acidophil hepatitis

Canine acidophil cell hepatitis was described only in Scotland nearly 40 years ago and was thought to be caused by a currently unidentified virus. The disease was experimentally reproduced via inoculation of serum or liver extracts from infected dogs. The diagnosis was based on histological findings of acute or chronic hepatitis and, importantly, scattered acidophils (dying hepatocytes).[3,4,56,57] Its current significance is unknown.

Protozoal causes of acute liver disease

Toxoplasma gondii

Toxoplasma has worldwide distribution. Dogs are intermediate hosts, and transmission can occur via ingestion of oocysts, tissue cysts, or vertical transmission. Respiratory, gastrointestinal, hepatic, cardiac, and neuromuscular involvement are most common in generalized cases. Diagnosis is by histopathology (focal to panlobular hepatic necrosis with identification of tachyzoites or bradyzoites) alongside serology.[3,4,28]

Neospora caninum

Dogs are definitive hosts for *N. caninum* infection, with deer and cattle considered intermediate hosts. *N. caninum* has worldwide distribution. Transmission is more common in puppies and young adults and is either transplacental or via consumption of tissue cysts from intermediate hosts, e.g., raw meat.[4,24] *N. caninum* has a tropism for neuromuscular tissues but can disseminate to the liver, leading to neutrophilic hemorrhagic coagulative necrosis with tachyzoites seen on histopathology. Other methods of diagnosis include serology, PCR, and IHC.[24,58]

Sarcocystis spp.

S. canis, *S. caninum*, and *S. svanai* are associated with canine hepatitis (necrosuppurative and eosinophilic described in one puppy) characterized by schizonts containing merozoites identified within the liver.[24,59,60] Worldwide distribution is reported.[4]

Hammondia spp.

The dog is the definitive host for *Hammondia* spp., particularly *H. heydorni*, which has been associated with diarrhea and, less commonly, acute neutrophilic hepatitis. Bile cytology and PCR can support the diagnosis. Interestingly, these dogs had positive *Toxoplasma* and *Neospora* serology despite negative *Toxoplasma* and *Neospora* PCR, suggesting a degree of cross-reactivity of serology between species.[22,24]

Hepatozoon canis

Hepatozoon canis is a worldwide protozoal infection, particularly prevalent in subtropical and temperate climates, transmitted via ingestion of the tick *Rhipicephalus sanguineus*, which leads to the release of sporozoites that disseminate via the gut and hematogenously target the bone marrow, spleen, and lymph nodes, and occasionally visceral organs, e.g., the liver. Diagnosis is based on the detection of gamonts in peripheral blood smears, and histological hepatic features are consistent with neutrophilic and mononuclear hepatitis with the presence of meronts.[3,4]

General approach to treatment of acute infectious liver disease

The goal of treatment is to treat the underlying etiology, if possible, and support liver function while trying to prevent or control the complications of ALF.[3] IV fluid therapy is recommended to rehydrate, replace fluid volume, increase ammonia excretion, and support dogs with concurrent AKI.[9] Hypoglycemia should be treated with IV dextrose. Antiemetic treatment (e.g., maropitant 0.5 mg/kg SC q24h) can be considered in nauseous and vomiting pets.

Treatment of bacterial acute liver disease

Empirical antibiotics should be chosen on their ability to concentrate in the bile and provide broad spectrum coverage for enteric Gram-negative bacteria and anaerobes.[1,35] For biliary tract infection, bile cytology has been shown to correlate with bacterial culture results, particularly in dogs who have received no prior antibiotics, so it could be used to initially guide therapy.[1,32] Treatment recommendations include a combination of fluoroquinolones, penicillin, and metronidazole or combining a fluoroquinolone with potentiated amoxicillin/clavulanate or clindamycin.[35] Resistance to potentiated amoxicillin/clavulanate and enrofloxacin have been reported in biliary isolates (namely *E. coli* and *Enterococcus*) from dogs, along with changing resistance patterns over time, highlighting the importance of obtaining culture and sensitivity and using antibiotics responsibly. The author recommends using potentiated amoxicillin/clavulanate as first-line therapy whilst awaiting culture and sensitivity results with a view to reserving fluoroquinolones for resistant infections following responsible antibiotic use guidelines.[1,35,36,61]

General approach to treatment of acute HE

The treatment of HE is covered in chapter 36 but will be briefly mentioned here in the context of acute HE. Warm water enemas can be used to physically reduce the number of urease-producing colonic bacteria, followed by lactulose retention enemas.[10] Due to the risk of aspiration with oral treatment in dogs with HE, oral lactulose is given only when stable.[10] Antibiotics prevent the production of gut-derived ammonia. 10-20 mg/kg amoxicillin IV/PO q8-12h should be considered in animals with acute HE with the additional benefit that the latter can be used to treat leptospirosis after obtaining diagnostic samples for PCR.[10] Patients who develop cerebral edema and intracranial hypertension (IH) as a result of acute HE may require methods to reduce intracranial pressure (ICP) including sedation or anesthesia; ventilation; head elevation to facilitate venous drainage; hypertonic saline and mannitol therapy.[10] Seizures should be treated as they can exacerbate IH and cause cerebral hypoxia.

Antioxidant and liver-supportive medications

Evidence of decreased glutathione concentrations suggestive of oxidative stress has been found in dogs with necroinflammatory liver disease[62] rationalizing treatment with antioxidants, including S-adenosyl methionine (SAMe) 20mg/kg PO q24h, silymarin (10 mg/kg PO q24h complexed with phosphatidylcholine), and vitamin E 10-15 IU/kg PO q24h. Ursodeoxycholic acid (UDCA; 10-15 mg/kg PO q24h) is a cytoprotective hydrophilic bile acid that can be used in ALD to treat extra- or intrahepatic cholestasis, and it may have a role in biliary elimination of infectious organisms.[63]

Prognosis

There is limited literature available to enable clinicians to estimate survival and outcome in pets with ALD. The long-term prognosis for acute hepatitis is better than chronic hepatitis, with an estimated median survival time of 34 months.[6] Due to the regenerative capacity of the liver, animals that survive the acute phase of ALD/ALF can recover completely without permanent liver injury and with normalization of liver enzymes and function.[6,64] However, in one case series, 5/12 dogs with acute hepatitis who underwent a repeat liver biopsy were identified as developing chronic hepatitis.[6] ALF is associated with a more guarded prognosis than ALD, with only 14% of dogs surviving to discharge compared to 71% of dogs with ALD.[8,15] Negative prognostic indicators in dogs with ALF include indicators of hepatic dysfunction (e.g., hyperbilirubinemia, hypoalbuminemia), ascites, and evidence of clinical bleeding. High serum ALT at presentation predicted survival in dogs with ALF, with speculation that survivors had more viable hepatocytes with subsequent greater ALT leakage.[8] Furthermore, a decline in sequential ALT concentrations is a good prognostic indicator in ALD.[3]

KEY POINTS

- Hepatobiliary infections can result from hematogenous spread in systemic infections, ascending infections through the biliary tract, or translocation of bacteria from the portal circulation.
- The etiology of acute infectious liver diseases can be bacterial, viral, fungal, protozoal, rickettsial, or parasitic.
- The treatment of acute infectious liver diseases is targeted at treating the underlying etiology, supporting the liver function, and preventing or controlling complications, e.g., hepatic encephalopathy.
- Dogs with a suspected infectious etiology should undergo specific infectious disease testing, including serology, PCR, culture, FISH, and IHC techniques, supported by cytology and histopathology.

References

1. Marsilio S, Marks SL. Hepatobiliary infections. In Sykes JE (editor). Infectious Diseases of the Dog and Cat 5th edition. St Louis, Elsevier, 2023.
2. Cullen JM, Stalker MJ. Liver and biliary system. In Maxie MG (editor). Jubb, Kennedy and Palmer's Pathology of Domestic Animals: Volume 2 6th edition. St Louis, Elsevier, 2016.
3. Johnson SE. Liver. In Washabau RJ, Day MJ (editors). Canine and Feline Gastroenterology. St Louis, Elsevier, 2013.
4. Kearns S. Infectious Hepatopathies in Dogs and Cats. *Top Companion Anim Med* 24:189-198, 2009.
5. Boomkens SY, Slump E, Egberik HF, et al. PCR screening for candidate etiological agents of canine hepatitis. *Vet Microbiol* 108:49-55, 2005.
6. Poldevaart JH, Favier RP, Penning LC, et al. Primary hepatitis in dogs: A retrospective review (2002-2006). *J Vet Intern Med* 23:72-80, 2009.
7. Thawley V. Acute liver injury and failure. *Vet Clin North Am Small Anim Pract* 47:617-630, 2017.
8. Lester C, Cooper J, Peters RM, et al. Retrospective evaluation of acute liver failure in dogs (1995-2012): 49 cases. *J Vet Emerg Crit Care (San Antonio)* 26:559-567, 2016.
9. Weingarten MA, Sande AA. Acute liver failure in dogs and cats. *J Vet Emerg Crit Care (San Antonio)* 25:455-473, 2015.
10. Lidbury JA, Cook AK, Steiner JM. Hepatic encephalopathy in dogs and cats. *J Vet Emerg Crit Care (San Antonio)* 26:471-487, 2016.
11. Kavanagh C, Shaw S, Webster CRL. Coagulation in hepatobiliary disease. *J Vet Emerg Crit Care (San Antonio)* 21:589-604, 2011.
12. Lawrence YA, Steiner JM. Laboratory evaluation of the liver. *Vet Clin North Am Small Anim Pract* 47:539-553, 2017.
13. Webster CRL. Hemostatic disorders associated with hepatobiliary disease. *Vet Clin N Am Small Anim Pract* 47:601-615, 2017.
14. Stravitz RT, Lisman T, Luketic VA, et al. Minimal effects of acute liver injury/acute liver failure on hemostasis as assessed by thromboelastography. *J Hepatol* 56:129-136, 2012.
15. Kelley D, Lester C, Shaw S, et al. Thromboelastographic evaluation of dogs with acute liver disease. *J Vet Intern Med* 29:1053-1062, 2015.
16. Feeney DA, Anderson KL, Ziegler LE, et al. Statistical relevance of ultrasonographic criteria in the assessment of diffuse liver disease in dogs and cats. *Am J Vet Res* 69:212-221, 2008.
17. Sykes JE, Hartmann K, Lunn KF, et al. 2010 ACVIM Small Animal Consensus Statement on Leptospirosis: Diagnosis, Epidemiology, Treatment, and Prevention. *J Vet Intern Med* 25:1-13, 2011.
18. Liffman R, Courtman N. Fine needle aspiration of abdominal organs: a review of current recommendations for achieving a diagnostic sample. *J Small Anim Pract* 58:599-609, 2017.
19. Leveille R, Partington BP, Biller DS, et al. Complications after ultrasound-guided biopsy of abdominal structures in dogs and cats: 246 cases (1984-1991). J Am Vet Med Assoc 203:413-415, 1993.
20. Reece J, Pavlick M, Penninck DG, et al. Hemorrhage and complications associated with percutaneous ultrasound-guided liver biopsy in dogs. *J Vet Intern Med* 34:2398-2404, 2020.
21. Bigge LA, Brown DJ, Penninck DG. Correlation between coagulation profile findings and bleeding complications after ultrasound-guided biopsies: 434 cases (1993-1996). *J Am Anim Hosp Assoc* 37:228-233, 2001.
22. Allan F, Blake D, Miller Z, et al. Biliary protozoa in a dog with acute cholangiohepatitis fed a raw food diet. *J Vet Intern Med* 36:2177-2180, 2022.
23. Patten PK, Rich LJ, Zaks K, et al. Cestode infection in 2 dogs: cytological findings in liver and a mesenteric lymph node. *Vet Clin Pathol* 42:103-108, 2013.
24. Irvine KL, Walker JM, Friedrichs KR. Sarcocystid organisms found in bile from a dog with acute hepatitis: A case report and review of intestinal

and hepatobiliary Sarcocystidae infections in dogs and cats. *Vet Clin Pathol* 45:57-65, 2016.
25. Weiss DJ, Blauvelt M, Aird B. Cytologic evaluation of inflammation in canine liver aspirates. *Vet Clin Pathol* 30:193-196, 2008.
26. Wang KY, Panciera DL, Al-Rukibat RK, et al. Accuracy of ultrasound-guided fine-needle aspiration of the liver and cytologic findings in dogs and cats: 97 cases (1990-2000). *J Am Vet Med Assoc* 224:75-78, 2004.
27. Roth L. Comparison of liver cytology and biopsy diagnoses in dogs and cats: 56 cases. *Vet Clin Pathol* 30:35-38, 2001.
28. Cullen JM, van den Ingh TSGAM, Van Winkle T, et al. Morphological classification of parenchymal disorders of the canine and feline liver. WSAVA Standards for Clinical and Histological Diagnosis of Canine and Feline Liver Disease. St Louis, Elsevier, 2006.
29. Cole TL, Center SA, Flood SN, et al. Diagnostic comparisons of needle and wedge biopsy specimens of the liver in dogs and cats. *J Am Vet Med Assoc* 220:1483-1490, 2002.
30. Niza MMRE, Ferreira AJA, Peleteiro MC, et al. Bacteriological study of the liver in dogs. *J Small Anim Pract* 45:401-404, 2004.
31. Dickerson V, Poses B, Hyndman P, et al. Outcomes in 38 dogs surgically treated for hepatic abscessation. *Vet Surg* 52:127-133, 2023.
32. Pashmakova MB, Piccione J, Bishop MA, et al. Agreement between microscopic examination and bacterial culture of bile samples for the detection of bactibilia in dogs and cats with hepatobiliary disease. *J Am Vet Med Assoc* 250:1007-1013, 2017.
33. Im J, Burney DP, McDonough SP, et al. Canine hepatitis associated with intrahepatic bacteria in three dogs. *J Am Anim Hosp Assoc* 54:65-70, 2018.
34. Farrar ET, Washabau RJ, Saunders HM. Hepatic abscesses in dogs: 14 cases (1982-1994). *J Am Vet Med Assoc* 208: 243-247, 1996.
35. Wagner KA, Hartmann FA, Trepanier LA. Bacterial culture results from liver, gallbladder, or bile in 248 dogs and cats evaluated for hepatobiliary disease: 1998-2003. *J Vet Intern Med* 21:417-424, 2007.
36. Tamborini A, Jahns H, McAllister H, et al. Bacterial cholangitis, cholecystitis, or both in dogs. *J Vet Intern Med* 30:1046-1055, 2016.
37. Giuliano A, Meiring T, Grant AJ, et al. Acute hepatic necrosis caused by *Salmonella enterica* serotype I 4,5,12:-:1,2 in a dog. *J Clin Microbiol* 53:3674-3476, 2015.
38. McCallum KE, Constantino-Cases F, Cullen JM, et al. Hepatic leptospiral infections in dogs without obvious renal involvement. *J Vet Intern Med* 33:141-150, 2019.
39. Schuller S, Moore GE, Sykes JE. Leptospirosis. In Sykes JE (editor). Infectious Diseases of the Dog and Cat 5th edition. St Louis, Elsevier, 2023.
40. Grooters AM, Sherding RG, Biller DS, et al. Hepatic abscesses associated with diabetes mellitus in two dogs. *J Vet Intern Med* 8:203-206, 1994.
41. Schwarz LA, Penninck DG, Leveille-Webster C. Hepatic abscesses in 13 dogs: a review of ultrasonographic findings clinical data and therapeutic options. *Vet Radiol Ultrasound* 39:357-365. 1998.
42. Lemetayer JD, Snead EC, Starrak GS, et al. Multiple liver abscesses in a dog secondary to the liver fluke *Metorchis conjunctus* treated by percutaneous transhepatic drainage and alcoholization. *Can Vet J* 57:605- 609, 2016.
43. Lord PF, Carb A, Prueter JC. Emphysematous hepatic abscess associated with trauma, necrotic hepatic nodular hyperplasia and adenoma in a dog: a case history report. *Vet Radiol* 23:46-49, 1982.
44. Love DN, Maddison JE, Finnimore PM, et al. Isolation of *Clostridium novyi* (*Cl. oedematiens*) from liver lesions in a dog with pancreatic acinar carcinoma. *J Small Anim Pract* 22:277-280, 1981.
45. Downs MO, Miller MA, Cross AR, et al. Liver lobe torsion and liver abscess in a dog. *J Am Vet Med Assoc* 5:678-680, 1998.
46. Zatelli A, Bonfanti U, Zini E, et al. Percutaneous drainage and alcoholization of hepatic abscesses in five dogs and a cat. *J Am Anim Hosp Assoc* 41:34-38, 2005.
47. Fox JG, Drolet R, Higgins R, et al. *Helicobacter canis* isolated from a dog liver with multifocal necrotizing hepatitis. *J Clin Microbiol* 34:2478-2482, 1996.
48. Takemura LS, Marcasso RA, Lorenzetti E, et al. Helicobacter infection in the hepatobiliary system: a possible association in dogs. *Brazilian J Microbiol* 50:297-305, 2019.
49. Jacobson SA, Ferro PJ, Navarro MA, et al. *Clostridium piliforme* and canine distemper virus coinfection in 2 domestic dog littermates and a gray fox kit. *J Vet Diagn Invest* 34:894-897, 2022.
50. Mylonakis ME, Kritsepi-Konstantinou M, Dumler JS, et al. Severe hepatitis associated with acute *Ehrlichia canis* infection in a dog. *J Vet Intern Med* 24:633-638, 2010.
51. Decaro N. Infectious canine hepatitis and feline adenovirus infection. In Sykes JE (editor). Infectious Diseases of the Dog and Cat 5th edition. St Louis, Elsevier, 2023.
52. Verin R, Forzan M, Schulze C, et al. Multicentric molecular and pathologic study on canine adenovirus type 1 in red foxes (*Vulpes vulpes*) in three European countries. *J Wildl Dis* 55:935-936, 2019.
53. Chouinard L, Martineau D, Forget C, et al. Use of polymerase chain reaction and immunohistochemistry for detection of canine adenovirus type 1 in formalin-fixed, paraffin-embedded liver of dogs with chronic hepatitis or cirrhosis. *J Vet Diagn Invest* 10:320-325, 1998.
54. Gadsden BJ, Maes RK, Wise AG, et al. Fatal canid herpesvirus 1 infection in an adult dog. *J Vet Diagn Invest* 24:604-607, 2012.
55. Malone EK, Ledbetter EC, Rassnick KM, et al. Disseminated canine herpesvirus-1 infection in an immunocompromised adult dog. *J Vet Intern Med* 24:965-968, 2010.
56. Jarrett WFH, O'Neil BW. A new transmissible agent causing acute hepatitis, chronic hepatitis and cirrhosis in dogs. *Vet Rec* 116:629-635, 1985.
57. Jarrett WFH, O'Neil BW, Lindholm I. Persistent hepatitis and chronic fibrosis induced by canine acidophil cell hepatitis virus. *Vet Rec* 120:234-235, 1987.
58. Fry DR, McSporran KD, Ellis JT, et al. Protozoal hepatitis associated with immunosuppressive therapy in a dog. *J Vet Intern Med* 23:366-368, 2009.
59. Dubey JP, Sykes JE, Shelton GD, et al. *Sarcocystis caninum* and *Sarcocystis svanai* n. spp. (Apicomplexa: Sarcocystidae) associated with severe myositis and hepatitis in the domesticated dog (*Canis familiaris*). *J Eukaryot Microbiol* 62: 307-317, 2014.
60. Allison R, Williams P, Lansdowne J, et al. Fatal hepatic sarcocystosis in a puppy with eosinophilia and eosinophilic peritoneal effusion. *Vet Clin Pathol* 35:353-357, 2006.
61. O'Neill EJ, Day MJ, Hall EJ, et al. Bacterial cholangitis/cholangiohepatitis with or without concurrent cholecystitis in four dogs. *J Small Anim Practice* 47:325-335, 2006.
62. Center SA, Warner KL, Erb HN. Liver glutathione concentrations in dogs and cats with naturally occurring liver disease. *Am J Vet Res* 63:1187-1197, 2002.
63. Webster CRL, Cooper J. Therapeutic use of cytoprotective agents in canine and feline hepatobiliary disease. *Vet Clin N Am Small Anim Pract* 39:631-652, 2009.
64. Kook PH, Baumstark M, Ruetten M. Clinical and histologic outcome in a dog surviving massive hepatic necrosis. *J Vet Intern Med* 33:879-884, 2019.

CHAPTER 33

Chronic hepatitis: copper-associated

Rommaneeya Leela-arporn
DVM, PhD

Cynthia RL Webster
DVM, DACVIM (SAIM)

Copper-associated chronic hepatitis (CuCH) is a common hepatic disorder that has been increasingly recognized in dogs over time.[1-4] It is caused by the accumulation of copper within hepatocytes. This accumulation leads to oxidative stress, cell death, and inflammation.[2] The progressive hepatic copper accumulation can ultimately cause liver dysfunction and result in chronic hepatitis, cirrhosis, and death from hepatic failure.[2] This chapter aims to provide veterinarians with practical insights into the clinical management of CuCH in dogs, including etiology, pathophysiology, clinical presentation, diagnostics, treatment options, monitoring, and prognosis.

Etiology

Copper is an essential trace mineral involved in a myriad of important reactions in the body. However, excess copper can elicit the generation of reactive oxygen species that can be cytotoxic.[2] Dietary copper is absorbed in the small intestines, mainly mediated by the copper transporter (Fig. 33.1). After being delivered to the liver via the portal circulation, a copper transporter on the hepatocyte basolateral membrane moves copper into the cytoplasm. Since free cytoplasmic copper is toxic, once in the hepatocyte, copper binds to one of several chaperone proteins. The chaperones deliver copper to intracellular trafficking proteins that either control its entry into the bloodstream or the eventual excretion of any excess in the bile. Two important proteins necessary for biliary excretion are ATP7B and COMMD1. ATP7B is a trans-Golgi protein that helps package copper for excretion. Mutations in ATP7B lead to copper excess in the liver and are the main cause of the human copper-associated hepatic disorder, Wilson's disease. The COMMD1 protein interacts with ATP7B, stabilizing its function. Mutation of COMMD1 leads to hepatic copper excess and CuCH but has only been described in Bedlington terriers.

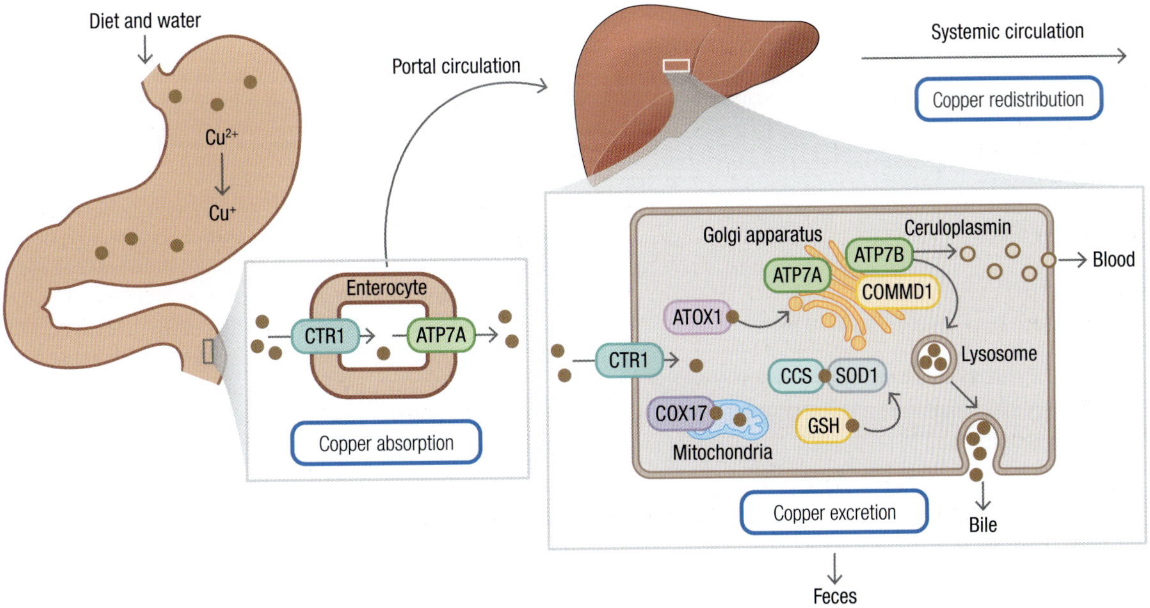

FIG. 33.1 Hepatic copper metabolism. Dietary copper is absorbed in the small intestines via the copper transporter (CTR1). ATP7A facilitates copper transport from the enterocyte to the liver via portal circulation. After being delivered to the liver, CTR1 on the hepatocyte basolateral membrane moves copper into the cytoplasm. Once in the hepatocyte, copper binds to one of several chaperone proteins (COX17, ATOX1, and CCS). The chaperones deliver copper to intracellular trafficking proteins (SOD1, ATP7A, ATP7B, and COMMD1) that either help redistribute to other tissues and organs via systemic circulation or excrete excess copper in the bile via proteins ATP7B and COMMD1. This figure was designed by the author (Rommaneeya Leela-arporn) and was created with BioRender.com.

An increase in hepatic copper is caused either by breed-specific hereditary genetic defects in copper handling or by a dietary copper excess in any dog breed, or often by a combination of genetic defects and dietary excess.[2,5] While hepatic copper accumulation has been noted as a consequence of cholestatic or inflammatory conditions in cats and humans,[2] it is generally accepted that these factors have a minimal effect in dogs with chronic hepatopathies,[2] because dogs are more resistant to hepatic copper accumulation from cholestasis unless copper uptake is concurrently increased.[2]

Hereditary copper-associated chronic hepatitis in dogs

Predisposed breeds with a hereditary component for CuCH include Labrador Retrievers, Bedlington Terriers, Doberman Pinschers, West Highland White Terriers, Dalmatians, and Cavalier King Charles Spaniels.[1,2,6] In some of these breeds, genetic mutations in copper transport genes have been identified. It should be emphasized that CuCH can occur in any dog breed despite breed predilections.[3]

In Bedlington Terriers, an autosomal recessive deletion in the gene coding for COMMD1 leads to the development of CuCH.[2] Genetic tests for the COMMD1 deletion and its microsatellite marker are used to screen for CuCH in this breed. However, a recent study has shown a marked reduction in the COMMD1 deletion over time facilitated by selective breeding enabled by the DNA screening for the defect, although it remains present in the breed.[7] Therefore, the genetic tests for CuCH in this breed lack sensitivity in homozygous negative dogs but remain specific to homozygous positive dogs for the COMMD1 deletion. Currently, this deletion has not been found in other breeds predisposed to CuCH, but the recent study revealed the COMMD1 deletion is no longer the primary cause of CuCH in Bedlington Terriers.[7] A mutation in copper transporter ATP7B has been associated with CuCH in Doberman Pinschers, Labrador Retrievers, and Cavalier King Charles Spaniels,[6,8,9] and interestingly, it appeared that the prevalence of ATP7B mutation associated with CuCH is increased in the Bedlington Terrier as well. Dogs homozygous for the mutation have a high incidence of excess hepatic copper accumulation. This mutation, however, only accounts for about 12% of the phenotype in Labradors and Dobermans,[8,10] and its contribution to disease is unknown in other breeds. This suggests that the genetic predisposition to CuCH is likely polygenic in most if not all, dog breeds, although the other genes involved have yet to be identified.

Dietary copper intake exceeding homeostatic regulatory mechanisms

An increased incidence of CuCH in dogs was recognized beginning in the late 1990s and correlates with the change in the type of copper premixes used in formulating dog foods in the US.[3-5]

In the mid to late 1990s, the National Research Council (NRC) and the Association of American Feed Control Officials (AAFCO) recommended the discontinuation of cupric oxide as a source of supplemental copper in commercial dog food in favor of more bioavailable forms, such as cupric sulfate or various forms of chelated copper.[3-6] The amount of copper in the base diet varies, and the increased bioavailability of copper in dog food led to a large variation in the total copper concentrations in dog foods, many of which exceeded the minimum allowances by 2-4 times or even more.[5] (See Table 40.1 in chapter 40 for minimal allowances). This problem was likely compounded by the advent of boutique diets containing ingredients with high copper content (e.g., salmon, organ meats, sweet potatoes, and chickpeas).

AAFCO has not established an upper limit for dietary copper intake in dogs, while the European Pet Food Industry Federation (FEDIAF) recently set this limit at 7 mg/1000 kcal (28 mg/kg dry matter [DM]) (see chapter 40 for more details) although they have identified individual diets exceeding this limit.

The copper content of a given pet food cannot be reliably determined by reading the label. Since there is no upper limit in the US, manufacturers add premixes to comply with AAFCO's minimum nutrient content recommendations without paying attention to the native copper already in the baseline diet (Fig. 33.2). The result is many dog foods are high in copper.

Pathophysiology

Normal hepatic copper concentrations for dogs are considered to be within a range of 120-400 parts per million (ppm) dry weight (DW).[1-4] An increased hepatic copper accumulation can be due to decreases in hepatic copper excretion in the bile, increased dietary copper intake, or both. In instances where the hepatic copper concentration exceeds the hepatocyte transport and copper-binding capacity, free copper causes oxidative stress and results in hepatocellular damage, cell death, and hepatic inflammation. The threshold copper concentration at which hepatic damage occurs in the dog has not been well documented. It is generally agreed that values greater than 1,000 ppm are toxic to the liver. However, variability in phenotype exists in that some dogs may have significant hepatic copper concentrations without evidence of hepatic damage, whereas others with lower hepatic copper concentrations (in the 600 to 1,000 ppm range) have evidence of hepatic damage. The threshold for hepatic copper injury is likely impacted by genetic, physiologic, and environmental factors[2] such as dietary concentrations, antioxidants, and other minerals, particularly zinc.

Clinical features

Dogs with CuCH are typically young to middle-aged and appear healthy with asymptomatic liver enzyme elevations before clinical signs develop at the later stage and progress to liver failure in the end-stage of the disease when a large portion of liver tissue is affected.[2] The duration of the asymptomatic period depends on several factors, including hepatic copper concentrations, genetic predisposition, and dietary copper intake, and can vary between breeds and individuals.[2] Initial clinical signs are nonspecific and commonly include anorexia, lethargy, nausea, vomiting, and weight loss. Signs of more progressive disease pointing toward liver failure include ascites, hepatic encephalopathy, coagulation disturbances, polyuria/polydipsia, and icterus.[2] These clinical signs, however, are not specific to copper-associated hepatitis. Rarely, dogs can present with an acute onset of signs compatible with acute liver injury/failure (hyperbilirubinemia, prolonged prothrombin time, and neurologic signs) when there is acute release of massive amounts of copper into the cytoplasm of hepatocytes. These dogs may also have copper excess in the blood, leading to a Coombs' negative hemolytic anemia.[2]

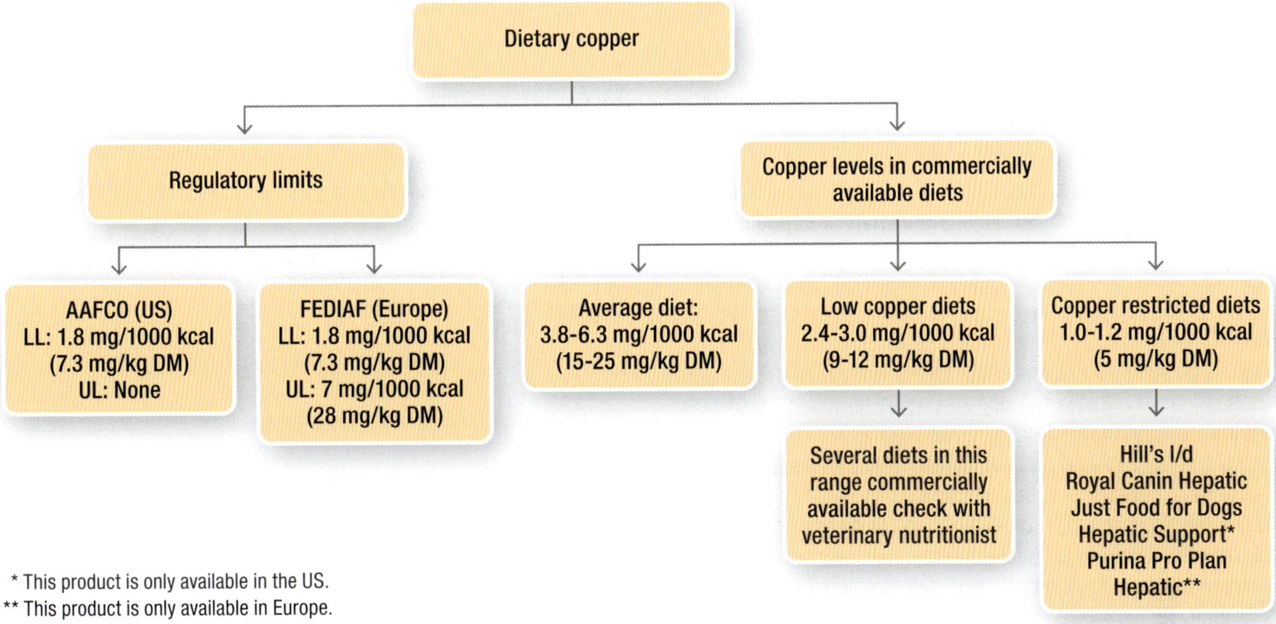

FIG. 33.2 Dietary copper allowance expressed on a dry matter (DM) and caloric basis. The Association of American Feed Control Officials (AAFCO) in the US and the European Pet Food Industry Federation (FEDIAF) set regulatory standards for the lower limits (LL) of copper in pet foods for dogs. FEDIAF also set an upper limit (UL). Dietary copper levels for average diets were derived from data collected by AAFCO. Only four restricted copper diets are commercially available. Several low-copper diets are commercially available; however, the pet food regulatory agencies have not defined a copper content that constitutes low dietary copper.

Clinicopathologic findings

Biochemical parameters

It is important to realize that an increased hepatic copper accumulation can be present with or without hepatocellular damage. Therefore, there are no parameters available that correlate with or predict hepatic copper accumulation.[2] Routine biochemical parameters can reveal elevated serum liver enzyme activity, but these alterations are not specific to CuCH. The most common biochemical parameter used for evaluating hepatocellular injury is serum alanine aminotransferase (ALT) activity. Elevation of ALT is often the first indicator for CuCH.[2]

In the later stage of the disease, when a significant amount of liver tissue is affected, other liver enzymes, including serum ALP, aspartate aminotransferase (AST), and γ-glutamyl transpeptidase (GGT) activity, can be elevated. In addition, serum biochemical parameters associated with liver function, including albumin, glucose, cholesterol, urea, total bilirubin, prothrombin, and partial thromboplastin times, may be abnormal in more advanced diseases.[2]

In dogs with end-stage liver disease or cirrhosis, serum liver enzyme activity may decrease or return to normal limits as damaged liver tissue is replaced with fibrous tissue.[2] Typically, the results of the complete blood counts are normal.

Urinalysis

Accumulation of copper in the liver can be accompanied by an acquired Fanconi-like syndrome associated with increased urinary copper excretion, resulting in copper deposition within the proximal renal tubular epithelium, causing tubular injury.[2,11] This acquired Fanconi-like syndrome is characterized by low urinary specific gravity, proteinuria, and normoglycemic glucosuria. It is transient and resolves on recovery from the acute injury. The presence of this syndrome in dogs with increased liver enzymes increases the index of suspicion for either acute leptospirosis or CuCH.

Genetic testing

Genetic testing for ATP7B mutations and the COMMD1 microsatellite marker is commercially available. Homozygous detection of the COMMD1 mutation in the Bedlington Terrier is diagnostic for copper toxicosis. However, as discussed earlier, Bedlington Terriers may be homozygous negative for this deletion and still have CuCH. Labradors and Dobermans that are homozygous for the ATP7B mutation appear to be at greater risk for developing copper accumulation in their liver, but the test is not diagnostic for copper toxicosis. Additionally, the lack of this particular gene mutation does not mean the dog will not develop CuCH, as the mutation is seen in only about 12% of the dogs with copper toxicosis.[8,10,12] Genetic testing is thus of limited usefulness in any breed for diagnosing CuCH, and a liver biopsy is usually necessary to confirm the disease.

Diagnostic imaging

While imaging modalities alone cannot definitively diagnose the presence of CuCH in dogs, they can provide valuable supplementary information during a comprehensive health assessment to rule out other causes of increased serum markers of hepatic damage. The changes seen on radiographs and ultrasound are those typically associated with chronic hepatitis of any etiology in the dog (see chapter 26 for more details).

Radiographs

Abdominal radiographs can be used to evaluate liver size, shape, opacity, and the presence of ascites. However, they are not sensitive to subtle changes in the liver parenchyma that accompany chronic hepatitis.

Ultrasonography

Ultrasonography is the preferred imaging modality for evaluating dogs with suspected CuCH, as it provides information regarding the size, shape, echogenicity, and echotexture of the parenchyma, as well as information on the biliary tract and main vessels.

Ultrasound findings in the liver in dogs with CuCH can be normal or only reveal subtle changes in echogenicity in the early stage of the disease.[2] A normal liver on ultrasound in a dog suspected of CuCH should never preclude the clinician from obtaining a liver biopsy.

In dogs with more advanced disease, ultrasonographic findings associated with chronic inflammation and remodeling may be seen (Fig. 33.3A), including a heterogeneous echotexture, irregular hypoechoic nodules, irregular margins, and microhepatica. Ultrasound evaluation may detect complications associated with late-stage disease, including portal vein thrombosis, portal hypertension, ascites, and multiple acquired portosystemic shunts.[2]

Other imaging modalities

The application of computed tomography (CT) and magnetic resonance imaging (MRI) for characterizing liver structure in dogs with CuCH has not been reported.

Cytology

Fine-needle aspiration of the hepatic parenchyma may have some value as a screening test in dogs with suspected CuCH. Cytological preparations can be stained with a specific copper stain (rhodanine), and the finding of many rhodanine-positive hepatocytes can be used as a noninvasive approach to increase the index of suspicion for CuCH.[13] However, it cannot make a definitive diagnosis of CuCH, as it has several limitations, including the inability to provide quantification of copper concentration or to evaluate the hepatic lobular copper distribution and accompanying inflammatory infiltrates or fibrosis.[2,13]

Liver biopsy acquisition

To confirm the diagnosis of CuCH, histopathology and liver biopsy remain the gold standard and are necessary in most cases. To provide representative samples, liver biopsies are best acquired as wedges at laparoscopy (Fig. 33.3B) or laparotomy[2] (see chapter 27 for more details on biopsy acquisition).

During the procedure, biopsy specimens should be obtained from multiple liver lobes as there can be considerable heterogenicity between lobes in terms of the amount of copper accumulated. Current recommendations are to acquire a minimum of five laparoscopic or surgical biopsy specimens from at least three liver lobes for histopathology (3), aerobic and anaerobic culture (1), and copper quantification (1). If percutaneous ultrasound-guided needle biopsy specimens are obtained, multiple biopsy specimens should be collected from more than one lobe, if possible. A 14G or 16G biopsy needle is recommended.[2]

Copper quantitative analysis using atomic absorption spectrometry requires approximately 20-40 mg of liver (wet weight) for the measurement. This amount equals one full-length 14G (2 cm long) needle biopsy specimen or half of a 5 mm laparoscopic biopsy specimen. A liver tissue sample obtained with a full-length 18G needle biopsy only provides 3-5 mg of liver tissue. Therefore, if submission of the 18G needle biopsy specimen for hepatic copper quantification, the result could be inaccurate and erroneously low.[2]

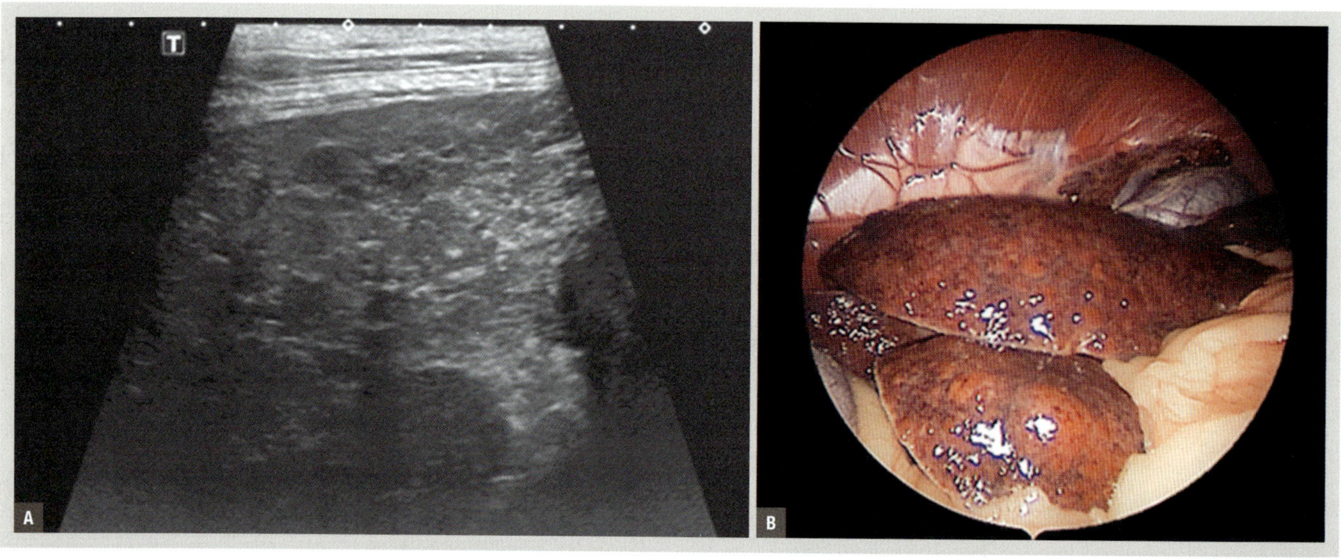

FIG. 33.3 (A) Hepatic ultrasonographic and (B) laparoscopic images of a dog with copper-associated chronic hepatitis with late-stage disease. (A) The liver has a heterogeneous echotexture with numerous hypoechoic nodules suggestive of chronic inflammation and remodeling. (B) At laparoscopy, the liver has an irregular margin, along with diffuse nodules in the liver lobes, representing hepatic fibrosis and regenerative nodules. Both figures are courtesy of Dr. Sarah Shropshire, Colorado State University.

Liver biopsy evaluation

A diagnosis of CuCH is made after assessing the liver biopsy (Table 33.1). Liver biopsies should be evaluated with at least three stains: 1) hematoxylin and eosin to access hepatic architecture and to localize and grade inflammation/degenerative changes, 2) Sirius red or trichrome to assess for fibrosis, and 3) rhodanine for assessment of the lobular location of copper and to obtain a semiquantitative score for the extent of copper accumulation.[2]

Affected hepatocytes and macrophages may accumulate copper in their cytoplasm, which manifests as granules staining orange-red with rhodanine (Fig. 33.4).[2] In dogs with CuCH, hepatic copper accumulation is usually most severe in the centrilobular regions. As the disease progresses, copper accumulation and accompanying hepatocyte degeneration and inflammation/fibrosis can spread to mid-zonal and portal regions, ultimately affecting hepatocytes in all zones, resulting in a cirrhotic liver. In some dogs with late-stage disease, it may be difficult for the pathologist to determine the lobular orientation of copper deposition, or the copper deposition may be marked but primarily periportal in orientation.

A semiquantitative subjective grading scale is recommended for rhodanine scoring of hepatic copper accumulation. This scoring system focuses on assessing the zonal location and the presence of copper granules in hepatocytes and macrophages, using a scale ranging from 0 to 5. Scores greater than 2 are abnormal.[2,4]

Atomic absorption spectroscopy is the gold standard for hepatic copper quantification and requires only a small amount (20-40 mg) of tissue for accurate determination.[2,4] Results of the analysis should be reported based on a dry weight (DW) basis. In dogs, normal hepatic copper concentrations are less than 400 ppm DW, while pathologic concentrations are greater than 1000 ppm DW[2] with a gray area in between. The diagnosis of CuCH is not always straightforward. A number of factors can confuse the interpretation of quantitative copper results, including lobe-to-lobe variability in the deposition of hepatic copper and the fact that regenerative nodules do not accumulate copper. In addition, fibrosis and parenchymal collapse can artifactually decrease the quantification in

TABLE 33.1 Diagnosis of copper-associated chronic hepatitis in dogs. DW, dry weight; ppm, parts per million.*

Category	Type of stain/tissue samples	Remarks
Histopathology	Hematoxylin and eosin	The presence of mixed inflammatory infiltrate is compatible with a diagnosis of chronic hepatitis with lesions concentrated in centrilobular hepatocytes.
	Sirius red or trichrome	Presence of fibrosis or cirrhotic changes
	Rhodanine	Positive histochemical rhodanine staining is most abundant in the centrilobular area. Semiquantitative scores greater than 2 compatibles with copper-associated disease (on a scale ranging from 0 to 5).
Copper quantification	Fresh tissue Frozen tissue Fixed or embedded in paraffin block	Hepatic copper concentrations greater than 1,000 ppm DW.*

*Some dogs with CuCH have lower hepatic copper concentrations between 600 and 1,000 ppm DW.

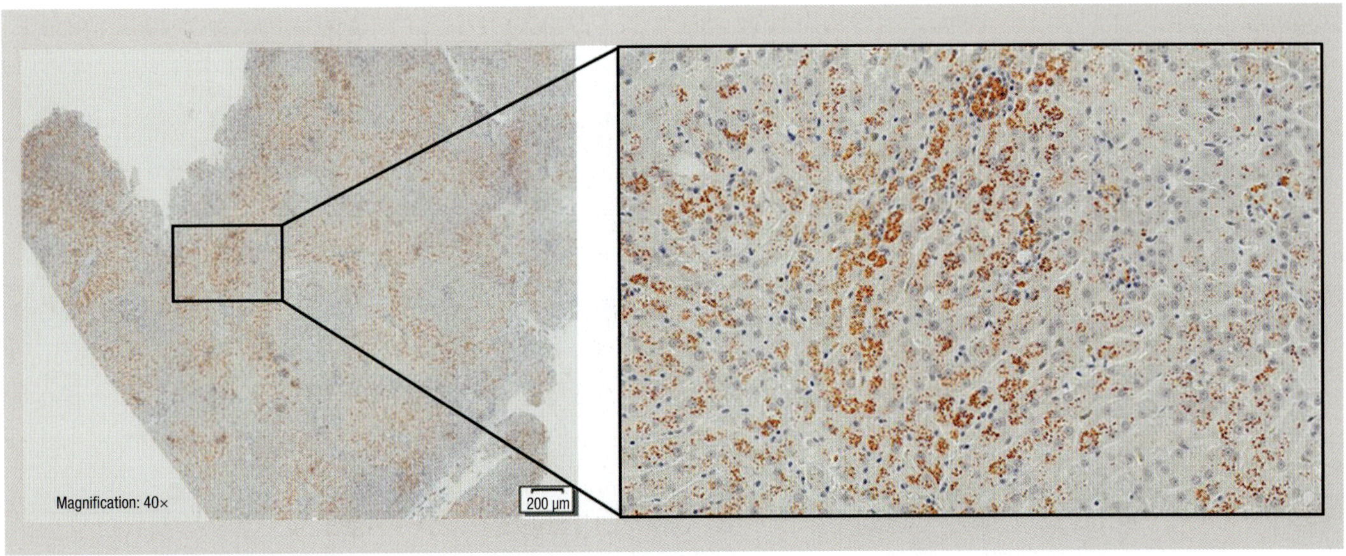

FIG. 33.4 Histochemical detection of copper in a hepatic biopsy. Staining of a hepatic biopsy with rhodanine reveals the presence of small red-orange granules representing hepatic copper accumulation in the centrilobular regions of the biopsy. Courtesy of Dr. Sarah Shropshire, Colorado State University.

dogs that have CuCH. In some of these cases where there is discordance between the semiquantitative and qualitative analysis of hepatic copper concentrations, digital copper quantification of rhodanine-stained biopsy sections may be helpful as this analysis can eliminate the lobe-to-lobe variation by evaluating multiple sections concurrently.[2] Alternatively, a histological block of tissue with a large amount of rhodanine staining could be sent for copper quantification.

In dogs where the hepatic copper quantification is the gray zone greater than 400 but less than 1,000 ppm DW, the clinician should search for other concurrent causes of chronic hepatitis (see chapter 34) and consider a trial period of treatment for CuCH to make a definitive diagnosis.

Biomarkers

At present, there are no blood or urine biomarkers that can be used in clinical practice for the definitive diagnosis of CuCH in dogs. The search for noninvasive biomarkers for hepatic copper status is under investigation.

Treatment

Treatment for CuCH involves copper chelation with D-penicillamine and restriction of dietary copper intake.[2] In addition, hepatoprotectants are recommended to counteract the oxidant damage from copper (Table 33.2).[2]

Copper chelation

None of the copper chelators used in veterinary practice are licensed for use in small animals, and the owner should give informed consent for off-label use. The most widely used copper chelator in clinical veterinary practice is D-penicillamine.[2] This medication binds hepatic copper, resulting in subsequent excretion in the urine.[2] In addition, D-penicillamine has mild anti-inflammatory and antifibrotic properties.[2] The treatment duration necessary to decopper the liver with D-penicillamine is dependent not only on quantitative copper concentrations in the liver at the start of treatment but also on individual factors in the dog that are not well understood, but it usually takes months. The most common side effect of D-penicillamine in dogs is gastrointestinal upset. Other side effects include skin eruptions, proteinuria, cytopenias, and the development of a vacuolar hepatopathy that can be accompanied by an increase in serum ALP activity. The bioavailability of D-penicillamine is decreased when administered with food, so it must be given on an empty stomach.[2] The current FDA-approved formulation to treat Wilson's disease in humans is prohibitively expensive in the US, so the drug must be formulated at a compounding pharmacy. The human drug is used in Europe, and the cost varies widely between pharmacies.

The dose of D-penicillamine that is currently used ranges from 10 to 15mg/kg PO q12h.[2] In order to avoid gastrointestinal side effects, it is recommended to titrate up to the full dose over a 2 to 3-week period. The concurrent use of antiemetics may be necessary. Some dogs may not be able to tolerate the full dose of D-penicillamine, and there is some anecdotal evidence to suggest that lower doses may also be effective in decoppering the liver, albeit at a much slower rate.

TABLE 33.2 Medications and supplements for treatment of copper-associated chronic hepatitis in dogs.*

Treatment	Mechanism of action	Dose	Adverse effects
D-penicillamine*	Chelates copper facilitating urinary excretion	10-15 mg/kg PO q12h on empty stomach	■ Nausea, vomiting, and hyporexia ■ Dermatological reaction ■ Proteinuria ■ Cytopenias ■ Vacuolar hepatopathy with increased serum ALP activity
Zinc*	Interferes with intestinal copper absorption by inducing intestinal metallothionein that binds copper, facilitating fecal excretion Induces hepatic metallothionein	8-10 mg/kg/day of elemental zinc on an empty stomach. Do not give concurrently with penicillamine.	■ Vomiting, hyporexia ■ Hemolytic anemia. Monitor serum levels to keep <800 μg/dL ■ Decoppers slowly best for maintenance therapy
Trientine*	Chelates copper	5-7.5 mg/kg PO q12h	■ Acute kidney injury
Ammonium tetrathiomolybdate*	Chelates copper	Approximately 0.5 mg/kg PO q6h	■ Vomiting, anorexia, hemolytic anemia. ■ Not commercially available
S-adenosylmethionine (SAMe)**	Antioxidant, which increases hepatic glutathione synthesis, promotes cell replication and regeneration, and controls production of inflammatory cytokines.	20 mg/kg PO q24h on an empty stomach	■ Rare but can include nausea
Vitamin E*	Antioxidant which has antifibrotic and anti-inflammatory effects	10 IU/kg PO q24h not to exceed 400 IU per dog, given with food to increase bioavailability	■ Well tolerated. Overdose can impair vitamin K activity and may increase risk of oxidative injury

*This medication or supplement is used in an extra-label manner. ** The dosage of this supplement is not FDA-approved and should be treated as extra-label.

Dogs that do not tolerate D-penicillamine, even on a lower dose, can be tried on less proven therapy. Zinc, which competes with intestinal uptake of copper, works very slowly to decopper the liver and thus should never be considered first-line therapy. The dose of zinc that results in successful decoppering of the liver has not been well characterized. Currently, 8-10 mg/kg/day of elemental zinc divided twice a day is recommended. Dosing is complicated by the fact that different zinc salts contain different amounts of zinc. Therefore, it is easiest to recommend zinc products that are sold by the amount of elemental zinc they contain. Zinc must be given on an empty stomach, which is again problematic as common side effects are stomach upset and vomiting. Serum zinc levels should be monitored to obtain concentrations above 200 µg/dL but below 800 µg/dL, the latter being a level at which hemolytic anemia may be seen. Zinc should not be given concurrently with penicillamine as they will negate each other's action.

Another chelator that has been used in dogs is trientine. Ammonium tetrathiomolybdate is also a copper chelator but is not currently commercially available. These two chelators can be considered as an alternative drug to decopper in dogs that are intolerant to penicillamine and zinc.

Restriction of copper uptake

A low copper diet is advised as a lifelong management strategy in any dog diagnosed with CuCH (Fig. 33.2).[2] In dogs with mildly increased hepatic copper concentration, dietary restriction alone may be enough to promote decoppering of the liver. However, some dogs will not respond to dietary restriction alone. It is hard to predict which dogs fall into this category, although there is some evidence in Labradors that dogs with higher hepatic copper values and those with evidence of a heritable component to their disorder are harder to decopper.

The current AAFCO and FEDIAF recommendations for minimum daily copper intake for maintenance adult canine diets is 1.8 mg/1000 kcal (Fig. 33.2).[2,5] Currently, there are four canine prescription diets that are copper-restricted at 1.1-1.2 mg/1000 kcal: Hill's Prescription Diet l/d and Royal Canin Hepatic (both available in the US and Europe), Just Food for Dogs Hepatic Support Low Fat (only available in the US), and Purina Pro Plan Veterinary Diet HP Hepatic (only available in Europe). The protein concentrations in the Hill's and Royal Canin diets are close to the minimum recommended by regulatory bodies (see chapter 40 for more detail), so close attention should be paid to muscle mass in dogs fed these diets, and they should not be given to growing, pregnant or lactating animals. If dogs do not find these diets palatable or have other dietary restrictions (e.g., low fat or novel ingredient diet), a veterinary nutritionist should be consulted for advice on other potential diets or home formulation of a balanced diet. Copper concentration of water should be less than 0.1 ppm.[2] If water copper concentrations exceed these limits, filters that remove metals or distilled bottled water can be used. High copper titbits and supplements should also be avoided. A careful dietary history will be necessary to make sure the owner is not inadvertently feeding these or giving supplements that contain an ingredient with high copper content (Table 33.3).

Hepatoprotectant therapy

During chelation treatment, hepatoprotective supplements with antioxidant properties, such as S-adenosylmethionine (SAMe) and vitamin E, should be used to counteract copper-associated oxidative liver injury.[2]

Monitoring treatment

To evaluate treatment efficacy, a repeat liver biopsy for qualitative and quantitative copper measurement should be performed.[2] A reasonable recheck interval for a repeat liver biopsy is somewhere between 6 months to a year after starting therapy. In reality, few owners will permit a second biopsy, and thus, most dogs are monitored by periodic assessment of serum ALT. If ALT does not normalize with therapy, it could be that the hepatic copper has not been effectively chelated or that another concurrent hepatic condition is present (such as immune-mediated hepatitis). A hepatic biopsy

TABLE 33.3 List of food ingredients containing low and moderate to high copper content.

Food category	Low copper content	Moderate to high copper content
Vegetables	Cucumber Green beans Brussel sprouts Celery Lettuce Broccoli Cauliflower Cabbage Fresh spinach Carrots	Cooked spinach Cooked kale Cooked broccoli rabe Cooked okra Sweet potato Potatoes with skin Mushroom Pumpkin Asparagus Green peas
Fruits	Apples Strawberries Blueberries Oranges Peaches Watermelon Cranberries	Bananas Mango Pears Pineapple Raspberries Coconut
Bread and grains	Pasta Rice Graham crackers	Wheat spaghetti Whole wheat crackers Brown or wild rice Chickpeas Quinoa Barley Flaxseed Buckwheat Lentils
Protein	Flounder Cod White meat turkey White meat chicken	Organ meat (liver) Beef Lamb Pork Dark meat turkey Dark meat chicken Peanut butter Shrimp Green-lipped mussels Salmon Crab Clams Duck Soybeans Peanuts
Fats, oils, and condiments	Oils Maple syrup	Molasses

with repeat histopathology and copper quantification is then necessary to determine the correct course of action.

There is limited information in the literature to determine which dogs can safely stop chelator therapy after successful decoppering of the liver. In dogs with relatively minor initial morphologic changes in the liver and modest increases in hepatic copper (less than 1,500 ppm), chelation therapy can be stopped 2 months after the normalization of serum ALT activity, and the dog monitored for relapse by reoccurrence of serum ALT activity elevations. In a dog that seemingly fails to respond to penicillamine, the owner should be questioned to make sure the bioavailability of the drug is not being compromised by being given with food and or with concurrent zinc supplementation and that they have been compliant with adherence to a copper-restricted diet. In some dogs, concurrent immune-mediated hepatitis may be present due to exposure to neoepitopes in the liver secondary to copper-mediated damage. These dogs may need immunomodulatory therapy. This diagnosis would require a rebiopsy with repeat histology and copper quantification.

Prognosis

The prognosis is generally good for dogs with early stages of CuCH that are started on appropriate treatment. In contrast, in dogs with late stages of disease in which cirrhosis and liver failure have been developed, the prognosis may be guarded, and many dogs do not present clinically until late in the disease process. However, there is a lack of studies looking at long-term follow-up in dogs with CuCH treated with chelation therapy and a restricted copper diet.

KEY POINTS

- Copper-associated chronic hepatitis is a common disorder in dogs, and its prevalence has increased over time.
- Excessive hepatic copper concentrations can arise from a hereditary defect, increased uptake of dietary copper, or a combination of both.
- Although certain dog breeds are predisposed to copper-associated chronic hepatitis, any breed can be affected.
- Clinical signs are often initially nonspecific and mild but can progress to end-stage disease and hepatic failure.
- The definitive diagnosis of copper-associated chronic hepatitis requires histologic evaluation of liver biopsies stained with rhodanine and quantitative assessment of hepatic copper concentrations.
- The most effective treatment strategies are copper chelation with D-penicillamine combined with feeding a copper-restricted diet and antioxidant support.
- Therapy is ideally monitored via repeat liver biopsy for qualitative and quantitative copper analyses, but if owners decline this, normalization of serum ALT activity is used as a surrogate noninvasive biomarker of treatment efficacy.

References

1. Ullal TV, Lakin S, Gallagher B, et al. Demographic and histopathologic features of dogs with abnormally high concentrations of hepatic copper. *J Vet Intern Med* 36(6):2016-2027, 2022.
2. Webster CRL, Center SA, Cullen JM, et al. ACVIM consensus statement on the diagnosis and treatment of chronic hepatitis in dogs. *J Vet Intern Med* 33(3):1173-1200, 2019.
3. Strickland JM, Buchweitz JP, Smedley RC, et al. Hepatic copper concentrations in 546 dogs (1982-2015). *J Vet Intern Med* 32(6):1943-1950, 2018.
4. Johnston AN, Center SA, McDonough SP, et al. Hepatic copper concentrations in labrador retrievers with and without chronic hepatitis: 72 cases (1980-2010). *J Am Vet Med Assoc* 242(1):372-380, 2013.
5. Center SA, Richter KP, Twedt DC, et al. Is it time to reconsider current guidelines for copper content in commercial dog foods? *J Am Vet Med Assoc* 258(4):357-364, 2021.
6. Nivy R, Kuzi S, Swinburne J, et al. Copper-associated chronic hepatitis in Cavalier King Charles spaniels. *Vet Rec* e3561, 2023.
7. Haywood S, Swinburne J, Schofield E, et al. Copper toxicosis in Bedlington terriers is associated with multiple independent genetic variants. *Vet Rec* 193(4):e2832, 2023.
8. Fieten H, Gill Y, Martin AJ, et al. The Menkes and Wilson disease genes counteract in copper toxicosis in Labrador retrievers: a new canine model for copper-metabolism disorders. *Dis Model Mech* 9(1):25-38, 2016.
9. Wu X, Mandigers PJJ, Watson AL, et al. Association of the canine atp7a and atp7b with hepatic copper accumulation in Doberman dogs. *J Vet Intern Med* 33(4):1646-1652, 2019.
10. Langlois DK, Nagler BSM, Smedley RC, et al. ATP7A, ATP7B, and RETN genotypes in Labrador Retrievers with and without copper-associated hepatopathy. *J Am Vet Med Assoc* 260(14):1-8, 2022.
11. Langlois DK, Smedley RC, Schall WD, et al. Acquired proximal renal tubular dysfunction in 9 labrador retrievers with copper-associated hepatitis (2006-2012). *J Vet Intern Med* 27(3):491-499, 2013.
12. Pindar S, Ramirez C. Predicting copper toxicosis: relationship between the ATP7A and ATP7B gene mutations and hepatic copper quantification in dogs. *Human Genetics* 138(5):541-546, 2019.
13. Moore AR, Medrano E, Coffey E, et al. Clinicopathological correlation and prevalence of increased copper in canine hepatic cytology. *J Am Anim Hosp Assoc* 55(1):8-13, 2019.

CHAPTER 34

Chronic hepatitis: idiopathic, autoimmune, and other non-copper-associated causes

Adam G. Gow
BVM&S, PhD,
DSAM, DECVIM-CA
(Internal Medicine),
FHEA, FRCVS

The World Small Animal Veterinary Association has defined chronic hepatitis (CH) as a histological diagnosis characterized by the presence of hepatocyte apoptosis or necrosis as well as an inflammatory infiltrate (see chapter 29).[1] As inflammation and hepatocellular death progress, fibrosis and regeneration occur, with resultant architectural disruption, influencing the clinical consequences. The inflammatory component may be predominantly composed of lymphocytes and plasma cells, may be granulomatous (defined as the presence of activated macrophages), or may have a neutrophilic component. "Chronic hepatitis" can therefore be subdivided based on the predominant inflammatory cells, which may direct investigation of potential underlying causes. Granulomatous hepatitis is uncommonly reported in the literature compared with lymphocytic-plasmacytic infiltration.[2,3] The disease can also be subclassified by a specific distribution of fibrosis known as lobular dissecting hepatitis (LDH), where fibrous bands between hepatocytes more markedly disrupt the lobar architecture. Although the signalment and clinical signs can increase or decrease the clinical suspicion of chronic hepatitis and potentially sub-types, a definitive diagnosis requires a biopsy.

Etiology

Initiation of inflammation in the liver can occur due to a multitude of potential causes: infectious, toxic, immune-mediated, and potentially metabolic. Accumulation of excess copper can also cause canine chronic hepatitis and is discussed in detail in chapter 33, so it will not be considered further here. Causes of initial acute hepatitis have the potential to progress to chronic disease (see chapters 31 and 32). Unfortunately, many cases of chronic hepatitis in dogs are considered idiopathic. Despite this, it is vitally important that potential underlying causes are thoroughly excluded, as treatment of idiopathic disease is a combination of attempting to control inflammation and symptomatic management of the consequences, whereas if an inciting cause is found, there is the potential for resolution.

Infection

In cases where there is a granulomatous or neutrophilic component to the inflammatory infiltrate, or there is evidence of other body system involvement, then the potential for an infectious cause should be evaluated. There are a large number of infectious organisms that have been reported to cause granulomatous hepatitis (Table 34.1). However, from small studies, cases of granulomatous hepatitis, particularly if pathology is confined to the liver, rarely have infectious organisms identified. These studies were retrospective and may have missed infectious causes as few cases were thoroughly screened, and some techniques lacked sensitivity.[2,3] It is important to rule out infections endemic to the region before commencing immunosuppressive treatment. These are most often bacterial, fungal, or protozoal. *Leishmania* spp. is an important rule-out in endemic areas. *Leptospira* spp. has been reported as causing chronic hepatitis without renal involvement, typically with a marked histiocytic response on histology. Diagnosis is challenging because *Leptospira* spp. is not identified with standard culture. Serum antibody titers, eubacterial fluorescent in situ hybridization, or PCR may be necessary for diagnosis.

Viral causes of canine chronic hepatitis appear to be rare, despite early reports of an "acidophil cell hepatitis virus", which was suggested to be the commonest cause of canine CH in Scotland at the time.[4] This contrasts with human hepatitis, where viral causes are common.[5] However, it remains possible that an unidentified virus causes some idiopathic cases of canine CH.

Toxins

Most toxins and drugs cause acute hepatitis (chapter 31), but some of these also have the potential to produce chronic injuries, such as carprofen, oxibendazole, amiodarone, aflatoxin, and cycasin.[6] Lomustine, phenobarbital, primidone, and phenytoin can cause

TABLE 34.1 Infectious organisms that may be associated with granulomatous hepatitis in the dog.*

Organisms		Infectious
Bacterial	*Rhodococcus equi*	Environmental bacteria associated with fatal pyogranulomatous hepatitis.[54]
	Mycobacterial infections (*M. avium* spp.)	Diagnosis: acid-fast cytology/histopathology, PCR, and culture.[54]
	Bartonella spp.	*B. henselae* and *B. clarridgeiae* associated with granulomatous hepatitis and peliosis hepatis.[54]
	Nocardia spp.	Diagnosis: suspicion on cytology and acid-fast staining. Definitive diagnosis requires culture and PCR.[54]
	Brucella canis	Diagnosis: serology, PCR, culture.[54]
	Leptospirosis	Has been detected by FISH and PCR in granulomatous hepatitis with no evidence of renal involvement.[55]
Fungal	*Histoplasma capsulatum*	Soil-borne pathogen endemic in the United States (US), causing primarily respiratory and gastrointestinal signs, but liver dissemination was reported. Diagnosis: cytological identification of yeast-like cells within macrophages.[54]
	Aspergillus spp. (*A. terreus* and *A. deflectus*)	Seen most often as part of multisystemic disseminated disease.[54]
	Prototheca zopfii	Algae found in US with primarily large intestinal and ocular involvement, with hemolymphatic dissemination to the liver.[54]
	Coccidioides immitis	Found in US, Central and South America. Pulmonary signs with dissemination to skin, axial skeleton, CNS, and abdominal viscera. Diagnosis: spherules on cytology/histopathology; serology.[54]
	Blastomyces dermatitidis	US and Canada. Transmitted by inhalation with dissemination to eyes, skin, bone, lymph nodes, and liver.[54]
	Cryptococcus neoformans	Inhalation primary mode of infection, rarely disseminated to liver.[4]
Protozoal	*Leishmania infantum*	Transmitted by the sandfly. Diagnosis: organisms on cytology/histopathology; serology; culture; PCR.[54]
	Hepatozoon americana[4]	Transmitted by *Amblyomma* tick; primary sites of infection cardiac and skeletal muscle. Diagnosis includes PCR.[54]
Parasitic	Visceral larval migrans	*Toxocara canis*, generally pulmonary signs predominate.[54]
	Echinococcus spp.	Alveolar echinococcus can produce cavitated hepatic masses. Diagnosis can be presumptive on ultrasound/CT and cytology of fluid. Histology/PCR for confirmation.[54]
	Dirofilaria immitis	Aberrant adults reported causing hepatic parenchyma granuloma in addition to more common clinical signs.[56]
	Schistosomiasis (*Heterobilharzia americana*)	Endemic in North America, intermediate host is water snail. Diagnosis may be fecal egg examination and cytology/histopathology.[54]

* Many of these cause multisystemic disease, with hepatitis being one of several organs affected. Relevant texts on infectious diseases and laboratories should be consulted on specific diagnostic testing. Copper accumulation, drug reactions, and neoplasia are also reported as potential causes of granulomatous hepatitis and should be considered.[2,3,6]
Adapted from an original table by Katie McCallum.

chronic hepatitis, more commonly as a primary event. Phenobarbital toxicity is important as it is commonly prescribed, used for long-term treatment, and induces hepatobiliary enzymes as a benign effect.[7] This makes deciding if hepatotoxicity is occurring in dogs on treatment more challenging, often relying on indicators of hepatic function, and as a result of this reduced sensitivity, phenobarbital-induced hepatitis may be picked up at a later stage. Phenobarbital toxicity appears dose and duration-dependent. As idiosyncratic drug reactions can occur, a full history of any recent drug administration is important in suspected hepatopathy cases, in addition to any food supplements or alternative therapies that may be used.

Metabolic

Copper-associated hepatitis is discussed in chapter 33. However, copper accumulation also appears to occur concurrently with other causes of chronic hepatitis, including immune-mediated, and in some cases, copper concentrations can be above 1000 µg/g dry weight. Therefore, it is important that each case is thoroughly evaluated, as discussed in chapter 33.

Other metabolic causes appear rare; one colony of German Shepherd dogs was reported with erythropoietic protoporphyria. American and English Cocker Spaniels with chronic hepatitis were reported in one study to have abnormal hepatic deposition of alpha-1 antitrypsin, although they differed from human alpha-1 antitrypsin deficiency in having normal serum concentrations.[8,9]

Immune-mediated

Autoimmune hepatitis is a defined entity in human hepatitis where there are diagnostic criteria, including the presence of interface hepatitis histologically, absence of other known triggers, identification of specific autoantibodies, and response to immunosuppressive medication.[10] In the dog, the occurrence of immune-mediated hepatitis is strongly suspected based on the presence of many of the human criteria in reported cases.[6,11] Consistent with other immune-mediated diseases, there is a female, as well as familial predisposition reported in CH. Associations with specific major histocompatibility complex class II haplotypes have been reported in the Dobermann Pinscher and English Springer Spaniel.[12,13] The presence of autoantibodies has also been reported in the

Dobermann Pinscher and a variety of breeds.[14,15] Lastly, many cases where other causes have been excluded respond to immunosuppressive treatment, such as corticosteroids or cyclosporine.[6,11] It is hoped that immunological testing can be developed and become commercially available to help achieve firm diagnostic criteria and make a definitive diagnosis. At present, this diagnosis is based on a combination of exclusion of other causes, supportive findings, and then response to treatment. Factors that may assist in a tentative clinical diagnosis are listed in Table 34.2.

Idiopathic

Studies show that many canine chronic hepatitis cases remain idiopathic. This likely reflects our limited ability to diagnose the cause as discussed in the previous categories (infectious, toxic, and autoimmune).

Pathophysiology

Once an inflammatory process is started in the parenchyma, generally identified in the periportal regions, there is amplifying of proinflammatory cytokines via Kupffer cell activation and hepatocyte necrosis, which in turn cause an increase in activated myofibroblasts within the hepatic parenchyma. Myofibroblasts are thought to mainly arise from stellate cells, normally quiescent vitamin A-storing cells in the space of Disse, which are activated by inflammation, lose their vitamin A, and transform into contractile, collagen-secreting cells. Potentially, additional myofibroblasts may originate from portal fibroblasts, bone marrow-derived mesenchymal cells, or epithelial to mesenchymal transformation of hepatocytes and cholangiocytes. Myofibroblasts produce collagen and extracellular matrix regardless of origin, leading to fibrosis. Disruption of hepatic architecture from a combination of inflammatory infiltrate, hepatocyte death, and fibrosis leads to intrahepatic cholestasis, and hydrophobic bile acids cause surrounding oxidative damage, further amplifying inflammation. Thus, the process becomes self-perpetuating. Disruption of hepatic architecture by fibrosis limits the ability of surviving hepatocytes to regenerate. Clinical signs are due to a combination of inflammation, fibrosis-producing portal hypertension as well as hepatic insufficiency/failure due to reduced hepatocyte mass.

Systemic consequences of chronic liver disease

The main systemic consequences of chronic liver disease are due to portal hypertension (PH), and at end-stage where there is insufficient hepatocyte mass to maintain liver function. Dogs may also suffer from clinically significant coagulopathies (see below and chapter 24) and from insufficient food intake resulting in protein-calorie malnutrition (see chapter 40 for more details of nutrition in liver disease)

Portal hypertension results from both architectural disruption of normally low resistance hepatic sinusoids by inflammation and fibrotic remodeling, and an increase in dynamic vascular tone due to oxidative damage and inflammatory mediators and myofibroblast contraction. This increase in portal pressure increases upstream splanchnic arterial flow, further contributing to portal pressure and resulting in increased blood volume in the splanchnic vasculature. This reduces effective circulating blood volume, causing renin-angiotensin-aldosterone system

TABLE 34.2 Factors that may increase the index of suspicion of immune-mediated hepatitis.*

- Lymphocytic infiltrate and hepatocyte apoptosis at the limiting plate (see chapter 29 for discussion of biopsy interpretation).
- Female*
- Known breed predisposition –English Springer Spaniel, Dobermann, Cocker Spaniels, Labrador Retriever*
- Familial history of chronic hepatitis where no cause identified
- No other cause identified
- Increased globulins
- Good response to immunosuppressive treatment

*Note that immune-mediated hepatitis can occur in either sex or any breed.

(RAAS) activation, increased antidiuretic hormone release, and increased cardiac output. These factors contribute to a further increase in PH. Increased portal pressure has a number of consequences: predisposing to ascites formation, development of acquired portosystemic shunting, and gastrointestinal ulceration.

Ascites

Increased hydrostatic pressure results in an increased rate of fluid transiting out of the splanchnic vascular bed. If this is higher than lymphatic uptake, ascites results, characterized as a protein-poor or, more commonly, protein-rich transudate. Hypoalbuminemia due to reduced hepatocyte production in advanced cases will potentiate ascites formation due to decreased oncotic pressure. The presence of ascites is a negative prognostic indicator in canine chronic hepatitis.[6] Clinically, it is noted by abdominal swelling (Fig. 34.1A) with a palpable fluid wave or during imaging. Large-volume ascites will contribute to morbidity, and in severe cases, restricts diaphragmatic movement and respiratory capacity. An acute presentation of ascites with abdominal pain and shock should warrant investigation for thrombosis development, particularly in the portal vein. Treatment is detailed later in this chapter. More details on the pathophysiology of ascites in liver disease are found in chapter 24, and the differential diagnoses of ascites are found in chapter 10.

Acquired portosystemic shunts

These are thought to develop from the recruitment of microscopic vessels or *de novo* angiogenesis. The stimulation is not only mechanical, as a result of the PH, but also via increased expression of vascular endothelial growth factors due to hypoxia and inflammation.[16] They connect the portal vein directly to the systemic circulation and are multiple and often tortuous. Their location and site of insertion are variable, making identification challenging. Common locations are around the left kidney, colonic/rectal, or splenic blood vessels. Abdominal ultrasound may identify these, but CT angiography is more sensitive (see chapter 26). These acquired portosystemic shunts result in very similar sequelae and clinical pathology abnormalities to congenital shunts, including hepatic encephalopathy (HE). This is often not recognized in older dogs, and it is important to maintain an index of suspicion for the development of hepatic encephalopathy in chronic hepatitis as low grades have subtle clinical signs and are easily attributed to general illness or ageing (see chapter 7 for more details on the differential diagnosis of hepatic encephalopathy). Medical management of HE with acquired shunts is similar to congenital cases, but bearing in mind that dogs with underlying chronic hepatitis are much more likely to be in negative nitrogen balance and require very careful dietary management (see chapters 36 and 40 for more details). Unlike congenital portosystemic shunts, attenuation is contraindicated due to the presence of PH.

Gastrointestinal ulceration/erosion

The effects of portal hypertension, increased splanchnic flow, inflammatory mediators, disturbances of coagulation status, and not least, if corticosteroids are used, make cases of CH at high risk of gastrointestinal ulceration/erosion (GUE).[17] This can be low-grade and contribute to morbidity with hyporexia, vomiting and anemia, or a potentially catastrophic event. As blood is extremely high in protein, gut bleeding, with subsequent digestion, releases large amounts of ammonia into the portal circulation, which will potentiate an encephalopathic crisis. The risk of GUE is increased with advanced disease. Monitoring for GUE includes teaching owners to recognize melena and hematochezia. It is also helpful to monitor trends in hematology and total protein. Both anemia and microcytosis can be a sign of chronic GI blood loss leading to iron deficiency but are not specific to this (see chapter 24).

Coagulopathy

As hepatocytes produce both pro- and anticoagulants as well as being the site of activation for vitamin K-dependent factors, the equilibrium of hemostasis can be altered unpredictably in chronic hepatitis. Testing specific parts of the clotting cascade will give information on that aspect, not whether there is a hypo- or hypercoagulable state overall. Cases may remain in balance because both pro- and anticoagulants are affected, but they are less able to cope with challenges. More global measures of hemostasis, such as thromboelastography (TEG), may provide a better picture of overall coagulation status. A small study of TEG in canine CH showed cases may be normocoagulable, hypercoagulable, and hypocoagulable.[18] Splanchnic thrombosis is recognized with advanced imaging in CH cases, although at low prevalence. It can contribute significantly to portal hypertension and worsening of ascites.[19] The use of corticosteroids is a risk factor for thrombosis. (See chapters 12 and 24 for more details on coagulation abnormalities in liver disease).

Clinical features

As the liver has a large structural and functional reserve capacity, CH is an insidious disease process where there may be significant ongoing hepatocyte loss and fibrosis with no clinical signs, and increases in liver enzyme activities may be detected incidentally. From postmortem studies, chronic hepatitis appears common, with one study reporting a 12% prevalence in older dogs.[20] In many of these cases, the disease may have been clinically insignificant during the animal's lifespan because of this hepatic reserve. It is important to note that a multitude of extrahepatic diseases can also impact upon the liver and cause increases in enzyme activity as a reactive or secondary event and distinguishing secondary (reactive) hepatitis from primary disease is an important part of the diagnostic workup. As hepatitis produces ongoing hepatocyte loss and architectural disruption progresses, signs are often initially nonspecific, such as lethargy, reduced appetite, GI signs, weight loss, and polyuria/polydipsia.[6] Gradually, as portal hypertension and hepatic insufficiency develop, more specific signs may become apparent, such as jaundice, ascites, or hepatic encephalopathy (Fig. 34.1). Even these may be insidious, or dogs may present apparently acutely due to decompensation. Cholestasis due to architectural disruption and hepatocyte loss leads to hyperbilirubinemia and jaundice. Portal hypertension (PH) occurs due to a combination of increased dynamic vascular tone, myofibroblast contraction, and mechanical obstruction due to inflammation and fibrosis. This increase in hydrostatic pressure can produce ascites as well as predisposing to gastrointestinal ulceration. Hepatic encephalopathy is more likely when acquired portosystemic shunting occurs due to portal hypertension, allowing portal blood into the systemic circulation. Clinical coagulopathy appears less frequent and in the late stage. The end stage of this loss of hepatocyte function and fibrosis is termed cirrhosis.

Lobular dissecting hepatitis, where banding of fibrosis is extensive and disease progression rapid, is more often reported in younger dogs than idiopathic CH, and ascites are common on presentation due to the effect of fibrosis on portal pressure.[21] It is unclear if LDH is a specific disease entity or a different response to a similar insult. Cases with granulomatous hepatitis may be more likely to present with overt clinical signs, including pyrexia and abdominal pain, but this can also be seen

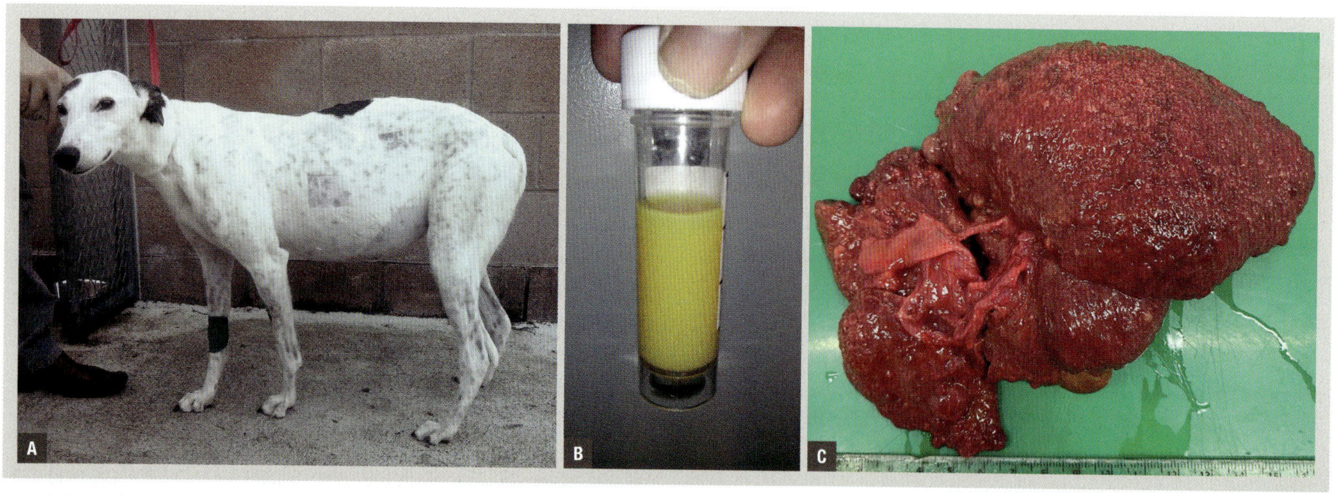

FIG. 34.1 (A) Crossbreed dog with ascites due to portal hypertension as a result of end-stage liver disease (cirrhosis). (B) Urine from the case with yellow opaque color as a result of hyperbilirubinuria and high concentrations of ammonium biurate crystals. After one month, the dog's clinical condition deteriorated acutely due to portal vein thrombosis, and the dog was euthanized. (C) Postmortem image of the cirrhotic liver from the same dog.

in cases of chronic hepatitis.[3,22] Granulomatous hepatitis may be only part of a multisystemic process, and additional body system signs may be present.

Due to the initial occult nature of the process and variability of clinical signs, the index of suspicion of chronic hepatitis is based upon considering multiple pieces of information from the history, clinical examination, and clinical pathology, as well as excluding extrahepatic diseases as potential causes of clinical signs and elevations in hepatobiliary enzymes.

Clinicopathological findings

Clinical pathology derangements can vary depending on the severity of inflammation as well as architectural and hepatic dysfunction (see chapters 24 and 25 for a detailed discussion of laboratory testing).

Serum biochemistry

Hepatocyte necrosis/apoptosis, as well as regeneration, can cause an increase in liver enzyme activity, and this may be the earliest indicator of chronic hepatitis. Increases in alanine aminotransferase (ALT) and aspartate aminotransferase (AST) usually appear first with then subsequent increase in alkaline phosphatase (ALP) and γ-glutaryl transferase (GGT) activities. Although increased hepatic enzymes are a relatively sensitive test for CH (85% ± 16% of published cases identified by the ACVIM Consensus Group had increased ALT), increases are extremely nonspecific. Reactive hepatopathy, endocrinopathies and drug induction can also increase enzyme activities.[6,7,23] The magnitude of the increase in enzyme activity does not relate to prognosis, low-grade hepatocyte necrosis/apoptosis may have been occurring over a long period of time where only moderate elevations in activity are identified, whereas conversely mild diffuse hepatocyte injury, for example, by hypoxia or edema, may cause marked elevation of hepatocellular enzymes. Furthermore, as hepatocyte loss continues and overall hepatocyte mass is decreased, it is possible for enzyme activities to fall within the reference range. Often, in these cases, markers of liver function, such as bile acid stimulation tests or bilirubin, would be abnormal. The approach to the dog with increased serum liver enzymes or bile acids is given in Algorithms 25.1 and 25.2, respectively.

Recently, microRNA-122 has been evaluated as an indicator of hepatocyte injury and appears more sensitive than ALT. However, further studies are required to assess this marker in clinically relevant cases.[24,25]

Markers of reduced liver function become abnormal once reserve capacity has been lost and are not sensitive to early disease. Hyperbilirubinemia is reported in approximately 50% of CH cases.[6] Decreased urea with hyperammonemia, hypoalbuminemia and reduced cholesterol are also indicators of later stage disease due to reduced hepatic synthetic capacity (see chapter 24 for more details). Bile acid stimulation testing would be sensitive when acquired portosystemic shunting has occurred. However, affected dogs also commonly have significant cholestasis (signified by hyperbilirubinemia), which prevents this test from being useful as cholestasis will also cause increased bile acids. More details on the approach to the dog with jaundice are found in chapter 8.

Urinalysis

Polyuria/polydipsia is common in chronic hepatitis with low urine specific gravity. Bilirubinemia will produce bilirubinuria, although up to 1+ bilirubin can be normal in concentrated urine, particularly in male dogs. Ammonium biurate crystals as a consequence of hyperammonemia may be seen in cirrhosis, generally where there are significant acquired portosystemic shunts. More details on urinalysis in liver disease are found in chapter 24.

Hematology

Hematological changes are nonspecific in chronic hepatitis and are described in detail in chapter 24. Anemia may be present, often nonregenerative, due to anemia of inflammatory disease. However, blood loss from gastrointestinal erosion/ulceration may cause regenerative anemia. Acanthocytes and target cells may be seen on a blood film examination due to altered lipid metabolism, but these morphological changes are neither sensitive nor specific for liver disease.[26] Leucocytosis with neutrophilia may be present due to the underlying inflammation, particularly in granulomatous hepatitis. A mild thrombocytopenia is commonly identified.

Diagnostic imaging findings

Imaging to investigate hepatic size and architecture can be helpful as well as assessing signs of portal hypertension, thrombi, and acquired portosystemic shunting (see chapter 26). Ultrasonography is more useful than radiography. Hepatic echogenicity is assessed relative to the spleen (liver normally hypoechoic). In chronic hepatitis, echogenicity is variable; it is most commonly reported to be increased, but it can be decreased, heterogenous, or nodular, or some studies report the majority of cases to be ultrasonographically normal.[27,28] Granulomatous hepatitis may be more often ultrasonographically abnormal, with hepatomegaly and the presence of nodules or hyperechoic bands.[3,28] Acquired shunts may be seen on ultrasound, although this may be challenging.

An end-stage cirrhotic liver may be small and nodular with irregular margins, although some dogs with cirrhosis have a normal hepatic ultrasound. No imaging findings are specific for chronic hepatitis as there is an overlap in appearance between disease processes as well as a large percentage of chronic hepatitis cases with no imaging abnormalities; therefore, imaging alone is never diagnostic.

Contrast CT should be most sensitive at assessing acquired shunts and thrombi, but this has not been reported in a significant number of dogs with CH.[29,30]

Histopathologic findings

Definitive diagnosis of canine chronic hepatitis requires liver biopsy and histopathology. To make the diagnosis, there should be the presence of hepatocyte apoptosis/necrosis as well as a lymphoplasmacytic or histiocytic inflammatory infiltrate with regeneration and fibrosis.[1] Granulomatous hepatitis is defined by the presence of focal aggregates of activated macrophages with an epithelioid appearance alongside lymphocytes, plasma cells, and variable fibroblasts and fibrosis.[31] Laparoscopy is recommended as the method which allows relatively large sample acquisition least invasively (see chapter 27 for more details), although wedge biopsies at laparotomy also give reliable samples. Needle biopsies tend to be smaller and less representative. As the severity of the disease can vary throughout the liver, the recommendation is that at least two lobes are sampled with a minimum of five biopsies. Samples should be submitted for standard histopathology, quantitative copper analysis, as well as aerobic and anaerobic culture. Consideration should be given to snap-freezing a sample if an underlying infectious disease is suspected. As well as standard hematoxylin and eosin (H&E), additional staining should be performed for copper as well as collagen (see chapter 29 for more details on histological sample handling). In cases where granulomatous or pyogranulomatous inflammation is identified on H&E, then further staining and testing for infectious organisms may be advisable (Table 34.1). In addition to the pathological diagnosis, it is important that the report scores cell type and degree of inflammation as well as fibrosis and copper staining location and copper semiquantitative score (see chapter 29 for more details on interpretation of biopsy reports).

Management of chronic hepatitis

Management of chronic hepatitis involves treatment of the cause whenever possible, together with supportive and symptomatic treatment as necessary. Please refer to Algorithm 34.1 for an approach to management.

Algorithm 34.1 Note 1 The most effective way of reducing and potentially reversing inflammation and fibrosis is to treat the underlying cause. Therefore, although many cases of chronic liver disease are idiopathic, where there is no specific treatment, it is important that cases where there is an underlying cause are not missed, such as hepatotoxic supplements or medications (like phenobarbital, lomustine or nonsteroidal anti-inflammatories).

Algorithm 34.1 Note 2 It is also important that copper-associated hepatitis, where inflammation is driven by copper deposition, is not overlooked. If the pathologist has not performed a copper stain on the biopsy and given a semiquantitative analysis, these should be requested (see chapter 33 for more details on diagnosis and treatment of copper-associated chronic hepatitis).

Algorithm 34.1 Note 3 In cases where there is a granulomatous or neutrophilic component to the inflammation, potential infectious diseases should be thoroughly investigated based upon endemic prevalence and travel history (Table 34.1), although some cases of granulomatous hepatitis appear idiopathic and respond to immunosuppressive treatment.[3]

Algorithm 34.1 Note 4 If an immune-mediated disease is suspected based on histology and ruling out other causes, then a trial of immunosuppressive medication, carefully monitored, is indicated. Immunosuppressives should never be used without histology as their use in infectious cases or animals with severe noninflammatory fibrosis, such as ductal plate malformation, is not only inappropriate but also potentially dangerous. Medications which may be used are detailed below.

Algorithm 34.1 Note 5 After potential inciting causes have been excluded as much as possible, treatment of chronic hepatitis can be divided into three main sections; hepatosupportive therapy to try and maintain existing hepatocytes as well as support any regenerative process, and symptomatic management of the consequences of chronic liver disease. Medication that is antifibrotic or ideally reverses fibrosis would be a holy grail as scarring affects function as well as the ability of the remaining hepatocytes to regenerate. However, no proven antifibrotic has yet been identified. Colchicine, which was previously used as an antifibrotic in canine CH, is not recommended due to a lack of evidence of efficacy, coupled with the high likelihood of side effects. At present, the evidence base for the medications currently used for canine liver disease is very limited. As a result, the potential benefits of medication need to be judged against the potential for side effects as well as the cost of the treatment for the owners. Nutrition is also a crucial cornerstone in managing chronic hepatitis cases, as discussed in chapter 40. Details of supportive treatment are found below.

Algorithm 34.1 Note 6 Clinical and clinicopathological monitoring of response to treatment is important. Noninvasive monitoring by repeat measurement of liver enzymes can be challenging, particularly if prednisolone treatment is used, as discussed below. Nonetheless, if enzymes increase markedly on treatment, the diagnosis should be reconsidered. The gold standard for monitoring response is a repeat liver biopsy, but this is rarely performed.

Immunosuppressive medication

Glucocorticoids (licensed for use in dogs)

Prednisolone has been the standard immunosuppressive treatment in canine chronic hepatitis and has the largest evidence base, although the retrospective nature and differing inclusion criteria of published studies make the evidence base still weak. Nonetheless, clinical, biochemical, and histopathological improvements are reported with the use of prednisolone in many dogs.[32-34] The difference in results between dogs and studies likely represents the difficulty in definitive diagnosis of immune-mediated hepatitis in dogs and underlines the importance of careful monitoring of clinical and biochemical response in treated animals. Reported doses also varied between immunosuppressive (2.2 mg/kg) and anti-inflammatory (0.5 mg/kg per day), but the ACVIM consensus group recommends starting with a dose of 2 mg/kg once a day.

The potentially beneficial action of prednisolone needs to be weighed against the risk of very significant adverse effects. particularly in dogs with extensive fibrosis and portal hypertension. The use of corticosteroids in the presence of gastrointestinal erosion/ulceration has the greatest potential to be catastrophic. As well as life-threatening gastrointestinal bleeding, this can also potentiate hepatic encephalopathy in dogs with acquired portosystemic shunts. This could be misinterpreted as a worsening of the liver disease when, in fact, it is iatrogenic. Other significant adverse effects are that they are catabolic and can significantly reduce muscle mass as well as cause fluid retention, which may exacerbate ascites. Glucocorticoids also predispose to hypercoagulability, and some chronic hepatitis cases will already be hypercoagulable. Another complicating factor in using glucocorticoids is that they will induce hepatic enzymes, particularly alkaline phosphatase, thus making it more difficult to monitor response to treatment with this drug noninvasively; see monitoring of the efficacy of immunosuppressive treatment below. The decision to treat with prednisolone should be carefully considered in each individual case and based upon biopsy results, which show a significant inflammatory infiltrate. The ACVIM consensus on treatment recommends a starting dose of prednisolone/prednisone at 2 mg/kg/day with the aim to taper to every other day treatment at 0.5 mg/kg. Other authors have suggested a 1 mg/kg dose, which could be titrated up if required in nonresponders.[35] In cases where there are concerns over the risk of side effects, particularly gastrointestinal hemorrhage (evidence of portal hypertension), it might be wiser to choose cyclosporine as a first-line treatment (see below) or use the lower end of the prednisolone dose range and titrate up if required. Alternatively, consideration could be given to adding a second immunosuppressive medication in the hope that this allows faster dose titration of glucocorticoid and maintenance

ALGORITHM 34.1

Approach to the treatment of chronic hepatitis.

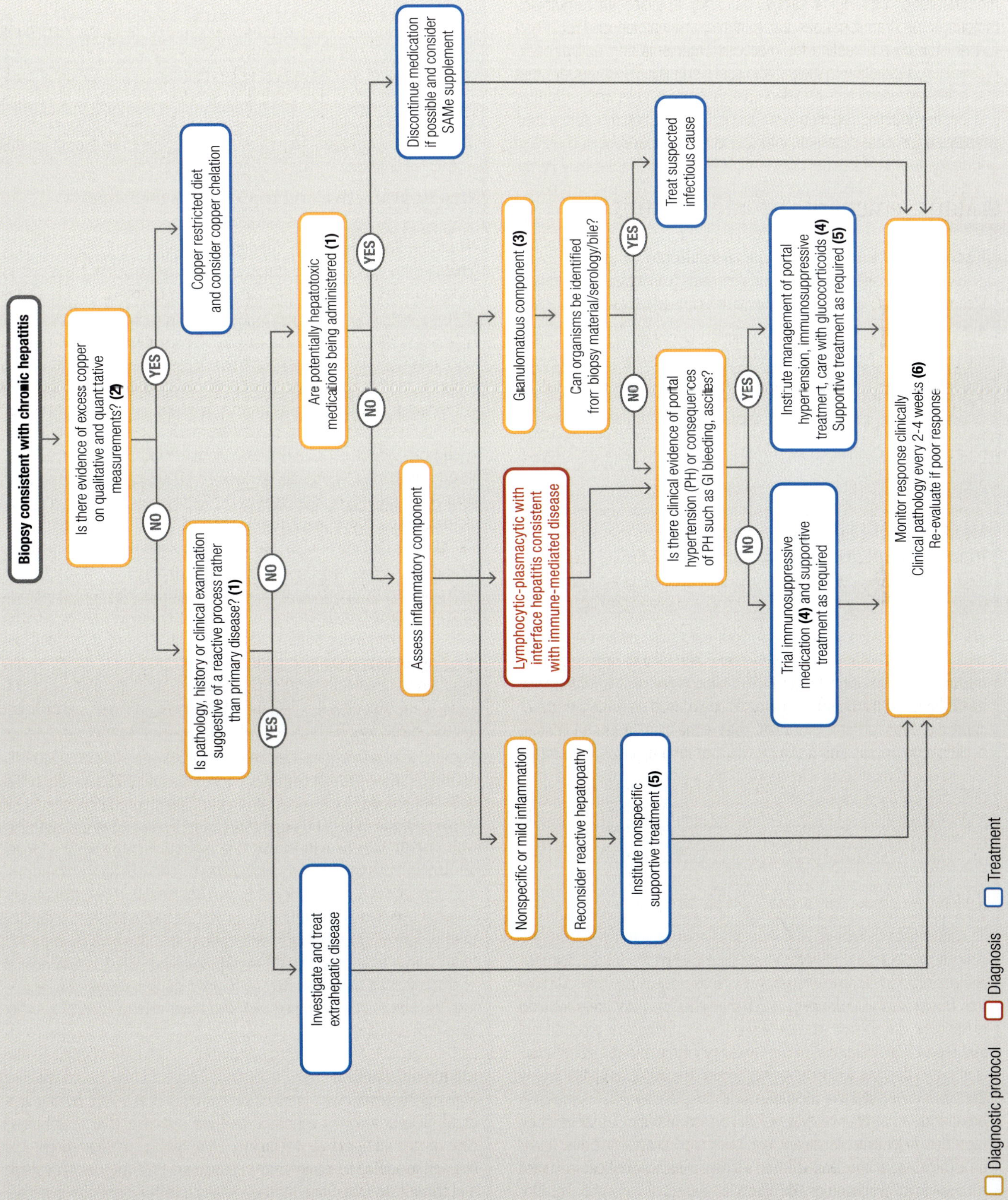

on the second drug to minimize adverse glucocorticoid effects. The use of dexamethasone has been recommended in cases where there is ascites present, as this drug has no mineralocorticoid activity.[6]

Cyclosporine (licensed for use in dogs for skin disease)

There is one case series of 48 dogs with idiopathic hepatitis treated with cyclosporine twice daily, where a good response was reported in 79% of dogs.[36] Common side effects are reduced appetite, vomiting, and diarrhea, as well as gingival hyperplasia. This could be considered as a single agent to avoid glucocorticoid side effects, particularly in dogs with suspected immune-mediated disease but marked fibrosis and portal hypertension.[6] Studies comparing cyclosporine and glucocorticoid efficacy in suspected immune-mediated hepatitis cases are needed. Cyclosporine may be the preferable option as it does not induce hepatobiliary enzymes and potentially has more benign side effects.

Mycophenolate (not licensed for use in dogs)

This has been used both in combination with prednisolone and also as a single agent at 10 mg/kg q12h initially.[6,37] Gastrointestinal side effects are most common.

Azathioprine (not licensed for use in dogs)

This has been reported anecdotally as another second-line treatment used at 2 mg/kg once daily for 14 days, then tapered to every second day with prednisolone.[6,38] However, it is reported to cause elevations of hepatobiliary enzymes and hepatotoxicity. Therefore, azathioprine may not be an ideal drug to select if there are the above alternatives.[39]

Monitoring the efficacy of immunosuppressive treatments

Monitoring response to treatment noninvasively is challenging, particularly as glucocorticoids induce hepatic enzymes. All hepatobiliary enzymes are affected by glucocorticoids from both induction and development of vacuolar hepatopathy. Generally, alkaline phosphatase and γ-glutaryl transferase activity are most affected, while alanine aminotransferase is less affected. Despite this, particularly if hepatobiliary enzymes are significantly increased prior to treatment, then serial monitoring can demonstrate a reduction in activity which can then be tracked as prednisolone is tapered.[32] If markers of liver function are abnormal at diagnosis, then these can also be tracked to assess if an improvement in function occurs. A marked rise in alanine aminotransferase after starting prednisolone or other immunosuppressive medication should trigger a reappraisal of other potential causes and tapering of the dose.

Repeat liver biopsy provides the most definitive evidence of control of the inflammatory infiltrate and stage of the disease process. This can be challenging to achieve as owners are understandably reluctant. Explaining the potential need for repeat biopsy when the initial diagnosis is discussed and the use of less invasive biopsy techniques (laparoscopy) may improve uptake. However, as serial biopsies are potentially required to monitor the disease process fully, this is difficult to recommend, and repeat biopsy is usually reserved for problematic cases. Many cases continue with long-term immunosuppressive treatment, partly due to the progressive nature of the disease and the difficulty of noninvasively monitoring what is occurring within the parenchyma. In these cases, the aim is to taper medication to the lowest apparent effective dose based on clinical signs and liver enzyme activity: ideally, every other day for corticosteroids to minimize side effects.

Supportive and symptomatic treatment

It is intuitive that the earlier cases of chronic hepatitis are diagnosed, then, the greater the remaining hepatic capacity, and if the disease can be controlled, the better the prognosis. This is true where the cause can be identified and effectively treated, such as copper storage disease and immune-mediated disease. Unfortunately, idiopathic disease may be progressive despite management, but immunosuppressive treatment has been shown to improve prognosis in a subset of cases, suggesting some are immune-mediated (see previous section).[6] In cases where the liver is cirrhotic or "end-stage" and inflammation is minimal, management is directed at controlling the clinical consequences of hepatic failure to improve quality of life and general benign hepatoprotective treatments.

Hepatoprotective and antioxidant measures

Ursodeoxycholic acid

This is a hydrophilic bile acid with many potential or theoretical benefits, including displacement of more hepatotoxic hydrophobic bile acids, choleretic, antiapoptotic, and antioxidant effects.[40] It is particularly indicated where there is cholestasis associated with chronic hepatitis and is generally well tolerated with occasionally nausea and diarrhea seen as side effects. It is used widely for choleretic effect as cholestasis is common and can potentially reduce injury from hydrophobic bile acids due to displacement. The dose is 15 mg/kg once daily with food.[6]

Antioxidants

No studies yet show the benefit of antioxidants in chronic hepatitis. However, inflammation, as well as necrosis, will produce oxidative damage, and there is evidence that some chronic hepatitis cases are depleted in hepatic antioxidants.[41] Therefore, various nutraceuticals are used in an attempt to preserve hepatocytes on this basis. They are generally well tolerated. The main disadvantages are the cost and additional effort in administration.

S-adenosylmethionine (SAMe)

This is produced by healthy hepatocytes from methionine and is a precursor in the pathway to glutathione (GSH) production. GSH is hepatoprotective by virtue of its antioxidant properties.[42] SAMe also regulates hepatocyte growth and has also been shown to be antiapoptotic.[42] In liver disease, it is possible that both SAMe and GSH concentrations may be reduced. One study has demonstrated reduced liver concentrations of GSH in a proportion of hepatitis/cirrhosis cases.[41] Various salts are available, with phytate salt thought to have the highest bioavailability. As these are generally classed as food supplements rather than pharmaceuticals, licensing and quality control can be variable, so reliable manufacturers who have data on concentration, as well as bioavailability, should be used. A dose of 20 mg/kg daily on an empty stomach is recommended.[6] Preparations may combine SAMe and silymarin. There is no evidence of efficacy in chronic liver disease, but one study assessing the hepatotoxicity of lomustine demonstrated a hepatoprotective effect of a SAMe/silymarin combination.[43]

Silymarin/silibinin

Phosphatidyl-complexed preparations improve bioavailability, but generally, bioavailability is poor, and half-life is very short. Therefore, it is unknown if any preparations achieve therapeutic concentrations. The dose of phosphatidyl-complexed ranges from 0.7-6 mg/kg once daily, and native extract, 4-8 mg/kg/day, divided into 2-3 doses.[6] The potential beneficial effects are antioxidant, antifibrotic, immunomodulatory, and choleretic.[6] Again, it is generally well tolerated, although it can inhibit cytochrome enzymes and P-glycoprotein transport. Thus, there is a theoretical risk of affecting concurrent drug metabolism.

Vitamin E

This can act as an intracellular antioxidant. There is one small study demonstrating that vitamin E supplementation in dogs with chronic hepatitis increased hepatic concentrations of vitamin E as well as increased antioxidant ability.[44] It is relatively cheap and very well tolerated; despite scant evidence base of clinical efficacy it is widely used. The dose is 10 IU/kg once daily with food up to a maximum of 400 IU/dog.[6]

Symptomatic management of the clinical consequences of chronic hepatitis

Ascites management

As increased vascular resistance is the cause of ascites, then ideally, the cause of this is targeted. Fibrosis is generally irreversible, and this is difficult to achieve unless increased vascular resistance is caused by inflammatory infiltrate, thrombosis, or dynamic vascular tone. Potentially, there are medications to target dynamic vascular tone, as well as constrict splanchnic vasculature, but to date, these are not reported in veterinary medicine, and there is no evidence of their efficacy. It is also unknown if treating portal hypertension prior to the development of ascites is beneficial. Although sodium-restricted diets have been recommended, these reduce palatability, so at least high-sodium foods should be avoided. Nutrition in chronic liver disease is covered in chapter 40. The mainstay of treatment of ascites is diuresis.

Diuretics

The aldosterone antagonist spironolactone is most commonly used. This directly counteracts the activation of RAAS, which is central to ascites formation. Experimentally, spironolactone has also been shown to reduce fibrosis and downregulate growth factors which potentiate angiogenesis and hypertension, potentially providing additional benefits.[45] The clinical efficacy is slow, with full effects not seen for up to 2 weeks. Standard initial dosing is 1-2 mg/kg q24h. If required, this can be titrated up every 4 days to 4 mg/kg. In cases where a more rapid effect is needed or control is not achieved, furosemide may be added (0.5-1 mg/kg/day).[6]

Monitoring diuretic use

Body weight is an easy objective measure of efficacy, aiming for a 0.5-1% reduction per day. Abdominal girth will also give an indication, and measuring this can be taught to owners. There is a risk of hypovolemia and electrolyte disturbances, particularly when furosemide is used, so PCV, total protein, creatinine, and electrolytes should be monitored. If ascites can be controlled, then the diuretic dose can often be tapered, potentially to spironolactone alone and every-other-day dosing.

Therapeutic drainage

In severe or refractory cases of ascites, particularly where there is respiratory capacity compromise, then therapeutic drainage can be considered, up to 50% of estimated volume. Diuretics should always be used if abdominocentesis is performed to try to minimize refilling. Sudden reduction in abdominal pressure will allow an increase in splanchnic blood capacity with the risk of circulatory collapse. If significant volumes need to be removed, then heart rate and blood pressure should be monitored during and after drainage. Intravenous crystalloids or colloids are often indicated to support circulating volume during drainage. There is a risk of significantly worsening hypoalbuminemia, particularly with high-volume paracentesis, and albumin should be checked prior to and 24 hours after drainage, and consideration should be given to intravenous replacement if it drops significantly.

Gastrointestinal ulceration/erosion management

Management of suspected GUE is with a combination of omeprazole (1 mg/kg q12h PO) and sucralfate (¼ to 1 g q8h PO). These should be used where there is evidence of active bleeding. There is evidence from healthy research dogs that prophylactic coadministration of omeprazole with prednisone at 2 mg/kg reduced endoscopic scoring of GUE compared to the use of prednisone in isolation.[46] However, in that study, diarrhea occurred more frequently in the omeprazole-treated group, and the authors did not recommend its use in dogs with diseases until further studies were undertaken. Proton pump inhibitors have been shown to increase the risk of decompensation and mortality in human cirrhotic patients. Therefore, the prophylactic use is not recommended in canine chronic hepatitis cases. Medications that can cause GUE should be avoided, particularly NSAIDs. Steroids can also precipitate GUE in animals with portal hypertension, as discussed above, so they should be avoided in high-risk animals unless absolutely necessary. GUE can also be precipitated or worsened by coagulopathy in CH. See Management of coagulopathies below.

Management of coagulopathies

Hypocoagulability criteria for assessing coagulation prior to biopsy are discussed in chapter 24. If no interventions are planned and there is no evidence of clinical bleeding, treating abnormal lab numbers is not required, particularly if lab assessment is selective, as pro- and anticoagulant factors produced by the liver are often equally affected. Two small studies suggest that the risk of bleeding that required clinical intervention after an ultrasound or laparoscopic biopsy is low (2-4%), and the risk of hemorrhage could not be predicted from prior coagulation testing.[47,48] Spontaneous bleeding is uncommon in CH, but potentially catastrophic gastrointestinal hemorrhage can occur, particularly in cirrhosis, due to the risk factors of PH, fragile rebalanced coagulation, and use of ulcerogenic drugs, particularly corticosteroids. If there is active bleeding, either spontaneous or after biopsy, management is generally to use fresh frozen plasma if PT and aPTT are prolonged or whole blood if red cell replacement is also needed. Many cases of CH are anemic, which may be a combination of anemia of inflammatory disease and chronic GUE bleeding. As a result, relatively small amounts of acute blood loss may result in clinical transfusion triggers where whole blood would be indicated.

Hypercoagulability

There is no evidence that treating the abnormal numbers is warranted for dogs in a hypercoagulable state. Treatment is recommended for cases where a thrombus is documented and thought to be clinically important (e.g., acute onset clinical signs or portal-vein thrombosis [PVT] contributing to PH). One study has shown improved survival of cases where anticoagulants were used in PVT. However, only about half of the cases had chronic liver disease.[49] The ideal anticoagulant regime is unknown. Clopidogrel has been recommended, and concurrent low molecular weight heparins have been used.[49,50] The author would advise against the use of rivaroxaban in chronic hepatitis at present, as the majority of the drug is metabolized by hepatocytes, and the dose/response is very variable in dogs with normal hepatic function.[51] Rivaroxaban is not recommended in humans with advanced liver disease, and it has been reported in rare cases to cause acute hepatocellular injury in humans.[52,53]

Prognosis with the treatment of canine chronic hepatitis

For cases where an underlying infectious organism is identified, then the prognosis will be variable depending on the severity of the disease and if hepatitis is just one of a constellation of multiorgan involvement. If the infectious organism can be cleared before there is end-stage cirrhosis, and the hepatic parenchyma can regenerate, the prognosis may be good. Likewise, the prognosis can be good with immune-mediated chronic hepatitis effectively treated and also with copper storage disease if it is diagnosed and treated before end stage (see chapter 33).

For idiopathic chronic hepatitis, the disease is often progressive, and although the current standard of care does appear to improve survival times. Ultimately, cases often die or are euthanized due to hepatic failure or complications because of portal hypertension.

Prognostic indicators

The parameters described below can also be used to provide a guide to prognosis, but it is important to remember that for the individual, CH prognosis is highly variable. This likely reflects differences between etiopathogenesis (which is unknown), severity of the disease when diagnosed, severity of inflammation and ongoing necrosis, and location of fibrosis and individual response to treatment. Additionally, although multiple biopsies should be obtained, they still may not represent the global disease process and may over or underestimate the severity of inflammation and stage of disease.

Histopathology

From retrospective studies, histopathological documentation of cirrhosis in dogs with CH gave a very poor prognosis with a mean survival of 23 days compared to the overall median survival of CH cases of 561 days.[6] Additionally, the diagnosis of lobular dissecting hepatitis gave a survival time of only 48 ± 38 days, although these case numbers were very small.[6] A small retrospective study of granulomatous hepatitis demonstrated a similar survival time (median 635 days) to lymphoplasmacytic idiopathic CH.[3]

Clinical and clinicopathological parameters

Clinicopathological prognostic parameters described from retrospective case series most likely reflect the fact that hepatic reserve capacity has been lost and the dog is in hepatic failure as well as potentially a proinflammatory state.[6] Negative prognostic indicators reported include increased PT and aPTT, thrombocytopenia, hypoalbuminemia, hyperbilirubinemia, hyperglobulinemia, and neutropenia. Ascites has been reported as a negative prognostic indicator likely reflecting the development of portal hypertension in more end-stage disease.

KEY POINTS

- Diagnosis of chronic hepatitis (CH) requires histopathological examination of samples from multiple liver lobes. It is defined by hepatocyte apoptosis or necrosis with an inflammatory infiltrate.
- Diagnostic imaging findings of the liver in CH cases are very variable, and cases can appear to have normal hepatic size and architecture.
- Potential CH cases should be thoroughly evaluated for potential underlying causes, which include toxins, infectious, immune-mediated, and metabolic. It is important that copper-associated disease is excluded as this requires specific management.
- Some cases of CH appear idiopathic. These may have an as-yet unrecognized etiology.
- Due to the large reserve capacity of the liver, cases with CH may be asymptomatic, and only an increase in hepatobiliary enzymes may be detected initially. Nonspecific signs include lethargy, reduced appetite/weight loss, vomiting, diarrhea and polyuria and polydipsia.
- More specific signs are seen because of hepatic insufficiency and portal hypertension: jaundice, ascites, gastrointestinal ulceration/erosion, and hepatic encephalopathy.
- The underlying cause of CH should be resolved or managed where identified (toxins, infectious organisms), or suspected (immune-mediated disease).
- Further management of CH cases involves general hepato-supportive measures such as ursodeoxycholic acid and antioxidants, as well as treating the consequences of portal hypertension.

References

1. van den Ingh TSGAM, Van Winkle T, Cullen JM, et al. Morphological classification of parenchymal disorders of the canine and feline liver: 2. Hepatocellular death, hepatitis, and cirrhosis. In Group WSAVALS, editors. WSAVA Standards for Clinical and Histological Diagnosis of Canine and Feline Liver Disease. Edinburgh, Saunders/Elsevier, 2006, pp. 117-124.
2. Hutchins RG, Breitschwerdt EB, Cullen JM, et al. Limited yield of diagnoses of intrahepatic infectious causes of canine granulomatous hepatitis from archival liver tissue. *J Vet Diagn Invest* 24:888-894, 2012.
3. Prentice KD, Callahan-Clark JE, Parry NM, et al. Characterization of clinical presentation, histological features, ultrasonographic findings, and survival in 29 dogs with granulomatous hepatitis. *J Vet Intern Med* 38(1):167-175, 2024.
4. Jarrett WF, O'Neil BW, Lindholm I. Persistent hepatitis and chronic fibrosis induced by canine acidophil cell hepatitis virus. *Vet Rec* 120:234-235, 1987.
5. Bexfield NH, Watson PJ, Heaney J, et al. Canine hepacivirus is not associated with chronic liver disease in dogs. *J Viral Hepat* 21:223-228, 2014.
6. Webster CRL, Center SA, Cullen JM, et al. ACVIM consensus statement on the diagnosis and treatment of chronic hepatitis in dogs. *J Vet Intern Med* 33:1173-1200, 2019.
7. Dayrell-Hart B, Steinberg SA, VanWinkle TJ, et al. Hepatotoxicity of phenobarbital in dogs: 18 cases (1985-1989). *J Am Vet Med Assoc* 199:1060-1066, 1991.
8. Kroeze EJ, Zentek J, Edixhoven-Bosdijk A, et al. Transient erythropoietic protoporphyria associated with chronic hepatitis and cirrhosis in a cohort of German Shepherd dogs. *Vet Rec* 158:120-124, 2006.
9. Sevelius E, Andersson M, Jonsson L. Hepatic accumulation of alpha-1-antitrypsin in chronic liver disease in the dog. *J Comp Pathol* 111:401-412, 1994.
10. Johnson PJ, McFarlane IG. Meeting report: International Autoimmune Hepatitis Group. *Hepatology* 18:998-1005, 1993.
11. Shropshire S, Ullal T. Diagnosis and treatment of immune-mediated and copper-associated chronic hepatitis. In ECVIM-CA Annual Congress Proceedings, Barcelona, 2023.
12. Bexfield NH, Watson PJ, Aguirre-Hernandez J, et al. DLA class II alleles and haplotypes are associated with risk for and protection from chronic hepatitis in the English Springer spaniel. *PLoS One* 7:e42584, 2012.
13. Speeti M, Stahls A, Meri S, et al. Upregulation of major histocompatibility complex class II antigens in hepatocytes in Doberman hepatitis. *Vet Immunol Immunopathol* 96:1-12, 2003.
14. Dyggve H, Jarva H, Spillmann T, et al. Identification of glyceraldehyde-3-phosphate and alcohol dehydrogenases as autoantigens in Doberman hepatitis. *Scand J Immunol* 86:156-164, 2017.
15. Weiss DJ, Armstrong PJ, Mruthyunjaya A. Anti-liver membrane protein antibodies in dogs with chronic hepatitis. *J Vet Intern Med* 9:267-271, 1995.
16. Coulon S, Heindryckx F, Geerts A, et al. Angiogenesis in chronic liver disease and its complications. *Liver Int* 31:146-162, 2011.
17. O'Kell AL, Gallagher AE, Cooke KL. Gastroduodenal ulceration in dogs with liver disease. *J Vet Intern Med* 36:986-992, 2022.
18. Fry W, Lester C, Etedali NM, et al. Thromboelastography in dogs with chronic hepatopathies. *J Vet Intern Med* 31:419-426, 2017.
19. Droes FC, Suchodolski JS, Steiner JM, et al. Prevalence of portal vein and splanchnic venous thrombosis in dogs with chronic hepatitis. *J Small Anim Pract* 64:375-383, 2023.
20. Watson PJ, Roulois AJ, Scase TJ, et al. Prevalence of hepatic lesions at post-mortem examination in dogs and association with pancreatitis. *J Small Anim Pract* 51:566-572, 2010.
21. van den Ingh TS, Rothuizen J. Lobular dissecting hepatitis in juvenile and young adult dogs. *J Vet Intern Med* 8:217-220, 1994.
22. Bexfield NH, Andres-Abdo C, Scase TJ, et al. Chronic hepatitis in the English springer spaniel: clinical presentation, histological description and outcome. *Vet Rec* 169:415, 2011.
23. Hall EJ, German AJ. Laboratory evaluation of hepatic disease. In Villiers E, Ristić J (editors). BSAVA Manual of Canine and Feline Clinical Pathology. British Small Animal Veterinary Association, 2016, pp. 237-261.
24. Oosthuyzen W, Ten Berg PWL, Francis B, et al. Sensitivity and specificity of microRNA-122 for liver disease in dogs. *J Vet Intern Med* 32:1637-1644, 2018.
25. Dirksen K, Verzijl T, van den Ingh TS, et al. Hepatocyte-derived microRNAs as sensitive serum biomarkers of hepatocellular injury in Labrador retrievers. *Vet J* 211:75-81, 2016.
26. Warry E, Bohn A, Emanuelli M, et al. Disease distribution in canine patients with acanthocytosis: 123 cases. *Vet Clin Pathol* 42:465-470, 2013.
27. Gaschen L. Update on hepatobiliary imaging. *Vet Clin North Am Small Anim Pract* 39:439-467, 2009.
28. Kemp SD, Panciera DL, Larson MM, et al. A comparison of hepatic sonographic features and histopathologic diagnosis in canine liver disease: 138 cases. *J Vet Intern Med* 27:806-813, 2013.
29. Hostnik ET, Parker VJ, Cullen JM. Computed tomography of lobular dissecting hepatitis in a young Golden Retriever. *J Am Anim Hosp Assoc* 55:e55203, 2019.
30. Bertolini G. Acquired portal collateral circulation in the dog and cat. *Vet Radiol Ultrasound* 51:25-33, 2010.
31. Van Winkle T, Cullen JM, van den Ingh TSGAM, et al. Morphological classification of parenchymal disorders of the canine and feline liver: 3. Hepatic abscesses and granulomas, hepatic metabolic storage disorders and miscellaneous conditions. In Group WSAVALS (editor). WSAVA Standards for Clinical and Histological Diagnosis of Canine and Feline Liver Disease. Edinburgh, Elsevier Saunders, 2006, pp.103-116.
32. Bayton W, Watson PJ, Bexfield NH. Prednisolone therapy for chronic hepatitis in English springer spaniels: a prospective study of 12 cases. *Vet Rec* 186:e21, 2020.
33. Strombeck DR, Miller LM, Harrold D. Effects of corticosteroid treatment on survival time in dogs with chronic hepatitis: 151 cases (1977-1985). *J Am Vet Med Assoc* 193:1109-1113, 1988.
34. Favier RP, Poldervaart JH, van den Ingh TS, et al. A retrospective study of oral prednisolone treatment in canine chronic hepatitis. *Vet Quart* 33:113-120, 2013.
35. Bexfield N. Canine idiopathic chronic hepatitis. *Vet Clin North Am Small Anim Pract* 47:645-663, 2017.
36. Ullal T, Ambrosini Y, Rao S, et al. Retrospective evaluation of cyclosporine in the treatment of presumed idiopathic chronic hepatitis in dogs. *J Vet Intern Med* 33:2046-2056, 2019.
37. Beehler MK, Kearns SA, Crouse ZJ. Mycophenolate mofetil as a treatment for presumed idiopathic chronic hepatitis in dogs: Six cases (2010-2022). *Vet Med Sci* 9:2527-2533, 2023.
38. Honeckman A. Current concepts in the treatment of canine chronic hepatitis. *Clin Tech Small Anim Pract* 18:239-244, 2003.
39. Wallisch K, Trepanier LA. Incidence, timing, and risk factors of azathioprine hepatotoxicosis in dogs. *J Vet Intern Med* 29:513-518, 2015.
40. Beuers U, Trauner M, Jansen P, et al. New paradigms in the treatment of hepatic cholestasis: from UDCA to FXR, PXR and beyond. *J Hepatol* 62:S25-37, 2015.
41. Center SA, Warner KL, Erb HN. Liver glutathione concentrations in dogs and cats with naturally occurring liver disease. *Am J Vet Res* 63:1187-1197, 2002.
42. Mato JM, Lu SC. Role of S-adenosyl-L-methionine in liver health and injury. *Hepatology* 45:1306-1312, 2007.
43. Skorupski KA, Hammond GM, Irish AM, et al. Prospective randomized clinical trial assessing the efficacy of Denamarin for prevention of CCNU-induced hepatopathy in tumor-bearing dogs. *J Vet Intern Med* 25:838-845, 2011.
44. Twedt D, Webb C, Tetrick MJJVIM. The effect of dietary vitamin E on the clinical laboratory and oxidant status of dogs with chronic hepatitis. *J Vet Intern Med* 17:418A, 2003.
45. Hsu SJ, Wang SS, Huo TI, et al. The impact of spironolactone on the severity of portal-systemic

collaterals and hepatic encephalopathy in cirrhotic rats. *J Pharmacol Exp Ther* 355:117-124, 2015.
46. Rak MB, Moyers TD, Price JM, et al. Clinicopathologic and gastrointestinal effects of administration of prednisone, prednisone with omeprazole, or prednisone with probiotics to dogs: A double-blind randomized trial. *J Vet Intern Med* 37:465-475, 2023.
47. Reece J, Pavlick M, Penninck DG, et al. Hemorrhage and complications associated with percutaneous ultrasound-guided liver biopsy in dogs. *J Vet Intern Med* 34:2398-2404, 2020.
48. Petre SL, McClaran JK, Bergman PJ, et al. Safety and efficacy of laparoscopic hepatic biopsy in dogs: 80 cases (2004-2009). *J Am Vet Med Assoc* 240:181-185, 2012.
49. Respess M, O'Toole TE, Taeymans O, et al. Portal vein thrombosis in 33 dogs: 1998-2011. *J Vet Intern Med* 26:230-237, 2012.
50. Webster CR. Hemostatic disorders associated with hepatobiliary disease. *Vet Clin North Am Small Anim Pract* 47:601-615, 2017.
51. Lynch AM, Ruterbories LK, Griffith EH, et al. Evaluation of point-of-care coagulation tests as alternatives to anti-Xa activity for monitoring the anticoagulant effects of rivaroxaban in healthy dogs. *J Vet Emerg Crit Care (San Antonio)* 31:18-24, 2021.
52. Licata A, Puccia F, Lombardo V, et al. Rivaroxaban-induced hepatotoxicity: review of the literature and report of new cases. *Eur J Gastroenterol Hepatol* 30:226-232, 2018.
53. Qamar A, Vaduganathan M, Greenberger NJ, et al. Oral anticoagulation in patients with liver disease. *J Am Coll Cardiol* 71:2162-2175, 2018.
54. Sykes JE. Greene's Infectious Diseases of the Dog and Cat. E-Book. Elsevier Health Sciences, 2022.
55. McCallum KE, Constantino-Casas F, Cullen JM, et al. Hepatic leptospiral infections in dogs without obvious renal involvement. *J Vet Intern Med* 33:141-150, 2019.
56. Goggin JM, Biller DS, Rost CM, et al. Ultrasonographic identification of *Dirofilaria immitis* in the aorta and liver of a dog. *J Am Vet Med Assoc* 210:1635-1637, 1997.

CHAPTER 35

Gallbladder and biliary tract diseases: mucoceles, biliary tract, and gallbladder infections

Ben Harris
MA, VetMB, CertSAM, FLS, DECVIM-CA (Internal Medicine), MRCVS

Function of the biliary system

The primary function of bile and its constituents is to facilitate the digestion and absorption of lipids. Further functions include the buffering of acids in the proximal duodenum and the excretion of metabolites and xenobiotics. Further details of the composition and function of bile are found in chapter 30.

Before secretion, bile acids are bound with taurine or glycine to form "conjugated bile acids" which allow them to be readily ionized to anions known as "bile salts". In their anionic state, they are not readily absorbed until they reach sodium-bile salt cotransporters in the distal small intestine, by which time they have fulfilled their function. The vast majority (>95%) of bile salts are reabsorbed in this way, entering the hepatic portal circulation and then being reabsorbed by the hepatocytes –known as "enterohepatic recirculation" of bile acids (Fig. 30.4). If liver function or portal blood flow is impaired then there may be a failure of reabsorption of bile acids from the portal blood, resulting in bile acids reaching the systemic circulation: these bile acids can be detected on biochemical laboratory tests, as a marker of hepatic function (see chapter 25).

Bile is continuously synthesized and secreted by hepatocytes and stored in the gallbladder during fasting periods. Feeding triggers gallbladder contraction and relaxation of the sphincter of Oddi at the duodenal papilla by the release of acetylcholine from cholinergic parasympathetic nerve fibers as well as cholecystokinin (CCK) and motilin from duodenal endocrine cells. The parasympathetic response is triggered by cephalic stimuli (smell, taste, expectation of food) and by gastric stretch. The endocrine release of CCK is triggered by the presence of amino acids, peptides, and lipids in the proximal duodenum. The presence of bile acids in the duodenum and in portal blood triggers gallbladder relaxation and inhibits further CCK release. Bile acids are detected by the farnesoid X receptor (FXR) in the ileum, triggering the expression of FGF-19, which suppresses bile acid synthesis and causes gallbladder relaxation,[1] inducing storage rather than secretion of bile. Bile and the biliary tree also offer some immunoprotective functions. In addition to digestive, buffering, and excretory functions, the detergent properties of bile also reduce the risk of ascending bacterial infections. The mechanical effect of bile flow and the valve that is the duodenal papilla serve to protect the biliary tree. Cholangiocytes also play a role in the T-cell response[2] in which pathogen-associated molecular patterns (PAMPs) such as lipopolysaccharide and other bacterial products entering the biliary tree trigger a cascade of inflammatory mediators. This inflammatory response may be maladaptive in some circumstances, triggering ductular proliferation and fibrosis such as is seen in primary sclerosing cholangitis in humans.[3,4]

Gallbladder structure and function

The gallbladder is situated between the right medial and quadrate lobes of the liver in dogs.

The canine gallbladder contains approximately 15 mL of bile in the fasting state. It serves not only to store bile but also alters its composition by reabsorption of water and a substantial proportion of electrolytes. This action results in stored bile being concentrated by a factor of several times compared to canalicular bile.

The gallbladder is innervated by both sympathetic and parasympathetic nerve fibers via the celiac and hepatic plexuses. The arterial blood supply is from the cystic artery, a branch of the left hepatic artery.

Most dogs have two separate pancreatic ducts opening at the minor duodenal papilla and separately from the bile duct opening (see chapter 17 for more detail).[5] This differs between cats and humans, where a single pancreatic duct joins the common bile duct before it reaches a common opening at the major duodenal papilla.

Bacterial cholangitis and cholecystitis

Definition and etiology

Cholangitis and cholecystitis are inflammation of the bile ducts and gallbladder, respectively; commonly in dogs, this is caused by bacterial infection –bacterial cholangitis and bacterial cholecystitis. The major route of biliary tract infections is direct ascending biliary infection involving enteric organisms, predisposed by altered bile flow or pathology at the duodenal papilla. This is supported by the fact that most infections detected in the hepatobiliary system in cats and dogs are of enteric origin: organisms such as *E. coli*, *Enterococcus* spp., *Bacteroides* spp., and *Clostridium* spp.[6,7]

Potential causes of altered bile flow include:

- Pancreatitis, causing swelling of the pancreas and tissues surrounding the common bile duct.
- Gallbladder mucocele.
- Infiltrative disease (neoplasia) of the duodenum at the duodenal papilla.

Less common causes include choleliths, biliary tract neoplasia, duodenal foreign bodies lodged at the duodenal papilla, or, very rarely, aberrant migration of roundworms.

A less well-characterized but potential route of biliary infection is by bacteria from portal blood returning from the intestines or from arterial blood from the systemic circulation. The presence of bacterial DNA in portal blood in normal dogs has been demonstrated,[8] but whether viable bacteria are present is unclear. The transit of viable bacteria into bile via the portal venous system has been demonstrated experimentally in cats: infusion of bacteria into the splenic vein of cats resulted in biliary excretion of those bacteria, and their presence was augmented in the case of biliary tract obstruction.[9] In the healthy liver, any bacteria reaching the liver are exposed to macrophages (Kupffer cells) in the hepatic sinusoids, triggering an immune response.[10]

There is evidence of higher concentrations of bacterial endotoxin in the portal blood of human patients with cirrhosis: endotoxin activity in blood is increased with more advanced disease, which reflects both the intestinal dysbiosis in hepatic disease and impaired hepatic immune mechanisms.[11]

Bacterial translocation of enteric bacteria has been demonstrated in 50% of healthy dogs undergoing general anesthesia and ovariohysterectomy by the culture of mesenteric lymph nodes.[12] Bacteria isolated from lymph nodes (including *Staphylococcus* spp., *Streptococcus* spp., *Bacillus* spp., *Enterococcus* spp., *E. coli*, *Salmonella* spp., *Pseudomonas* spp.) were not demonstrated in peripheral blood samples from the same individuals. In none of these patients were bacteria detected in portal blood.

The true prevalence of bacterial cholangitis in dogs is difficult to determine as published data are based either on studies including animals undergoing investigation of hepatobiliary disease or on a study of repeated sampling of six healthy dogs and six dogs with iatrogenic hypercortisolism. In this latter study, two of 42 bile samples from six healthy dogs yielded a positive bacterial culture.[13] Both organisms isolated were of enteric origin (*Enterococcus* spp. and *E. coli*). In a study including dogs with suspected bacterial cholangitis, 19% of 208 canine bile samples (from 202 dogs) were culture-positive. In another study of patients with hepatobiliary disease, 28% of 46 dogs were culture-positive.[14]

Subclinical bactibilia has been demonstrated in rescue shelter dogs.[15] The presence of bactibilia in these dogs was associated with histological lesions, including cholecystitis, but this was also seen in dogs with no cytologic or bacteriologic evidence of bactobilia.

Clinical presentation of bacterial cholangitis

In dogs with culture-positive cholangitis/cholecystitis, common clinical signs include vomiting, anorexia, lethargy, and jaundice.[6,16,17] In these studies, no more than 30% of the dogs were pyrexic at presentation, and in some case series, only a little more than half of the dogs were jaundiced.[6] Apart from jaundice, these clinical signs are common in various gastrointestinal and systemic diseases and are nonspecific. This illustrates the importance of further investigation of patients with gastrointestinal signs that do not resolve acutely with supportive care.

On clinical examination, dogs with bacterial cholangitis may exhibit pyrexia and signs of abdominal pain.

Clinicopathological findings in bacterial cholangitis

Blood biochemical changes in the majority of cases include increased alkaline phosphatase (ALP) and alanine aminotransferase (ALT) concentrations, with hyperbilirubinemia with or without other indicators of cholestasis such as hypercholesterolemia. Neutrophilia is commonly present, with a left shift (band neutrophils) and toxic changes in some cases.[6] Though coagulation times are infrequently affected, testing these is advisable if sampling is planned.

Diagnostic imaging in bacterial cholangitis

The most common modality for diagnostic imaging of the biliary tract, and that with generally the greatest diagnostic yield, is ultrasound. Ultrasonography allows noninvasive visual assessment and measurement of the biliary tract and surrounding structures, as well as guiding sampling (cholecystocentesis). Importantly, in acutely unwell patients, repeated focal examinations can be performed to objectively monitor the progress of the patient or lesion (e.g., biliary tract dilation) on a regular –even daily– basis. More details of diagnostic imaging of the biliary tract are found in chapter 26. Ultrasound findings in dogs with positive bacterial culture of bile include thickening of the gallbladder wall, mucosal hyperplasia, and bile sludge.[18,19] An abnormal ultrasound appearance of the gallbladder has a high sensitivity (81%) for bile infection. A normal ultrasonographic appearance of the gallbladder has a negative predictive value for a positive bile culture of 88% in dogs.[18] Thickening of the gallbladder or common bile duct should prompt sampling for bacterial culture and cytology.

Other diagnostic procedures

Diagnosis of bacterial cholangitis or cholecystitis requires culture of bile and in some instances liver tissue. Cytological evidence of neutrophilic inflammation in bile samples, including intracytoplasmic bacteria, strengthens the diagnosis.

In a study of 248 dogs undergoing investigation for hepatobiliary disease, positive cultures were more readily obtained from bile than from liver tissue: in patients that had both liver and bile cultures performed, bile yielded positive culture in 32% of patients, but the liver was positive in only 5%.[14]

Gram-negative aerobes represented nearly half of all organisms cultured in this study, with Gram-positive aerobes, including *Enterococcus* spp., making up another quarter of the isolates.

Cholecystocentesis has been demonstrated to be safe in cats and dogs[19-21] with a complication rate of less than 3.5%. Complications may include peritoneal hemorrhage, intraluminal hemorrhage, or bile peritonitis. Cardiorespiratory arrest has been documented in some cases: 1% in a study including 300 cholecystocentesis events in 201 dogs and 51 cats.[21]
Cholecystocentesis can be performed at laparotomy or laparoscopy with visualization of the gallbladder or by percutaneous ultrasound guidance. In this latter situation, the needle is directed through liver tissue into the gallbladder as the apposition of the liver to the gallbladder wall may reduce the risk of bile leakage. See chapters 26 and 27 for more details of bile aspiration under ultrasound guidance or at surgery or laparoscopy.
Histology of the liver or gallbladder wall may demonstrate acute neutrophilic inflammation, potentially with accompanying longer-standing changes such as mononuclear inflammation and fibrotic changes (see chapter 29). Biliary tract infections induce not only a fibrotic response but also a proliferation of bile duct epithelium.[22]

Treatment of bacterial cholangitis/cholecystitis

Having submitted bile (and/or liver) samples for culture and antimicrobial susceptibility testing, patients with bacterial cholangitis/cholecystitis should be started on antibiotics. Antimicrobial resistance is common in hepatobiliary infections.[23] *E. coli* and other coliform bacteria cultured from bile or liver demonstrated resistance to amoxicillin-clavulanate in up to 50% of isolates.[6,14] Therefore, antimicrobial selection should preferably be based on culture and susceptibility results rather than empirical choice. In patients at risk of, or demonstrating signs of sepsis, an initial antibiotic may be necessary pending culture results. Considering the responsibility of veterinarians for antimicrobial stewardship, an initial choice of antibiotic should be licensed, reach effective concentrations within the biliary tract, and should not be an antibiotic reserved for resistant infections or for restricted use only. Despite the known resistance of many isolates in vitro to beta-lactams and considering the inducible resistance of *E. coli* to fluoroquinolones, the author's favored empirical choice of antibiotic for cholangitis pending culture is amoxicillin-clavulanate.
Additional supportive treatment includes opioid analgesia, intravenous fluid therapy, ursodeoxycholic acid, silybin, and S-adenosylmethionine.

Prognosis

Where underlying predisposing causes or reasons for persistence are also addressed if present, the prognosis of bacterial cholangitis/cholecystitis is fair to good. More challenging cases include those with multi-resistant bacterial isolates, patients presenting in sepsis, and those with perpetuating factors such as cholelithiasis.

Gallbladder mucocele

Definition and etiology

Gallbladder mucocele (GBM) is an accumulation of solidified mucus in the gallbladder lumen, accompanied by cystic mucinous hyperplasia of the gallbladder wall.[24] The accumulation of mucus causes distension of the gallbladder and exerts pressure on the mucosal surface, which eventually causes gallbladder wall necrosis and rupture (Fig. 35.1).
Reasons for the accumulation of the mucus are uncertain, but there is a clear breed association in Shetland Sheepdogs,[25] Border Terriers,[26] Miniature Schnauzers,[27] Cocker Spaniels,[28] and some other breeds.[29]

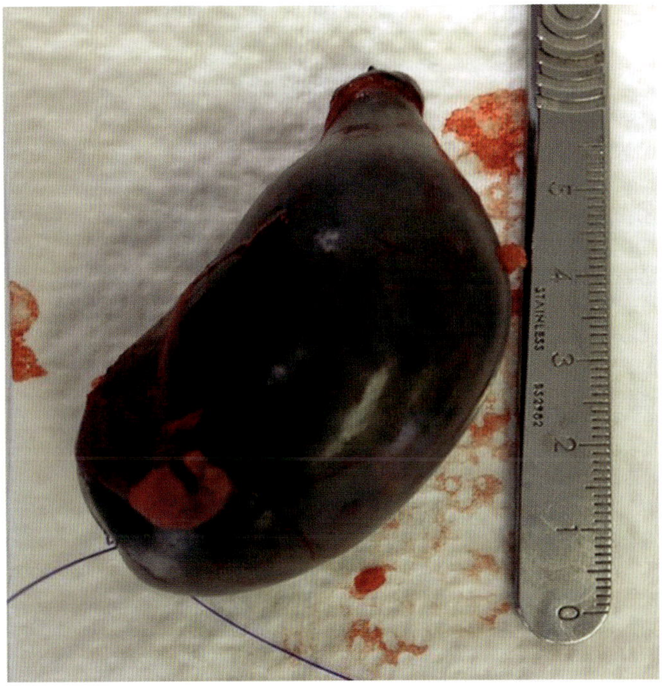

FIG. 35.1 Gallbladder containing a mucocele removed at surgery.

Some studies have suggested a genetic cause with a mutation in ABCB4 in Shetland Sheepdogs.[30] However, further association studies have indicated that, while this may be a factor in developing GBM, this is not a stand-alone cause.[31]
Endocrinopathies certainly show a strong association with GBM, with an odds ratio of 29 for developing GBM in dogs with hyperadrenocorticism[24,32,33] and a three-fold increased risk in hypothyroid dogs.[24,34] Hyperlipidemia also appears to be associated.[33] Corticosteroids change mucin composition and reduce the rate of gallbladder emptying in dogs[35] although the actual mechanism predisposing to mucocele is unclear. An ultrastructural study of mucoceles demonstrated that the gallbladder epithelium adopts a mucin-secretory phenotype and that there is a seven-fold increase of the ratio of Muc5a to Muc5b, as well as defective unfolding of mucins after secretion.[36] This results in marked changes in the physical properties of gallbladder mucus. These changes may result from altered epithelial electrolyte, acid-base or fluid handling.[36] Infrared spectroscopic analysis of the mucus in GBM has shown a similar composition to that of biliary sludge, suggesting that GBM may be the end-stage of progression of biliary sludge.[37]
Gallbladder mucoceles increase in prevalence with age, which may reflect their insidious development.[38]

Clinical presentation

Clinical signs of GBM may not be apparent until late in the course of the disease –30% of dogs are asymptomatic at the time of diagnosis.[24] The most common signs include vomiting, reduced appetite, and lethargy, which are seen in more than 75% of symptomatic dogs.[29,38] Abdominal pain and visible jaundice were only reported in 17% and 10%, respectively, in the largest retrospective study of more than 1,000 dogs with GBM.[39] Some patients may have concurrent clinical signs associated with endocrinopathies, such as polyuria, polydipsia, polyphagia, or weight gain.

Clinicopathological findings

Hematologic changes are nonspecific and generally relate to the inflammatory state of neutrophilia, lymphopenia, and monocytosis. Blood smear examination is likely to reveal left-shift neutrophilia in patients with concurrent bacterial cholangitis or gallbladder rupture and septic peritonitis.

Blood biochemistry may reveal indicators of cholestasis such as hypercholesterolemia, and total bilirubin concentrations are increased by 50 to 80%.[26,40-42] Alkaline phosphatase is increased in 63 to 97% and GGT in 60-85%.[26,40-42] Alanine aminotransferase is increased in more than 90% of mucocele patients.[26]

Diagnostic imaging

Abdominal ultrasound is the imaging modality of choice for GBM. The defining feature of GBM is the filling of the GB with echoic, immobile bile. With time, the bile becomes organized and develops striations extending from the center of the accumulation of bile towards the gallbladder mucosa, eventually creating a stellate appearance reminiscent of a short axis section of kiwi fruit. Other findings can include gallbladder wall thickening, dilatation of the extrahepatic bile duct, and extension of the echoic bile into the cystic duct and common bile duct. See chapter 26 for examples of ultrasound images.

In cases of GB rupture, discontinuity of the GB wall may be appreciated, as well as pericholecystic fluid or hyperechoic mesenteric fat. Occasionally a conglomeration of mucocele material may be found in the abdominal cavity. The sensitivity of ultrasound for GB rupture in a study of 219 dogs was only 56%.[39]

Other diagnostic procedures

Cholecystocentesis is contraindicated in GBM because of the risk of rupture of the impaired GB wall. Diagnostic testing for endocrinopathies may be performed, but in clinically unwell patients, this may be best delayed until they are clinically stable, which may be after surgery.

Abdominocentesis should be performed if free abdominal fluid is present. The basic analysis includes cytology to assess for bilirubin crystals (indicating bile leakage), inflammatory changes (neutrophilia), and evidence of abdominal sepsis (toxic neutrophils, intracytoplasmic bacteria). Comparison of glucose concentration in abdominal fluid and blood is a useful confirmatory test for a septic abdomen: a difference of >1 mmol/L (blood > fluid) has 100% sensitivity and specificity for a septic abdomen.[43]

Treatment and prognosis

Cholecystectomy is the treatment of choice for gallbladder mucocele, but mortality rates within the first 2 weeks after surgery have been reported to be between 7 and 40%.[28,42,44] Negative prognostic indicators include increased total bilirubin, presence of clinical signs at the time of surgery, owner recognition of jaundice, hyperadrenocorticism, postoperative increased venous lactate concentration, and immediate postoperative hypotension.[29,44] The time from onset of clinical signs to surgery, time from ultrasound detection to surgery, and the comorbidities of diabetes mellitus, hypothyroidism, or bacterial cholecystitis appear to have no impact on survival.[29,39,45] Conflicting evidence has shown a significant negative impact or no impact on the prognosis of bile leakage prior to surgery.[39,42] Median survival times of dogs with GBM that were managed medically were significantly shorter than those having surgery.[46]

Dogs with gallbladder rupture are more likely to have increased venous lactate,[40] and ultrasonographic findings of pericholecystic fluid or pericholecystic reactive changes.[42] However, abdominal ultrasound has poor sensitivity for the detection of gallbladder rupture.[39] Most studies report reduced survival with ultrasonographic evidence of gallbladder rupture, but one study showed a surprising increased survival in this group of dogs.[47] However, in that study, ultrasound overestimated the actual presence of biliary rupture found at surgery but may have prompted a more aggressive clinical approach in all those cases.

Postoperative hypernatremia has been demonstrated in more than 50% of canine cholecystectomy patients; development of hypernatremia within 6 hours of surgery and sodium of more than 160 mmol/L are associated with worse outcomes.[48]

At the time of cholecystectomy, liver biopsies should be taken and submitted along with sections of the gallbladder wall for histology and bacterial culture. Many patients, including those that had normal appetite prior to surgery, will be inappetent following surgery, so a feeding tube, such as an esophagostomy tube should be placed at the time of surgery. In patients with significant ileus, a surgically placed gastric feeding tube may be advisable as an alternative.

Postsurgical pancreatitis is a common complication following cholecystectomy; attention should be paid to analgesia and an appropriate low-fat diet (see chapters 22 and 23 for more details).

Gallbladder sludge

Gallbladder sludge (GBS) is a description used for the presence of echogenic luminal material within the gallbladder seen on ultrasound. The constituents of GBS are generally mucin, cholesterol, calcium salts, proteins, glycoproteins, and cellular debris. GBS is generally nonshadowing on ultrasound but can contain echogenic specks of mineralized material, and in patients with a high mineral content may cause some distal acoustic shadowing (see chapter 26).

Gallbladder sludge in dogs has often been regarded as an incidental finding,[49,50] although it is generally considered abnormal in cats.[51-53] The prevalence of GBS in dogs presenting for abdominal ultrasound for any reason at veterinary hospitals has been documented as between 35% and 67%.[49,54,55] This hospital population clearly still does not reflect the true prevalence of GBS in healthy patients. In a study comparing healthy dogs with dogs with hepatobiliary disease and dogs with nonhepatobiliary disease, there was no significant difference in the prevalence of GBS between the groups.

GBS may occur due to changes in gallbladder motility, allowing sedimentation of material, or due to mucus hypersecretion.[54] Dogs with GBS have been shown to have gallbladder distention and reduced gallbladder emptying fraction postprandially.[56,57] Corticosteroid therapy has been shown to negatively affect gallbladder emptying as well as reduce the mucin content of bile.[35] Hyperlipidemic dogs have reduced gallbladder emptying regardless of fasting or feeding,[58] and dogs with hyperadrenocorticism or hypothyroidism are more likely to have GBS.[55] Despite this, a prospective study of a period of iatrogenic hypercortisolism did not induce GBS in dogs.[59]

GBS may be described as gravity-dependent (mobile) or non-gravity-dependent (immobile) and may progress from one to the other with time. Serial assessment of GBS in dogs has shown that it is not a transient finding but may progress over time to become more voluminous or non-gravity-dependent.[54] Some dogs with non-gravity-dependent sludge may progress to gallbladder mucocele (GBM): over a period of more than 12 months, 20 of 154 dogs with GBS developed GBM.[60] In most this was preceded by a change from gravity-dependent to non-gravity-dependent sludge, which suggests a continuum between these stages.

The composition of sludge examined by infrared spectroscopy has been shown to have a similar mucin content to gallbladder content in GBM.[37] Biochemical analysis of gravity-dependent and non-gravity-dependent sludge and GBM revealed a lower concentration of secondary hydrophobic bile acids in non-gravity-dependent sludge and GBM,[61] but this may simply reflect the reduced storage of secondary bile acids from enterohepatic reabsorption in patients with reduced gallbladder motility. Hydrophobic bile acids do trigger gallbladder mucosal fluid and chloride ion secretion; a reduced concentration of these bile acids or alteration of a bile acid receptor may alter the response.[61]

Sampling or bacterial culture of gallbladder sludge is not warranted in patients that display no related clinical signs and no abnormality of hepatobiliary parameters. 10% of samples of bile sludge from dogs yielded a positive bacterial culture,[37] but whether this is a secondary infection facilitated by biliary stasis, or whether the infection is a contributory factor to GBS formation is uncertain.[28]

Cholelithiasis

Definition and etiology

Choleliths are uncommon in dogs, with a prevalence of approximately 1% in populations of patients having abdominal ultrasound at referral hospitals.[62,63] More than 92% of choleliths are found in the gallbladder,[64] with the remainder mostly within the common bile duct and relatively few within the intrahepatic bile ducts. The composition of canine choleliths includes calcium carbonate, cholesterol, and bilirubin.[63,64]

Clinical presentation

52.6% to 87% of canine choleliths are asymptomatic incidental findings.[62,64] Despite this, choleliths are not regarded as a normal finding: their presence indicates altered bile composition or altered bile flow, so further investigation may be warranted. Potential underlying factors include bacterial cholecystitis, altered biliary outflow, and hypercholesterolemia.[65] In a study of canine cholelithiasis, 75% of dogs yielded a positive bacterial culture of bile.[66] Reasons for symptomatic presentation of choleliths include bile duct obstruction, pain related to cholecystitis, or systemic effects of bacterial cholecystitis (fever, signs of sepsis). In patients exhibiting clinical signs of cholelithiasis, the most common signs are lethargy, anorexia, vomiting, icterus, and abdominal pain.[62,64]

Clinicopathological findings

Clinicopathologic findings include increased ALP, ALT, and GGT, which tend to be higher in symptomatic patients.[64]

Diagnostic imaging

The ultrasound appearance of choleliths is of rounded, echogenic, gravity-dependent luminal structures with distal acoustic shadowing. The degree of acoustic shadowing depends upon the mineral content and density of the cholelith[67] (see chapter 26).

Some choleliths with significant mineral content are radiodense and appear as mineral opacities on abdominal radiographs.

Treatment

Asymptomatic nonobstructive choleliths may be treated medically by using a choleretic agent such as ursodeoxycholic acid (UDCA), which may result in dissolution in some patients.[64,68] Symptomatic patients without biliary tract obstruction may require antibiotics based on bacterial culture of a cholecystocentesis sample and supportive management such as intravenous fluids and analgesia. In a study of canine cholelithiasis, fewer than 7% of dogs developed complications within a 2-year period.[62] This lends further confidence to medical management of choleliths in an attempt to dissolve them rather than surgical intervention. A recent study demonstrated the dissolution of canine choleliths in 50% (4/8) of medically managed patients receiving UCDA.[64] The exception to this is in the case of bile duct obstruction, which necessitates surgery.

Ursodeoxycholic acid (UCDA) is commonly prescribed to treat cholestatic disease in humans and dogs. It is a hydrophilic bile acid that reduces the toxicity of hydrophobic bile acids on hepatocyte and cholangiocyte cell membranes and mitochondria and reduces hepatocyte apoptosis stimulated by the accumulation of hydrophobic bile acids in cholestasis. UCDA exerts its protective effects by physical displacement of hydrophobic bile acids, removing harmful hydrophilic bile acids from hepatocytes by stimulating secretion from the canalicular membranes, as well as by effects on the composition of phospholipid-rich micelles in bile.[70]

UCDA also reduces the absorption of cholesterol from the intestine, which may assist in preventing or reducing cholelithiasis. It simulates bicarbonate secretion into bile and is thus choleretic, which, together with the dilutional effects on hydrophobic bile acids, may also assist with the dissolution of choleliths and delay or prevent GBM formation.

UCDA is not licensed for use in dogs but is widely used, and side effects are uncommon. Mild gastrointestinal side effects are seen in some dogs. It is an unconjugated bile acid that is passively absorbed from the small intestine and requires conjugation to glycine or taurine in the liver to its active form before excretion in the bile. It undergoes hepatic recirculation by efficient reabsorption by the sodium-dependent bile acid transporter in the distal ileum. This recirculation explains why it is the total daily dose and not the dosing interval, which is important. Ingested UCDA is solubilized in micelles with bile acids and phospholipids, and passive absorption is reduced in the absence of small intestinal bile acids, which will reduce its effectiveness in biliary obstruction.

KEY POINTS

- Bacterial cholangitis/cholecystitis can present with nonspecific gastrointestinal signs.
- Fewer than 30% of patients with cholangitis/cholecystitis are febrile at presentation.
- Bacteria implicated in cholangitis are generally of enteric origin, which reflects ascending bacterial infection due to altered impaired bile flow.
- Many bacteria in cholangitis have resistance to commonly used antibiotics; treatment choices should be based upon antimicrobial susceptibility testing, with appropriate antibiotic stewardship.
- Gallbladder mucocele is a surgical condition but of gradual onset. In asymptomatic patients without gallbladder rupture, surgery can be electively scheduled.
- Mobile gallbladder sludge is an incidental finding in dogs requiring no treatment; immobile sludge may progress to gallbladder mucocele formation and should be treated with choleretic agents (ursodeoxycholic acid).
- Nonobstructive choleliths have a low complication rate and may be managed medically long-term.

References

1. Matsubara T, Li F, Gonzalez FJ. FXR signaling in the enterohepatic system. *Mol Cell Endocrinol* 368:17-29, 2013.
2. Mehrfeld C, Zenner S, Kornek M, Lukacs-Kornek V. The contribution of non-professional antigen-presenting cells to immunity and tolerance in the liver. *Front Immunol* 28:9:635, 2018.
3. Maroni L, Ninfole E, Pinto C, Benedetti A, Marzioni M. Gut-liver axis and inflammasome activation in cholangiocyte pathophysiology. *Cells* 9(3):736, 2020.
4. Cai X, Tacke F, Guillot A, Liu H. Cholangiokines: undervalued modulators in the hepatic microenvironment. *Front Immunol* 14:1192840, 2023.
5. Penninck D, D'Anjou MA. Pancreas. In: Penninck D, D'Anjou MA (editors). Atlas of Small Animal Ultrasonography 2nd edition. Oxford, John Wiley & Sons, 2015, pp. 309-330.
6. Tamborini A, Jahns H, McAllister H, Kent A, Harris B, Procoli F, et al. Bacterial cholangitis, cholecystitis, or both in dogs. *J Vet Intern Med* 30(4):1046-1055, 2016.
7. Wagner KA, Hartmann FA, Trepanier LA. Bacterial culture results from liver, gallbladder, or bile in 248 dogs and cats evaluated for hepatobiliary disease: 1998-2003. *J Vet Intern Med* 21(3):417-424, 2007.
8. Scarsella E, Meineri G, Sandri M, Ganz HH, Stefanon B. Characterization of the blood microbiome and comparison with the fecal microbiome in healthy dogs and dogs with gastrointestinal disease. *Vet Sci* 10(4):277, 2023.
9. Sung JY, Shaffer EA, Olson ME, Leung JWC, Lam K, Costerton JW. Bacterial invasion of the biliary system by way of the portal venous system. *Hepatology* 14(2):313-337, 1991.
10. Crispe IN. The liver as a lymphoid organ. *Annu Rev Immunol* 27(1):147-163, 2009.
11. Fukui H. Leaky gut and gut-liver axis in liver cirrhosis: clinical studies update. *Gut Liver* 15(5):666-676, 2021.
12. Dahlinger J, Marks SL, Hirsh DC. Prevalence and identity of translocating bacteria in healthy dogs. *J Vet Intern Med* 11(6):319-322, 1997.
13. Kook PH, Schellenberg S, Grest P, Reusch CE, Corboz L, Glaus TM. Microbiologic evaluation of gallbladder bile of healthy dogs and dogs with iatrogenic hypercortisolism: a pilot study. *J Vet Intern Med* 24(1):224-228, 2010.
14. Wagner KA, Hartmann FA, Trepanier LA. Bacterial culture results from liver, gallbladder, or bile in 248 dogs and cats evaluated for hepatobiliary disease: 1998-2003. *J Vet Intern Med* 21(3):417-424, 2007.
15. Verwey E, Gal A, Kettner F, Botha WJ, Pazzi P. Prevalence of subclinical bactibilia in apparently healthy shelter dogs. *J Small Anim Pract* 62(11):948-958, 2021.
16. O'Neill EJ, Day MJ, Hall EJ, Holden DJ, Murphy KF, Barr FJ, et al. Bacterial cholangitis/cholangiohepatitis with or without concurrent cholecystitis in four dogs. *J Small Anim Pract* 47(6):325-335, 2006.
17. Harrison JL, Turek BJ, Brown DC, Bradley C, Callahan Clark J. Cholangitis and cholangiohepatitis in dogs: a descriptive study of 54 cases based on histopathologic diagnosis (2004-2014). *J Vet Intern Med* 32(1):172-180, 2018.
18. Schiborra F, McConnell JF, Maddox TW. Percutaneous ultrasound-guided cholecystocentesis: complications and association of ultrasonographic findings with bile culture results. *J Small Anim Pract* 58(7):389-394, 2017.
19. Policelli Smith R, Gookin JL, Smolski W, Di Cicco MF, Correa M, Seiler GS. Association between gallbladder ultrasound findings and bacterial culture of bile in 70 cats and 202 dogs. *J Vet Intern Med* 31(5):1451-1458, 2017.
20. Webb CB. Evidence-based medicine ultrasound-guided percutaneous cholecystocentesis in the cat. *Vet Clin North Am Small Anim Pract* 50(5):1123-1134, 2020.
21. Schiborra F, Mcconnell JF, Maddox TW. Percutaneous ultrasound-guided cholecystocentesis: complications and association of ultrasonographic findings with bile culture results. *J Small Anim Pract* 58:389-394, 2017.
22. Ohta T, Nagakawa T, Tsukioka Y, Sanada H, Miyazaki I, Terada T. Proliferative activity of bile duct epithelium after bacterial infection in dogs. *Scand J Gastroenterol* 27(10):845-851,1992.
23. Sposato A, Cordisco M, de Ruvo G, Ferro S, Raineri RA, Trotta A, et al. Multidrug resistant Enterococcus faecium isolate from cholangitis/cholecystitis in a dog. *Vet Med Sci* 8(4):1366-1372, 2022.
24. Cornejo L, Webster CR. Canine gallbladder mucoceles. *Comp Cont Educ Pract Vet* 27(12): 912-928, 2005.
25. Aguirre AL, Center SA, Randolph JE, Yeager AE, Keegan AM, Harvey HJ, et al. Gallbladder disease in Shetland Sheepdogs: 38 Cases (1995-2005). *J Am Vet Med Assoc* 231(1):79-88, 2007.
26. Allerton F, Swinbourne F, Barker L, Black V, Kathrani A, Tivers M, et al. Gall bladder mucoceles in Border terriers. *J Vet Intern Med* 32(5):1618-1628, 2018.
27. Saunders H, Thornton LA, Burchell R. Medical and surgical management of gallbladder sludge and mucocoele development in a Miniature Schnauzer. *Int J Vet Sci Med* 5(1):75-80, 2017.
28. Besso JG, Wrigley RH, Gliatto JM, Webster CRL. Ultrasonographic appearance and clinical findings in 14 dogs with gallbladder mucocele. *Vet Radiol Ultrasound* 41(3):261-271, 2000.

29. Jaffey JA, Pavlick M, Webster CR, Moore GE, McDaniel KA, Blois SL, et al. Effect of clinical signs, endocrinopathies, timing of surgery, hyperlipidemia, and hyperbilirubinemia on outcome in dogs with gallbladder mucocele. *Vet J* 251, 2019.
30. Mealey KL, Minch JD, White SN, Snekvik KR, Mattoon JS. An insertion mutation in ABCB4 is associated with gallbladder mucocele formation in dogs. *Comp Hepatol* 9:6, 2010.
31. Cullen JM, Willson CJ, Minch JD, Kimbrough CL, Mealey KL. Lack of association of ABCB4 insertion mutation with gallbladder mucoceles in dogs. *J Vet Diagn Invest* 26(3):434-436, 2014.
32. Kim KH, Han SM, Jeon KO, Kim HT, Li Q, Ryu MO, et al. Clinical relationship between cholestatic disease and pituitary-dependent hyperadrenocorticism in dogs: A retrospective case series. *J Vet Intern Med* 31(2):335-342, 2017.
33. Kutsunai M, Kanemoto H, Fukushima K, Fujino Y, Ohno K, Tsujimoto H. The association between gall bladder mucoceles and hyperlipidaemia in dogs: A retrospective case control study. *Vet Journal* 199(1):76-79, 2014.
34. Aicher KM, Cullen JM, Seiler GS, Lunn KF, Mathews KG, Gookin JL. Investigation of adrenal and thyroid gland dysfunction in dogs with ultrasonographic diagnosis of gallbladder mucocele formation. *PLoS One* 14(2), 2019.
35. Nagahara T, Ohno K, Kanemoto H, Kakimoto T, Fukushima K, Goto-Koshino Y, et al. Effect of prednisolone administration on gallbladder emptying rate and gallbladder bile composition in dogs. *Am J Vet Res* 79(10):1050-1056, 2018.
36. Kesimer M, Cullen J, Cao R, Radicioni G, Mathews KG, Seiler G, et al. Excess secretion of gel-forming mucins and associated innate defense proteins with defective mucin un-packaging underpin gallbladder mucocele formation in dogs. *PLoS One* 10(9), 2015.
37. Mizutani S, Torisu S, Kaneko Y, Yamamoto S, Fujimoto S, Ong BHE, et al. Retrospective analysis of canine gallbladder contents in biliary sludge and gallbladder mucoceles. *J Vet Med Sci* 79(2):366-374, 2017.
38. Galley M, Lang J, Mitchell M, Fletcher J. Article Factors affecting survival in 516 dogs that underwent cholecystectomy for the treatment of gallbladder mucocele. *Can Vet J* 63, 2022.
39. Jaffey JA, Graham A, VanEerde E, Hostnik E, Alvarez W, Arango J, et al. Gallbladder mucocele: variables associated with outcome and the utility of ultrasonography to identify gallbladder rupture in 219 dogs (2007-2016). *J Vet Intern Med* 32(1):195-200, 2018.
40. Pike FS, Berg J, King NW, Penninck DG, Webster CRL. Gallbladder mucocele in dogs: 30 cases (2000-2002). *J Am Vet Med Assoc* 224(10):1615-1622, 2004.
41. Youn G, Waschak MJ, Kunkel KAR, Gerard PD. Outcome of elective cholecystectomy for the treatment of gallbladder disease in dogs. *J Am Vet Med Assoc* 252(8):970-975, 2018.
42. Crews LJ, Feeney DA, Jessen CR, Rose ND, Matise I. Clinical, ultrasonographic, and laboratory findings associated with gallbladder disease and rupture in dogs: 45 cases (1997-2007). *J Am Vet Med Assoc* 234(3):359-366, 2009.
43. Bonczynski JJ, Ludwig LL, Barton LJ, Loar A, Peterson ME. Comparison of peritoneal fluid and peripheral blood pH, bicarbonate, glucose, and lactate concentration as a diagnostic tool for septic peritonitis in dogs and cats. *Vet Surg* 32(2):161-166, 2003.
44. Malek S, Sinclair E, Hosgood G, Moens NMM, Baily T, Boston SE. Clinical findings and prognostic factors for dogs undergoing cholecystectomy for gall bladder mucocele. *Vet Surg* 42(4):418-426, 2013.
45. Rogers E, Jaffey JA, Graham A, Hostnik ET, Jacobs C, Fox-Alvarez W, et al. Prevalence and impact of cholecystitis on outcome in dogs with gallbladder mucocele. *J Vet Emerg Crit Care* 30(1):97-101, 2020.
46. Parkanzky M, Grimes J, Schmiedt C, Secrest I Scott, Bugbee I Andrew. Long-term survival of dogs treated for gallbladder mucocele by cholecystectomy, medical management, or both. *J Vet Intern Med* 33(5):2057-2066, 2019.
47. Parkanzky M, Grimes J, Schmiedt C, Secrest S, Bugbee A. Long-term survival of dogs treated for gallbladder mucocele by cholecystectomy, medical management, or both. *J Vet Intern Med* 33(5):2057-2066, 2019.
48. Brunori L, Dolan C, Elias Santo-Domingo N. Occurrence and clinical relevance of postoperative hypernatremia in dogs undergoing cholecystectomy. *J Vet Intern Med* 37(6):2171-2177, 2023.
49. Secchi P, Pöppl AG, Ilha A, Kunert Filho HC, Lima FES, García AB, et al. Prevalence, risk factors, and biochemical markers in dogs with ultrasound-diagnosed biliary sludge. *Res Vet Sci* 93(3):1185-1189, 2012.
50. Mannion P (editor). The Liver and Spleen. Diagnostic Ultrasound in Small Animal Practice. Wiley Blackwell, 2007, pp. 50-80.
51. Griffin S. Feline abdominal ultrasonography: What's normal? What's abnormal? The pancreas. *J Feline Med Surg* 22(3):241-259, 2020.
52. Harran N, -André D'anjou M, Dunn M, Beauchamp G. Gallbladder sludge on ultrasound is predictive of increased liver enzymes and total bilirubin in cats. *Can Vet J* 52, 2011.
53. Villm J, DeMonaco S, Larson M. Prevalence of gallbladder sludge and associated abnormalities in cats undergoing abdominal ultrasound. *Vet Radiol Ultrasound* 63(5):601-608, 2022.
54. Demonaco SM, Grant DC, Larson MM, Panciera DL, Leib MS. Spontaneous course of biliary sludge over 12 months in dogs with ultrasonographically identified biliary sludge. *J Vet Intern Med* 30(3):771-778, 2016.
55. Cook AK, Jambhekar A V, Dylewski AM. Gallbladder sludge in dogs: Ultrasonographic and clinical findings in 200 patients. *J Am Anim Hosp Assoc* 52(3):125-131, 2016.
56. Viljoen AD, Tamborini A, Watson PJ, Bexfield NH. Clinical characteristics and histology of cholecystectomised dogs with nongravity-dependent biliary sludge: 16 cases (2014-2019). *J Small Anim Pract* 62(6):478-488, 2021.
57. Tsukagoshi T, Ohno K, Tsukamoto A, Fukushima K, Takahashi M, Nakashima K, et al. Decreased gallbladder emptying in dogs with biliary sludge or gallbladder mucocele. *Vet Radiol Ultrasound* 53(1):84-91, 2012.
58. Villm JA, DeMonaco SM, Panciera DL, Larson MM, Bolton TA. Evaluation of gallbladder motility assessed by ultrasonography in dogs with hyperlipidemia. *J Vet Intern Med* 37(3):968-975, 2023.
59. Kook PH, Schellenberg S, Rentsch KM, Reusch CE, Glaus TM. Effects of iatrogenic hypercortisolism on gallbladder sludge formation and biochemical bile constituents in dogs. *Vet J* 191(2):225-230, 2012.
60. Butler T, Bexfield N, Dor C, Fantaconi N, Heinsoo I, Kelly D, et al. A multicenter retrospective study assessing progression of biliary sludge in dogs using ultrasonography. *J Vet Intern Med* 36(3):976-985, 2022.
61. Kakimoto T, Kanemoto H, Fukushima K, Ohno K, Tsujimoto H. Bile acid composition of gallbladder contents in dogs with gallbladder mucocele and biliary sludge. *Am J Vet Res* 78(2):223-229, 2017.
62. Ward PM, Brown K, Hammond G, Parkin T, Bouyssou S, Coia M, et al. Cholelithiasis in the dog: prevalence, clinical presentation, and outcome. *J Am Anim Hosp Assoc* 56(3):152-158, 2020.
63. Brunet A, Duperrier-Simond C, Amoyal S, Benchekroun G, Hernandez J, Lecot L, et al. Prevalence and clinical relevance of cholelithiasis in cats: A multicenter retrospective study of 98 cases. *J Vet Intern Med* 37(6):2157-2170, 2023.
64. Allan F, Watson PJ, McCallum KE. Clinical features and outcomes in 38 dogs with cholelithiasis receiving conservative or surgical management. *J Vet Intern Med* 35(6):2730-2742, 2021.
65. Lee S, Kweon O kyeong, Kim WH. Associations between serum leptin levels, hyperlipidemia, and cholelithiasis in dogs. *PLoS One* 12(10), 2017.
66. Kirpensteijn J, Fingland RB, Ulrich T, Sikkema DA, Allen SW. Cholelithiasis in dogs: 29 cases (1980-1990). *J Am Vet Med Assoc* 202(7):1137-1142, 1993.
67. Larson MM, Mattoon JS, Lawrence Y, Sellon RK. Liver. In: Mattoon JS, Sellon RK, Berry CR (editors). Small Animal Diagnostic Ultrasound 4th edition. St Louis, Elsevier, 2020.
68. Allan F, McCallum KE, Genain MA, Harris BJ, Watson PJ. Dissolution of cholelithiasis in a cavalier king charles spaniel receiving conservative management with ursodeoxycholic acid. *J Am Vet Med Assoc* 202(7):1137-1142, 1993.
69. Paumgartner G, Beuers U. Ursodeoxycholic acid in cholestatic liver disease: mechanisms of action and therapeutic use revisited. *Hepatology* 36(3):525-531, 2002.
70. Heuman DM, Bajaj RS, Lin Q. Adsorption of mixtures of bile salt taurine conjugates to lecithin-cholesterol membranes: implications for bile salt toxicity and cytoprotection. *J Lipid Res* 37:562-573, 1996.

CHAPTER 36

Congenital vascular diseases

Michael S. Tivers
BVSc, PhD, CertSAS, DECVS, MRCVS

There are three congenital vascular diseases seen in dogs: congenital portosystemic shunts (CPSS), hepatic arteriovenous malformations (HAVM), and primary portal vein hypoplasia (PPVH)/microvascular dysplasia (MVD). These conditions are differential diagnoses for one another and have some similarities but also significant, very important differences. It is also possible to have more than one concurrently. The most common and best-researched condition is CPSS.

Disease definition

Congenital portosystemic shunts

A CPSS is an aberrant blood vessel that forms a communication between the portal and the systemic venous systems. The shunt represents a failure of the normal development of the venous system in the fetus. The precise embryogenesis is unknown and may vary depending on the specific type of shunt. The abnormal vessel can lie outside the liver (extrahepatic) or within the hepatic parenchyma (intrahepatic). Extrahepatic CPSS (EHCPSS) are more common than intrahepatic CPSS (IHCPSS) and have a relatively wide variety of morphologies. However, they all connect a tributary of the extrahepatic portal vein to either the caudal vena cava, phrenic vein, or azygous vein.[1] IHCPSS originate from an intrahepatic portal vein branch and typically insert on a hepatic vein or the caudal vena cava. They are traditionally characterized by their location within the liver into left, central, and right divisional shunts, although the precise anatomy is more complex than this.[2] Some, but not all, left divisional shunts are patent ductus venosus (PDV).

Hepatic arteriovenous malformation

HAVM is typically a direct communication between a branch of the hepatic artery and the portal vein in the form of multiple vessels. HAVM has been called hepatic arteriovenous fistula, but a malformation is more correct as there are multiple communications/vessels. An HAVM allows blood to flow directly from the high-pressure arterial system into the low-pressure portal system. This causes blood to flow away from the liver (hepatofugal flow) and causes portal hypertension. Portal hypertension causes the formation of multiple acquired shunts (MAS) to relieve the pressure. HAVMs are relatively rare, particularly compared with CPSS and PVH.

Primary portal vein hypoplasia

Primary portal vein hypoplasia is a complicated congenital liver disease and can take two forms clinically based on whether portal hypertension is present. It seems likely that these two forms are closely related.

Primary portal vein hypoplasia without hypertension (PVH) has also been referred to as microvascular dysplasia (MVD). This condition is due to the arrested development of the terminal portal vein branches, resulting in small or absent portal veins in the smaller portal triads (often described as a "pollard willow" pattern). Reduction in the parallel pathways for flow in the portal vasculature should increase resistance and thus pressure in the portal vein, but in PVH without hypertension, it is thought blood is shunted from the portal to systemic systems at the microscopic level within the liver, protecting against portal hypertension. Histopathology of the affected liver demonstrates signs of portal hypoperfusion (small or absent intrahepatic portal vessels, endothelial hyperplasia, atrophic hepatocytes, small lobules, and variable amounts of fibrosis). These changes are typical of portal hypoperfusion and, thus, the same as those seen with CPSS. Signs of portal vein hypoperfusion without a macroscopic shunting vessel confirm a diagnosis of PVH. Dogs with CPSS likely have a variable degree of concurrent PVH, but this is impossible to characterize further.

PVH also occurs with concurrent portal hypertension (PVH-PH), and this has been referred to previously as idiopathic noncirrhotic portal hypertension. Importantly, liver cirrhosis is not a feature of this condition, although in some cases, there is concurrent congenital hepatic fibrosis, which presents in a similar way to cirrhosis (see chapter 37). In PVH-PH, it is thought that intrahepatic shunting fails to occur, resulting in portal hypertension and, hence, MAS development. Histopathology of affected livers is consistent with portal vein hypoperfusion and indistinguishable from PVH and CPSS.

Clinical presentation/features

Congenital portosystemic shunts

CPSS are relatively uncommon in dogs, but certain pedigree breeds are over-represented, suggesting it is a hereditary condition. This has been shown in Yorkshire Terriers, Cairn Terriers, Maltese Terriers, Irish Wolfhounds, and Australian Cattle dogs, whilst other breeds such as West Highland White Terriers and Labrador Retrievers also appear to be predisposed. A study of dogs at a North American teaching hospital found that a CPSS was diagnosed in 0.18% of dogs seen.[3] In a study of the occurrence of CPSS in pedigree dog breeds in the UK, the prevalence varied from 0.1-2.9%.[4] EHCPSS are typically found in small breed dogs (terriers in particular) but can be seen in larger breeds. Nearly all IHCPSS are seen in large breed dogs.

The presence of a CPSS allows blood from the gastrointestinal tract to bypass the liver and enter the systemic circulation directly. Portal blood carries oxygen, nutrients, and hormones (see chapter 30), without which the liver is not stimulated to develop normally and is hypoplastic with reduced function. Animals have clinical signs associated with both portosystemic shunting of toxins of gut origin and effective hepatic insufficiency. The amount of blood shunting past the liver and, hence, the degree of hepatic development is variable between animals, and this results in a variety of clinical signs both in terms of type and severity. Due to the congenital nature of the condition, most dogs will show clinical signs as puppies, and they are typically diagnosed between 6 weeks and 6 months of age. These dogs are typically small and underweight, particularly when compared to litter mates. However, dogs can appear normal when juvenile and develop clinical signs when mature. It is also possible for dogs to be diagnosed as adults without obvious clinical signs, for example, when a routine blood test picks up increased bile acids. In one study of 2,400 dogs, 27% were older than 2 years of age at the time of diagnosis of their shunt.[3] Decision-making for apparently normal dogs can be challenging.

Clinical signs can affect the neurological, gastrointestinal, and urinary systems (Table 36.1). Neurological signs are most common and are related to hepatic encephalopathy (HE). HE is a syndrome related to the build-up of toxins in the blood, and signs can vary in type and severity. The pathophysiology of HE is very complicated, but ammonia is one of the most important and readily measured factors. Many others are involved, including inflammation, aromatic amino acids (phenylalanine, tyrosine, tryptophan, and methionine), central nervous system inhibitors (γ-aminobutyric acid [GABA] and GABA receptors), mercaptans, and short-chain fatty acids. See chapter 7 for more details. It is likely that factors act synergistically and that this process differs in each individual and may result in the variety of signs seen.

Urinary tract signs are due to ammonium urate urolithiasis because of impairment of hepatic metabolism of ammonia. Stones can be found in both the upper and lower urinary tract and can cause urethral obstruction or recurrent urinary tract infection.

Dogs can be seen as emergencies with very severe HE causing coma or seizures or with urethral obstruction due to ammonium urate stones in male animals.

It is thought that the morphology of EHCPSS can affect the severity of clinical signs.[5] Portoazygous and portophrenic CPSS insert between the liver and diaphragm and intermittent compression of the shunt during respiration or with distension of the stomach with food may reduce the amount of shunting. Dogs with these morphologies can show reduced severity of clinical signs and are, therefore, more likely to be older at the time of diagnosis.

TABLE 36.1 Common clinical signs seen in dogs with congenital portosystemic shunts (CPSS).

Affected system	Clinical sign
Neurologic (hepatic encephalopathy)	■ Lethargy ■ Abnormal behavior ■ Reduced mentation ■ Head pressing ■ Ataxia ■ Wandering/circling ■ Tremors ■ Blindness ■ Coma ■ Seizures
Gastrointestinal	■ Diarrhea ■ Vomiting ■ Evidence of gastrointestinal bleeding: melena ■ Pica
Urinary tract (related to ammonium urate urolithiasis)	■ Hematuria ■ Pollakiuria ■ Dysuria ■ Stranguria
Other	■ Small stature ■ Failure to gain weight/poor body condition ■ Intolerance to sedative/anesthetic agents ■ Polyuria/polydipsia

Hepatic arteriovenous malformation

HAVM has been reported in a variety of breeds, suggesting no specific breed predisposition. Dogs with HAVM typically show clinical signs at a young age. Signs can be acute or chronic, including lethargy, vomiting, diarrhea, ascites, poor growth/weight gain, and neurological signs of HE (although with less frequency compared to CPSS). Ascites is seen in 75% of dogs and is a pure transudate (protein concentration of <2.5g/dL). A flow murmur may be detectable on auscultation of the cranial abdomen (abdominal bruit).

Primary portal vein hypoplasia

PVH has been shown to be hereditary in Cairn Terriers, and Yorkshire Terriers are predisposed. The overlap in predisposed breeds with EH-CPSS is interesting and may suggest a common hereditary cause. Dogs with PVH have similar but less severe signs to CPSS, including those affecting the neurological (HE), gastrointestinal, and urinary systems. Some animals may not show obvious signs, and the condition is typically identified at a later stage than CPSS, with dogs often being mature at diagnosis.

Dogs with PVH-PH are normally pedigree breeds and typically greater than 10 kg. Dogs with PVH-PH are more severely affected compared to those with PVH, and most are less than 4 years old at presentation. They can show signs of ascites, polyuria/polydipsia, gastrointestinal abnormalities, HE, stunted growth, and weight loss.

Clinicopathological findings

Congenital portosystemic shunts

Changes in routine biochemistry, hematology, and urinalysis are relatively nonspecific but can show certain abnormalities characteristic of a CPSS (Table 36.2).

Dogs with CPSS often have increases in clotting times (activated partial thromboplastin time and prothrombin time).[6] However, one study using thromboelastography showed that 9/21 dogs were hypercoagulable, whereas 12/21 were normocoagulable.[7]

Although routine blood tests may be useful, liver function tests are essential to investigate a suspected CPSS. Serum bile acids are recommended as they are accurate and convenient. Preprandial bile acids have a sensitivity of 90-98% and a specificity of 58-68%.[8] In comparison, dynamic bile acids (pre- and postprandial samples) have an excellent sensitivity of 100% for CPSS.[8] A dynamic test is always recommended as, occasionally, dogs with CPSS can have a normal preprandial result. Because of the lack of specificity, diagnostic imaging is then necessary to demonstrate a CPSS (see below).

TABLE 36.2 Common abnormalities on routine complete blood count (CBC), biochemistry profile, and urinalysis in dogs with congenital portosystemic shunts (CPSS).

Test	Abnormality
Complete blood count (CBC)	■ Microcytosis ■ Anemia
Biochemistry	■ Hypoalbuminemia ■ Decreased blood urea nitrogen ■ Hypoglycemia ■ Hypocholesterolemia ■ Increased liver enzymes (ALP and ALT)
Urinalysis	■ Decreased urine specific gravity ■ Ammonium biurate crystalluria

ALP, alkaline phosphatase; ALT, alanine aminotransferase.

Resting plasma ammonia is an alternative test with a sensitivity of 81-98% and specificity of 86-90%.[8] However, ammonia is very labile, and measurement may not be readily available. Nevertheless, a high ammonia raises the suspicion of a CPSS.

Hepatic arteriovenous malformation

Dogs with HAVM have similar clinicopathological changes to those with CPSS, including microcytic anemia, hypoalbuminemia, and increased liver enzymes. Plasma ammonia and pre- and postprandial bile acids are increased, consistent with acquired portosystemic shunting due to portal hypertension.

Primary portal vein hypoplasia

Dogs with PVH typically have normal biochemistry and hematology. Increased dynamic bile acids may be the only abnormality.

Dogs with PVH-PH have clinicopathological changes consistent with hepatic dysfunction, portal hypertension, and acquired portosystemic shunting, including microcytosis, mild anemia, increased liver enzymes, hypoalbuminemia, decreased urea and increased bile acids and ammonia.

Diagnostic imaging findings

Congenital portosystemic shunts

Diagnostic imaging is used to confirm the diagnosis by identifying the CPSS. This also allows differentiation from other conditions, such as PVH or HAVM. Imaging will also yield important information on the location and morphology of the shunt, which will help guide treatment. Imaging may be less important for dogs where surgical management is not possible or desired by the owner, as it may not change the treatment.

Computed tomography angiography (CTA) provides excellent and detailed information on the morphology of the shunt and intrahepatic portal vasculature development and is therefore considered the gold standard imaging technique[9] (Fig. 36.1). CTA is minimally invasive and has been shown to be safe to perform prior to surgery.[10] However, it is relatively expensive and does require heavy sedation or anesthesia.

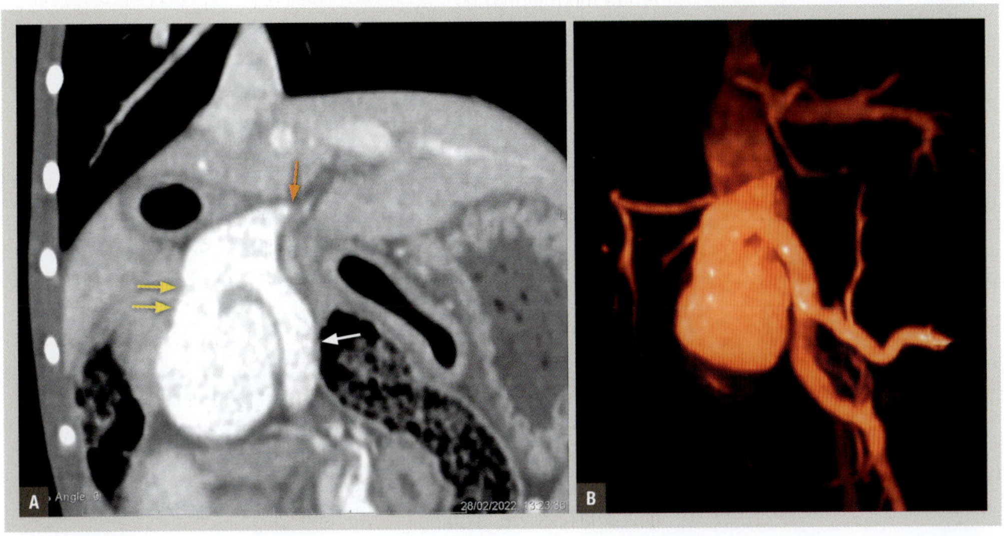

FIG. 36.1 Reconstructed computed tomography angiography (CTA) images showing a right divisional intrahepatic congenital portosystemic shunt (IHCPSS). The image on the left has been reconstructed in the dorsal plane and shows the portal vein (white arrow) and the right portal vein branch (two yellow arrows) entering the shunt, which appears as a large, dilated vessel. The left portal vein branch can also be seen (orange arrow). The image on the right shows a three-dimensional reconstruction of the shunt.

Abdominal ultrasound is also commonly used and has the advantage of being more convenient than CTA. It can be used to confirm the presence of a CPSS and will provide some information on the morphology. In many instances, this is sufficient to confirm a diagnosis and allow surgical planning. However, ultrasound is very operator-dependent, and therefore the accuracy is variable.

The author uses ultrasound as the first-line imaging technique in dogs with suspected CPSS. With an experienced operator, ultrasound can confirm the presence of a shunt and whether it is extrahepatic or intrahepatic. CTA is recommended for dogs with an IHCPSS or when ultrasound was not able to identify a vascular abnormality.

Intraoperative mesenteric portovenography (IOMP) under fluoroscopic guidance can be used during the surgical management of a CPSS (Fig. 36.2). It provides detailed information on the morphology of the shunt, although less than that from CTA.[9] IOMP can be used to confirm accurate identification of the shunt and the optimal location of attenuation. It also provides information about the degree of intrahepatic portal development and rules out a second CPSS or multiple acquired shunts. IOMP may be particularly useful in dogs that have not had CTA,[9] and the author performs this in all dogs with shunts during surgery.

Hepatic arteriovenous malformation

Doppler ultrasonography can be used to diagnose an HAVM, but CTA is recommended to obtain more information on the precise nature of the abnormality, particularly if considering surgery. IOMP can also be used during surgical treatment.

Primary portal vein hypoplasia

Dogs with PVH have a relatively normal liver and portal vasculature anatomy on imaging (including ultrasound, CTA, and IOMP). However, these techniques will help to rule out a CPSS.

For dogs with PVH-PH, ultrasound may show a small liver, ascites, and MAS. More detail on MAS and liver size can be revealed with CTA or IOMP, although this information may not be necessary as only medical management is possible with this condition.

Treatment

Congenital portosystemic shunts

Medical management

Dogs with CPSS can be managed with medical treatment or surgery. Medical management consists of strategies to control HE by reducing the amount of ammonia absorbed from the gastrointestinal tract. Ammonia is produced in the gastrointestinal tract by urease-positive gut bacteria metabolizing amino acids derived from dietary protein. It is also produced as a byproduct of the enterocyte metabolism of glutamine. Gastric urease-positive *Helicobacter* spp. may also contribute to ammonia production. The CPSS allows the ammonia (and other toxins) that would normally be metabolized by the liver to enter the systemic circulation, causing HE. Medical management can involve dietary modification, lactulose, and antimicrobials. Ideally, treatment should start with dietary modification as the sole treatment, and then lactulose can be added as needed. Due to increasing concerns over antimicrobial resistance, these should be reserved for dogs that do not respond adequately to diet and lactulose. Studies have shown that diet and lactulose are adequate for the medical management of their CPSS in most dogs.[11,12] Modification of dietary protein is very important for managing HE. However, protein restriction is problematic in dogs with CPSS, particularly as most are growing puppies. Therefore, protein levels should meet the dog's requirements without being excessive. More details are found in chapter 40. Therefore, a hydrolyzed soya-based diet balanced for growth is preferred (e.g., Purina ProPlan Veterinary Diet HA or Royal Canin Canine Hypoallergenic) as it will cause less ammonia production whilst providing all the essential nutrients for growth. Lactulose is a nonabsorbable, synthetic disaccharide (fructose-galactose) that is hydrolyzed by colonic bacteria to lactic, acetic, and formic acids. These organic acids reduce the pH of the colonic contents, trapping free ammonia (NH_3) as ammonium (NH_4^+) ions that cannot be absorbed. This, coupled with the osmotic laxative effect, reduces the amount of ammonia absorbed from the gastrointestinal tract. Lactulose is given at a dose of 0.5-1.0 mL/kg orally every 8-12 hours, and it is titrated to give 2-3 soft stools daily. Antimicrobials are used to reduce the urease-positive

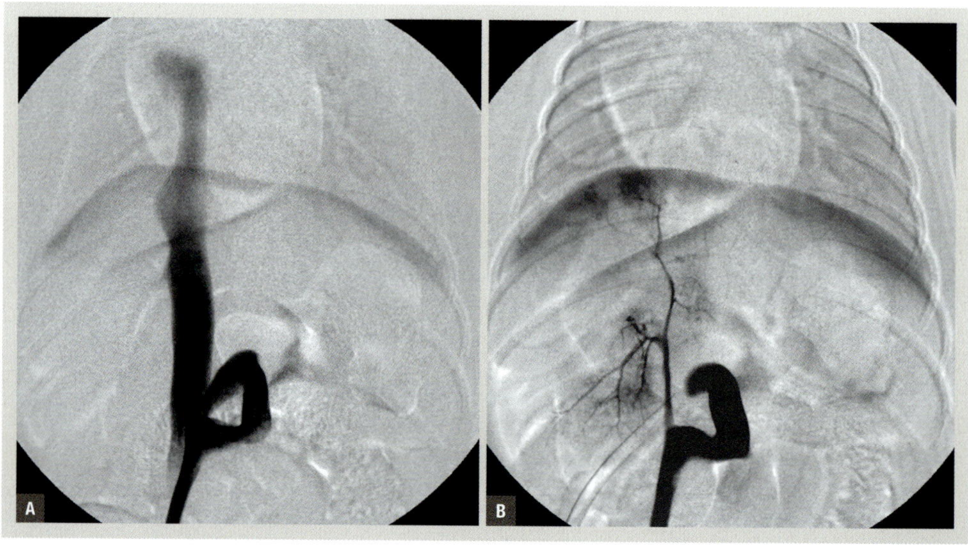

FIG. 36.2 Two ventrodorsal intraoperative mesenteric portovenography (IOMP) images from a Miniature Schnauzer with an extrahepatic congenital portosystemic shunt (EHCPSS). The images are orientated so that cranial is at the top. Contrast has been injected through a jejunal vein under fluoroscopic guidance with digital subtraction. The image on the left shows a portovenogram with flow into the caudal vena cava with no intrahepatic portal blood flow. The image on the right is a repeat portovenogram after temporary complete occlusion of the shunting vessel. Note the increased opacification of the liver and the lack of contrast flow through the abnormal vessel. However, the intrahepatic portal vasculature is not well developed, and this dog was unable to tolerate a complete attenuation of the shunt. Therefore, an ameroid constrictor was placed.

gut bacteria implicated in the production of ammonia, although there is no good evidence for their efficacy in this context. Ampicillin, amoxicillin, metronidazole, and neomycin have all been used in dogs. The author no longer uses antimicrobials in the management of HE in dogs with CPSS. Dogs with evidence of gastrointestinal hemorrhage should be treated with antacids and gastroprotectants such as omeprazole and sucralfate. Dogs with intermittent seizures that do not respond to medical treatment of HE should be started on antiseizure medication such as levetiracetam. If seizures are refractory to this treatment, then phenobarbital may be considered. However, as phenobarbital is metabolized by the liver, it should be used at a minimal dose and closely monitored. See chapter 7 for more details on seizure management.

Dogs can be seen as emergencies with severe HE resulting in collapse, coma, or status epilepticus (Fig. 36.3). Deterioration in signs of HE can be caused by various factors, including increased dietary protein, gastrointestinal hemorrhage, constipation, metabolic alkalosis, hypokalemia, hypoglycemia, and dehydration. A minimum database, including serum electrolytes and blood glucose, should be performed to check for exacerbating factors or other causes of collapse or seizure. The dog should be treated with intravenous fluid therapy with appropriate supplementation to correct any hypoperfusion, dehydration, or metabolic abnormalities. Medical therapy should be started as described above with lactulose and possibly antimicrobials, although it may not be possible to administer drugs orally if the animal is in a coma or seizing. Lactulose can be given as a retention enema. There is potential controversy about the use of diazepam to treat seizures in dogs with CPSS due to concerns about increased γ-aminobutyric acid (GABA) and GABA receptors in HE. Diazepam can be given as a first-line treatment for seizures, but dogs that do not respond should be treated with levetiracetam, propofol, or phenobarbital intravenously. See chapter 7 for more details of seizure management. Once stable, the dog can be transitioned to oral medication, and antibiotics are withdrawn if they have been used (see above). Dogs with severe HE can develop cerebral edema, which may worsen neurological signs. This may respond to a single bolus of mannitol, although this should not be used in severely dehydrated or hypoperfused animals (see chapter 7 for more details of emergency treatment of suspected increased intracranial pressure).

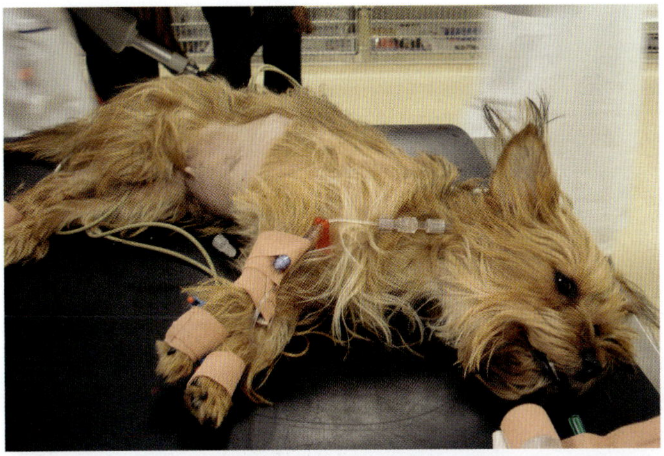

FIG. 36.3 Image of a crossbreed dog with severe hepatic encephalopathy (HE) secondary to an extrahepatic congenital portosystemic shunt (EHCPSS). The dog is collapsed and obtunded. The dog responded well to medical management of HE.

Decision-making

Medical management can be used as the sole treatment for dogs with CPSS, but it only manages the clinical signs and does not treat the underlying cause. In this sense, it is very much a way of managing the problem rather than resolving it. Some dogs can do well with medical management, but there is a risk of recurrence of clinical signs, and surgery results in a better outcome in terms of length and quality of life. A prospective study assessed the long-term outcome for 97 dogs treated surgically and 27 dogs managed medically.[13] Surgically treated dogs had a significantly improved survival rate and a lower frequency of clinical signs compared with those managed medically. Another study of 78 dogs with CPSS found good improvements in the owner-reported quality of life and clinical signs with medical management alone.[12] Nevertheless, 54% of dogs died or were put to sleep for reasons related to their CPSS.

Overall, surgical management is recommended for dogs with CPSS, but as outlined below, there is a risk associated with surgery, and this is an expensive referral procedure. Medical management may be preferred for dogs where surgical treatment is not feasible for clinical or financial reasons or where the owner considers the risks associated with surgery to be unacceptable.

In some instances, animals mildly affected or without obvious clinical signs are diagnosed with a CPSS. This can happen in mature animals, and they may be diagnosed incidentally on the results of a routine blood test or imaging for other reasons. These animals can represent something of a conundrum as the risk/benefit of surgery may not be clear. In addition, the risk associated with surgery may be increased in older animals.[14] The author believes that dogs with CPSS are not normal, even if they appear to be. CPSS is a congenital disease, and dogs may have subclinical HE, which is difficult to appreciate. Therefore, these dogs would benefit from surgical correction of their shunt, but this must be weighed against the risks of morbidity and mortality and the financial costs involved.

Surgical management

Surgical management aims to attenuate the CPSS to improve hepatic portal blood flow, ideally to normal. An improvement in portal flow should result in improved liver function and, hence, resolution of clinical signs. Several surgical techniques have been recommended for the treatment of CPSS, including suture ligation, aneroid constrictors (AC), thin film (cellophane) bands (TFB), and endovascular coils. Medical management is vital for stabilizing dogs prior to surgery, with 2 to 4 weeks of medical treatment recommended.

Originally, CPSS were treated with suture ligation (with silk or polypropylene) (Fig. 36.4). However, in many dogs, the liver is small with an underdeveloped portal vasculature, and this prohibits acute complete closure due to portal hypertension. Temporary occlusion of the shunt allows intraoperative subjective and objective assessment of portal pressure changes, and this, along with portal flow on IOMP, can be used to determine whether a dog will tolerate a complete ligation. Those that cannot tolerate complete closure can be treated with partial ligation, but these dogs will have persistent shunting through the shunt, with concerns over persistent or recurrent clinical signs. Further surgery has been recommended for dogs treated with partial ligation, and this is associated with a good rate of complete closure (in two procedures).[15,16] However, this approach has been superseded by gradual attenuation devices or a hybrid approach (see below).

Gradual attenuation devices are preferred by many surgeons for CPSS attenuation as they overcome concerns over portal hypertension and the inability to completely close the shunt acutely. Such devices include AC and TFB

(Fig. 36.5). Polyacrylic acid-silicone gradual occlusion devices (PAS-OD) have also been described, but limited information is available. These devices are placed around the CPSS and will gradually close the vessel over a period of weeks. Both TFB and AC are relatively easy to use and have been associated with a good outcome (see below). However, once placed, there is no control over how quickly they occlude the vessel or the completeness of closure. Gradual attenuation devices can result in persistent shunting if the shunt does not fully close or in MAS if the closure is too rapid. For dogs with EHCPSS, a persistent shunting rate of 24.1% after AC[17] and 30.06-37.5% after TFB have been reported.[18-20]

IHCPSS can be treated via an open surgical approach and suture ligation, AC and TFB as for EHCPSS (Fig. 36.6). Placement of a hydraulic occluder has also been described, and this device allows greater control over gradual attenuation, but the technique has not been widely adopted. As they are located within the liver parenchyma, IHCPSS are technically more difficult to access for occlusion. The ligation site or device placement can be the hepatic vein draining the shunt, the portal vein branch supplying the shunt, or the abnormal vessel itself. Open surgery for IHCPSS has been associated with a relatively high rate of morbidity and mortality compared with EHCPSS.

Therefore, coil embolization via interventional radiology has been developed to reduce the complications associated with open surgery in dogs with IHCPSS.[21] This is performed via a jugular catheter and under fluoroscopic guidance. A stent is placed in the vena cava, and then coils are placed into the shunt (the stent prevents them from migrating). The coils provide acute partial shunt closure via thrombosis, and further occlusion may occur with time. Coil embolization has the advantage of being minimally invasive compared with surgery, and this is associated with a lower rate of complications. However, it may be harder to achieve full closure of the shunt; therefore, persistent shunting may be expected in a proportion of dogs.[21] It is typically more expensive than open surgery. This technique has been used in dogs with EHCPSS, but reports are limited, and it may not offer significant advantages over open surgery for this type of shunt.

A good compromise between ligation and gradual attenuation devices is a hybrid approach, which has been recently described.[22] Dogs are assessed intraoperatively, and those that can tolerate temporary complete attenuation are treated with a complete acute ligation of the shunt (with polypropylene suture). For dogs that cannot tolerate complete attenuation, a gradual attenuation device (either AC or TFB) is placed. The author uses this approach for both EHCPSS and IHCPSS. When using an AC or TFB, the author will also place a length of loose suture material around the shunt vessel to allow further surgical attenuation at a subsequent surgery if the device fails to close the shunt completely.

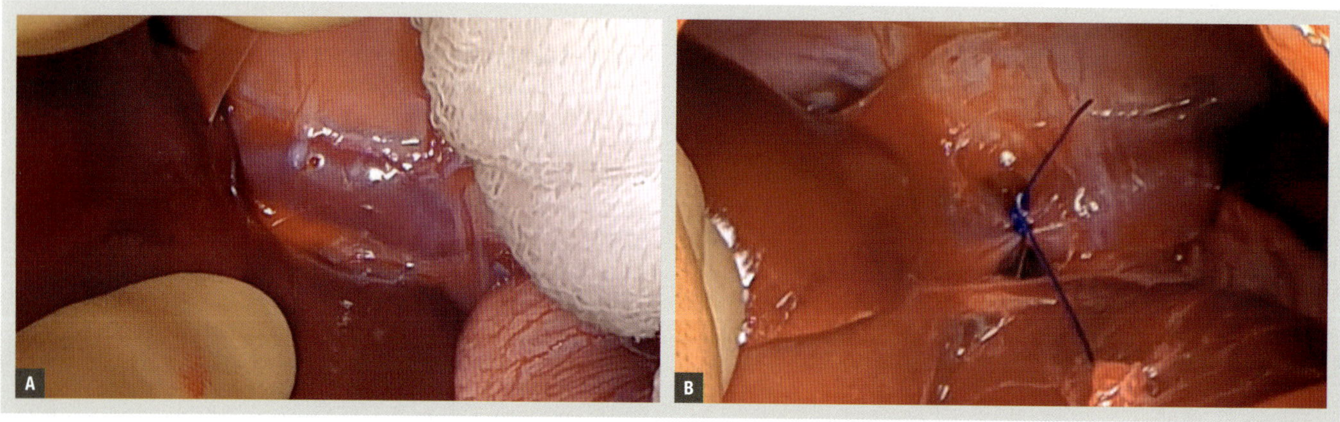

FIG. 36.4 Intraoperative images of a portophrenic extrahepatic congenital portosystemic shunt (EHCPSS). The images show the enlarged phrenic vein closely associated with the diaphragm. In the image on the right, the vessel has been fully ligated with polypropylene suture.

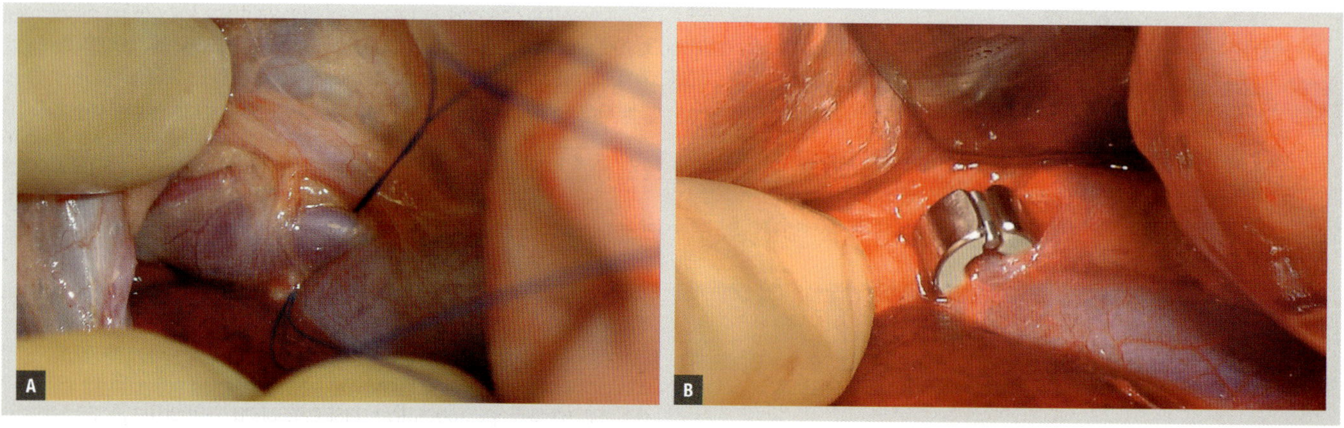

FIG. 36.5 Intraoperative images of a portocaval extrahepatic congenital portosystemic shunt (EHCPSS). This is the shunt represented in Fig. 36.3. (A) Two lengths of suture have been passed around the shunt vessel adjacent to its insertion on the vena cava. (B) An ameroid constrictor (AC) has been placed around the shunt vessel.

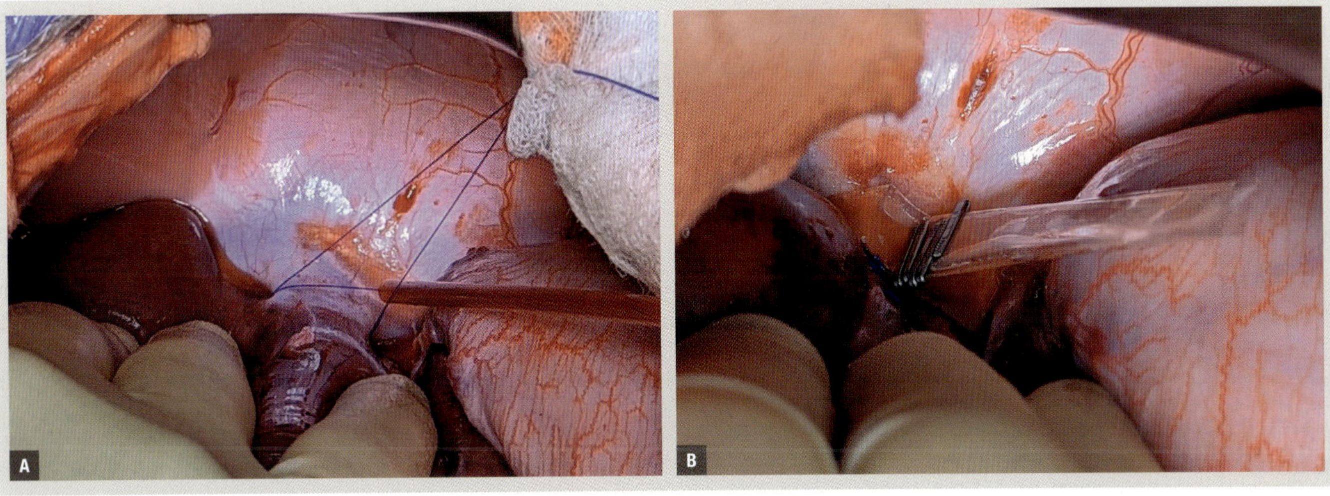

FIG. 36.6 Intraoperative images of a left divisional intrahepatic congenital portosystemic shunt (IHCPSS). (A) Two lengths of suture have been passed around the shunt vessel adjacent to its insertion on the vena cava. The red tubing is used to create a Rummel tourniquet to temporarily occlude the vessel. (B) A cellophane band has been placed around the vessel. The cellophane will be cut shorter prior to the closure of the abdomen.

Hepatic arteriovenous malformation

Most HAVM are confined to a single liver lobe, although two lobes can be affected (Fig. 36.7). Reported treatments include liver lobectomy, ligation of the artery supplying the malformation or embolization of the HAVM with glue (23).

Primary portal vein hypoplasia

Dogs with PVH or PVH-PH should be managed medically with treatment for HE, including diet and lactulose. Antimicrobials are usually not necessary and should be avoided (see above). Symptomatic treatment of portal hypertension will also be necessary in some cases with diuretic treatment of ascites, as detailed in chapter 34.

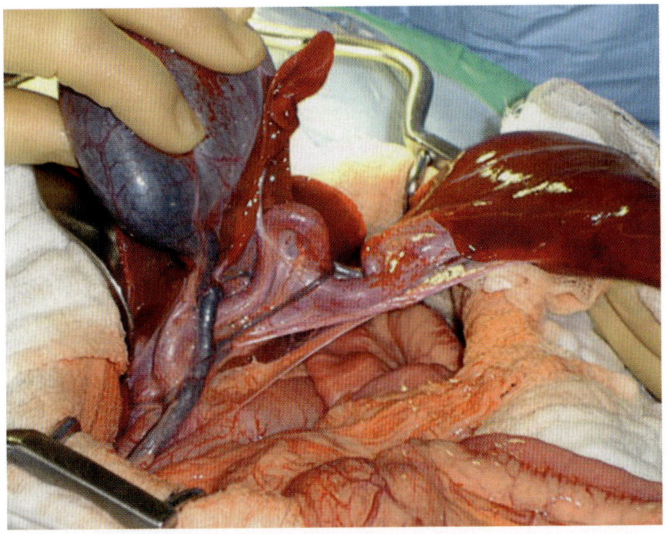

FIG. 36.7 Image of a hepatic arteriovenous malformation (HAVM) at exploratory laparotomy in a 6-month-old Labrador Retriever.

Prognosis

Congenital portosystemic shunts

Surgical complications

Complications of CPSS surgery include perioperative hypoglycemia, hemorrhage, portal hypertension, postoperative gastrointestinal bleeding, and postattenuation neurological signs (PANS).

CPSS dogs can be hypoglycemic. Therefore, it is important for blood glucose to be monitored during surgery and supplemented as needed. Bleeding can occur during dissection of the shunt, but this is very uncommon in EHCPSS. Portal hypertension can occur postoperatively if there is excessive attenuation of the shunt with suture ligation or due to sudden kinking with an AC. Fortunately, due to the widespread use of gradual attenuation devices and with careful intraoperative assessment with suture ligation, significant portal hypertension is a very rare complication. PANS is the most important postoperative complication in dogs with EHCPSS but can also occur in dogs with IHCPSS, although apparently less frequently. The etiology of PANS is unknown, but it is not directly caused by HE or hypoglycemia. It is hypothesized that it could be influenced by postoperative changes in false neurotransmitters and toxins associated with HE. Signs associated with PANS can vary in type and severity, including mild tremors, ataxia, behavioral changes, blindness, and seizures. Signs typically occur within 72 hours of surgery and can be seen with all surgical techniques. PANS has been reported in 1.6-27.3% of dogs with CPSS, with seizures in 0-18.2% of dogs with EHCPSS and 0-14.3% of dogs with IHCPSS.[24] Severe PANS, particularly seizures, can be challenging to treat, and this is the most common cause of mortality in dogs with EHCPSS. Unfortunately, evidence suggests that using antiepileptic medications (e.g., levetiracetam) prior to surgery does not reduce the incidence of PANS.[24] Increasing age and the presence of signs of HE immediately before surgery have been shown to be significant risk factors for PANS.[14] Both open surgery and endovascular coiling for IHCPSS have been associated with postoperative gastrointestinal hemorrhage, and this is a common cause of morbidity and mortality.[15,21] The cause of the hemorrhage is unclear but may be related to portal hypertension. One study

TABLE 36.3 Reported perioperative and postoperative mortality for surgical treatment of extrahepatic and intrahepatic congenital portosystemic shunts (CPSS) in dogs. The data is taken from the largest and most recent studies.

Technique	Mortality for extrahepatic CPSS		Mortality for intrahepatic CPSS	
	Number of dogs in study	Percentage mortality	Number of dogs in study	Percentage mortality
Suture ligation	49-66[25,26]	2.0-28.8%	17-55[15,25,27,28]	5.9-22.6%
Ameroid constrictor	23-206[17,19,20,29]	2.6-7.3%	9-11[28,30]	0-9.1%
Thin film band	23-95[19,20,29,31]	0.0-11.8%	11-31[31,32]	3.2-27.3%
Intravascular coil	Only studies with <10 dogs	–	25-95[21,32,33]	0-7.4%

found that the use of nonsteroidal anti-inflammatory drugs (NSAIDs) was associated with mortality in dogs having surgery for IHCPSS.[15] The author avoids the use of NSAIDs in dogs with CPSS.

The surgical mortality rate for CPSS is shown in Table 36.3.

Outcome following surgery

Successful surgery redirects portal blood flow to the liver (either acutely or gradually), and this leads to improvements in portal vasculature and liver volume due to liver regeneration.[34,35] Liver function is improved, and hence, clinical signs improve or resolve. A good clinical response should be mirrored by improvements in clinicopathological parameters, including dynamic bile acids. Long-term outcome following successful surgery is very good and superior to medical management alone. A good to excellent outcome is reported following surgery in 52.0-100% of dogs with EHCPSS and 70.0-100% of dogs with IHCPSS. However, direct comparison between studies is difficult due to variations in outcome measures and definitions of outcome categories. The different treatment options have advantages and disadvantages, but all can result in a good outcome. The evidence base for comparing treatment options for both EHCPSS and IHCPSS is very weak.[36-38] One review suggested that AC is superior to TFB in leading to EHCPSS closure, but the evidence is not strong.[38] Further research should focus on prospective comparative studies to determine the best treatment, although recruiting an adequate number of dogs is likely to remain a challenge.

Postoperatively, dogs should be assessed with hematology, biochemistry, and dynamic bile acids to assess their response to surgery. The author repeats blood tests at approximately two months after surgery, but when a gradual attenuation device has been used, it may take longer for a full response to be seen. Dogs are typically kept on medical management until blood tests show an improvement in liver function, but reducing or stopping medical management can be considered earlier in dogs treated with complete acute closure of their shunt. Ideally, a good clinical response is associated with the resolution of clinicopathological abnormalities. Significantly increased bile acids following surgery suggest persistent shunting, and this should be investigated further, particularly if ongoing or recurrent clinical signs are present. Some dogs can have a persistent mild increase in bile acids following complete shunt attenuation and a good clinical outcome.[39] This is probably due to concurrent PVH but could also represent mild subclinical persistent shunting.

Significant persistent shunting can occur following surgery and may be associated with ongoing or recurrent clinical signs. This can be due to continued flow through the shunt due to incomplete attenuation, either due to the failure of a gradual attenuation device to fully close the shunt or in dogs treated with partial ligation. Persistent shunting can also be due to the development of MAS in dogs that have developed portal hypertension following rapid closure by a gradual attenuation device or excessive acute attenuation. A study of dogs with EHCPSS treated with AC found evidence of persistent shunting in 28/116 dogs (24.1%) on scintigraphy at 4-14 weeks following surgery.[17] This study found that dogs with no evidence of persistent shunting on scintigraphy were 10.7 times more likely to have a good outcome long-term. Intuitively, dogs that have all shunting abolished should have a better outcome than those with ongoing portal blood bypassing the liver, and this is supported by this data. Therefore, dogs with clinical or clinicopathological evidence of persistent shunting should ideally have further imaging. CTA is the most accurate, but ultrasound may be useful in the first instance to check for obvious flow in the CPSS or MAS. Animals with persistent flow through the CPSS (and no MAS) are likely to benefit from further surgery to provide more attenuation, and the author routinely leaves a loose length of suture material around the shunt to facilitate this when necessary. Further surgery to attenuate the CPSS in the presence of MAS is not likely to be beneficial. Owners may be reluctant to consider further imaging or surgery in dogs with a good clinical response. Long-term medical management can be used in dogs with persistent shunting, whether through the CPSS or MAS. Nevertheless, some dogs have a good outcome despite persistent shunting, and it is unclear how much shunting is clinically acceptable.

Hepatic arteriovenous malformation

Based on a very small number of dogs, glue embolization is safer than surgery with a better long-term outcome.[23] Although surgery/embolization can be significantly beneficial, many dogs will have persistent shunting through pre-existing MAS. Approximately 75% of dogs require ongoing medical management. Overall, the prognosis for HAVM is not as good as that for CPSS or PVH.

Primary portal vein hypoplasia

Although there is no surgical treatment, the prognosis for the medical management of PVH is excellent. Dogs do very well and much better than CPSS dogs managed with medicine alone. In one study, 92% of dogs had a good long-term survival rate or died of unrelated causes.[40]

The prognosis for dogs with PVH-PH is relatively good. In one study, a good outcome was reported in 13/19 dogs (68%), with 4/19 dogs (21%) euthanized due to the condition and 2/19 dogs (11%) for other reasons.[41] Interestingly, three of the dogs were euthanized due to duodenal ulceration.

KEY POINTS

Congenital portosystemic shunts

- Surgical management is recommended for most dogs with CPSS and is associated with a better long-term outcome than medical management alone.
- Whilst outcomes are typically very good, there is risk associated with surgery.
- Medical management is indicated for dogs that do not have surgery for financial or other reasons, and some dogs do well long-term.
- Dogs should be stabilized with medical management prior to surgery.
- Persistent shunting can occur following surgery, but dogs are normally significantly improved. It is unclear how much persistent shunting is "acceptable" for a good long-term outcome.

Hepatic arteriovenous malformation

- This is a very rare and variable condition.
- Embolization of the HAVM via interventional radiology is the recommended treatment for most dogs.
- Most dogs will still require ongoing medical management after surgery.

Primary portal vein hypoplasia

- PVH has an excellent prognosis with medical management.
- The prognosis for PVH-PH is not as good as that for PVH, and animals will need ongoing management.

References

1. White RN, Parry AT, Shales C. Implications of shunt morphology for the surgical management of extrahepatic portosystemic shunts. *Aust Vet J* 96(11):433-441, 2018.
2. Walsh ND, Porter IR, Miller AV, Fischetti AJ, Cheong SH, Scrivani PV. Canine intrahepatic portosystemic shunts: interlobar and intralobar classifications. *Vet Radiol Ultrasound* 64(4):646-660, 2023.
3. Tobias KM, Rohrbach BW. Association of breed with the diagnosis of congenital portosystemic shunts in dogs: 2,400 cases (1980-2002). *J Am Vet Med Assoc* 223(11):1636-1639, 2003.
4. Asher L, Diesel G, Summers JF, McGreevy PD, Collins LM. Inherited defects in pedigree dogs. Part 1: disorders related to breed standards. *Vet J* 182(3):402-411, 2009.
5. Kraun MB, Nelson LL, Hauptman JG, Nelson NC. Analysis of the relationship of extrahepatic portosystemic shunt morphology with clinical variables in dogs: 53 cases (2009-2012). *J Am Vet Med Assoc* 245(5):540-549, 2014.
6. Kummeling A, Teske E, Rothuizen J, Van Sluijs FJ. Coagulation profiles in dogs with congenital portosystemic shunts before and after surgical attenuation. *J Vet Intern Med* 20(6):1319-1326, 2006.
7. Kelley D, Lester C, DeLaforcade A, Webster CR. Thromboelastographic evaluation of dogs with congenital portosystemic shunts. *J Vet Intern Med* 27(5):1262-1267, 2013.
8. Devriendt N, Serrano G, Paepe D, de Rooster H. Liver function tests in dogs with congenital portosystemic shunts and their potential to determine persistent shunting after surgical attenuation. *Vet J* 261:105478, 2020.
9. Parry AT, White RN. Comparison of computed tomographic angiography and intraoperative mesenteric portovenography for extrahepatic portosystemic shunts. *J Small Anim Pract* 58(1):49-55, 2017.
10. Brunson BW, Case JB, Ellison GW, Fox-Alvarez WA, Kim SE, Winter M, et al. Evaluation of surgical outcome, complications, and mortality in dogs undergoing preoperative computed tomography angiography for diagnosis of an extrahepatic portosystemic shunt: 124 cases (2005-2014). *Can Vet J* 57(1):59-64, 2016.
11. Serrano G, Devriendt N, de Rooster H, Paepe D. Comparison of diet, lactulose, and metronidazole combinations in the control of pre-surgical clinical signs in dogs with congenital extrahepatic portosystemic shunts. *J Vet Intern Med* 36(4):1258-1266, 2022.
12. Favier RP, de Graaf E, Corbee RJ, Kummeling A. Outcome of non-surgical dietary treatment with or without lactulose in dogs with congenital portosystemic shunts. *Vet Quart* 40(1):108-114, 2020.
13. Greenhalgh SN, Reeve JA, Johnstone T, Goodfellow MR, Dunning MD, O'Neill EJ, et al. Long-term survival and quality of life in dogs with clinical signs associated with a congenital portosystemic shunt after surgical or medical treatment. *J Am Vet Med Assoc* 245(5):527-533, 2014.
14. Strickland R, Tivers MS, Adamantos SE, Harcourt-Brown TR, Fowkes RC, Lipscomb VJ. Incidence and risk factors for neurological signs after attenuation of single congenital portosystemic shunts in 253 dogs. *Vet Surg* 47(6):745-755, 2018.
15. Tivers MS, Lipscomb VJ, Bristow P, Brockman DJ. Intrahepatic congenital portosystemic shunts in dogs: short- and long-term outcome of suture attenuation. *J Small Anim Pract* 59(4):201-210, 2018.
16. Lee KC, Lipscomb VJ, Lamb CR, Gregory SP, Guitian J, Brockman DJ. Association of portovenographic findings with outcome in dogs receiving surgical treatment for single congenital portosystemic shunts: 45 cases (2000-2004). *J Am Vet Med Assoc* 229(7):1122-1129, 2006.
17. Falls EL, Milovancev M, Hunt GB, Daniel L, Mehl ML, Schmiedt CW. Long-term outcome after surgical ameroid ring constrictor placement for treatment of single extrahepatic portosystemic shunts in dogs. *Vet Surg* 42(8):951-957, 2013.
18. Landon BP, Abraham LA, Charles JA. Use of transcolonic portal scintigraphy to evaluate efficacy of cellophane banding of congenital extrahepatic portosystemic shunts in 16 dogs. *Aust Vet J* 86(5):169-79; quiz CE1, 2008.
19. Matiasovic M, Chanoit GPA, Meakin LB, Tivers MS. Outcomes of dogs treated for extrahepatic

congenital portosystemic shunts with thin film banding or ameroid ring constrictor. *Vet Surg* 49(1):160-171, 2020.

20. Traverson M, Lussier B, Huneault L, Gatineau M. Comparative outcomes between ameroid ring constrictor and cellophane banding for treatment of single congenital extrahepatic portosystemic shunts in 49 dogs (1998-2012). *Vet Surg* 47(2):179-187, 2018.
21. Weisse C, Berent AC, Todd K, Solomon JA, Cope C. Endovascular evaluation and treatment of intrahepatic portosystemic shunts in dogs: 100 cases (2001-2011). *J Am Vet Med Assoc* 244(1):78-94, 2014.
22. Lipscomb V, Cassie C, Ritchie B, Greenhalgh S, Tivers M. Prospective study comparing outcome following complete polypropylene suture ligation versus partial thin film band attenuation of congenital portosystemic shunts in dogs. *Vet Sci* 10(7), 2023.
23. Chanoit G, Kyles AE, Weisse C, Hardie EM. Surgical and interventional radiographic treatment of dogs with hepatic arteriovenous fistulae. *Vet Surg* 36(3):199-209, 2007.
24. Mullins RA, Escribano Carrera A, Anderson DM, Billet JP, Brissot H, Broome C, et al. Postattenuation neurologic signs after surgical attenuation of congenital portosystemic shunts in dogs: A review. *Vet Surg* 51(1):23-33, 2022.
25. Kummeling A, Van Sluijs FJ, Rothuizen J. Prognostic implications of the degree of shunt narrowing and of the portal vein diameter in dogs with congenital portosystemic shunts. *Vet Surg* 33(1):17-24, 2004.
26. Hunt GB, Hughes J. Outcomes after extrahepatic portosystemic shunt ligation in 49 dogs. *Aust Vet J* 77(5):303-307, 1999.
27. White RN, Burton CA, McEvoy FJ. Surgical treatment of intrahepatic portosystemic shunts in 45 dogs. *Vet Rec* 142(14):358-365, 1998.
28. Mehl ML, Kyles AE, Case JB, Kass PH, Zwingenberger A, Gregory CR. Surgical management of left-divisional intrahepatic portosystemic shunts: outcome after partial ligation of, or ameroid ring constrictor placement on, the left hepatic vein in twenty-eight dogs (1995-2005). *Vet Surg* 36(1):21-30, 2007.
29. Otomo A, Singh A, Jeong J, Dobberstein R, Lundhild A, Peter E, et al. Long-term clinical outcomes of dogs with single congenital extrahepatic portosystemic shunts attenuated with thin film banding or ameroid ring constrictors. *Vet Surg* 49(3):436-44, 2020.
30. Bright SR, Williams JM, Niles JD. Outcomes of intrahepatic portosystemic shunts occluded with ameroid constrictors in nine dogs and one cat. *Vet Surg* 35(3):300-309, 2006.
31. Hunt GB, Kummeling A, Tisdall PL, Marchevsky AM, Liptak JM, Youmans KR, et al. Outcomes of cellophane banding for congenital portosystemic shunts in 106 dogs and 5 cats. *Vet Surg* 33(1):25-31, 2004.
32. Case JB, Marvel SJ, Stiles MC, Maisenbacher HW, Toskich BB, Smeak DD, Monnet EL. Outcomes of cellophane banding or percutaneous transvenous coil embolization of canine intrahepatic portosystemic shunts. *Vet Surg* 47(S1):059-066, 2018.
33. Culp WTN, Zwingenberger AL, Giuffrida MA, Wisner ER, Hunt GB, Steffey MA, et al. Prospective evaluation of outcome of dogs with intrahepatic portosystemic shunts treated via percutaneous transvenous coil embolization. *Vet Surg* 47(1):74-85, 2018.
34. Kummeling A, Vrakking DJ, Rothuizen J, Gerritsen KM, van Sluijs FJ. Hepatic volume measurements in dogs with extrahepatic congenital portosystemic shunts before and after surgical attenuation. *J Vet Intern Med* 24(1):114-119, 2010.
35. Tivers MS, Lipscomb VJ, Smith KC, Wheeler-Jones CP, House AK. Markers of hepatic regeneration associated with surgical attenuation of congenital portosystemic shunts in dogs. *Vet J* 200(2):305-311, 2014.
36. Tivers MS, Upjohn MM, House AK, Brockman DJ, Lipscomb VJ. Treatment of extrahepatic congenital portosystemic shunts in dogs –what is the evidence base? *J Small Anim Pract* 53(1):3-11, 2012.
37. Tivers MS, Lipscomb VJ, Brockman DJ. Treatment of intrahepatic congenital portosystemic shunts in dogs: a systematic review. *J Small Anim Pract* 58(9):485-94, 2017.
38. Serrano G, Charalambous M, Devriendt N, de Rooster H, Mortier F, Paepe D. Treatment of congenital extrahepatic portosystemic shunts in dogs: A systematic review and meta-analysis. *J Vet Intern Med* 33(5):1865-1879, 2019.
39. Bristow P, Tivers M, Packer R, Brockman D, Ortiz V, Newson K, Lipscomb V. Long-term serum bile acid concentrations in 51 dogs after complete extrahepatic congenital portosystemic shunt ligation. *J Small Anim Pract* 58(8):454-460, 2017.
40. Christiansen JS, Hottinger HA, Allen L, Phillips L, Aronson LR. Hepatic microvascular dysplasia in dogs: A retrospective study of 24 cases (1987-1995). *J Am Anim Hosp Assoc* 36(5):385-389, 2000.
41. Bunch SE, Johnson SE, Cullen JM. Idiopathic noncirrhotic portal hypertension in dogs: 33 cases (1982-1998). *J Am Vet Med Assoc* 218(3):392-329, 2001.

CHAPTER 37

Other congenital liver diseases: ductal plate and gallbladder disorders

Andre J. Kortum
BVSc, MANZCVS(SAM), SFHEA, DECVIM-CA (Internal Medicine), MRCVS

While hepatic vascular abnormalities in dogs and cats are frequently documented, far less attention has been given to congenital biliary disorders. Under normal circumstances, the development of the biliary tree is a tightly controlled and intricate process, and precisely coordinated remodeling of the ductal plate—a sheet of embryonic biliary precursor cells encircling the portal vasculature—gives rise to an intricate network of bile ducts and ductules. However, disruptions in this process result in a spectrum of pathological abnormalities collectively known as "ductal plate malformations" (DPM), which may manifest individually or in combination depending upon the regions and extent of the biliary tree impacted.[1-6] In addition, disorders of extrahepatic biliary tract development, such as gallbladder atresia, are also occasionally encountered. Whilst most congenital biliary disorders are considered rare in dogs, it is possible that their importance may be underestimated as many share clinical and histopathological similarities with other causes of chronic hepatobiliary disease.[4]

Normal biliary tract development

Knowledge of normal biliary tract development is valuable in understanding the pathophysiology and characteristics of biliary malformations. Whilst this has been primarily studied in humans and rodent embryos, the process is relatively well conserved across species, with the liver and biliary tract arising from a ventral outpouching, known as the hepatic diverticulum or "liver bud" of the embryonic cranial foregut.[1,7–9] As development continues, this hepatic diverticulum further divides into a cranial (*pars hepatica*) and caudal part (*pars cystica*), which ultimately form the liver parenchyma and extrahepatic biliary tract, respectively.

The caudal bud of the hepatic diverticulum progressively lengthens and develops another outpouching, giving rise to the primitive gallbladder, cystic duct, and common bile duct (ductus choledochus).[1,7–9] In addition, a further bud arises from the common bile duct, which subsequently fuses with the dorsal bud of the developing pancreas.

Unlike the common bile duct and cystic duct, the hepatic ducts are derived from the cranial part of the hepatic diverticulum; however, despite their differing origins luminal continuity of the biliary tree is thought to be maintained throughout its development.[7,10] The hepatic ducts originally arise from a single, broad, funnel-like structure within the cranial bud, which ultimately subdivides and differentiates into numerous individual ducts.[7,8,10] In addition, sprouts of endodermal cells develop from its outer surface, interdigitating with endothelium-lined spaces connected with the capillary plexus of the vitelline veins and giving rise to the characteristic hepatic architecture of alternating hepatic cords and venous sinusoids.[1,8,9]

Based on studies in humans and rodent embryos, intrahepatic biliary development is thought to start later in gestation, initially occurring in the hilar region and later progressing centrifugally in a predictable and organized fashion to the periphery of the liver.[1,7,11] The intrahepatic ducts are believed to arise from periportal hepatoblasts, which undergo biliary cell differentiation as a result of periportal gradients of activin/transforming growth factor-beta (TGFβ) and other influences (e.g., hepatocyte nuclear factor 6 [HNF6] and Notch and Wnt signaling).[7,8,11] The portal veins consequently become surrounded by a cuff of biliary cells, which subsequently duplicate to form a double-layered sleeve known as the "ductal plate" (Fig. 37.1).

Extensive remodeling of this structure results in the formation of tubular dilatations, which ultimately become incorporated into the surrounding periportal mesenchyme as individualized bile ducts.[1,7,8] Under normal circumstances, other redundant parts of the ductal plate either involute or differentiate back into periportal hepatocytes; however, thin epithelial channels remain, providing continuity between the primitive intrahepatic ducts and the developing biliary canalicular network.[7]

The ductal plates are also believed to influence the development of the adjacent intrahepatic arterial vessels, leading to a synergistic relationship between the developing portal, biliary, and arterial components of the portal triads, which is key in the development of the lobular architecture of the liver.[7,8]

Development and classification of ductal plate malformations

Rather than a single entity, DPM might be more accurately regarded as a broad categorization encompassing a wide array of developmental abnormalities of biliary development.[3,5] Essentially, the term "ductal plate malformation" denotes the absence of adequate remodeling of the ductal plate, resulting in the persistence of embryonic bile duct structures.[1,7,12] The consequences and phenotypic manifestations of DPM vary depending on the level of the biliary tree affected and the extent of ductal plate remodeling that has occurred.[1,3,5,13]

In cases where remodeling is entirely absent, biliary vessels may appear histologically as ring-like luminal structures encircling a central fibrovascular axis, whereas incomplete remodeling may give rise to C-shaped structures or interrupted circles of curved bile duct lumina. Progressive dilation of these structures can also lead to the formation of cyst-like lesions (Fig. 37.1).[1,7,13]

Furthermore, DPM is often accompanied by abnormal portal vein development where the vascular tree forms as a dense network of narrow vessels that has been likened to the appearance of a pollarded willow tree.[1,7] Consequently, whilst portal areas often appear subjectively enlarged, these areas represent the fusion of multiple adjacent portal tracts, each containing multiple hypoplastic portal vessels surrounded by incompletely remodeled bile ducts.[1,5,7]

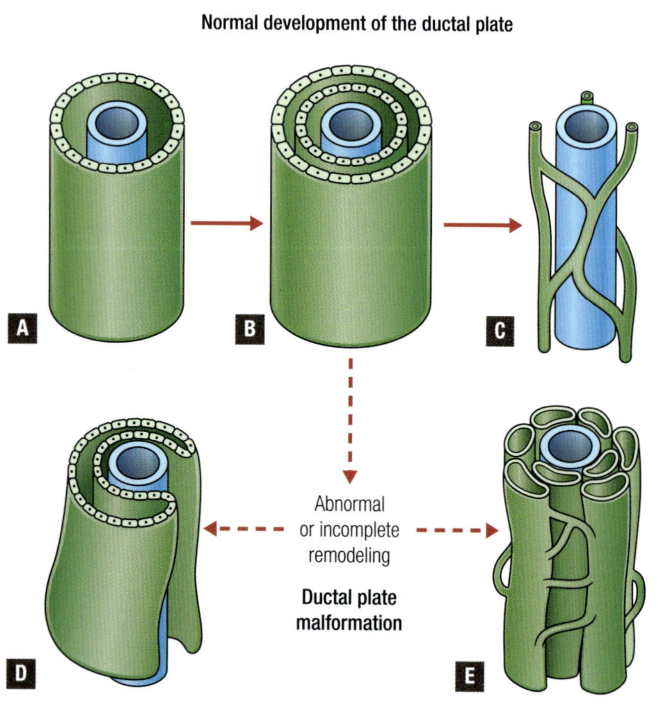

FIG. 37.1 (A-C) Illustration of normal ductal plate development and (D, E) ductal plate malformation. (A) A single layer of biliary precursor cells initially forms around the developing portal vein, which later differentiates into a double-layered ductal plate with a slit-like lumen (B). (C) Complex remodeling of this structure normally results in a periportal network of fine bile ducts; however, derangements in this process can lead to large, dilated bile duct structures or numerous, irregularly shaped bile ducts with abnormal branching. Courtesy of Ettinger SJ, Feldman EC, Etienne Côté E (editors). Textbook of Veterinary Internal Medicine, Elsevier, 2024.

In addition, DPM may also affect the larger branches of the intrahepatic biliary tree, and some also consider developmental abnormalities of the extrahepatic biliary tract, such as choledochal cysts, as part of the spectrum of DPM disorders.[4,14-17]

Although the precise genetic and molecular pathogenesis of DPM remains ill-defined, it is believed that defective formation and function of primary cilia on the apical cholangiocyte membrane, as well as abnormalities in various transcriptional regulators (e.g., HNF6, HNF1B, and SOX9) and signaling pathways (e.g., TGF-β, Notch, and Wnt), may play a significant role in the development of these conditions.[8,11] Furthermore, studies in rodents have suggested that DPM is likely to be a common endpoint resulting from a range of genetic or biochemical defects affecting biliary development.[12] Consequently, DPMs have traditionally been broadly classified as follows based on histological appearance and the level of the biliary tree affected:[1,3,4,13,15,17]

- Diseases of the small intrahepatic ducts, e.g., congenital hepatic fibrosis and Von Meyenburg complexes.
- Diseases of the medium-sized ducts, e.g., polycystic liver disease.
- Diseases of the extrahepatic or large intrahepatic bile ducts, e.g., Caroli's disease or syndrome and choledochal cysts.

Each entity may occur independently, but it is not uncommon for different types of DPMs to coexist, as is seen in Caroli's syndrome, where dilation of the large intrahepatic ducts (Caroli's disease) is accompanied by congenital hepatic fibrosis. It has been suggested that these complex phenotypes may occur commonly in dogs, and, in general, the pattern of lesions appears to be less clearly defined than in people. Consequently, it has been proposed that the term "ductal plate malformation" should be used to encompass all phenotypes within this spectrum, with specific disease terminologies reserved for cases with distinct histological abnormalities.[1,3,5] In addition, other congenital biliary disorders, such as gallbladder agenesis, as well as hepatic and vascular malformations, renal cystic lesions, and peritoneopericardial diaphragmatic hernias, are commonly associated with DPM, indicating an interrelationship between these anomalies.[5,18,19]

Diseases of the small intrahepatic ducts

Congenital hepatic fibrosis

Definition and etiology

Congenital hepatic fibrosis (CHF) is attributed to abnormal ductal plate remodeling of small interlobular bile ducts and is histologically characterized by periportal fibrosis and irregular bile ducts.[1-3] In many cases, these changes are also accompanied by hypoplastic portal vein branches, suggesting concurrent malformation of the portal vascular tree.[1,3,20,21] The fibrosis is generally progressive, and portal hypertension often ultimately occurs in affected patients.[20,21]

Whilst best described in humans, CHF also occurs in dogs and various other species.[5,20] The cause and inheritance in animals are unknown, but in people, it is inherited as an autosomal recessive disorder and, similar to other ductal plate malformations, causative mutations impacting the formation and function of the primary cilium are suspected.[5,15,17,21] In support of this theory, CHF may occur concurrently with other DPMs (e.g., Caroli's disease or polycystic liver disease) and other conditions, such as autosomal dominant polycystic kidney disease, suspected to have a similar pathogenesis.[1,5,21]

Clinical presentation

Affected dogs often present at a young age (2 months-2 years) with signs relating to portal hypertension such as ascites, anorexia, vomiting, and neurological signs; however, the clinical presentation can be varied and complicated by the concurrent presence of other DPMs and other congenital abnormalities.[5,20,22] A firm liver and other findings associated with portal hypertension, such as ascites, may also be noted on clinical examination.[20] An important differential diagnosis is cirrhosis, which may present with similar clinical signs and laboratory and diagnostic imaging changes. Histological confirmation is therefore important to avoid misdiagnosis because the treatment and prognosis of the two conditions are different, as described below.

In humans, latent and cholangitic forms are also described, although it is unclear whether such presentations occur in other species.[21]

Clinicopathological findings

Changes in hematology and biochemistry are often mild and nonspecific; however, elevations in cholestatic and hepatocellular enzymes may be noted. Most cases are not hyperbilirubinemic; however, increased serum bile acids or hyperammonemia levels may indicate the presence of acquired portosystemic shunting (APSS).[5,20,22]

Diagnostic imaging findings

On abdominal ultrasound, the liver may have a relatively normal appearance or appear increased or decreased in size with variably hyperechoic or heterogeneous parenchyma. Ascites and acquired portosystemic shunts may also be noted if advanced fibrosis and portal hypertension are present.[15,20]

Although CT and MRI are valuable for the diagnosis of congenital hepatic fibrosis in people, the hepatic changes in affected dogs have not yet been described.[15,17] Nonetheless, advanced imaging may facilitate the detection of vascular abnormalities, such as APSS in advanced cases.

In some cases, concurrent evidence of other DPMs or other congenital anomalies (e.g., gallbladder agenesis, liver lobe or vascular malformations, cystic renal disease, or pericardioperitoneal diaphragmatic hernia) may be observed.[5,18,19,21]

Other diagnostic procedures

Definitive diagnosis of CHF relies on histopathological examination, which typically reveals diffuse and often severe periportal to bridging fibrosis containing numerous small and irregular bile ducts, reduced portal venous vasculature, and hyperplastic arterioles (Fig. 37.2).[2,20,21]

Care should be taken to distinguish these changes from those of cirrhosis, lobular dissecting hepatitis, congenital hepatic vascular abnormalities, and extrahepatic biliary obstruction (Table 37.1). However, the numerous and irregular bile duct profiles in the relative absence of concurrent inflammatory changes, cholestasis, or nodular regeneration are indicative of CHF.[2,20,22] Immunohistochemistry with cytokeratin-19 and Ki 67 can also be used to confirm the biliary origin of the ducts and exclude active cholangiocyte proliferation, respectively, as seen with ductular reactions secondary to other hepatobiliary diseases.[5,18,19]

The histological appearance of CHF in dogs may be more variable than in people, with many dogs displaying complex histopathological changes reflecting a mixture of DPM phenotypes and other developmental abnormalities.[3,5] For example, in a study of 30 young, unrelated Boxer dogs with a diverse spectrum of DPM phenotypes, marked fibrosis with increased numbers of small bile ducts and reduced portal vein profiles were documented in all cases, but only 37% and fulfilled criteria for CHF and 7% for Caroli's syndrome, and many had variable saccular dilation of the larger bile ducts and various other hepatobiliary malformations.[5]

Treatment

Given the differences in the pathogenesis of fibrosis in CHF compared with necroinflammatory liver disease, anti-inflammatory and antifibrotic treatments are ineffective in preventing or slowing disease progression.[19] Whilst liver transplantation is the preferred treatment for humans with advanced disease or signs of liver failure, treatment of affected dogs is limited to symptomatic treatment of secondary complications, including hepatic encephalopathy and ascites (see chapters 34, 36, and 40 for more details of dietary and drug treatment of these complications).[4,20,21] The efficacy of hepatic antioxidants and choleretics is uncertain.

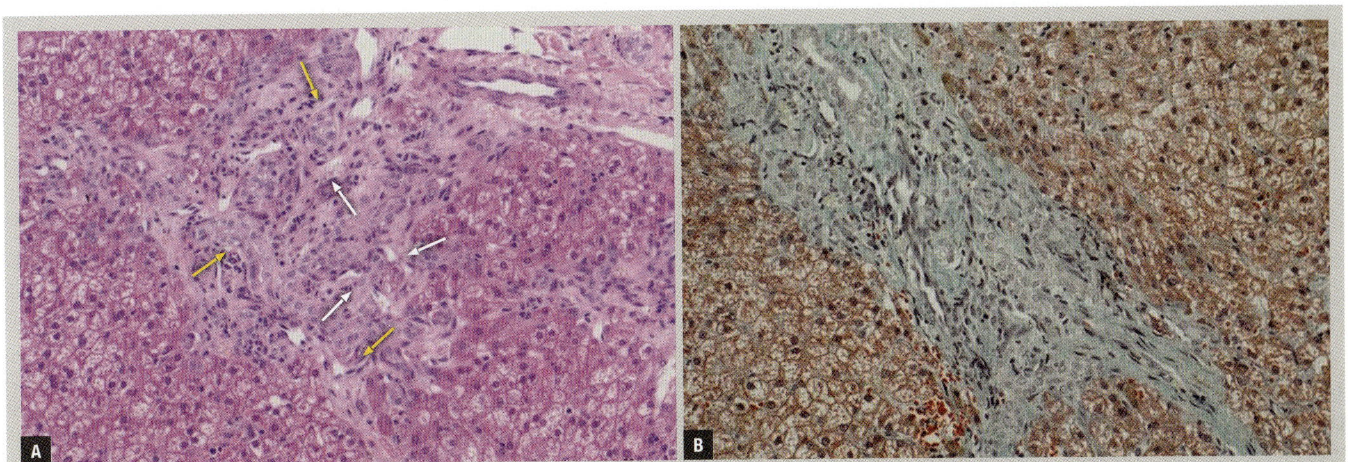

FIG. 37.2 (A) Liver histopathology from an 18-month-old mixed breed dog with suspected congenital hepatic fibrosis showing biliary hyperplasia and tortuosity (yellow arrows) and reduced portal vein profiles (white arrows) (hematoxylin and eosin stain). (B) Liver histology from the same dog as (A) showing portal bridging fibrosis stained green (Masson's trichrome stain). Courtesy of Fernando Constantino-Casas. Anatomical Pathology, Department of Veterinary Medicine, University of Cambridge, UK.

TABLE 37.1 Clinical and diagnostic features of congenital hepatic fibrosis compared with other causes of hepatic fibrosis.

Congenital hepatic fibrosis	Chronic hepatitis/cirrhosis	Lobular dissecting hepatitis	Chronic EHBDO/cholangitis
Presentation: ■ Typically young dogs ■ Clinical signs are variable and often nonspecific. Ascites, vomiting, anorexia, and neurological signs may occur if portal hypertension present.	**Presentation:** ■ Wide age range, typically middle-aged to older dogs ■ Clinical signs variable and often nonspecific; ascites, icterus, neurological signs, coagulopathy may occur with advanced disease	**Presentation:** ■ Typically young dogs ■ Clinical signs variable and often nonspecific; 80% present with ascites and icterus, diarrhea, neurological signs, coagulopathy may occur.	**Presentation:** ■ Any age and breed ■ Clinical signs nonspecific, including vomiting, lethargy, inappetence, icterus, abdominal pain, pyrexia.
Laboratory and imaging changes: ■ Variable, often mild increases in liver enzymes ■ Hyperbilirubinemia uncommon, but APSS may cause elevated bile acids and ammonia ■ Imaging appearance variable – liver may be increased, normal, or decreased in size with hyperechoic or heterogeneous parenchyma. Ascites and/or APSS may be noted if portal hypertension is present.	**Laboratory and imaging changes:** ■ Variable (mild to marked) increases in liver enzymes ■ Hyperbilirubinemia, increased bile acids, hyperammonemia, reduced albumin, urea and/or cholesterol may seen with advanced disease ■ Imaging appearance variable, but liver size often reduced with hyperechoic parenchyma and architectural distortion. Ascites and/or APSS may be noted if portal hypertension is present.	**Laboratory and imaging changes:** ■ Variable (mild to marked) increases in liver enzymes ■ Reduced urea, hyperbilirubinemia and increased bile acids/ hyperammonemia common; reduced urea and/or cholesterol may also occur ■ Imaging appearance variable, but liver size often normal-reduced with smooth surface and few regenerative nodules. Ascites and/or APSS are common.	**Laboratory and imaging changes:** ■ Variable (mild to marked) increases in liver enzymes, particularly ALP and GGT ■ Hyperbilirubinemia and hypercholesterolemia common ■ Biliary tract distension (especially with obstruction); echogenic gallbladder/ luminal content. Liver enlargement with increased/mixed echogenicity may be noted. ■ Neutrophilic bile and/or bactibilia or positive culture with cholangitis
Histological features: ■ Progressive, diffuse portal-portal bridging fibrosis ■ Marked increase of small often irregular bile duct profiles ■ Reduction of portal vein branches ■ Minimal to absent inflammation ■ Minimal to absent hepatocyte apoptosis or necrosis ■ Lack of nodular regeneration ■ Bile ducts positive for cytokeratin 19 and negative for Ki67 on IHC	**Histological features:** ■ Periportal progressing to portal-portal bridging fibrosis ■ Hepatocyte apoptosis or necrosis ■ Inflammatory infiltrates (portal, multifocal, zonal, or panlobular) ■ Nodular hepatocyte regeneration resulting in architectural distortion ■ Variable increase in bile duct profiles ■ Bile ducts positive for cytokeratin 19 and Ki67 on IHC	**Histological features:** ■ Distortion of lobular architecture with fibrosis (reticular fibers) dissecting around single or small groups of hepatocytes ■ Mild lobular inflammation and hepatocellular apoptosis/necrosis. ■ Variable increase in bile duct profiles and cholestasis ■ Bile ducts positive for cytokeratin 19 and Ki67 on IHC	**Histological features:** ■ Variable increases in bile duct profiles ■ Cholestasis, duct dilation and tortuosity, and/or periductular edema and inflammation with obstruction ■ Inflammation centered on bile ducts and/or epithelial destruction, periportal hepatitis in cholangitis ■ Periportal progressing to portal-portal bridging fibrosis ■ Bile ducts positive for cytokeratin 19 and Ki67 on IHC

Prognosis

The prognosis for CHF is variable, depending on its severity, progression, and the presence of comorbidities, including other DPMs and developmental abnormalities. Whilst some dogs succumb to liver failure in early life, others may survive until middle age or beyond.[5,19,20] Advanced fibrosis and signs of portal hypertension are generally considered to be negative prognostic indicators; however, survival times of several years have been reported even in these severely affected cases.[5,19] Unfortunately, the factors underlying disease progression are unknown.

Von Meyenburg complexes

Definition and etiology

Von Meyenburg complexes (VMCs), or biliary hamartomas, are benign, nodular lesions that are rarely identified within the liver parenchyma. They are believed to originate from the abnormal remodeling of peripheral interlobular bile ducts during later stages of biliary development and have been described in various species, including dogs.[1-3,15,17]

Clinical presentation

VMCs are typically diagnosed as incidental imaging or necropsy findings in otherwise asymptomatic patients. Mild clinical signs, including abdominal discomfort, fever, weight loss, and jaundice, are described in some humans with VMCs; however, it is unknown if similar consequences arise in dogs.[23]

Clinicopathological findings

Hematology, biochemistry, and liver function testing are typically unremarkable; however, mild, nonspecific elevations in ALT, AST, GGT, and ALP may occasionally occur.[23]

Diagnostic imaging

On abdominal ultrasound and other imaging modalities (e.g., CT or MRI), VMCs appear as variably sized nodular cystic lesions, which may occur as single or multiple lesions. In humans, they commonly occur multifocally with a relatively uniform size, usually less than 1.5 cm; however, their appearance in dogs may be more variable and has not been well characterized.[2,15,17] Similar to other DPMs, VMCs may occur alone or in conjunction with other DPMs or developmental anomalies.[1,3]

Other diagnostic procedures

Histology is required for definitive diagnosis of VMC and differentiation from other etiologies, including primary or metastatic neoplasia, abscessation, and simple liver cysts. This typically documents focal collections of disordered, irregular, and frequently dilated bile ducts embedded within a dense fibrous stroma.[1-3,24]

Treatment and prognosis

No specific treatment is typically required, and given their benign nature, the prognosis is usually excellent. Whilst malignant transformation is a rare complication of VMCs in people, it is unknown whether the same risk exists in other species.[4,23]

Diseases of medium-sized intrahepatic ducts

Polycystic liver disease

Definition and etiology

Polycystic liver diseases (PLD) are a group of genetic disorders characterized by the progressive replacement of liver parenchyma with fluid-filled cysts.[11] While primarily described in humans, these conditions have also been observed in various species, including dogs.[24-27] The cysts are believed to result from ductal plate malformation of the medium-sized intrahepatic bile ducts, where the ductal plate cells continue to proliferate instead of involuting after disconnection from the biliary tree.[11,17] Concurrent congenital hepatic fibrosis or other DPMs may also occur if other stages of biliary development are affected.[1]

Various mutations affecting the normal formation or function of the primary cilium have been implicated in causing PLD.[11] Because primary cilia also play a crucial role in the normal development of other structures (e.g., the renal tubules), many also cause cystic abnormalities in other organs.[11,28] In people, PLD is usually associated with autosomal dominant polycystic kidney disease (ADPKD) resulting from mutations in PKD1 or PKD2 genes that encode polycystin, a transmembrane protein essential for normal ciliary function.[11,28,29] PKD1 mutation has also been identified as a cause of ADPKD in Persian cats and related breeds, many of whom also have cystic abnormalities in the liver and other organs.[30-32] PLD is also reported to occur rarely in dogs, both in combination with renal cysts and occurring as an isolated hepatobiliary pathology.[24-27] This might suggest that other causes of human PLD, such as autosomal recessive polycystic kidney disease and autosomal dominant polycystic liver disease, also occur in dogs; however, the causative mutations in this species have not been investigated.

Clinical presentation

The clinical consequences of PLD vary depending on factors such as the number, size, growth rate, and location of hepatic cysts, as well as the presence of coexisting liver and other visceral pathologies.

In dogs, PLD can have a particularly variable presentation. Whilst some cases may be asymptomatic and identified incidentally on abdominal imaging or postmortem, severe and diffuse polycystic liver and renal disease has been described in Cairn Terriers and White Highland White Terriers, culminating in organomegaly and hepatic failure by 6 weeks of age.[24-26] Whilst this diverse presentation may reflect different etiologies, the genetic basis of the condition in dogs has not been well-defined; therefore, it has been suggested that PLD in this species should be subclassified according to age of presentation into juvenile or adult forms.[2] Whilst ADPKD is described in Bull Terriers, the concurrent occurrence of PLD with this condition has not yet been reported.[33,34] Nonetheless, this may reflect the limited number of canine cases documented in the literature.

Clinicopathological findings

Variable elevations in ALT, AST, ALP, and GGT may be seen in serum biochemistry in affected dogs.[26] In severe, diffuse disease, evidence of liver dysfunction may also be noted, such as elevated fasting and postprandial bile acids, hypoalbuminemia, or reduced serum urea. Whilst concurrent AKPKD and PLD have not been reported in the dog, evaluation of PKD1 mutation status might be considered in Bull Terriers with concurrent hepatic and renal cystic changes.[34]

Diagnostic imaging findings

Abdominal ultrasound typically documents multiple, thin-walled, anechoic, or fluid-filled cysts within the hepatic parenchyma, which are distinguishable from Caroli's disease in that they do not communicate with the biliary tract.[26] Similar findings are also observed on CT or MRI, which are frequently used to establish the diagnosis in people.[16,17] The number and size of cysts may vary considerably, ranging from a few millimeters to several centimeters in diameter, and other lesions may also be noted in the kidneys and other organs.[24-26]

Other diagnostic procedures

Whilst the diagnosis in asymptomatic patients is often based on imaging findings, histopathology is required to conclusively rule out other potential etiologies, including parasitic/hydatid cysts or cystadenoma, and to assess the presence of concurrent CHF or other DPMs.[1,2] Cyst aspiration is generally not recommended as it provides limited diagnostic value and poses a risk of infection or cyst rupture.

Treatment

Treatment of clinically affected dogs is usually symptomatic and supportive, including management of concurrent chronic kidney disease if present. While somatostatin analogs have been suggested to reduce the cyst growth rate in humans, their efficacy in animals remains unexplored.[29] Percutaneous drainage of cysts is generally not practical and ineffective. However, cyst fenestration or partial hepatectomy are described in people for the management of localized cysts causing biliary or vascular compression.[29] Considering the risk of familial transmission demonstrated in other species, breeding from animals with PLD should be discouraged.

Prognosis

The prognosis for dogs with PLD is variable depending on disease severity, rate of progression, and the presence of comorbidities such as concurrent polycystic renal changes and other DPMs or biliary anomalies.[24-26] Whilst some cases follow a relatively benign course, others may succumb to hepatic failure at a young age due to severe and diffuse polycystic pathology.[24-26,29] Complications seen in humans with PLD, such as cyst infection, rupture, torsion, and hemorrhage, may conceivably occur but have not been reported in dogs.[29]

Diseases of extrahepatic and large intrahepatic ducts

Caroli's disease and Caroli's syndrome

Definition and etiology

Caroli's disease and Caroli's syndrome, first described by the French physician Jacques Caroli in 1958, represent two distinct variants characterized by multifocal, segmental dilatation of the large intrahepatic bile ducts.[35] The less common form, known as Caroli's disease, is defined by bile duct dilation in the absence of other hepatic abnormalities, while the more common variant, Caroli's syndrome, is associated with congenital hepatic fibrosis.[1,35,36] Caroli's disease is also classified as a type V cholechodal cyst according to the Todani classification.[16,37] Both syndromes are considered rare causes of hepatobiliary disease in humans and have also been observed in dogs and other species.[5,19,36,38-42]

The pathogenesis of both phenotypes is believed to involve disordered ductal plate remodeling, with Caroli's disease affecting the earlier forming, large intrahepatic bile ducts and Caroli's syndrome involving both the large and small intrahepatic ducts.[1,3,36] The exact genetic and molecular mechanisms are not fully understood; however, most cases in humans are inherited in an autosomal recessive manner, suggesting a genetic basis. Mutations in the polycystic kidney and hepatic disease 1 (PKHD1) gene, which encodes a cilial protein called fibrocystin, are considered a potential cause, particularly due to the frequent coexistence of autosomal recessive polycystic kidney disease (ARPKD).[28,43] Nonetheless, the causal relationship between these genetic mutations and Caroli's disease/syndrome, as well as the potential contribution of other factors, remains uncertain. No genetic studies have been performed in other species although cystic renal disease also appears to be a common concurrence in dogs.[38,39,42]

Clinical presentation

Similar to the presentation in humans, dogs affected by Caroli's disease and Caroli's syndrome may exhibit symptoms at a young age or remain asymptomatic for several years, with reported ages at diagnosis spanning from 6 months to 6 years.[5,38,39,41,42] Gender and breed predilections are unknown in dogs, but gender distribution is reported to be equal in humans.[40]

The clinical presentation is variable depending on the extent and severity of biliary dilation and hepatic fibrosis, as well as the presence of comorbidities such as chronic kidney disease (CKD). Commonly reported clinical signs in severely affected dogs include vomiting, polyuria/polydipsia, ascites, anorexia, weight loss, jaundice, and neurological symptoms, although patients with milder degrees of hepatic fibrosis or isolated intrahepatic duct dilation (i.e., Caroli's disease) may have milder signs or even be asymptomatic.[38,39,41,42]

Liver enlargement, jaundice, ascites, and/or pyrexia may be noted on clinical examination but are inconsistently present. While recurrent cholecystitis and cholelithiasis are common complications in humans, they appear to be less frequently encountered in dogs, and presenting signs and examination findings usually relate to portal hypertension and impaired liver function due to advanced hepatic fibrosis.[38,41,44] Although this is also a recognized sequala in humans with Caroli's syndrome, it is considered a late complication; therefore, it is possible that the milder signs of disease described in people with the condition, such as low-grade abdominal pain and pyrexia, are underrecognized in dogs.[36]

Clinicopathological findings

In affected dogs, serum biochemistry and hematology tests often reveal variable increases in ALP, GGT, ALT, AST, bile acids, and bilirubin, as well as leukocytosis and nonregenerative anemia.[38,39,41,42] Additionally, azotemia and isosthenuria may be identified in cases with concurrent chronic kidney disease.

Diagnostic imaging findings

Abdominal imaging, such as ultrasonography or CT, typically documents the presence of multiple cystic dilations of intrahepatic bile ducts, which exhibit communication with the biliary tree (Fig. 37.3).

Additional findings such as cyst calcification and evidence of comorbidities like portal hypertension, renal cysts, portosystemic shunts (PSS), or cholelithiasis may also be noted.[38-41] On CT, the identification of a contrast-enhancing fibrovascular bundle within the center of dilated intrahepatic bile ducts (known as the central dot sign) is suggested to be pathognomonic in humans and has also been reported in dogs.[36,40,41] While magnetic resonance cholangiopancreatography (MRCP), endoscopic retrograde cholangiopancreatography (ERCP), or percutaneous transhepatic cholangiography are considered the diagnostic modalities of choice in humans, they are rarely available or performed in dogs.[16,17,36,40]

Other diagnostic procedures

Although clinical evidence of portal hypertension and compatible imaging findings may be suggestive of Caroli's syndrome, a liver biopsy is required for a definitive diagnosis. In patients with Caroli's syndrome, this documents the concurrent presence of congenital hepatic fibrosis and allows reliable differentiation from cases with Caroli's disease.[2,5,38]

Treatment

Ursodeoxycholic acid and antibiotics are often recommended in humans to address concurrent cholelithiasis and ascending biliary infections, and similar management is indicated in dogs with these complications (see chapter 35 for more details on treating biliary tract infections).[36,40]

In patients presenting with clinical signs suggestive of cholangitis (e.g., vomiting, inappetence, lethargy, abdominal pain, icterus), gallbladder aspiration for cytology and culture should ideally be performed to confirm the diagnosis and inform antibiotic treatment. However, many dogs are diagnosed at a late stage with diffuse and advanced disease, at which point treatment is largely supportive, focusing on symptomatic treatment of portal hypertension and other associated complications (see chapter 34 for details of treatment of portal hypertension).[38,41]

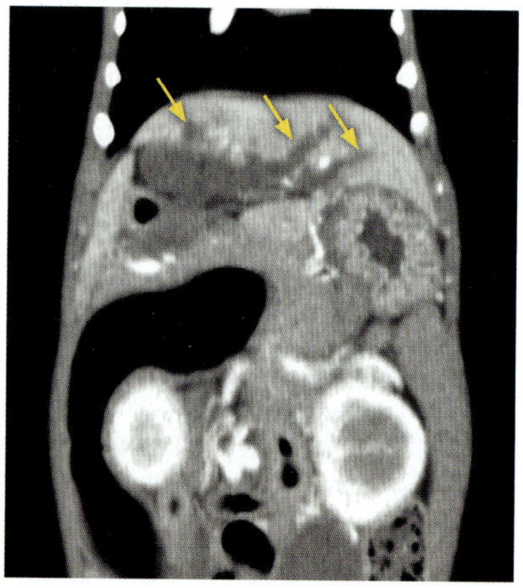

FIG. 37.3 Computed tomography, dorsal plane multiplanar reconstruction of hypoattenuating non-contrast-enhancing dilated intrahepatic bile ducts (arrows) in a 5-month-old Dachshund with complex ductal plate malformation. Courtesy of Marie-Aude Genain. Diagnostic Imaging, Department of Veterinary Medicine, University of Cambridge, UK.

Surgical resection or liver transplantation is often recommended for affected human patients, given the potential risks of severe complications, including recurrent cholangitis, cholelithiasis, and malignancy.[36,40,44] Whether these same complications occur in dogs is unknown; however, partial hepatectomy or liver lobectomy may be considered a viable and potentially curative option for dogs with localized disease.

Prognosis

As most reported cases in dogs have been diagnosed at a late stage of disease, the prognosis for animals diagnosed at an earlier stage is unknown. However, it is likely the disease progression and outcome are influenced by the extent and severity of biliary malformation and hepatic fibrosis and the presence of secondary complications or comorbidities. Successful conservative management has been reported in dogs over a follow-up period of 5 months; however, signs of portal hypertension, severe hepatic fibrosis, and recurrent cholangitis/cholangiohepatitis are likely to be negative prognostic indicators.[38,41] Whether the increased risk of malignancy described in people also applies to dogs is currently unknown.

Gallbladder agenesis

Definition and etiology

Gallbladder agenesis is a rare biliary anomaly characterized by the absence of the gallbladder without atresia of the extrahepatic biliary system. It is best described in humans but also occurs in other species, including dogs.[5,18,19,45-49] Although not considered a DPM, it is also considered to result from disordered biliary development; however, it differs from the former in arising from a failure of differentiation of the hepatic diverticulum or its caudal bud (*pars cystica*) rather than the more peripheral ductal plates. In humans, familial and genetic factors are thought to lead to failure of vacuolation of the *pars cystica*, although earlier failure of development of the hepatic diverticulum may explain the concurrent occurrence of liver lobe malformations often observed in dogs.[6,18,48] Considering the similarities in their pathophysiology, it is perhaps unsurprising that gallbladder agenesis is often accompanied by DPM and other hepatobiliary anomalies.[5,18,19,45,46,48]

Clinical presentation

The condition has been most commonly reported in young, small-breed dogs, with Chihuahuas appearing to be overrepresented.[6,18,45-48] Many patients are asymptomatic, although clinical signs, including vomiting, anorexia, diarrhea, lethargy, and seizures, can occur in approximately half of the patients, usually relating to concurrent DPMs (particularly congenital hepatic fibrosis) and secondary complications. Similarly, physical examination is typically unremarkable in affected patients, although ascites and neurological signs may be noted if concurrent liver disease resulting in portal hypertension and APSS is present.[18,46-49] Abdominal pain resulting from dysfunction of the sphincter of Oddi and biliary dyskinesia is reported in people but may be challenging to detect in dogs.[50]

Clinicopathological findings

Variable increases in liver enzymes are seen in most affected patients, with ALT being most commonly and markedly elevated.[18,48] Variable increases in fasting and postprandial bile acid concentrations are not uncommon and may relate to cholestasis, altered bile acid kinetics, or the frequent concurrence of DPM.[18] Otherwise, clinicopathological testing, including evaluation of serum bilirubin, is typically unremarkable unless concurrent liver pathology resulting in impaired liver function is present.[18,48,49]

Diagnostic imaging findings

On abdominal ultrasound, the gallbladder is not detectable or occasionally vestigial in size (gallbladder hypoplasia). Many patients also have evidence of common bile duct dilation and evidence of concurrent hepatopathy, such as hyper- or hypoechogenicity of the liver parenchyma with irregular margination. Concurrent malformation of the liver lobes and evidence of portal hypertension and APSS are also reported to be common findings in affected dogs.[18]

Similar changes are also observed on CT or CT cholangiography, which may be particularly valuable in the identification of common bile duct dilation and APSS and in ruling out biliary obstruction (Fig. 37.4).[18,48]

Other diagnostic findings

Gross examination at laparotomy or laparoscopy confirms agenesis or hypoplasia of the gallbladder and other concurrent abnormalities, including liver lobe malformations (most commonly of the quadrate lobe), liver adhesions and capsule abnormalities, and APSS (Fig. 37.5).[18,45,47]

Liver biopsy should be considered, particularly in patients with signs of concurrent hepatopathy, as DPM resembling CHF is reported to occur in over 90% of cases.[18]

Treatment

Treatment is primarily focused on the management of comorbidities, in particular, portal hypertension resulting from DPM. Conversely, uncomplicated cases may require no specific treatment because the absence of a gallbladder alone should not cause a clinical problem. UDCA is commonly prescribed; however, its value is unknown.[18,48,49]

Prognosis

The prognosis is largely dependent on the presence and severity of concurrent conditions such as DPM. The presence of portal hypertension and APSS are considered negative prognostic indicators; however, many dogs have a favorable prognosis, with 95% remaining alive over a median follow-up period of 570 days (range 4-3379 days).[18]

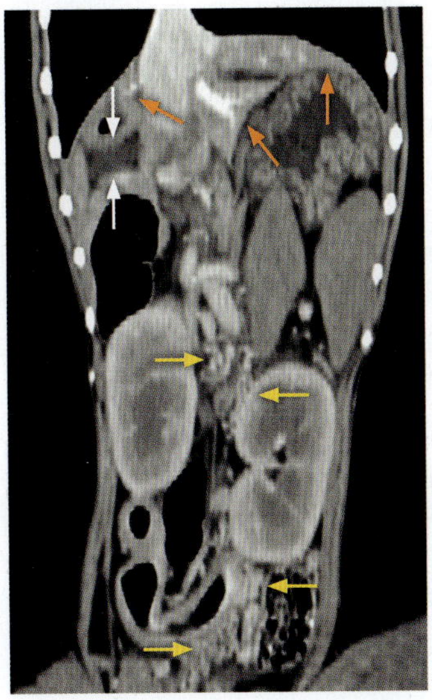

FIG. 37.4 Dorsal plane CT image from an 8-month-old Whippet with gallbladder agenesis, extrahepatic bile duct dilation (white arrows), microhepatia (orange arrows), and acquired portosystemic shunting vessels secondary to portal hypertension (yellow arrows). Courtesy of Kate Shumway, VetCT, and Federica Manna, Bath Vet Referrals, UK.

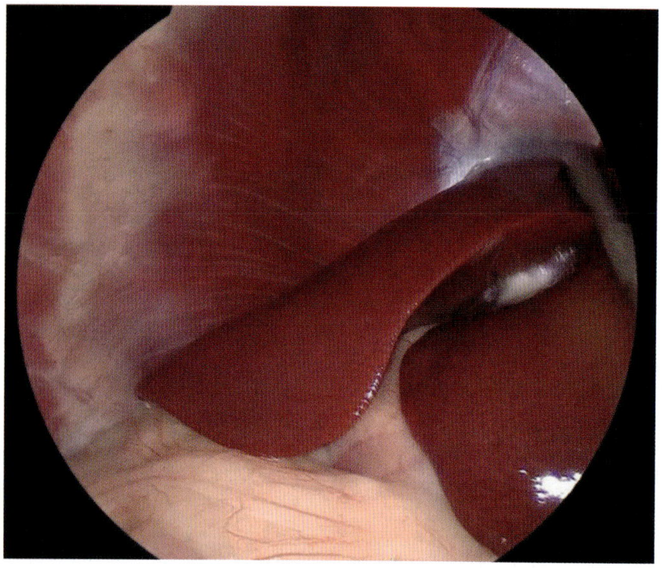

FIG. 37.5 Laparoscopic image from an 18-month-old mixed-breed dog with gallbladder agenesis depicting the right liver lobes and absence of a gallbladder at its normal location. Despite the normal size and appearance of the liver, histopathology documented concurrent changes consistent with congenital hepatic fibrosis. Courtesy of Akash Alexander, Soft Tissue Surgery, Department of Veterinary Medicine, University of Cambridge, UK.

Other extrahepatic biliary anomalies

Choledochal cysts (CC) are rare biliary anomalies characterized by dilated extrahepatic and/or intrahepatic ducts. Predominantly described in humans and cats, they have also been reproduced experimentally in young dogs and may conceivably occur in this species.[37,51-54] Despite resembling cysts, the term is a misnomer as continuity with the biliary system is maintained.[37,52] The etiology is debated, with some considering them part of the spectrum of DPMs, while others propose that anomalous connection of pancreatic and common bile ducts leads to chronic inflammation and progressive dilation.[16,17,37] CCs are subcategorized based on their appearance according to the Todani classification system, with fusiform dilatations of the extrahepatic bile duct (type Ic CCs) occurring most commonly.[52-55] Presentation and diagnostic findings often relate to complications such as cholangitis/choledochitis and cholelithiasis, but they may also be identified incidentally.[16,52-54,56] Treatment and prognosis are dependent on CC complexity and presence/severity of secondary complications; however, successful outcomes in cats are reported both with surgical and medical management.[52-54] Malignant transformation is a recognized complication in humans; however, it is unclear if this sequela also occurs in other species.[56]

A range of other extrahepatic biliary anomalies have been scarcely reported in dogs, including biliary atresia, umbilicobiliary fistula/communication and anomalous bile duct morphology, and septate or mispositioned gallbladder.[6,57-60] Consequences of these malformations and the need for intervention depend on the degree of resulting biliary obstruction and predisposition to secondary complications. Whilst biliary atresia usually presents in early life with signs relating to complete biliary obstruction (e.g., jaundice, acholic feces, vitamin K deficiency, biliary tract distension) and necessitates biliary diversion, milder abnormalities such as septate gallbladder may have minimal or no clinical consequence.[57,58]

KEY POINTS

- Ductal plate and other biliary malformations arise as a consequence of aberrant biliary development. Although considered rare, they may be under-recognized and should be considered as differential diagnoses, particularly for young dogs presenting with signs of hepatobiliary disease.
- Ductal plate malformations encompass a spectrum of disorders resulting from abnormal remodeling of the ductal plate—a double-layered sleeve of biliary precursor cells surrounding the developing portal vein—which is key to bile duct development. The resulting phenotypes depend on the stage of development affected and the extent to which the biliary tree is impacted.
- DPM disorders are conventionally subdivided into separate diseases such as congenital hepatic fibrosis, Caroli's disease or syndrome, polycystic liver disease, or Von Meyenburg complexes; however, mixed phenotypes also commonly occur in dogs.
- Other biliary malformations, such as gallbladder agenesis, are also occasionally encountered and are often associated with concurrent DPM and other malformations.
- Diagnostic imaging is often valuable in the diagnosis of malformations affecting the extrahepatic tree or larger intrahepatic bile duct; however, liver histology is required to confirm DPM affecting the smaller ducts, such as congenital hepatic fibrosis and Von Meyenburg complexes.
- Treatment is typically supportive, and prognosis depends on the severity and extent of the affected biliary tract. In general, signs of functional impairment (e.g., relating to portal hypertension and acquired portosystemic shunting) are usually associated with a poorer prognosis.

References

1. Desmet VJ. Congenital diseases of intrahepatic bile ducts: variations on the theme "ductal plate malformation". *Hepatology* 16(4):1069-1083, 1992.
2. van den Ingh TSGAM, Cullen JM, Twedt DC, Van Winkle T, Desmet VJ, Rothuizen J. Morphological classification of biliary disorders of the canine and feline liver. In WSAVA Liver Standardisation Group, editor. WSAVA Standards for Clinical and Histological Diagnosis of Canine and Feline Liver Diseases. Philadelphia, Elsevier Ltd., 2006, pp. 61-74.
3. Cullen JM. Summary of the World Small Animal Veterinary Association Standardization Committee Guide to Classification of Liver Disease in Dogs and Cats. *Vet Clin North Am Small Anim Pract* 39(3):395-418, 2009.
4. Center S. Ductal plate malformation (congenital hepatic fibrosis). In Tilley L, Smith F (editors). Blackwell's Five-Minute Veterinary Consult: Canine and Feline 6th edition. Ames, Iowa, Wiley Blackwell, 2016, pp. 413-415.
5. Pillai S, Center SA, McDonough SP, Demarco J, Pintar J, Henderson AK, et al. Ductal plate malformation in the liver of Boxer dogs: clinical and histological features. *Vet Pathol* 53(3):602-613 2016.
6. Jaffey JA. Canine hepatobiliary anatomy, physiology and congenital disorders. *J Small Anim Pract* 63(2):95-103, 2022.
7. Roskams T, Desmet V. Embryology of extra- and intrahepatic bile ducts, the ductal plate. *Anat Rec* 291(6):628-635, 2008.
8. Raynaud P, Carpentier R, Antoniou A, Lemaigre FP. Biliary differentiation and bile duct morphogenesis in development and disease. *Int J Biochem Cell Biol* 43(2):245-256, 2011.
9. McGeady T., Quinn P., FitzPatrick E, Ryan M, Kilroy D, Lonergan P. Digestive system. In Veterinary Embryology 2nd edition. Chichester, UK, Wiley Blackwell, 2017, pp. 214-231.
10. Tan CEL, Moscoso GJ. The developing human biliary system at the porta hepatis level between 29 days and 8 weeks of gestation: A way to understanding biliary atresia. Part 1. *Pathol Int* 44(8):587-599, 1994.
11. Wills ES, Roepman R, Drenth JPH. Polycystic liver disease: Ductal plate malformation and the primary cilium. *Trends Mol Med* 20(5):261-270, 2014.
12. Raynaud P, Tate J, Callens C, Cordi S, Vandersmissen P, Carpentier R, et al. A classification of ductal plate malformations based on distinct pathogenic mechanisms of biliary dysmorphogenesis. *Hepatology* 53(6):1959-1966, 2011.
13. Desmet VJ. Pathogenesis of ductal plate abnormalities. *Mayo Clin Proc* 73(1):80-89, 1998.
14. Summerfield JA, Nagafuchi Y, Sherlock S, Cadafalch J, Scheuer PJ. Hepatobiliary fibropolycystic diseases. A clinical and histological review of 51 patients. *J Hepatol* 2(2):141-156, 1986.
15. Venkatanarasimha N, Thomas R, Armstrong EM, Shirley JF, Fox BM, Jackson SA. Imaging features of ductal plate malformations in adults. *Clin Radiol* 66(11):1086-1093, 2011.
16. Sureka B, Rastogi A, Bihari C, Bharathy KGS, Sood V, Alam S. Imaging in ductal plate malformations. *Indian J Radiol Imaging* 27(1):6-12, 2017.
17. Mamone G, Carollo V, Cortis K, Aquilina S, Liotta R, Miraglia R. Magnetic resonance imaging of fibropolycystic liver disease: the spectrum of ductal plate malformations. *Abdom Radiol* 44(6):2156-2171, 2019.
18. Sato K, Sakai M, Hayakawa S, Sakamoto Y, Kagawa Y, Kutara K, et al. Gallbladder Agenesis in 17 Dogs: 2006–2016. *J Vet Intern Med* 32(1):188-194, 2018.
19. Seibert LM, Center SA, Randolph JF, Miller ML, Miller AD, Choi E, et al. Relationships between congenital peritoneopericardial diaphragmatic hernia or congenital central diaphragmatic hernia and ductal plate malformations in dogs and cats. *J Am Vet Med Assoc* 259(9):1009-1024, 2021.
20. Brown DL, van Winkle T, Cecere T, Rushton S, Brachelente C, Cullen JM. Congenital hepatic fibrosis in 5 dogs. *Vet Pathol* 47(1):102-107, 2010.
21. Shorbagi A, Bayraktar Y. Experience of a single center with congenital hepatic fibrosis: A review of the literature. *World J Gastroenterol* 16:683-690, 2010.
22. Eulenberg VM, Lidbury JA. Hepatic fibrosis in dogs. *J Vet Intern Med* 32(1):26-41, 2018.
23. Sheikh AAE, Nguyen AP, Leyba K, Javed N, Shah S, Deradke A, et al. Biliary duct hamartomas: A systematic review. *Cureus* 26;14(5):e25361, 2022.
24. Van Den Ingh TSGAM, Rothuizen J. Congenital cystic disease of the liver in seven dogs. *J Comp Pathol* 95(3):405-414, 1985.
25. McKenna SC, Carpenter JL. Polycystic disease of the kidney and liver in the Cairn Terrier. *Vet Pathol* 17(4):436-442, 1980.
26. McAloose D, Casal M, Patterson DF, Dambach DM. Polycystic kidney and liver disease in two related West Highland White Terrier litters. *Vet Pathol* 35(1):77-81, 1998.
27. Hirose N, Uchida K, Kanemoto H, Ohno K, Chambers JK, Nakayama H. A retrospective histopathological survey on canine and feline liver diseases at the University of Tokyo between 2006 and 2012. *J Vet Med Sci* 76(7):1015-1020, 2014.
28. Housset, C. Cystic liver diseases. Genetics and cell biology. *Gastroenterologie Clinique et Biologique* 29(8-9):861-869, 2005.
29. Patel A, Chapman AB, Mikolajczyk AE. A practical approach to polycystic liver disease. *Clin Liver Dis* 14(5):176-179, 2019.
30. Biller DS, DiBartola SP, Eaton KA, Pflueger S, Wellman ML, Radin MJ. Inheritance of polycystic kidney disease in Persian cats. *J Hered* 87(1):1-5, 1996.
31. Eaton KA, Biller DS, DiBartola SP, Radin MJ, Wellman ML. Autosomal dominant polycystic kidney disease in Persian and Persian-cross cats. *Vet Pathol* 34(2):117-126, 1997.
32. Lyons LA, Biller DS, Erdman CA, Lipinski MJ, Young AE, Roe BA, et al. Feline polycystic kidney disease mutation identified in PKD1. *J Am Soc Nephrol* 15(10):2548-2555, 2004.
33. O'Leary CA, Mackay BM, Malik R, Edmondston JE, Robinson WF, Huxtable CR. Polycystic kidney disease in Bull Terriers: An autosomal dominant inherited disorder. *Aust Vet J* 77(6):361-366, 1999.
34. Gharahkhani P, O'Leary CA, Kyaw-Tanner M, Sturm RA, Duffy DL. A non-synonymous mutation in the canine Pkd1 gene is associated with autosomal dominant polycystic kidney disease in Bull Terriers. *PLoS One* 6(7):e22455, 2011.
35. Caroli J, Soupault R, Kossakowski J, Plocker L, Paradowska. Congenital polycystic dilation of the intrahepatic bile ducts; attempt at classification. *Sem Hop* 18(34):488-495, 1958.
36. Ananthakrishnan AN, Saeian K. Caroli's disease: Identification and treatment strategy. *Current Gastroenterol Rep* 9:151-155, 2007.
37. Singham J, Yoshida EM, Scudamore CH. Choledochal cysts part 1 of 3: Classification and pathogenesis. *Can J Surg* 52(5):434-440, 2009.
38. Görlinger S, Rothuizen J, Bunch S, Van Den Ingh TSGAM. Congenital dilatation of the bile ducts (Caroli's disease) in young dogs. *J Vet Intern Med* 17(1):28-32, 2003.
39. Last RD, Hill JM, Roach M, Kaldenberg T. Congenital dilation of the large and segmental intrahepatic bile ducts (Caroli's disease) in two Golden retriever littermates. *J S Afr Vet Assoc* 77(4):210-214, 2006.
40. Yonem O, Bayraktar Y. Clinical characteristics of Caroli's disease. *World J Gastroenterol* 13(13), 2007.
41. Serrano G, Mortier F, Bosseler L, Taylor O, Paepe D. Diagnosis of Caroli syndrome in a crossbreed dog. *Vet Rec Case Reports* 6(2):e000576, 2018.
42. Helgert ND, Sula MM. Caroli syndrome in a 6-year-old Rottweiler dog. *J Comp Pathol* 167:1-5, 2019.
43. Hao X, Liu S, Dong Q, Zhang H, Zhao J, Su L. Whole exome sequencing identifies recessive PKHD1 mutations in a Chinese twin family with Caroli disease. *PLoS One* 9(4):e92661, 2014.
44. Kassahun WT, Kahn T, Wittekind C, Mössner J, Caca K, Hauss J, et al. Caroli's disease: Liver resection and liver transplantation. Experience in 33 patients. *Surgery* 138(5):888-898, 2005.
45. Liptak JM, Swinney GR, Rothwell TLW, Hunt GB. Aplasia of the gallbladder in a dog. *J Small Anim Pract* 41(4):175-177, 2000.
46. Kamishina H, Katayama M, Okamura Y, Sasaki J, Chiba S, Goryo M, et al. Gallbladder agenesis in a Chihuahua. *J Vet Med Sci* 72(7):959-962, 2010.
47. Austin B, Tillson DM, Kuhnt LA. Gallbladder Agenesis in a Maltese Dog. *J Am Anim Hosp Assoc* 42(4):308-311, 2006.
48. Kelly D, Moreno-Aguado B, Lamb V. Gallbladder agenesis in a dog: clinicopathological, histopathology, and computed tomography findings. *J Am Anim Hosp Assoc* 55(6):E556-E02, 2019.

49. Gojska-Zygner O, Galanty M, Degorska B, Frymus J, Zygner W. Congenital gallbladder agenesis in a 9-month-old Bull Terrier. *Vet Med* 66 (7):305-312, 2021.
50. Thant PC, Gupta A. Agenesis of gallbladder—an unexpected absence in laparoscopy. *J Surg Case Rep* 2023(4):rjad214, 2023.
51. Kato T, Asakura Y, Kasai M. An attempt to produce choledochal cyst in puppies. *J Pediatr Surg* 9(4):509-513, 1974.
52. Spain HN, Penninck DG, Webster CR, Daure E, Jennings SH. Ultrasonographic and clinicopathologic features of segmental dilatations of the common bile duct in four cats. *J Feline Med Surg Open Reports* 3(1):2055116917716881, 2017.
53. Best EJ, Bush DJ, Dye C. Suspected choledochal cyst in a domestic shorthair cat. *J Feline Med Surg* 12(10):814-817, 2010.
54. Grand JG, Doucet M, Albaric O, Bureau S. Cyst of the common bile duct in a cat. *Aust Vet J* 88(7):268-271, 2010.
55. Todani T, Watanabe Y, Narusue M, Tabuchi K, Okajima K. Congenital bile duct cysts. Classification, operative procedures, and review of thirty-seven cases including cancer arising from choledochal cyst. *Am J Surg* 134(2):263-9, 1977.
56. Ronnekleiv-Kelly SM, Soares KC, Ejaz A, Pawlik TM. Management of choledochal cysts. *Curr Opin Gastroenterol* 32(3):1, 2016.
57. Thiel C, Vet M, Ecvs D, Steinbach S, Acvim D, Schmidt M, et al. Extrahepatic biliary atresia in a 4-week-old Pug. *Vet Surg* 44(1):35-40, 2015.
58. Lange E, Beaudu-Lange C. Canine multi-septate gall bladders in Bull Terrier puppies: first description and follow up of the most affected one. *Rev Vétérinaire Clin* 53(4):129-133, 2018.
59. Kim MJ, Kang SC, Kim JH, Oh HJ, Kim GA, Jo YK, et al. Ectopic liver and gallbladder in a cloned dog: possible nonheritable anomaly. *Theriogenology* 84(6):995-1002, 2015.
60. Wong HE, Cullen JM, Vilà-González M, Pittaway R, Desmet VJ, Gillian TD. Patent hepatic ciliated foregut remnant resulting in an umbilicobiliary sinus tract, with gallbladder agenesis, in an 8-week-old male French Bulldog. *J Vet Diagnostic Investig* 35(2):196-200, 2023.

CHAPTER 38

Canine vacuolar hepatopathies, hepatocutaneous syndrome, and amyloidosis

Sharon Kuzi
DVM, DECVIM-CA
(Internal Medicine)

Vacuolar hepatopathies

Definition and etiology

Vacuolar hepatopathy (VH) is an umbrella term encompassing the most common metabolic liver disorders in dogs, characterized by vacuolated hepatocytes. Hepatocellular swelling due to accumulation of fat or glycogen, comprising the most common types of VH, is a pattern of mostly reversible liver cell injury.[1] Hepatocellular vacuoles may also result from water accumulation (cloudy swelling) when injured hepatocytes are unable to maintain ionic and fluid homeostasis.[1] Vacuolar hepatopathies are mostly considered a secondary phenomenon associated with endocrinopathies such as diabetes mellitus (DM), hypothyroidism, and hyperadrenocorticism (HAC). VHs can also result from toxicities and deficiencies (e.g., aflatoxicosis and congenital cobalamin deficiency), hepatic congestion (e.g., congestive right-sided heart failure), inflammatory hepatobiliary diseases, portosystemic shunting, and dyslipidemias.[2,3] Lysosomal storage diseases can also cause VH, although mostly manifesting neurologic and skeletal clinical signs (listed in Table 8.1 in the WSAVA Standards for Clinical and Histological Diagnosis of Canine and Feline Liver Diseases).[1] Table 38.1 lists the varied causes of VH. Vacuolar hepatopathies are usually benign, but they suggest the presence of other primary diseases, which are usually outside the liver. Furthermore, progression to hepatic dysfunction and predisposition to hepatocellular carcinoma have been reported, justifying a thorough diagnostic, monitoring, and treatment plan.[4,5]

TABLE 38.1 Causes of vacuolar hepatopathy in dogs.

Type of vacuolar hepatopathy*	Potential etiology
Glycogen-associated vacuolar hepatopathy/"steroid hepatopathy" and cloudy changes	■ Endocrinopathy (e.g., typical and atypical hyperadrenocorticism, diabetes mellitus) ■ Any chronic stress/acute and chronic illness (causing hypercortisolemia or involving the liver) ■ Glycogen-like vacuolar hepatopathy of the Scottish Terrier ■ Nutrient deficiencies (e.g., vitamin B_{12}) ■ Drug-induced/other hepatotoxicity (e.g., D-penicillamine) ■ Inflammatory hepatobiliary diseases ■ Portosystemic shunting ■ Liver congestion (e.g., right-sided congestive heart failure) ■ Aminoaciduric canine hypoaminoacidemic hepatopathy syndrome
Hepatic steatosis	■ Endocrinopathy (e.g., hypothyroidism, diabetes mellitus) ■ Dyslipidemia/hypertriglyceridemia ■ Obesity ■ Hepatotoxicity (e.g., aflatoxicosis, tetracycline idiosyncratic toxicity)
Specific metabolite accumulation	■ Lysosomal storage disease (e.g., cholesterol ester storage disease in Fox Terriers)

* Combined changes (i.e., both lipid and glycogen accumulation) may be present in some diseases (e.g., DM)

Main types of vacuolar hepatopathies in dogs

Glycogen-associated vacuolar hepatopathy: "steroid hepatopathy"

Glycogen accumulation is the most common form of VH in dogs, mostly associated with increased levels of endogenous or exogenous steroids.[5] Steroid hepatopathy (SH) can be secondary to various acute and chronic diseases, probably due to stress-induced hypercortisolemia. Other steroid hormones (progestins and aldosterone) and drugs (e.g., D-penicillamine) may also induce SH.[1] Increases in serum alkaline phosphatase activity (ALP), sometimes thousands-fold the upper reference interval, are common due largely to the steroid-induced but also the biliary isoenzyme (see chapter 25 for more details). While HAC may be the cause, SH is not a pathognomonic finding in HAC, and hypercortisolemia was not demonstrated in 45% of dogs with SH in one study.[5] Therefore, cortisol assays should only be performed when clinical signs (e.g., polyuria and polydipsia) and other changes in the biochemistry (e.g., hypercholesterolemia) are noted. Typically, hepatocytes are swollen with glycogen, appearing as clear cytoplasm and strands of eosinophilic cytoplasm without displacement of the nucleus (Fig. 38.1).[1,6] Occasionally, marginated neutrophils in small blood vessels and sporadic foci of extramedullary hematopoiesis can be seen in histology samples.[1,6] SH has been considered benign in the majority of dogs. However, hepatic remodeling and carcinoma have been reported,[4,5] warranting a comprehensive diagnostic approach and monitoring of clinicopathologic and imaging findings that might suggest the development of a more severe liver parenchymatic injury (e.g., elevated alanine aminotransferase [ALT] activities, and progressive elevation in ALP activities), functional liver failure (e.g., decreased albumin, cholesterol, and urea serum concentrations), or malignant transformation.

Glycogen-like vacuolar hepatopathy of the Scottish Terrier

Scottish Terriers are reportedly predisposed to a breed-specific glycogen-associated VH, characterized by a moderate to marked elevation in serum ALP, a milder increase in ALT activity, and an increased risk of developing hepatocellular carcinoma at an older age (median >8 years).[4,7] The pathogenesis is poorly understood, but associations with increased steroid hormones are documented. While typical HAC is usually ruled out by low-dose dexamethasone suppression testing and urine cortisol:creatinine ratios within reference intervals, clinical signs suggestive of HAC are noted in nearly half the dogs. Increases in progesterone and androstenedione, post-ACTH stimulation concentrations, are commonly reported. Affected dogs have a poor response to cortisol-lowering medical treatments, including severe side effects with mitotane or ketoconazole and lack of efficacy of trilostane, supporting the lack of typical HAC. Nevertheless, data is limited to a small number of treated dogs. Common sonographic hepatic changes include nonspecific mottled or coarse hepatic parenchyma. The presence of hypoechoic nodules may indicate progression to a degenerative lesion and occasionally malignant transformation.[4] Adrenal glands are enlarged in a minority (26%) of cases, and gallbladder mucocele is diagnosed in 16% of dogs. A small number of dogs have small nodular livers and decreases in portal flow, suggestive of portal hypertension. Thus, SH in Scottish Terrier dogs may range from subclinical disease to liver failure or malignancy. The magnitude of liver enzyme elevations is neither discriminatory nor predictive of specific disease phenotypes. Monitoring of progressive increases in ALP and sonographic changes is recommended in affected dogs, as these changes might indicate malignant transformation or mucocele development, necessitating medical or surgical intervention.

Hepatic steatosis

Accumulation of fat within hepatocytes is interchangeably termed "steatosis", "lipidosis" or "fatty change". Steatosis is the preferred term, as it is used in human medicine and toxicology textbooks while also allowing differentiation between hepatic steatosis in dogs and the clinical hepatic lipidosis syndrome in cats.[1] Deposition of fat within hepatocytes is associated with endocrinopathies (i.e., DM, HAC, and hypothyroidism), toxic hepatocyte injury (e.g., aflatoxicosis and tetracycline toxicity), congenital portosystemic shunts, or primary and secondary disorders of fat metabolism.[2] Histologically, microvesicular or macrovesicular steatosis patterns are described (Fig. 38.2). In addition to hepatic steatosis, hyperlipidemia is associated with gallbladder distention and dysmotility in dogs. Thus, it may contribute to bile retention, cholelithiasis formation, and the development of gallbladder mucocele.[8]

Histologically, steatosis in dogs shows some resemblance to nonalcoholic fatty liver disease in humans, a common liver disease ranging from benign hepatic steatosis to steatohepatitis, cirrhosis, and hepatocellular carcinoma.[9] NAFLD is primarily associated with overnutrition, obesity, and metabolic syndrome (insulin-resistant type 2 DM, hypertension, and dyslipidemias).[9] Although obesity in dogs can induce insulin resistance, hyperlipidemia, and increased liver enzyme activities, secondary fat accumulation in the liver is not well documented.[10-13] Obesity-related metabolic changes in dogs are likely mostly benign, and NAFLD and its inflammatory and neoplastic consequences have not been described in dogs.[14]

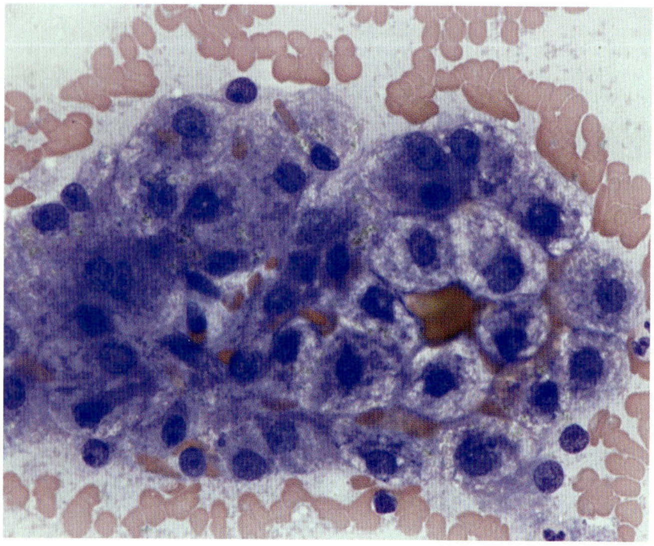

FIG. 38.1 Cytology of an aspirate of canine liver showing steroid (glycogen) hepatopathy. The hepatocytes have mild to moderate rarefactive nonlipid vacuolar changes. These have indistinct, feathery clearings, resulting in the appearance of thinner cytoplasmic density. These also demonstrate mild anisocytosis and mild anisokaryosis. Magnification ×60. Modified Wright's stain.

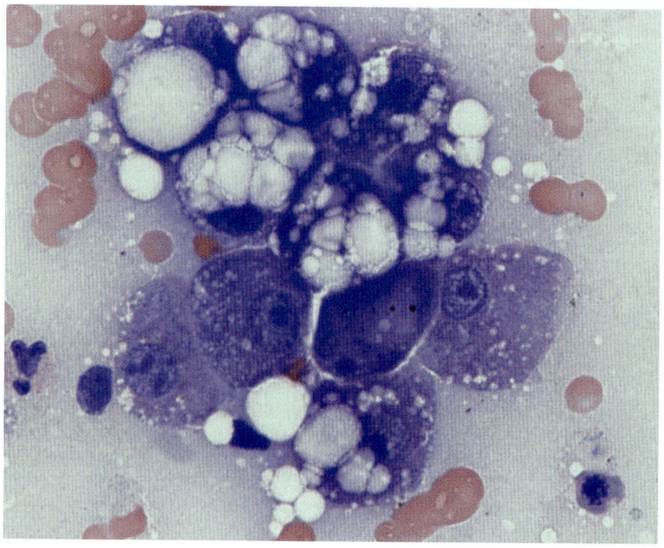

FIG. 38.2 Cytology of an aspirate of canine liver showing lipid hepatopathy. The hepatocytes have moderate to marked lipid vacuolar changes, including microvesicular (discrete vacuoles, smaller than the cell's nucleus) and macrovesicular lipid vacuolation (variably sized discrete vacuoles, larger than the cell's often displaced nucleus). These are seen adjacent to a few hepatocytes with minimal to no lipid vacuolar changes and one hepatocyte containing a small amount of black bile pigment. Magnification ×100. Modified Wright's stain.

Familial hypertriglyceridemia of Miniature Schnauzers

Miniature Schnauzers are predisposed to hypertriglyceridemia, documented in 32.8% of dogs.[15] Pancreatitis, hepatic steatosis, and gallbladder mucoceles are common secondary complications of familial hypertriglyceridemia (FHTG).[2] In one study, reduced expression of genes involved in hepatic cholesterol trafficking was found, potentially delaying hepatic clearance of dietary fats. This metabolic disturbance worsens with age, and indeed, >75% of hypertriglyceridemic Miniature Schnauzers were >9 years old. However, a study of mutations in lipoprotein lipase (LPL) and apolipoprotein C-II genes did not distinguish hyper- from normotriglyceridemic dogs.[16]

Diagnosis of canine vacuolar hepatopathies

Dogs with VH may present clinical signs associated with their primary disease (e.g., polyuria and polydipsia in HAC and DM) or may be detected during routine health checks with no apparent clinical changes.

Algorithm 38.1 outlines the workup of these cases.

Algorithm 38.1 Note 1 Increased alkaline phosphatase (ALP) activity is the most common finding in dogs with all VH types, with or without clear evidence of GC excess.[5] Other laboratory abnormalities are caused by the primary underlying disease.

Algorithm 38.1 Note 2 Although abdominal ultrasound findings are nonspecific, a diffusely hyperechoic liver or the presence of hypoechoic hepatic nodule(s) <3 cm in diameter was moderately predictive of VH.[17] Several obstacles may hinder the ability to recognize diffuse echogenic changes, including the occurrence of focal fatty sparing, which appears as a hypoechoic lesion within an apparently normal liver when it is actually a relatively normal liver surrounded by steatosis. Combining biochemistry and sonographic findings had poor diagnostic accuracy (50%) for VH.[18]

Algorithm 38.1 Note 3 Cytology has moderate to high sensitivity in detecting VH. Overinterpretation of subtle changes might lead to a false positive diagnosis, as mild vacuolation of a minority of hepatocytes represents normal physiologic metabolic activity.[3] Cytology may also be falsely negative if there are focal liver lesions. Well-delineated clear cytoplasmic vacuoles usually represent lipids, while indistinct vacuoles may represent glycogen (Figs. 38.1 and 38.2).

Algorithm 38.1 Note 4 Histological findings include cellular distention, increased fragility, and ballooning degeneration. Special stains differentiate between lipid and glycogen accumulation (e.g., periodic acid-Schiff for glycogen and oil red O for fat).[1] Lipid is lost in routine formalin-fixed section processing, causing fat to appear as clear cytoplasmic vacuoles; thus, frozen sections are required to demonstrate fat with special stains. Severe VH may cause diffuse hepatic remodeling with hepatocellular necrosis, inflammation, possible cirrhosis, portal hypertension, hepatic insufficiency, or malignancy.[4,5]

Algorithm 38.1 Note 5 Computed tomography attenuation values for normal canine liver range between 60 and 70 HU. Fatty infiltration is diagnosed when hepatic attenuation is decreased, and a single study described negative hepatic attenuation in a dog diagnosed with mixed hepatic glycogen and lipid accumulation, secondary to concurrent Cushing's syndrome and DM.[19] Computed tomography is not routinely required for diagnosis of VH, but it may be indicated with progressive elevations of ALP activities, and/or nodular hepatic lesions, to help detect malignant transformation.

Additional current and future diagnostic modalities

Micro-RNAs (MiRNA) are short, noncoding, naturally occurring RNA molecules that act as regulators of target genes involved in lipid homeostasis within hepatocytes. MiRNA expression has been shown to be markedly disrupted in hepatic steatosis and fibrosis, and specific MiRNAs may serve as noninvasive biomarkers of different hepatobiliary diseases. Hepatocyte-derived *Canis familiaris* (cfa)-microRNAs MiRNA-122, -34a, and -21 expression was significantly upregulated in dogs with liver steatosis or fibrosis and secondary cholelithiasis compared to healthy control dogs. Hepatocyte-derived cfa-MiRNA-21 expression was significantly higher in dogs with hepatic fibrosis and had the diagnostic power to differentiate hepatic steatosis from fibrosis with a ROC AUC = 0.98.[20] Commercial applications are yet to be developed.

Serum metabolomic profiles in dogs with various liver diseases were investigated in a single study, and distinct metabolomic phenotypes differed between dogs with congenital portosystemic shunts and dogs with increased hepatobiliary enzyme activities in a predictive manner. These included differences in branched-chain amino acid and fatty acid concentrations and lipoprotein profiles.[21] However, histopathological diagnoses were not available in all dogs with elevated serum liver enzyme activities. Thus, neither congenital nor acquired liver vascular abnormalities could not have been ruled out. While this approach is not commercially available at present, in the future, metabolic alterations may be used as diagnostic and therapeutic targets in different metabolic liver diseases.

Treatment of canine vacuolar hepatopathies

When possible, treatment of VH should primarily target primary disease conditions which led to secondary VH. S-adenosylmethionine (20 mg/kg PO q24h) may be beneficial in SH, given the reduction in glutathione reported in dogs with SH.[23,24] Treatments including low-fat diets, chitosan, and omega-3 unsaturated fatty acids supplementation may aid in decreasing both hyperlipidemia and weight, which may be potentially beneficial in decreasing hepatic steatosis.

Micronized, nanocrystal formulation of fenofibrate was effective in normalization of hypertriglyceridemia and hypercholesterolemia and significantly reducing ALP activities in hyperlipidemic dogs. A median dose of 6.4 mg/kg PO q24h (range, 2.2-13.5), using a dose-escalation protocol, was effective within 3-9 weeks.[25]

Hepatocutaneous syndrome

Hepatocutaneous syndrome (also known as superficial necrolytic dermatitis, metabolic epidermal necrosis, necrolytic migratory erythema, and aminoaciduric canine hypoaminoacidemic hepatopathy syndrome) is an uncommon, severe hepatopathy, usually accompanied by skin lesions. This syndrome is associated with decreases in circulating amino acid concentrations and excess loss of amino acids via the urine. Thus, it is termed "aminoaciduric canine hypoaminoacidemic hepatopathy syndrome" (ACHES).[26-29] ACHES is associated with several metabolic conditions in dogs, including glucagonomas (usually metastatic),

ALGORITHM 38.1

Diagnostic approach to canine vacuolar hepatopathies.

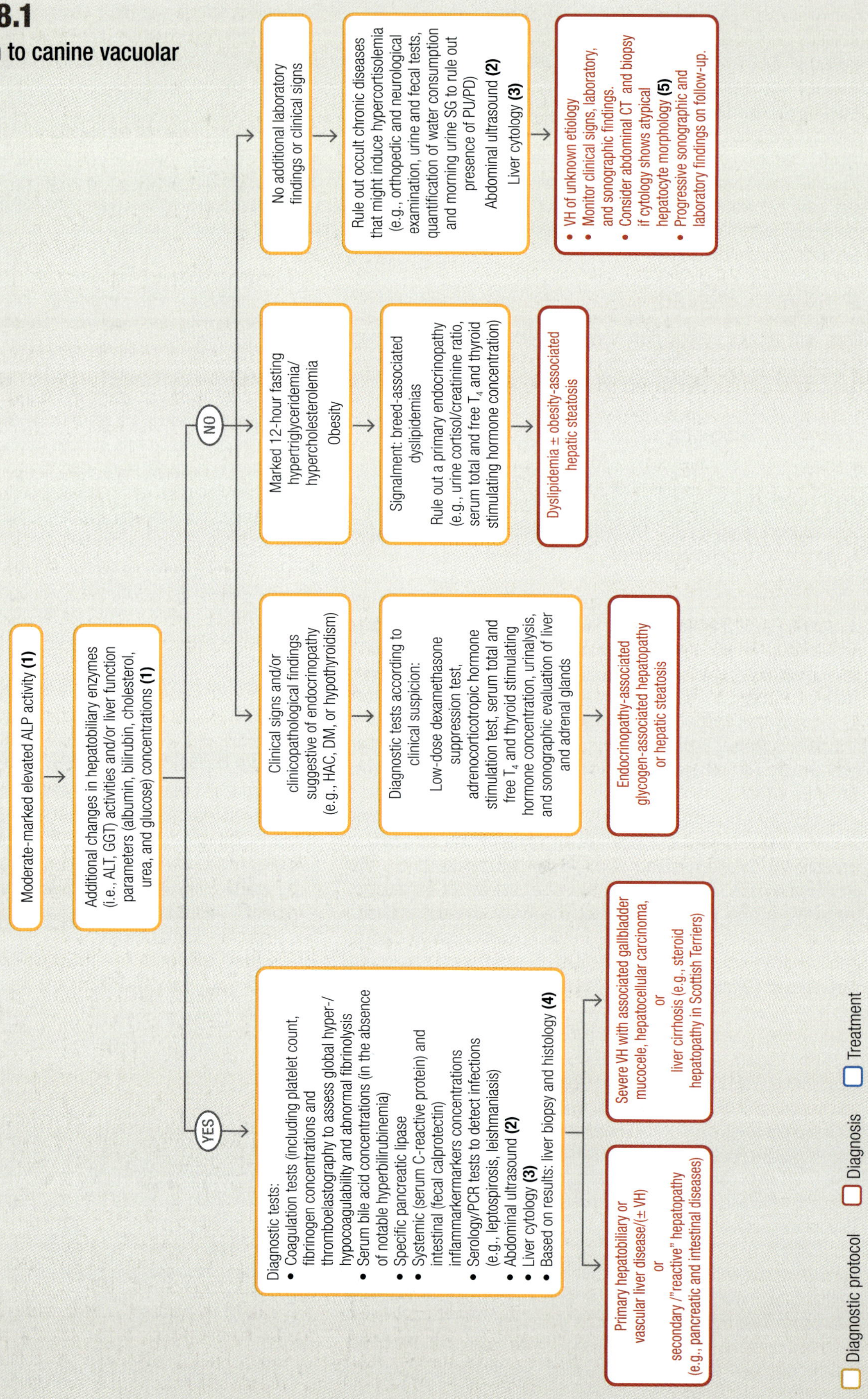

insulinoma, and prolonged phenobarbital treatment. A heritable component was suspected in affected Shih Tzus.[30,31] However, in most dogs with ACHES, the cause is unknown.[26] Amino acid, zinc, fatty acid, and B vitamin deficiencies are associated with skin lesions and may develop due to upregulated hepatic metabolic activity, driven by glucagon and other unidentified stimuli.[28,32]

Clinical presentations

ACHES has been reported most commonly in older small breed dogs with a median age of 8-10 years.[26,30] Skin lesions include hyperkeratotic, erythematous, crusting lesions, mainly on the extremities (paw pads, nose, periorbital, and perianal regions), around the genitals, and on pressure points. The lesions may be painful, with fissures and secondary infections. The presence and severity of skin lesions vary, and ACHES with initial clinicopathologic and sonographic hepatic changes and later skin involvement were reported in 73% of dogs.[26] Signs of DM were reported in 25-40% of dogs with ACHES, although the DM often develops later in the disease course. Increased glucagon secretion is thought to cause marked insulin resistance and DM. Although some dogs with DM have normal glucagon concentrations, the latter might be inappropriate in the context of hypoaminoacidemia.[26] Clinical signs that are associated with liver disease or metastatic neoplasia (e.g., glucagonoma) are uncommon.

Diagnosis of hepatocutaneous syndrome

Diagnosis is made on the basis of skin and/or liver histology, combined with the typical appearance of the liver on imaging.[29] Plasma and urine amino acid profiling is a noninvasive method for disease confirmation. Hypoaminoacidemia was present in all dogs with ACHES when measured, with significant deficiencies in plasma concentrations of alanine, glutamine, glycine, lysine, proline, and threonine.[26] Complementary aminoaciduria is also a key characteristic of ACHES.[27] Elevations of ALP and ALT activities are common, and hypoalbuminemia is reported in approximately half of cases. Hyperglycemia and glucosuria are present in cases with DM. Anemia and microcytosis were reportedly associated with the presence and severity of skin lesions.[26] Ultrasound of the liver demonstrates a "honeycomb" (or, more accurately, "Swiss cheese") appearance, with variably sized, hypoechoic nodules surrounded by hyperechoic borders.[33] Histologically, nodular areas of normal hepatocytes surrounded by zones of collapsed parenchyma with vacuolated hepatocytes correspond to the sonographic image. Skin biopsies show parakeratotic hyperkeratosis with inter- and intracellular edema, which results in a typical "red, white, and blue" appearance on hematoxylin and eosin-stained skin sections. A primary pancreatic mass and metastases may be visible on ultrasound, but histology and immunohistochemistry are necessary to classify the tumor type.

Prognosis and treatment

ACHES carries a poor prognosis in most dogs, with death or euthanasia often reported within 6 months of diagnosis. Treatment of a primary cause (i.e., removal of a pancreatic tumor, octreotide injections, or replacement of phenobarbital with other antiepileptic) is important, but in most cases, where no underlying cause is identified, treatment is supportive. A high-quality, digestible, high-protein diet administers ample amino acid supplementation. Protein content approximating 50% of metabolizable energy, unless contraindicated by other disease conditions, is recommended. Additional suggested supplementations of proline (500 mg daily), lysine (500-1000 mg daily), arginine/ornithine (500-750 mg daily each), and glutathione (500-1000 mg daily) are also reported.[26] A daily egg yolk addition and extra zinc and essential fatty acids supplements may be beneficial. Administering weekly parenteral amino acid treatment has been reported, but the efficacy of this approach has not been widely investigated.[34] Supportive treatment of skin lesions should include appropriate antibiotics and antimycotics for secondary infections, topical shampoos, and analgesia. The use of corticosteroids should be avoided because of the risk of precipitating DM.

Hepatic amyloidosis in dogs

Amyloid deposition in the liver of dogs usually refers to serum amyloid-associated protein deposition secondary to chronic inflammation or tissue destruction.[35] The latter processes lead to liver production of the acute phase protein serum amyloid A (SAA). Amyloid is an extracellular matrix of SAA protein fibrils with a characteristic appearance of crossed β-pleated sheet conformation on electron microscopy. Histologically, it appears as a deposition of hyaline eosinophilic material in the space of Disse, with frequent concurrent atrophy of adjacent hepatocytes and dilation of sinusoids. The amyloid deposition may have a diffuse, zonal, or multifocal parenchymal distribution and may be accompanied by deposition of amyloid in the walls of vessels and the portal and perivenular connective tissue.[35] The presence of amyloidosis can sometimes be detected with liver cytology as amorphous, pink material interspersed among hepatocytes. Differential diagnoses for pink extracellular matrix include amyloid, osteoid, chondroid, and collagen. Thus, special stains (Congo red or Stokes) may be needed to identify the presence of amyloid in either cytology or histology samples. With extensive hepatic amyloid accumulation, the liver becomes markedly enlarged and fragile, and intrahepatic hemorrhage, as well as spontaneous or biopsy-induced liver rupture and hemoabdomen, may occur.[36] Various primary chronic inflammatory and infectious diseases have been reported associated with amyloidosis of the liver (and other organs) in dogs, including leishmaniasis, cyclic hematopoiesis in gray Collie dogs, and blastomycosis. The commonest cause of canine amyloidosis is familial Shar Pei fever syndrome.

Familial Shar Pei fever syndrome, swollen hock syndrome, or Shar Pei autoinflammatory disease

Some Shar Pei dogs suffer from this syndrome, manifested with recurrent bouts of fever, vesicular hyaluronosis, and various inflammatory conditions, including arthritis, dermatitis, otitis, and inflammatory chronic enteropathies.[37] Some dogs develop amyloidosis, mostly involving the kidneys and liver. Familial Shar Pei fever syndrome, swollen hock syndrome, or Shar Pei autoinflammatory disease (SPAID) has a suspected incomplete dominant mode of inheritance, and episodic fever occurs in up to 23-53% of Shar Pei dogs, usually beginning before 18 months of age, although adult-onset episodes may be seen.[38] A missense variant in oncoprotein murine double minute (Mdm2) binding protein (MTBP) related to proinflammatory processes via the MTBP-MDM2 pathway is associated with SPAID. The MTBP missense variant is also associated with increased hyaluronan synthase 2 (HAS2) expression, the driver of long-chain hyaluronan (HA) synthesis. The elevated expression of HAS2 results in hereditary cutaneous hyaluronanosis, which causes the breed's heavily thickened and wrinkled skin and the "meat mouth" (padded muzzle) appearance. Hyaluronan overproduction and resultant degradation products create a "danger-associated molecular pattern" signal, which triggers an immune response and inflammation.[39] It was also found that there is a role for copy number variants (CNVs) in the heredity of SPAID through the disruption of HAS2 gene expression. An increased copy number of the "meat mouth" (16.1) variant, especially harboring CNV 16.1 allele 5, results in a duplication upstream of HAS2 on chromosome 13, increased expression of HAS2 and SPAID. While these discoveries shed light on the pathophysiology of SPAID, there are still discrepancies (e.g., SPAID-affected "bone mouth" Shar Pei types and hyaluronic acid accumulation in SPAID-unaffected dogs) which suggest that the inflammatory processes in SPAID are complex, and other genetic variants play a role in disease development.

Diagnosis of Shar Pei autoinflammatory disease

PCR blood testing for analysis of the 16.1 Kb copy number variant, the allele associated with SPAID, is available, and double carriers of allele 5 are eight times more likely to suffer from SPAID compared with non-carriers. Results are reported as "copy number variant", with higher risk associated with a higher number of variant copies.[39] Testing for the MTBP missense mutation is also available and can be used to identify whether an individual is homozygous or heterozygous for the mutant genotype; dogs with the homozygous mutant genotype above the age of 6 years old were all affected by SPAID, and Shar Peis with a heterozygous genotype had a 2.13-fold increased risk of developing SPAID.[40] Nevertheless, neither test may detect all affected dogs or dogs at risk, and diagnosis is usually made based on the clinical findings, specifically pyrexia, without a specific cause. Lethargy, hyporexia, joint or muzzle swelling, and vomiting are additionally commonly reported.[38] While renal amyloidosis is more commonly reported, hepatic amyloidosis is also described.[41,42] The clinical presentation of the hepatic form varies and might include nonspecific clinical signs (i.e., anorexia, weight loss, and lethargy), as well as icterus and hemoabdomen secondary to rupture of the liver.

Treatment of Shar Pei autoinflammatory disease

Many of the recommendations for treating SPAID are based on anecdotes or extrapolated from the management of the phenotypically similar condition of familial Mediterranean fever (FMF) in humans. The antifibrotic drug colchicine has been shown to reduce the frequency, severity, and duration of fever episodes in FMF patients and could theoretically block amyloid deposition and SAA synthesis, downregulate inflammatory pathways, and modulate innate immunity. However, colchicine treatment lacks good evidence based on this condition and has a narrow therapeutic index, with gastrointestinal adverse effects being common in dogs. In humans, colchicine is associated with severe adverse effects, including myelosuppression, neuromuscular toxicity, and rhabdomyolysis, and these more severe adverse effects may also be relevant in veterinary medicine. In a large retrospective study, nonsteroidal anti-inflammatory drugs (NSAIDs) were prescribed to 73% of febrile Shar Peis, repeated as needed.[38] Although a logical treatment choice due to their inhibition of interleukin-6 and antipyretic effect, cautious NSAID use is advocated in a breed predisposed to kidney disease and gastroenteropathies. Colchicine was prescribed in 19% of affected dogs. According to owners, there was a reduction in the frequency of fever episodes in 70% of dogs treated with colchicine, and 50% demonstrated a reduction in the severity of episodes. Therefore, despite the small number (10) of treated dogs, colchicine was associated with minimal adverse effects and improved quality of life in affected dogs.[38] The median dose prescribed was 0.06 mg/kg per day (range 0.01 to 0.33 mg/kg per day). Self-limiting diarrhea was documented in 4 out of 10 dogs undergoing colchicine therapy. However, this did not result in cessation of treatment, and no other adverse effects were reported. Nevertheless, blood tests were not performed following commencing of colchicine treatment, and myelosuppression might have occurred.

Prognosis of Shar Pei autoinflammatory disease

Data on prognosis is limited. Renal amyloidosis and azotemia are associated with early death (median age of 4.5 years; range, 2 to 9 years) compared to dogs without renal disease (median age, 6 years; range, 1 to 11 years).[38] Only a few case reports of dogs with hepatic amyloidosis are available, where concurrent renal amyloidosis was not the major disease process, and the owners did not opt for immediate euthanasia. In one dog, euthanasia due to repeated cholestatic, icteric episodes was performed 33 months after diagnosis, and a second dog was alive for <2 years following diagnosis. Both dogs were treated with colchicine.[41]

KEY POINTS

- Canine vacuolar hepatopathy (VH) encompasses glycogen ("steroid hepatopathy") and lipid ("hepatic steatosis") accumulation in hepatocytes, as well as hydropic cellular injury.
- In most cases, VH is a secondary phenomenon, necessitating diagnostic investigation into the potential primary causes.
- Infrequently, specific disease conditions may be present, some with a clear etiology (e.g., lysosomal storage diseases) and some with partially known pathophysiology (e.g., hepatocutaneous syndrome).
- Canine steroid hepatopathy or hepatic steatosis are usually benign conditions, commonly manifested by increased serum ALP activities and nonspecific liver sonographic changes. In a few cases, parenchymal remodeling, malignant transformation, gallbladder mucocele, and rarely, liver failure and portal hypertension can occur.
- If no treatable primary disease is identified and there are significant increases in liver enzyme activities, changes in liver function indices, and sonographic changes (i.e., increase in liver nodule size and texture) between follow-ups, a broader investigation is warranted, such as advanced imaging (e.g., computed tomography) and liver biopsies.
- Treatment of vacuolar hepatopathy is aimed at the primary disease. Evidence of the utility of treatments aimed at reducing hepatocellular vacuolation and damage is lacking, but supportive, antioxidative treatment may be beneficial. For steatosis, low-fat diets, omega-three fatty acids, and lipid-lowering drugs (e.g., fenofibrate) may be beneficial.
- Prognosis with VH is dependent on the primary disease and presence of sequelae such as hepatocellular carcinoma or gallbladder mucocele.
- Hepatocutaneous syndrome, also known as aminoaciduric canine hypoaminoacidemic hepatopathy syndrome (ACHES), is an uncommon, severe hepatopathy, usually accompanied by skin lesions. The syndrome is associated with decreases in circulating amino acid concentrations and excess loss of amino acids via the urine.
- ACHES is associated with glucagonoma, insulinoma, prolonged phenobarbital treatment, and a suspected heritable component in Shih Tzus. However, in most dogs, the cause is unknown.
- Clinical signs in ACHES include skin lesions with hyperkeratotic, erythematous, crusting lesions, mainly on the extremities, around the genitals, and pressure points. The lesions may appear later in the disease course. Diabetes mellitus (DM) develops in 25-40% of dogs with ACHES, usually also in later disease stages.
- Diagnosis of ACHES is based on skin and/or liver histology, combined with the typical "Swiss cheese" sonographic liver appearance. Hypoaminoacidemia and complementary aminoaciduria are key characteristics of ACHES. Routine blood tests may reveal increased ALP and ALT activities, hypoalbuminemia, hyperglycemia, and glucosuria in cases with DM.
- Treatment of ACHES where no underlying cause is identified is supportive, with supplementation of amino acids and treatment of skin lesions targeting secondary bacterial and mycotic infections and providing analgesia.
- ACHES carries a poor prognosis in most dogs, with death or euthanasia often reported within 6 months of diagnosis, but intensive supportive treatment was associated with longer survival of individual dogs.
- Hepatic amyloidosis develops due to serum amyloid-A (SAA) protein deposition in the space of Disse, walls of vessels, and in the portal and perivenular connective tissue, leading to atrophy of adjacent hepatocytes, cholestasis, increased parenchymatic fragility, and risk of rupture and abdominal bleeding.
- Increased amyloid production and SAA deposition may be secondary to any chronic inflammation or tissue destruction, but the commonest cause of canine amyloidosis is familial Shar Pei fever syndrome, also termed "swollen hock syndrome", or "Shar Pei autoinflammatory disease" (SPAID).
- SPAID affects 23-53% of Shar Pei dogs, usually beginning before 18 months of age. The syndrome is manifested with recurrent bouts of fever, vesicular hyaluronosis, and various inflammatory conditions, including arthritis, dermatitis, otitis, and inflammatory chronic enteropathies. Lethargy, hyporexia, joint or muzzle swelling, and vomiting are also common. SPAID may lead to amyloidosis of organs, most commonly affecting the kidneys and, less commonly, the liver. Anorexia, weight loss, lethargy, icterus, and hemoabdomen were described in dogs affected with hepatic amyloidosis.
- SPAID is associated with excessive hyaluronic acid production and the consequent skin mucinosis typical of the breed; nevertheless, only some of the potentially associated hereditary perturbations are known. Genetic tests are available, but while results are indicative of disease risk, they might miss dogs affected by different mutations.
- Treatment of SPAID is based on supportive and antipyretic treatment with NSAIDs. The use of colchicine may be beneficial in reducing the frequency and severity of fever episodes and could theoretically block amyloid deposition, but evidence is lacking, and side effects (ranging from mostly mild gastrointestinal signs to potentially severe but infrequent myelosuppression) may occur.
- While renal amyloidosis is associated with an early death, data on prognosis in dogs with liver amyloidosis is limited. Two dogs treated with colchicine survived for 33 and <24 months.

References

1. Van Winkle TCJ, Van den Ingh SGAMT, Charles JA, Desmet VJ. Morphological classification of parenchymal disorders of the canine and feline liver: 3. Hepatic abscesses and granulomas, hepatic metabolic storage disorders, and miscellaneous conditions. In Rothuizen J BS, Charles JA, Cullen JM, Desmet VJ, Szatmári V, Twedt DC, Van den Ingh SGAMT, Van Winkle T, editors. WSAVA Standards for Clinical and Histological Diagnosis of Canine and Feline Liver Diseases. WSAVA Liver Standardization Group, W.B. Saunders, 2006, pp. 103-116.
2. Watson P. Canine breed-specific hepatopathies. *Vet Clin North Am Small Anim Pract* 47:665-682, 2017.
3. Stockhaus C, Van Den Ingh T, Rothuizen J, et al. A multistep approach in the cytologic evaluation of liver biopsy samples of dogs with hepatic diseases. *Vet Pathol* 41:461-470, 2004.
4. Cortright CC, Center SA, Randolph JF, et al. Clinical features of progressive vacuolar hepatopathy in Scottish Terriers with and without hepatocellular carcinoma: 114 cases (1980-2013). *J Am Vet Med Assoc* 245:797-808, 2014.
5. Sepesy LM, Center SA, Randolph JF, et al. Vacuolar hepatopathy in dogs: 336 cases (1993-2005). *J Am Vet Med Assoc* 229:246-252, 2006.
6. Fittschen C, Bellamy JE. Prednisone-induced morphologic and chemical changes in the liver of dogs. *Vet Pathol* 21:399-406, 1984.
7. Peyron C, Lecoindre P, Chevallier M, et al. Vacuolar hepatopathy in 43 French Scottish Terriers: A morphological study. *Rev Med Vét* 166:176-184, 2015.
8. Villm JA, DeMonaco SM, Panciera DL, et al. Evaluation of gallbladder motility assessed by ultrasonography in dogs with hyperlipidemia. *J Vet Intern Med* 37:968-975, 2023.
9. Rinella ME. Nonalcoholic fatty liver disease: a systematic review. *J Am Med Assoc* 313:2263-2273, 2015.
10. ribuddharatana TKY, Sribhen K, Sribhen C. Biochemical alterations and their relationships with the metabolic syndrome components in canine obesity. *Kasetsart J Natural Science* 4:622-628, 2011.
11. Tvarijonaviciute A, Baric-Rafaj R, Horvatic A, et al. Identification of changes in serum analytes and possible metabolic pathways associated with canine obesity-related metabolic dysfunction. *Vet J* 244:251-259, 2019.
12. Belotta AF, Teixeira CR, Padovani CR, et al. Sonographic evaluation of liver hemodynamic indices in overweight and obese dogs. *J Vet Intern Med* 32:181-187, 2018.
13. Weeth LP. Other risks/possible benefits of obesity. *Vet Clin North Am Small Anim Pract* 46:843-853, 2016.
14. Chandler M, Cunningham S, Lund EM, et al. Obesity and associated comorbidities in people and companion animals: A One Health perspective. *J Comp Pathol* 156:296-309, 2017.
15. Xenoulis PG, Suchodolski JS, Levinski MD, et al. Investigation of hypertriglyceridemia in healthy Miniature Schnauzers. *J Vet Intern Med* 21:1224-1230, 2007.
16. Xenoulis PG, Suchodolski JS, Ruaux CG, et al. Association between serum triglyceride and canine pancreatic lipase immunoreactivity concentrations in miniature schnauzers. *J Am Anim Hosp Assoc* 46:229-234, 2010.
17. Guillot M, Danjou MA, Alexander K, et al. Can sonographic findings predict the results of liver aspirates in dogs with suspected liver disease? *Vet Radiol Ultrasound* 50:513-518, 2009.
18. Feeney DA, Anderson KL, Ziegler LE, et al. Statistical relevance of ultrasonographic criteria in the assessment of diffuse liver disease in dogs and cats. *Am J Vet Res* 69:212-221, 2008.
19. Carloni A, Paninarova M, Cavina D, et al. Negative hepatic computed tomographic attenuation pattern in a dog with vacuolar hepatopathy and hepatic fat accumulation secondary to Cushing's syndrome. *Vet Radiol Ultrasound* 60:E54-E57, 2019.
20. El-Sebaey AM, Abramov PN. Hepatocyte-derived canine familiaris-microRNAs as serum biomarkers of hepatic steatosis or fibrosis as implicated in the pathogenesis of canine cholecystolithiasis. *Vet Clin Pathol* 50 Suppl 1:37-46, 2022.
21. Imbery CA, Dieterle F, Ottka C, et al. Metabolomic serum abnormalities in dogs with hepatopathies. *Sci Rep* 12:5329, 2022.
22. Lin LS, Chung CS. Novel contrast agent Visphere© is feasible for contrast-enhanced ultrasonography in dogs. *Vet Radiol Ultrasound* 61:461-470, 2020.
23. Center SA, Warner KL, McCabe J, et al. Evaluation of the influence of S-adenosylmethionine on systemic and hepatic effects of prednisolone in dogs. *Am J Vet Res* 66:330-341, 2005.
24. Center SA, Warner KL, Erb HN. Liver glutathione concentrations in dogs and cats with naturally occurring liver disease. *Am J Vet Res* 63:1187-1197, 2002.
25. Munro MJL, Hulsebosch SE, Marks SL, et al. Efficacy of a micronized, nanocrystal fenofibrate formulation in the treatment of hyperlipidemia in dogs. *J Vet Intern Med* 35:1733-1742, 2021.
26. Loftus JP, Center SA, Astor M, et al. Clinical features and amino acid profiles of dogs with hepatocutaneous syndrome or hepatocutaneous-associated hepatopathy. *J Vet Intern Med* 36(1):97-105, 2022.
27. Loftus JP, Center SA, Lucy JM, et al. Characterization of aminoaciduria and hypoaminoacidemia in dogs with hepatocutaneous syndrome. *Am J Vet Res* 78:735-744, 2017.
28. Outerbridge CA, Marks SL, Rogers QR. Plasma amino acid concentrations in 36 dogs with histologically confirmed superficial necrolytic dermatitis. *Vet Dermatol* 13:177-186, 2002.
29. DeMarle KB, Webster CRL, Penninck D, et al. Approach to the diagnosis of hepatocutaneous syndrome in dogs: A retrospective study and literature review. *J Am Anim Hosp Assoc* 57:15-25, 2021.
30. March PA, Hillier A, Weisbrode SE, et al. Superficial necrolytic dermatitis in 11 dogs with a history of phenobarbital administration (1995-2002). *J Vet Intern Med* 18:65-74, 2004.
31. Hall-Fonte DL, Center SA, McDonough SP, et al. Hepatocutaneous syndrome in Shih Tzus: 31 cases (1996-2014). *J Am Vet Med Assoc* 248:802-813, 2016.
32. Cave TA, Evans H, Hargreaves J, et al. Metabolic epidermal necrosis in a dog associated with pancreatic adenocarcinoma, hyperglucagonaemia, hyperinsulinaemia and hypoaminoacidaemia. *J Small Anim Pract* 48:522-526, 2007.
33. Jacobson LS, Kirberger RM, Nesbit JW. Hepatic ultrasonography and pathological findings in dogs with hepatocutaneous syndrome: new concepts. *J Vet Intern Med* 9:399-404, 1995.
34. Jaffey JA, Backus RC, Sprinkle M, et al. Successful long-term management of canine superficial necrolytic dermatitis with amino acid infusions and nutritionally balanced home-made diet modification. *Front Vet Sci* 7:28, 2020.
35. World Small Animal Veterinary Association. Liver Standardization G, Routhuizen J, World Small Animal Veterinary Association. Liver Standardization G. WSAVA standards for clinical and histological diagnosis of canine and feline liver disease. Edinburgh, New York, Saunders/Elsevier, 2006.
36. Olsson M, Meadows JR, Truve K, et al. A novel unstable duplication upstream of HAS2 predisposes to a breed-defining skin phenotype and a periodic fever syndrome in Chinese Shar-Pei dogs. *PLoS Genet* 7:e1001332, 2011.
37. Olsson M, Tintle L, Kierczak M, et al. Thorough investigation of a canine autoinflammatory disease (AID) confirms one main risk locus and suggests a modifier locus for amyloidosis. *PLoS One* 8:e75242, 2013.
38. Work M, Scudder C, Bergum Hjellegjerde K, et al. A survey on Shar Pei autoinflammatory disease in the United Kingdom. *J Small Anim Pract* 64:401-408, 2023.
39. Olsson M, Kierczak M, Karlsson A, et al. Absolute quantification reveals the stable transmission of a high copy number variant linked to autoinflammatory disease. *BMC Genomics* 17:299, 2016.
40. Metzger J, Nolte A, Uhde AK, et al. Whole genome sequencing identifies missense mutation in MTBP in Shar-Pei affected with Autoinflammatory Disease (SPAID). *BMC Genomics* 18:348, 2017.
41. Loeven KO. Hepatic amyloidosis in two Chinese Shar Pei dogs. *J Am Vet Med Assoc* 204:1212-1216, 1994.
42. Flatland B, Moore RR, Wolf CM, et al. Liver aspirate from a Shar Pei dog. *Vet Clin Pathol* 36:105-108, 2007.

CHAPTER 39

Liver tumors in dogs

Luca Schiavo
DVM, DECVIM-CA (Oncology)

Jane M. Dobson
MA, DVetMed, DECVIM-CA (Oncology and Radiation Oncology)

Incidence and risk factors

Incidence

Liver tumors are uncommon in dogs, accounting for 0.6-1.3% of all neoplasms in this species.[1] The most common primary tumor in dogs is hepatocellular carcinoma (HCC), accounting for 50% to 80% of primary hepatic tumors, followed by cholangiocellular carcinoma, accounting for 9% to 41% of the cases.[3] These two tumors represent most primary hepatic neoplasia, with neuroendocrine, mesenchymal, and mixed tumors generally uncommon.[2,4] More commonly, the liver represents a site for metastatic disease. It has been estimated that hepatic metastases are approximately three times more common than primary neoplasia.[5] In a previous survey, lymphoma was the most common secondary tumor in the liver, followed by hemangiosarcoma.[6] In the same study, pancreatic carcinoma was the most common epithelial metastatic neoplasia.[6]

Risk factors

Age

Most dogs and cats diagnosed with malignant hepatobiliary tumors are older than 10 years.[7] HCC has a peak at 12 years. The mean age of dogs with cholangiocellular carcinoma is reported to be 11.4 years.[2] Patients with carcinoids usually present younger, with an increased risk noted at 7 years.[8]

Breed

No breed predispositions have been found in dogs with hepatic tumors. However, some breeds seem to be overrepresented.[4] Welsh Corgis, Beagles, and Miniature Schnauzers seem at increased risk of developing HCC, while the Labrador Retriever appears to have a higher risk of developing cholangiocellular carcinomas.[9] No breed predisposition was found in dogs with carcinoids.[4]

Sex

A direct link between sex hormones and the development of hepatic neoplasia has not been identified. However, male dogs seem predisposed to developing HCC, cholangiocarcinoma, and mesenchymal neoplasia, while female dogs seem prone to developing biliary carcinomas.[8,10] No sex predisposition was found in dogs with carcinoids.[4]

Metabolic diseases

Due to the liver's vital role as a regulator of the body's metabolism, several links have been found between endocrine disorders and the development of HCC. HCC was diagnosed in 34% of Scottish Terriers with progressive vacuolar hepatopathy.[11] In a large study that analyzed epidemiological data in dogs with HCC, hyperadrenocorticism was the most common concurrent disease.[9] In this study, the odds of hyperadrenocorticism in dogs with HCC were 4.13 higher than those of the reference population.[9] In another study, 20% of dogs with HCC were diagnosed with additional tumors, which were more commonly benign and endocrine in origin.[2] In a recent study, hepatic copper concentrations were increased in dogs with HCC compared to the control population, suggesting a potential link between hepatic copper concentrations and the development of HCC, but the nature of the relationship between copper and the tumor was not determined.[12]

Infectious causes

In human medicine, several correlations have been found between infectious agents such as Herpesviridae, Hepatitis B and C viruses, and *Helicobacter* spp. and the development of hepatocellular tumors.[13] In feline medicine, a suspected association between Hepadnavirus and HCC has been suggested.[14] However, no convincing association has been found in dogs between infectious diseases and the development of hepatic neoplasia.[4] In people, trematode infestation is a risk factor for developing biliary carcinoma.[15] In dogs, most patients with biliary carcinoma have no evidence of concurrent fluke infestations, so it seems unlikely to be a predisposing factor.[10]

Classification and biological behavior

Classification of liver tumors can be based on their tissue of origin and morphology (Table 39.1).

TABLE 39.1 Summary of the biological behavior and epidemiological data of the most common primary liver tumors in dogs. Mesenchymal neoplasia has been omitted due to the paucity of data and heterogenicity of the disease.

Tumor type	Cell of origin	Breeds predisposed	Sex predisposed	Morphology	Intrahepatic vs. extrahepatic	Rate of metastasis
Hepatocellular carcinoma	Epithelial hepatic cells	■ Welsh Corgi ■ Beagle ■ Miniature Schnauzer	Male	■ Massive (50%-83%) ■ Nodular (16%-29%) ■ Diffused (10%-19%)	Intrahepatic	■ 25%-61% ■ Massive form (0%-37%) ■ Nodular and diffuse (93%-100%)
Biliary carcinoma	Biliary epithelium	■ Labrador	Female	■ Nodular 57% ■ Diffuse (17%-54%) ■ Massive (27%-46%)	Intrahepatic (extrahepatic lesions are relatively common)	■ 60%-88%
Cholangio-carcinoma	Bipotential hepatic progenitor cells	–	Male	■ Massive (100%)	Intrahepatic	■ 71%
Carcinoids	Neuroectodermal cells	–	–	■ Diffuse (67%) ■ Nodular (33%)	Intrahepatic (extrahepatic cases reported)	■ 93%-100%

Morphology and origin

Liver tumors can be classified as massive, nodular, or diffuse based on their morphology. Massive liver tumors are defined as a single tumor involving only one liver lobe; nodular tumors include multiple tumors affecting one or more liver lobes; diffuse tumors show multifocal or coalescing changes affecting all the liver lobes or effacing the liver parenchyma.[7] Potentially, any histological subtype can present with any of these morphologies. However, HCCs typically have a massive morphology, while bile duct tumors and sarcomas have a nodular appearance. Carcinoids usually present as a diffuse tumor.

Liver tumors can be further characterized as intrahepatic and extrahepatic. Intrahepatic tumors develop within the liver parenchyma, while extrahepatic tumors involve the biliary tree within the hepatoduodenal ligament.[16]

Tissue of origin

Based on the tissue of origin, hepatic tumors can be divided into hepatocellular tumors, bile duct tumors, carcinoids, and sarcomas.

Hepatocellular tumors

These include hepatic adenoma, HCC, and hepatoblastoma.[7] These tumors arise from the epithelium of the liver parenchyma, except for hepatoblastomas, which arise from the putative pluripotent stem cells of the liver.[17] HCC is the most common canine epithelial neoplasia, followed by hepatocellular adenomas. Hepatoblastoma is a rare tumor with just a few cases reported.[18] Morphologically, HCC can present as massive, nodular, or diffuse. The massive form is the most common (50-83% of cases), followed by the nodular (16%-29%) and the diffuse (10-19%).[7,18] The left liver lobe is most commonly affected (64%-68%), followed by the central liver lobe (17%-20%) and the right liver lobe (12%-18%).[19,20] HCC is locally aggressive with a relatively low rate of metastasis, which has been reported between 25% and 61%.[4] The morphology of the tumor is strongly associated with the metastatic potential. Massive HCCs have a low metastatic potential (0%-37%), while nodular or diffuse tumors have a high metastatic rate (93%-100%).[2,21] Intrahepatic metastases are the most common, with only 8% of cases having metastasis in other organs.[4] The locoregional lymph nodes, the peritoneum, and the lungs represent the most common site of extrahepatic metastasis.[2,3] Other reported sites of metastasis include the heart, kidneys, adrenal glands, pancreas, intestines, spleen, and urinary bladder.[18]

Tumors of the bile ducts

Two tumor types can arise from the biliary tract in dogs: biliary (cholangiocellular) carcinoma and biliary (cholangiocellular) adenoma. In dogs, the malignant subtype is more common than the benign counterpart.[4] These tumors can be intrahepatic, extrahepatic, or arise from the gallbladder. However, tumors arising from the intrahepatic biliary system are more common than extrahepatic biliary tumors.[2-4] Tumors arising from the gallbladder are rare.[18] In contrast to HCC, nodular morphology is the most common (57%), followed by diffuse (17%-54%) and massive (27%-46%).[8] Cholangiocellular carcinoma is a locally and systemically aggressive neoplasia with a high predisposition to develop local and distant metastases.[7] Metastases are present in 60% to 88% of patients with biliary carcinoma, with locoregional lymph nodes and lungs being the most common site for metastases. Additionally, these tumors might disseminate through the entire body, but carcinomatosis is not a common feature.[4]

Cholangiocarcinoma

Cholangiocarcinoma represents approximately 1.8% of all primary tumors of the liver.[2,8] They are characterized by a mixed cytological and histological appearance between hepatocellular and cholangiocellular tumors.[2,8] Their origin is not completely clear, but they likely originate from the canals of Hering.[22] Only a small number of dogs with cholangiocarcinoma have been reported. In a recent study on 14 dogs the tumor was massive in all cases, and preoperative staging showed the presence of suspected intrahepatic metastatic disease in 3 of the 14 cases and metastasis to the locoregional lymph nodes in 3. No dogs had evidence of pulmonary metastatic disease.[8]

Neuroendocrine tumors (hepatic carcinoids)

Hepatic carcinoids are extremely rare in dogs, with only 3 cases reported in a study of 106 dogs with primary liver neoplasia.[22] These tumors originate from neuroectodermal tissue, or amine precursor uptake and decarboxylation (APUD) cells distributed along the biliary tract.[4,23] Hepatic carcinoids are usually intrahepatic, with only a few cases of extrahepatic tumors reported.[2,23] Morphologically, they are usually diffuse (67%) or nodular (33%), with no cases reported of massive tumors.[23] They have markedly aggressive behavior locally and systemically, with metastases reported in between 93% and 100% of cases.[2,18] Due to the diffuse nature of the disease, metastases can develop in virtually any part of the body, with lesions in the liver, spleen, peritoneum, regional lymph nodes, lungs, and pancreas reported.[23]

Mesenchymal tumors

Primary mesenchymal tumors of the liver are extremely rare. Some studies report that up to 13% of primary hepatic tumors are mesenchymal in origin, but in a study of 106 cases of primary liver tumors, none of them was a primary mesenchymal neoplasia.[2,22] Leiomyosarcoma has been reported as the most common primary hepatic mesenchymal tumor in dogs by some authors,[2] whereas other authors suggest that hemangiosarcoma is the most common.[4] However, only 4% to 6% of the hemangiosarcomas affecting the liver are primary in origin, with the rest being metastatic.[24] Other primary mesenchymal tumors of the liver reported in dogs include fibrosarcomas, osteosarcomas, mesenchymomas, and rhabdomyosarcomas.[4] Due to the limited literature regarding these tumors and their different histological origins, there is very little information about their biological behavior, but they generally present with a nodular morphology.[25] Primary hemangiosarcomas of the liver are aggressive, with the majority of patients showing invasion of the surrounding tissues and metastases, both intrahepatic and extrahepatic, at the time of diagnosis.[4]

History and clinical signs

Clinical signs in patients with liver neoplasia are generally nonspecific. Approximately half of dogs with hepatobiliary neoplasia have no clinical signs at presentation, and the mass is found incidentally or during investigations of raised liver enzymes.[3,26] Most clinical signs are due to the mass effect of the neoplasia, and hepatic tumors rarely cause organ insufficiency.[18] In the authors' experience, organ insufficiency is most common in infiltrative tumors (e.g., lymphoma or mast cell tumors). In dogs presenting with clinical signs, inappetence, lethargy, and weight loss are the most common symptoms, present in 40% to 50% of cases.[8,20] Hepatomegaly is a common clinical sign, with a cranial abdominal mass palpable in 50% to 75% of dogs.[2,25] This finding can be misleading. Hepatomegaly is a nonspecific finding, while the inability to feel an abdominal mass might be due to the tumor's location or to the nodular diffuse morphology of the neoplasia.[3,25]

Other common clinical signs include vomiting, polyuria/polydipsia, pyrexia, and ascites.[7]

Although rare, weakness and neurological signs such as ataxia and seizure might develop. The pathophysiology of neurological symptoms is likely multifactorial, and possible underlying causes include hepatic encephalopathy and hypoglycemia.[25,27] Brain metastases have not been reported in canine patients with hepatocellular carcinoma.[4] Icterus is more common in dogs with extrahepatic bile duct carcinomas and diffuse neuroendocrine tumors.[18] Approximately 10% to 40% of patients with cholangiocellular carcinoma are jaundiced.[4] In a recent study in dogs with icterus, primary neoplastic liver disease was considered the cause in 13 of the 83 cases.[28] Gastrointestinal signs and lethargy are the more common clinical signs in dogs with cholangiocarcinoma.[8]

Diagnosis

Laboratory testing

Most clinicopathological abnormalities in dogs with liver tumors are largely nonspecific, and they overlap with other liver diseases.

Hematology and coagulation profile

Anemia is one of the most common hematological changes in dogs with liver tumors and is present in 35% to 55% of cases. It is usually mild and poorly regenerative. Several factors might contribute to the anemia, including RBC destruction or sequestration and the inflammation caused by chronic disease.[7] Neutrophilic leukocytosis is reported in 60% to 90% of cases of hepatic neoplasia, likely due to large areas of intratumoral necrosis and chronic inflammation.[7]

Thrombocytosis is a common finding in patients with HCC, and it is present in more than 50% of dogs.[29] The mechanism is not clear, but the causes postulated include the proinflammatory status of the patient, ectopic production of thrombopoietin, and iron deficiency.[25] Prolonged coagulation times are present in approximately 20% of dogs with liver tumors; however, these are rarely clinically relevant.[30]

In people, one of the most common complications following hepatectomy is portal vein or pulmonary thromboembolism.[31] In a recent study in dogs, TEG value and fibrinogen indicated a hypercoagulable state in patients with liver neoplasia compared to control dogs.[32] Interestingly, these dogs remained hypercoagulable for up to 14 days following surgical resection of the mass.[32]

Biochemistry

Elevation of liver enzymes is the most common biochemical change in dogs with hepatic neoplasia, found in more than 90% of patients.[33] These changes are not specific, and there is no correlation between the extent of the disease and the degree of liver enzyme elevation.[4,20] However, some patterns have been reported. For example, once a diagnosis of hepatic neoplasia has been made, an AST-to-ALT ratio of less than one suggests HCC or carcinoma of the bile duct, while a ratio of more than 1 is more often found in patients with neuroendocrine tumors or sarcomas.[2] Another study found that alkaline phosphatase (ALP) is more often and highly elevated and that bilirubin is more commonly elevated in patients with hepatic neoplasia compared to vacuolar hepatopathy with or without inflammation (termed "degenerative liver disease" by the author).[33] Albumin concentration is reportedly low, 7% to 48% of patients with hepatic tumors.[20,33] Hypoglycemia is an uncommon paraneoplastic syndrome noted in patients with hepatocellular neoplasia.[4] The underlying mechanism of hypoglycemia appears to be due to the production of insulin-like growth factor 2 (IGF-2) and may also involve excessive consumption of glucose by the neoplasia.[34]

Other markers

An increase in lactate dehydrogenase (LDH) levels has been reported in 50 to 75% of dogs with hepatic neoplasia, particularly carcinomatosis.[2] Alpha-fetoprotein (AFP), a serum glycoprotein produced by the fetus and during neoplastic and regenerative processes, is commonly used in humans for the diagnosis and monitoring of hepatic tumors.[3,35] In dogs, the serum concentration of AFP is elevated in approximately 75% of dogs with HCC and 50% with biliary carcinoma. However, its clinical use is limited because it is also often elevated in non-neoplastic diseases of the liver.[36]

Diagnostic imaging

Assessment of the primary mass

Diagnostic imaging is essential in the initial diagnosis and treatment planning of hepatic neoplasia. More details can be found in chapter 26.
Abdominal radiographs are helpful to evaluate the morphologic abnormalities in size, shape, and position and for the presence of mineralization of the liver.[37] A hepatic mass can be detected by an alteration in the hepatic margin or a localized displacement of the surrounding organs.[38]
Abdominal radiographs are not specific for diagnosing a malignant process in the liver. Mineralization of the biliary tree has been reported in bile duct carcinoma,[18] but this can also occur in nonmalignant diseases and normal dogs.[39]
Ultrasound gives more information than radiographs but is not specific in distinguishing between neoplastic and non-neoplastic diseases affecting the liver and between different tumors due to the overlap in their ultrasonographic presentation.[40] Liver tumors have variable ultrasonographic appearances ranging from a single, localized hyperechoic lesion to multiple hypoechoic nodules affecting the entire liver parenchyma.[41] Cystic appearance has been reported, particularly in neoplastic processes involving the biliary tree.[37]
Contrast-enhanced ultrasound (CEUS) has also been investigated to assess hepatic neoplasia in dogs with significant overlapping features between various tumors.[40]
Abdominal ultrasound can be helpful in the presurgical assessment of single hepatic masses. A small number of canine studies have highlighted that this technique is quite specific but poorly sensitive in accurately locating single hepatic masses.[42,43] Interestingly, in these studies, the diagnostic accuracy was higher for masses arising from the left division of the liver (sensitivity 55%-90%; specificity 72%-98%) compared to tumors arising from the right (sensitivity 55%-65%; specificity 89%-93%) and central (sensitivity 29%-33%; specificity 87%-93%) division of the liver.[42,43] The concurrent presence of non-neoplastic liver pathology might reduce the diagnostic accuracy of ultrasound in predicting the location of the mass.[42] Despite these limitations, ultrasound remains extremely useful in assessing the size of the mass and its relationship with adjacent anatomic structures.[44]
Advanced imaging, particularly computed tomography (CT) scan, is increasingly used to assess hepatic masses (Figs. 39.1A and 39.1B). There are controversies regarding the ability of CT scans to help distinguish between different neoplastic processes with an overall accuracy in the prediction of malignancy reported between 62% and 92%. The difference in these results is likely due to technical differences between studies. Compared to ultrasound, a CT scan was found to have the greatest precision in predicting the correct location of hepatic masses, with an overall accuracy between 84% and 93%.[43] CT was more specific than sensitive in predicting the location of hepatic masses, with higher sensitivity and specificity for tumors arising from the left division than the right and central divisions.[43]
In the author's opinion, a CT scan is helpful but not mandatory in the preoperative assessment of patients with hepatic malignancies. Despite its high diagnostic accuracy, sometimes the intraoperative appearance of the mass does not reflect the imaging appearance, and surgery should be attempted unless multifocal lesions are present.
MRI is the diagnostic method of choice in people with hepatic neoplasia but is not widely used in dogs. MRI would be likely to provide superior soft tissue detail than a CT scan,[3] but only small studies have been performed in dogs to date.

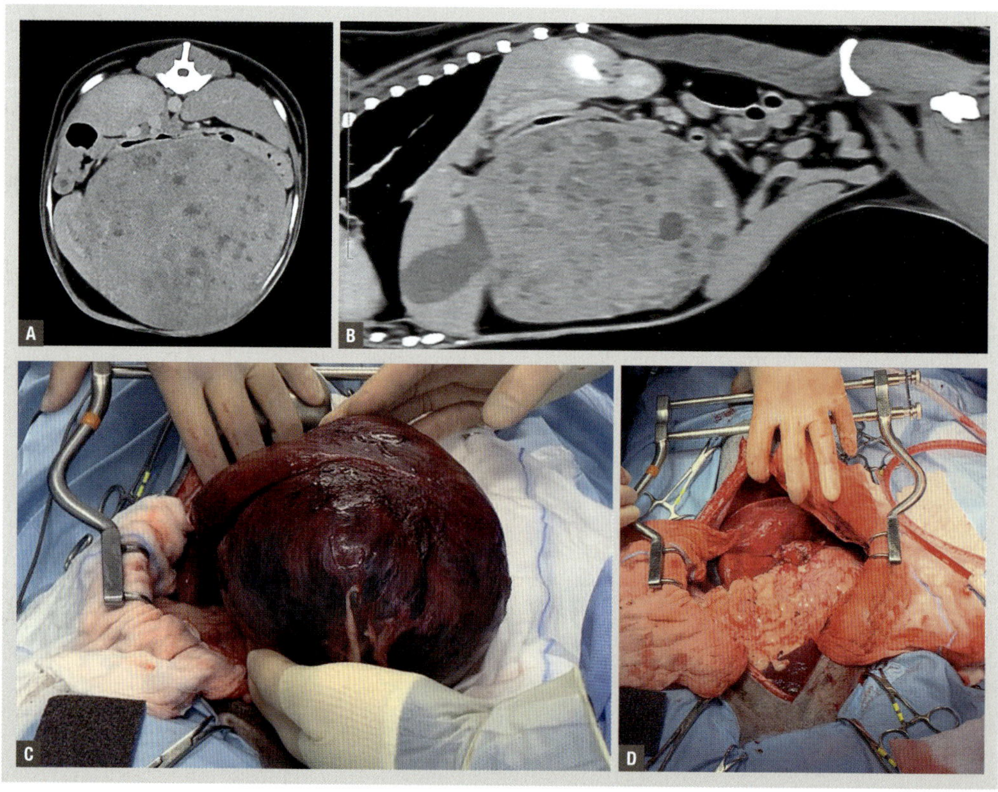

FIG. 39.1 (A) Transversal and (B) sagittal CT scan of the abdomen of a dog with a massive hepatocellular carcinoma. The mass was arising from the left division of the liver and occupying most of the abdominal cavity, causing caudal displacement of the other organs. (C) In the bottom line, intraoperative pictures of the large mass and (D) the abdominal cavity following the surgery. Images from the archive of Davies Veterinary Specialists (Hitchin, UK).

Staging

Hepatic tumors tend to be locally aggressive, and they can metastasize within the hepatic parenchyma, within the abdomen and, less commonly, to the lungs. The presence of abdominal metastases can be detected during the assessment of the primary tumor. Despite their low incidence, thoracic metastases should be assessed by three-view thoracic radiographs or, alternatively, via a CT scan of the thorax preoperatively.

Tissue sampling

Diagnostic imaging alone cannot differentiate a tumor from benign nodular hyperplasia nor assess histological type or malignancy of liver masses, and tissue sampling is required for a definitive diagnosis. In some cases, obtaining a preoperative cytological or histological diagnosis of the mass is essential, while surgery might provide diagnosis and treatment in the case of single solitary masses.[3] The author recommends careful evaluation of the coagulation profile in dogs with liver masses prior to biopsy or surgery despite the low incidence of clinical coagulation abnormalities in patients with liver tumors.

Cytology

Cytology is usually the first diagnostic tool in suspected hepatic neoplasia. Cytological samples are generally obtained by ultrasound guidance. The technique is relatively safe, with complications reported in 2.7% of cases with a very low risk of severe complications.[45] Cytology is not accurate in diagnosing hepatic diseases in dogs, with an overall agreement with histopathology ranging from 22% to 30%.[45,46] However, the positive predictive value of cytology in diagnosing a neoplastic process is relatively high (88%-91%),[45,47] so if cytology identifies a tumor, it is present, whereas a negative cytology does not rule out neoplasia. The sensitivity for the detection of hepatic neoplasia is nearly double for round cell neoplasms (60%), compared to HCC (35%) and sarcomas (17%).[47]

Histology and immunohistochemistry

Histological samples can be obtained by percutaneous ultrasound-guidance, laparoscopically or surgically. Tissue biopsy is not routinely used for the preoperative assessment of single liver masses, as an excisional biopsy can provide both treatment and diagnosis. Ultrasound-guided Tru-Cut liver biopsy can provide adequate tissue samples for definitive diagnosis in 83.3% to 96.3% of liver samples.[48] However, this procedure has a potentially high risk of complications, with a reported rate of bleeding in up to 40% for ultrasound-guided biopsy compared to 2%-5% for patients undergoing a laparoscopic liver biopsy, so laparoscopy would be preferred if the mass is accessible.[48,49]

Histology with standard stains is usually diagnostic, and immunohistochemistry is rarely required for the assessment of liver neoplasia in dogs. Keratin (K) 19 is a protein typically expressed by hepatic progenitor cells (HPCs) and cholangiocytes but not hepatocytes.[50] In human medicine, K19 expression in more than 5% of cells has been strongly correlated with the outcome in patients with liver tumors.[50] The protein was expressed in approximately 12% of dogs with hepatocellular tumors, and its expression was associated with the aggressiveness of the neoplasia and outcome.[51] Even if K19 staining might have prognostic value, it is not routinely used in dogs with hepatocellular tumors.

Treatment

Surgery

Liver lobectomy is the treatment of choice for massive hepatocellular carcinomas and bile duct carcinomas that have not metastasized. Even when metastases are present, in some cases, palliative removal/debulking of a massive tumor can give clinical relief and help in controlling the paraneoplastic syndromes.[25,34] Different techniques have been reported, including surgical staplers, bipolar vessel sealant, or mass ligation.[52] The latter is not recommended in tumors affecting the central or the right division of the liver or in tumors with a wide base.[52] A full discussion of surgical techniques is beyond the scope of this book.

Preoperative planning of the surgery is essential. Recent studies have analyzed intraoperative near-infrared (NIR) fluorescence imaging with indocyanine green (ICG). The technique is based on the IV administration of ICG, which is selectively taken up by the hepatocytes, which emit fluorescence when exposed to the near-infrared machine.[53] The intraoperative use of this technique in dogs helped to identify the margins of neoplastic lesions affecting the liver with a sensitivity and specificity of 100% and 77.3%, respectively.[53] No differences in the uptake in different tumors were found.[53]

Intraoperative complications during liver lobectomy are reported in 13% to 29% of cases.[19,20,54] Bleeding is the most common surgical complication, but vascular compromise, hypoglycemia, and decreased hepatic function postoperatively have been reported.[20]

Historically, right-sided tumors have been described as more challenging to resect due to the relation of the right-sided liver lobes to the vena cava,[7,20] although controversially, in a recent study, no increase in the rate of complications was found in dogs with right-sided or central liver tumors.[19]

Intraoperative mortality is relatively low, with up to 5% of intraoperative deaths reported in liver lobectomies for massive HCC.[20]

Chemotherapy

Hepatic tumors are chemoresistant, with less than 25% response rates reported in people.[18] In dogs, gemcitabine (300-450 mg\m^2 weekly) has been used as either a neoadjuvant or adjuvant treatment in dogs with HCC of various morphology.[55] The treatment was generally well tolerated, and the median survival time in that study was 983 days.[55] The author concluded that the use of gemcitabine over liver lobectomy alone did not improve survival in patients with incompletely resected neoplasia.[55]

Other case reports or small case series reported using toceranib phosphate, mitoxantrone, and sorafenib.[56-58] In the authors' opinion, the data is too limited to recommend the use of chemotherapy in patients with nonresectable HCC.

Emerging treatment modalities

In recent years, significant efforts have been made to find alternative treatment options for these tumors.

In humans, transarterial embolization (TAE) and transarterial chemoembolization (TACE) are essential components of treatment for nonresectable hepatocellular neoplasia. These treatments are based on the delivery of embolic agents or chemotherapeutics directly into the feeding artery of the tumor to cause ischemic necrosis (embolization) or to achieve a high local concentration of chemotherapeutics reducing systemic exposure (chemoembolization).[59] In dogs, using these treatments for patients with nonresectable hepatocellular tumors led to a median survival time of 337 days.[60] Despite these promising results, the rate of complications was high, with minor complications reported in 30% of patients and major complications in 11%.[60]

The use of radiation therapy in managing hepatic neoplasia has historically been limited due to the low tolerance of the normal liver to radiation.[61] However, with the advent of more precise, 3D conformal machines, the possibility to spare normal tissue has grown, and in humans, radiation therapy has been used with good results. In a study of 6 dogs, treatment with radiation therapy showed promising results and was well tolerated in 5 of 6 patients, suggesting this may be a treatment for the future.[61]

Prognosis

The prognosis for dogs with liver neoplasia is variable, depending on the histological subtype, the tumor morphology, the presence of metastases, and the possibility of surgically removing the mass.

Hepatocellular tumors

The prognosis for patients with HCC is strongly correlated with the possibility of surgically resecting the mass. The median survival time in patients with massive hepatocellular carcinoma treated with surgery was up to 1,836 days compared with 270 days for patients treated medically, with 15.4 times increased risk of dying for tumor-related causes for the latter.[20,29] The location of the primary tumor seems correlated with the prognosis in dogs with massive hepatocellular carcinoma. Dogs with left-sided, central, and right-sided tumors have median survival times of 1,460, 795, or 365 days, respectively.[20] Likely, this difference is due to the perioperative mortality due to their location rather than a true aggressiveness of the neoplasia. Other reported negative prognostic factors include high serum ALT, AST, and increased ALP\AST and ALT\AST ratios.[20] Surprisingly, neither tumor size nor completeness of excision was prognostic in two independent studies, supporting the value of incomplete excision (debulking) surgery.[20,62] Up to 1 to 3% of cases recur after surgical resection.[20] No predictive factors were found in a recent study that analyzed the risk of reoccurrence of hepatic neoplasia.[19] Additionally, no increase in survival time was found between patients undergoing a second surgical resection compared to patients managed conservatively.[19] Prognosis is poor for patients with nodular or diffuse hepatocellular neoplasia due to the impossibility of performing surgical resection. As mentioned previously, embolization and chemoembolization are emerging treatments. In the study evaluating the use of gemcitabine, the prognosis for patients with nodular and diffuse disease was 983 and 113 days, respectively.[55]

Bile duct tumors

Carcinomas of the bile ducts are highly aggressive, with most tumors presenting with a nodular or diffuse pattern. Even in the presence of single masses, the prognosis following surgical resection is usually less than 6 months due to the high rate of metastatic disease.[63] Septic bile peritonitis, elevated partial thromboplastin time, and elevated creatinine concentration are negative prognostic factors in dogs undergoing surgery for extrahepatic biliary neoplasia.[64]

Mixed hepatocellular and bile duct tumors

There is limited information regarding prognosis in dogs with hepatocellular cholangiocarcinoma. In a study of 14 cases, the median survival time was 700 days following surgical resection, similar to patients with HCC and longer than with bile duct tumors.[8] The high expression of cholangiocellular markers was not prognostic in this study.[8]

Neuroendocrine tumors

Neuroendocrine tumors are highly aggressive, with a reported metastatic rate of up to 93% at presentation and up to 100% during the disease. Currently, there are no effective treatments for patients with this malignancy; therefore, the prognosis is extremely poor.[18]

Sarcomas

Due to the different sarcomas that can affect the liver, it is difficult to define a specific prognosis for these patients. Dogs with hemangiosarcoma usually have a high rate of metastases at presentation; however, due to the low number of cases reported, it is difficult to have a defined prognosis.[4]

KEY POINTS

- Liver tumors are uncommon in dogs.
- Tumors can have different morphology and histological origin, but massive hepatocellular carcinoma represents most tumors.
- Clinical, hematological, and biochemical changes are nonspecific and overlap with other liver diseases.
- Ultrasound is the first-line imaging modality. A CT scan might be helpful to plan the surgical approach.
- Cytology has a poor sensitivity in diagnosing liver tumors, and histopathology is often necessary.
- Surgery is the treatment of choice, and chemotherapy is not effective for these neoplasms.
- The prognosis is generally good for patients with massive hepatocellular carcinomas undergoing surgery. It is poor for cholangiocellular carcinomas and carcinoids.

References

1. Gibson EA, Goldman RE, Culp WTN. Comparative oncology: management of hepatic neoplasia in humans and dogs. *Vet Sci* 9(9), 2022.
2. Patnaik AK, Hurvitz AI, Lieberman PH. Canine hepatic neoplasms: a clinicopathologic study. *Vet Pathol* 17(5):553-564, 1980.
3. Ettinger SJ, Feldman EC, Côté E. Textbook of Veterinary Internal Medicine-Inkling E-Book. Elsevier Health Sciences, 2016.
4. Cullen JM. Tumors of the liver and gallbladder. In Meuten DJ (editor). Tumors in Domestic Animals 5th edition. John Wiley and Sons Ltd, 2016, pp. 602-631.
5. Aloia A, Bosch RV, Saches S, Zaidan L, Hernandez-Blazquez FJ, Cogliati B. Retrospective study of hepatic neoplasms in dogs (1999-2012). *Braz J Vet Pathol* 5(3):146-149, 2012.
6. Trigo FJ, Thompson H, Breeze RG, Nash AS. The pathology of liver tumours in the dog. *J Comp Pathol* 92(1):21-39, 1982.
7. Selmic LE. Hepatobiliary neoplasia. *Vet Clin North Am Small Anim Pract* 47(3):725-735, 2017.
8. Terai K, Ishigaki K, Kagawa Y, Okada K, Yoshida O, Sakurai N, et al. Clinical, diagnostic, and pathologic features and surgical outcomes of combined hepatocellular-cholangiocarcinoma in dogs: 14 cases (2009-2021). *J Am Vet Med Assoc* 260(13):1668-1674, 2022.
9. Leela-Arporn R, Ohta H, Nagata N, Sasaoka K, Tamura M, Dermlim A, et al. Epidemiology of massive hepatocellular carcinoma in dogs: A 4-year retrospective study. *Vet J* 248:74-78, 2019.
10. Hayes HM, Morin MM, Rubenstein DA. Canine biliary carcinoma: epidemiological comparisons with man. *J Comp Pathol* 93(1):99-107, 1983.
11. Cortright CC, Center SA, Randolph JF, McDonough SP, Fecteau KA, Warner KL, et al. Clinical features of progressive vacuolar hepatopathy in Scottish Terriers with and without hepatocellular carcinoma: 114 cases (1980-2013). *J Am Vet Med Assoc* 245(7):797-808, 2014.
12. Harro CC, Smedley RC, Buchweitz JP, Langlois DK. Hepatic copper and other trace mineral concentrations in dogs with hepatocellular carcinoma. *J Vet Intern Med* 33(5):2193-2199, 2019.
13. Hokuto D, Sho M, Yamato I, Yasuda S, Obara S, Nomi T, et al. Clinical impact of herpesvirus entry mediator expression in human hepatocellular carcinoma. *Eur J Cancer* 51(2):157-165, 2015.
14. Pesavento PA, Jackson K, Hampson TSTT, Munday JS, Barrs VR, Beatty JA. A novel Hepadnavirus is associated with chronic hepatitis and hepatocellular carcinoma in cats. *Viruses* 11(10), 2019.
15. Kapatkin A, Mullen H, Matthiesen D, Patnaik A. Leiomyosarcoma in dogs: 44 cases (1983-1988). *J Am Vet Med Assoc* 201(7):1077-1079, 1992.
16. Cardinale V, Semeraro R, Torrice A, Gatto M, Napoli C, Bragazzi MC, et al. Intra-hepatic and extra-hepatic cholangiocarcinoma: new insight into epidemiology and risk factors. *World J Gastrointest Oncol* 2(11):407-416, 2010.
17. Shiga A, Shirota K, Shida T, Yamada T, Nomura Y. Hepatoblastoma in a dog. *J Vet Med Sci* 59(12):1167-1170, 1997.
18. Vail DM, Thamm DH, Liptak JM. Withrow and MacEwen's Small Animal Clinical Oncology. E-Book, Elsevier Health Sciences, 2019.
19. Lapsley JM, Wavreille V, Barry S, Dornbusch JA, Chen C, Leeper H, et al. Risk factors and outcome in dogs with recurrent massive hepatocellular carcinoma: A Veterinary Society of Surgical Oncology case-control study. *Vet Comp Oncol* 20(3):697-709, 2022.
20. Liptak JM, Dernell WS, Monnet E, Powers BE, Bachand AM, Kenney JG, et al. Massive hepatocellular carcinoma in dogs: 48 cases (1992-2002). *J Am Vet Med Assoc* 225(8):1225-1230, 2004.
21. Patnaik AK, Hurvitz AI, Lieberman PH, Johnson GF. Canine hepatocellular carcinoma. *Vet Pathol* 18(4):427-438, 1981.
22. van Sprundel RG, van den Ingh TS, Guscetti F, Kershaw O, Kanemoto H, van Gils HM, et al. Classification of primary hepatic tumours in the dog. *Vet J* 197(3):596-606, 2013.
23. Patnaik A, Lieberman P, Hurvitz A, Johnson G. Canine hepatic carcinoids. *Vet Pathol* 18(4):445-453, 1981.
24. Brown NO, Patnaik AK, MacEwen EG. Canine hemangiosarcoma: retrospective analysis of 104 cases. *J Am Vet Med Assoc* 186(1):56-58, 1985.
25. Liptak JM, MVetClinStud F, Dernell WS, Withrow SJ. Liver tumors in cats and dogs. *Sarcoma* 36(64):0, 2004
26. Strombeck DR. Clinicopathologic features of primary and metastatic neoplastic disease of the liver in dogs. *J Am Vet Med Assoc* 173(3):267-269, 1978.
27. Leifer CE, Peterson ME, Matus RE, Patnaik AK. Hypoglycemia associated with nonislet cell tumor in 13 dogs. *J Am Vet Med Assoc* 186(1):53-55, 1985.
28. Andrade MC, Oliveira LB, Santos ÁF, Moreira MV, Pierezan F, Ecco R. Differential diagnoses in 83 dogs with icterus. *Pesquisa Veterinária Brasileira* 40:451-465, 2020.
29. Liptak J, Dernell W, Monnet E. Massive hepatocellular carcinoma: surgical outcome in 40 dogs. *Proc Vet Cancer Soc Conf*, 2002.
30. Badylak SF, Dodds WJ, Van Vleet JF. Plasma coagulation factor abnormalities in dogs with naturally occurring hepatic disease. *Am J Vet Res* 44(12):2336-2340, 1983.
31. Tzeng C-W, Katz M, Fleming J, Pisters P, Lee J, Abdalla E, et al. Risk of venous thromboembolism outweighs post-hepatectomy bleeding complications: analysis of 5651 National Surgical Quality Improvement Program patients. *HPB (Oxford)* 14(8):506-513, 2012.
32. Fontes GS, Wavreille VA, Lapsley JM, Cooper ES, Guillaumin J, Selmic LE. Thromboelastographic results and hypercoagulability in dogs with surgically treated hepatocellular adenoma and carcinoma: A Veterinary Society of Surgical Oncology prospective study. *Vet Comp Oncol*, 2023. Online ahead of print.
33. Neumann S. Comparison of blood parameters in degenerative liver disease and liver neoplasia in dogs. *Comp Clin Pathol* 12:206-210, 2004.
34. Tamura K, Ishigaki K, Yoshida O, Terai K, Iizuka K, Sakurai N, et al. Glucoregulatory factors in canine hepatocellular carcinoma and leiomyosarcoma with non-islet cell tumour hypoglycaemia. *Res Vet Sci* 152:640-646, 2022.
35. Kitao S, Yamada T, Ishikawa T, Madarame H, Furuichi M, Neo S, et al. Alpha-fetoprotein in serum and tumor tissues in dogs with hepatocellular carcinoma. *J Vet Diagn Invest* 18(3):291-295, 2006.
36. Yamada T, Fujita M, Kitao S, Ashida Y, Nishizono K, Tsuchiya R, et al. Serum alpha-fetoprotein values in dogs with various hepatic diseases. *J Vet Med Sci* 61(6):657-659, 1999.
37. Kumar V, Kumar A, Varshney AC, Tyagi SP, Kanwar MS, Sharma SK. Diagnostic imaging of canine hepatobiliary affections: A review. *Vet Med Int* 2012:672107, 2012.
38. Partington BP, Biller DS. Hepatic imaging with radiology and ultrasound. *Vet Clin Small Anim Pract* 25(2):305-335, 1995.
39. Genain MA, Barbosa A, Herrtage M, Watson P. Clinical relevance of radiographic linear branching mineral opacities in the canine liver. *J Small Anim Pract* 59(7):432-437, 2018.
40. Burti S, Zotti A, Rubini G, Orlandi R, Bargellini P, Bonsembiante F, et al. Contrast-enhanced ultrasound features of malignant focal liver masses in dogs. *Sci Rep* 10(1):6076, 2020.
41. Whiteley MB, Feeney DA, Whiteley LO, Hardy RM. Ultrasonographic appearance of primary and metastatic canine hepatic tumors. A review of 48 cases. *J Ultrasound Med* 8(11):621-630, 1989.
42. Wormser C, Reetz JA, Giuffrida MA. Diagnostic accuracy of ultrasound to predict the location of solitary hepatic masses in dogs. *Vet Surg* 45(2):208-213, 2016.
43. Cheney DM, Coleman MC, Voges AK, Thieman Mankin KM, Griffin JF. Ultrasonographic and CT accuracy in localising surgical- or necropsy-confirmed solitary hepatic masses in dogs. *J Small Anim Pract* 60(5):274-279, 2019.
44. Griebie ER, David FH, Ober CP, Feeney DA, Anderson KL, Wuenschmann A, et al. Evaluation of canine hepatic masses by use of triphasic computed tomography and B-mode, color flow, power, and pulsed-wave Doppler ultrasonography and correlation with histopathologic classification. *Am J Vet Res* 78(11):1273-1283, 2017.
45. Cray M, Hokamp J, Abrams B, Husbands BD, Grimes JA, Gleason H, et al. Clinical utility of cytology from preoperative percutaneous fine needle aspirates of solitary liver masses in 220 dogs: A retrospective study (2009-2019). *J Am Anim Hosp Assoc* 59(1):12-19, 2023.

46. Wang KY, Panciera DL, Al-Rukibat RK, Radi ZA. Accuracy of ultrasound-guided fine-needle aspiration of the liver and cytologic findings in dogs and cats: 97 cases (1990-2000). *J Am Vet Med Assoc* 224(1):75-78, 2004.
47. Bahr KL, Sharkey LC, Murakami T, Feeney DA. Accuracy of US-guided FNA of focal liver lesions in dogs: 140 cases (2005-2008). *J Am Anim Hosp Assoc* 49(3):190-196, 2013.
48. Vasanjee SC, Bubenik LJ, Hosgood G, Bauer R. Evaluation of hemorrhage, sample size, and collateral damage for five hepatic biopsy methods in dogs. *Vet Surg* 35(1):86-93, 2006.
49. McDevitt HL, Mayhew PD, Giuffrida MA, Brown DC, Culp WT, Runge JJ. Short-term clinical outcome of laparoscopic liver biopsy in dogs: 106 cases (2003-2013). *J Am Vet Med Assoc* 248(1):83-90, 2016.
50. Durnez A, Verslype C, Nevens F, Fevery J, Aerts R, Pirenne J, et al. The clinicopathological and prognostic relevance of cytokeratin 7 and 19 expression in hepatocellular carcinoma. A possible progenitor cell origin. *Histopathology* 49(2):138-151, 2006.
51. van Sprundel RG, van den Ingh TS, Desmet VJ, Katoonizadeh A, Penning LC, Rothuizen J, et al. Keratin 19 marks poor differentiation and a more aggressive behaviour in canine and human hepatocellular tumours. *Comp Hepatol* 9(1):4, 2010.
52. Slatter DH (editor). Textbook of Small Animal Surgery 3rd edition. Philadelphia, Saunders, 2003.
53. Sakurai N, Ishigaki K, Terai K, Heishima T, Okada K, Yoshida O, et al. Clinical impact of near-infrared fluorescence imaging with indocyanine green on surgical treatment for hepatic masses in dogs. *BMC Vet Res* 18(1):374, 2022.
54. Kinsey JR, Gilson SD, Hauptman J, Mehler SJ, May LR. Factors associated with long-term survival in dogs undergoing liver lobectomy as treatment for liver tumors. *Can Vet J* 56(6):598-604, 2015.
55. Elpiner AK, Brodsky EM, Hazzah TN, Post GS. Single-agent gemcitabine chemotherapy in dogs with hepatocellular carcinomas. *Vet Comp Oncol* 9(4):260-268, 2011.
56. Marconato L, Sabattini S, Marisi G, Rossi F, Leone VF, Casadei-Gardini A. Sorafenib for the treatment of unresectable hepatocellular carcinoma: preliminary toxicity and activity data in dogs. *Cancers (Basel)* 12(5), 2020.
57. Kim SW, Choi JW, Kim JM, Yoon HY, Bae K, Yoon KA, et al. Case report: toceranib as adjuvant chemotherapy in a dog with incompletely resected combined hepatocellular-cholangiocarcinoma. *Front Vet Sci* 9:963390, 2022.
58. Ogilvie GK, Obradovich JE, Elmslie RE, Vail DM, Moore AS, Straw RC, et al. Efficacy of mitoxantrone against various neoplasms in dogs. *J Am Vet Med Assoc* 198(9):1618-2821, 1991.
59. Zhou X, Tang Z, Wang J, Lin P, Chen Z, Lv L, et al. Doxorubicin-eluting beads versus conventional transarterial chemoembolization for the treatment of hepatocellular carcinoma: a meta-analysis. *Int J Clin Exp Med* 7(11):3892-3903, 2014.
60. Rogatko CP, Weisse C, Schwarz T, Berent AC, Diniz MA. Drug-eluting bead chemoembolization for the treatment of nonresectable hepatic carcinoma in dogs: A prospective clinical trial. *J Vet Intern Med* 35(3):1487-1495, 2021.
61. Mori T, Ito Y, Kawabe M, Iwasaki R, Sakai H, Murakami M, et al. Three-dimensional conformal radiation therapy for inoperable massive hepatocellular carcinoma in six dogs. *J Small Anim Pract* 56(7):441-445, 2015.
62. Moyer J, Lopez DJ, Balkman CE, Sumner JP. Factors associated with survival in dogs with a histopathological diagnosis of hepatocellular carcinoma: 94 cases (2007-2018). *Open Vet J* 11(1):144-153, 2021.
63. Fry P, Rest J. Partial hepatectomy in two dogs. *J Small Anim Pract* 34(4):192-195, 1993.
64. Mehler SJ, Mayhew PD, Drobatz KJ, Holt DE. Variables associated with outcome in dogs undergoing extrahepatic biliary surgery: 60 cases (1988-2002). *Vet Surg* 33(6):644-649, 2004.

CHAPTER 40

Nutrition for acute and chronic liver disease

Becca Leung
BSc, BVSc, PhD,
DACVIM-CA (Nutrition)

As described in earlier chapters, the liver is a vital organ that plays numerous roles in the body. As one of the key players in digestion, metabolism, and the storage of nutrients, liver dysfunction can lead to sequelae of malnutrition and metabolic derangement. The nutritional goals in patients with liver disease are thus to support their nutritional status, minimize ongoing damage to the liver, encourage regeneration of hepatocytes, and reduce the clinical signs associated with dysfunction.

General nutritional considerations should be made for all patients with hepatic disease. This includes performing a nutritional assessment on every patient at every visit.[1] Measuring body weight, body condition score (BCS), and muscle condition score (MCS) gives an indication of the current nutritional status of a patient and allows for more accurate monitoring over time. In addition, monitoring MCS can help identify patients with cachexia, sarcopenia, or those in a state of negative nitrogen balance due to improper nutrition.

Furthermore, as there are several etiologies of hepatic disease, additional attention to specific nutrients may need to be paid for each patient. Most commercial hepatic diets are designed to help in the management of hepatic encephalopathy (HE) and copper storage toxicosis. However, the nutritional considerations for these diseases will not be appropriate in all cases of hepatic disease.

Energy requirements

Malnutrition is a nutritional state that results from a lack (or excess) of intake or uptake of nutrients that leads to an alteration of the body, which reduces physical and mental function and impairs clinical outcome.[2] The prevalence of malnutrition in veterinary patients with hepatic disease is not known; however, it is recognized in 20-50% of human patients with liver cirrhosis and is associated with an increased risk of infections, hepatic encephalopathy, and mortality.[3] Hyporexia or anorexia during illness occurs due to an altered neuronal control of appetite as the result of the anorexigenic effects of inflammatory cytokines, interleukin-1, and tumor necrosis factor-α.[4,5] Assisted feeding through enteral or partial parenteral methods is necessary to prevent malnutrition, and patients who are considered at risk for malnutrition should be closely monitored.[6] Cases of acute disease can be at less risk of malnutrition compared to cases of chronic disease, but these patients still need to be closely monitored. Malnutrition is common overall in hospitalized veterinary patients and can occur after a few days of hospitalization.[7] In addition, studies have demonstrated a positive outcome when implementing early enteral nutritional support in hospitalized veterinary patients.[8-10] A discussion on calculating energy requirements and methods of assisted feeding for hospitalized patients can be found in chapter 22.

Protein

Dietary proteins provide both essential and nonessential amino acids and are needed in adequate amounts to maintain muscle mass and promote protein synthesis. In humans, having low muscle mass was associated with an increased risk of hepatic encephalopathy.[11] The same association has not been found in dogs. However, an increase in circulating ammonia concentrations was found to be predictive of hepatic encephalopathy in dogs with congenital portosystemic shunts (CPSS).[12] Sources of ammonia and the effects of liver dysfunction on ammonia metabolism are summarized in Fig. 40.1 and Fig. 40.2, respectively. Ammonia generation is thought to be largely driven by the small and large intestines.[13] Enterocytes utilize glutamine as their primary source of energy and convert glutamine to ammonia and glutamate. In addition, the production of ammonia from bacterial fermentation of undigested protein or blood reaching the colon also contributes to circulating concentrations.[14] Muscle acts as an important ammonia "sink" by increasing glutamine synthesis during times of hyperammonemia.[15] As such, a sufficient intake of calories and protein in order to preserve lean mass is thought to be important in patients with hepatic disease to reduce the risk of hepatic encephalopathy and, equally, excessive dietary protein restriction leading to negative nitrogen balance and the loss of muscle mass might increase the risk of increased circulating ammonia and hepatic encephalopathy in patients.

Therefore, current recommendations are to feed enough protein to maintain nitrogen balance in patients. Determining exactly how much to feed to achieve a positive nitrogen balance of individual patients would be key; however, this can be difficult to do in a hospital setting. In humans with liver cirrhosis, the recommendation is to feed a higher protein requirement than the recommended daily allowance for healthy individuals.[3] However, dogs with experimentally induced shunts were found to have similar protein requirements to clinically healthy dogs.[16] Therefore, dogs with liver disease may not have a drastically higher protein requirement than healthy dogs, although we do not know how naturally occurring disease and chronicity could affect this. For example, dogs with cirrhosis and acquired portosystemic shunts might have different protein requirements to dogs with previously normal livers and those with experimentally produced shunts.

Commercial hepatic support-type diets contain protein concentrations that are above the recommended allowance for healthy dogs and cats, according to the National Research Council (NRC), and close to the minimum requirements set by the Association of American Feed Control Officials (AAFCO) and European Pet Food Industry Federation (FEDIAF) (Table 40.1). The recommendation by the NRC was established using highly digestible proteins and is similar to the types of proteins found in hepatic diets, whereas AAFCO and FEDIAF take into account that most diets will not always be formulated with highly digestible proteins. While feeding higher quantities of protein to preserve muscle mass in these patients is tempting, it is prudent to remember that protein eaten above what is required to maintain nitrogen balance is catabolized to produce energy. The liver is the principal site for amino acid metabolism and the conversion of the resulting metabolite, ammonia, into urea. Therefore, feeding excess protein above what is necessary can be ineffective and may even be detrimental, particularly in animals with hepatic encephalopathy, so care should be exercised.

While the quantity of protein fed is important, so is the source of the protein. A diet containing soy isolate was associated with lower plasma ammonia concentrations in dogs with CPSS compared to a diet with similar protein concentrations but using animal-derived protein ingredients.[17] Current recommendations in both humans and veterinary patients are to give diets containing highly digestible proteins (such as soy isolate) and proteins with a low concentration of nonprotein nitrogen (such as dairy and egg).[3] Feeding highly digestible proteins will reduce the amount of nondigested proteins entering the colon and undergoing microbial fermentation to ammonia. In addition, vegetable protein sources tend to contain more fibers, which are beneficial in reducing colonic ammonia absorption (see the indigestible carbohydrates section below). Vegetable proteins also contain less sulfur-containing amino acids than animal proteins. Intestinal microbes metabolize these amino acids to mercaptans and indoles, which are thought to contribute to the development of hepatic encephalopathy.[18] Just like in dogs, a reduction in ammonia concentrations, in addition to improvements in hepatic encephalopathy scores, have been described in humans fed diets containing vegetable proteins compared to animal proteins.[19]

Another consideration for the protein source is its amino acid composition. Diets should contain all essential amino acids in appropriate quantities to address irreversible losses (for example, protein loss through the epithelia) even when there is no net change in body protein mass. In addition, an alteration in the branched-chain amino acids (BCAA) to aromatic amino acids (AAA) has been described in both human and veterinary patients with liver disease, and an increase in AAA has been proposed to predispose to hepatic encephalopathy. These amino acids share the same transporter across the blood-brain barrier, and it is hypothesized that a rise in AAA leads to an increase in precursors that cause a "false" dopaminergic effect and reduce dopamine synthesis through a negative feedback loop.[20] Supplementing a diet with BCAAs may help balance the ratio of BCAAs to AAAs, in addition to stimulating protein synthesis and reducing muscle loss. The efficacy of BCAA supplementation in reducing hepatic encephalopathy and muscle loss is still uncertain in humans, with some studies showing a benefit while others do not.[21] Far fewer studies have been performed on veterinary patients, with minimal to no benefits found to date.[22] Plasma BCAAs were found to be decreased in dogs with portocaval shunts.[23] However, while improvements in this ratio occurred following the closure of PSS, clinical improvements were already noted from medical treatment alone using hepatic support-type diets with lactulose and/or antibiotics when the ratio was still inversed presurgery.[24] As such, more studies are needed to determine if BCAA supplementation should be recommended in patients with hepatic disease.

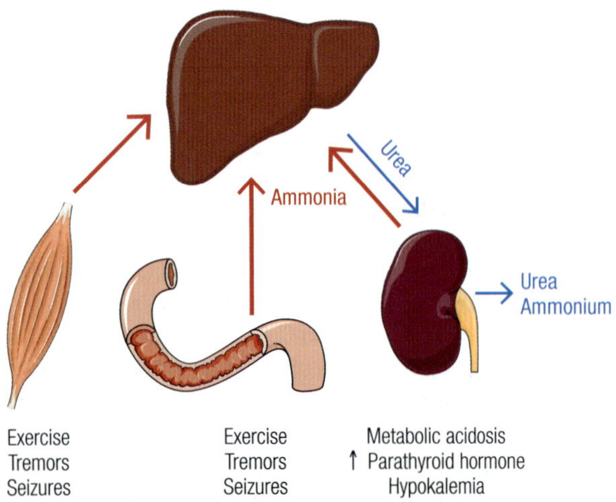

FIG. 40.1 Ammonia metabolism with a functioning liver.

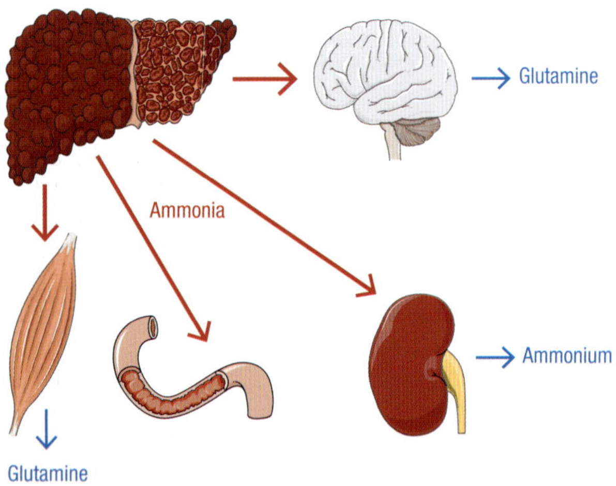

FIG. 40.2 Ammonia metabolism with liver dysfunction (for example, portosystemic shunt or severe disease).

TABLE 40.1 Requirements established by the NRC, AAFCO, and FEDIAF and profiles of commercially available canine diets that might be used in liver disease.*

	Protein (g/1,000 kcal)	Fat (g/1,000 kcal)	Dietary fibre (g/1,000 kcal)	Copper (mg/1,000 kcal)	Zinc (mg/1,000 kcal)	Sodium (g/1,000 kcal)
NRC recommended allowance	25	13.8	–	1.5	15	0.2
AAFCO minimum requirements	45	13.8	–	1.8	20	0.2
FEDIAF minimum requirements**	45	13.8	–	1.8	18	0.25
Commercial diets:						
Royal Canin Hepatic dry	40.9	40.9	17.9	0.77	43	0.51
Royal Canin Hepatic wet	45.9	28.3	17.0	1.20	25	0.57
Royal Canin Hypoallergenic dry	51.5	46.6	13.7	3.70	42	0.98
Hill's Prescription Diet l/d dry	42.0	53.0	15.0	0.58	70	0.44
Hill's Prescription Diet l/d wet	41.0	56.0	17.0	1.0	60	0.50
Hill's Prescription Diet k/d chicken dry	36.0	49.0	13.0	Undeclared	Undeclared	0.41
Hill's Prescription Diet k/d chicken stew	37.0	53.0	22.0	Undeclared	Undeclared	0.45
Purina Veterinary Diet Gastroenteric dry	66.7	30.9	19.3	4.0	68	1.2
Purina Veterinary Diet Gastroenteric chicken wet	93.3	46.7	18.4	4.1	59	1.0
Purina Veterinary Diet HA Hydrolyzed dry	53.6	26.5	11.6	4.4	80	0.90

* Values are based on company product guides and may change. Please consult directly with the company for the latest information.
** Using a maintenance energy calculation with a factor of 110.

With these aspects in mind and taking into consideration the quantity and quality of the proteins, it is reasonable to start with commercially available hepatic support-type diets in patients with hepatic encephalopathy. Feeding smaller meals multiple times a day can also improve protein digestion and absorption and improve overall nitrogen balance.[3,25] After signs are controlled, the level of dietary protein can be gradually increased whilst carefully monitoring clinical signs, body and muscle condition, and, in the longer term, serum albumin concentration, although this may be influenced by disease progression. Other commercial diets, which contain higher concentrations of highly digestible, high-quality proteins, such as gastrointestinal and recovery-type diets and those containing hydrolyzed proteins, could be used (Table 40.1). In addition, homemade recipes tailored to the individual patients and formulated by a boarded veterinary nutritionist can also be helpful in some cases.

Fat

Dietary fat is important as a source of essential fatty acids, fat-soluble vitamins A, D, E, and K, steroids, eicosanoids, phospholipids, and sphingolipids. It also increases the energy density of a diet and reduces the total volume needed to be eaten to meet energy requirements. This can be particularly helpful in patients who need assisted feeding. Dietary fat is also a driver of intake in healthy dogs, so providing a higher-fat diet could help increase the palatability of a diet.[26] However, dietary fat may need restriction in cases of hyperlipidemia and patients with cholestatic disease.

Dietary fats can also be a source of polyunsaturated, long-chain fatty acids, such as eicosapentaenoic acid (EPA) and docosahexaenoic acid (DHA), which have several biological functions, including the modulation of inflammatory pathways.[27-29] In a rodent model of hepatic injury, enriching a diet with EPA and DHA improved survival rates compared to control mice who were given a standard diet.[30] In dogs with primary hepatitis, an association was found between the presence of systemic inflammation and a poorer clinical outcome.[31] It is unknown if reducing systemic inflammation could improve outcomes for veterinary patients with hepatic diseases, but supplementing with EPA and DHA may be worth considering.

Ketones are metabolites of fat that are produced during extended fasting or starvation. Ketogenesis occurs mainly in hepatocytes and intestinal epithelial cells but is also reported in other tissues at lower rates.[32,33] The importance of ketones in sparing glucose during starvation is clear. However, other benefits of ketones are starting to emerge, including their role as a signal molecule and epigenetic regulator, which has been shown to be protective following hepatic injury.[34] Its therapeutic use in veterinary medicine is unknown to date, but it remains an interesting ongoing area of research.

Digestible and nondigestible carbohydrates

Digestible carbohydrates can be provided as small units (such as sugars) or as more complex molecules (such as starches and glycogen). The main function of these carbohydrates is to provide a source of energy for organisms. The liver has an important function in the metabolism of digestible carbohydrates, and so when there is dysfunction, this can lead to derangement of glucose metabolism and subsequent hyper- or hypoglycemia. Hyperglycemia has been reported in cases of hepatocutaneous syndrome and when assisted feeding is performed too aggressively.[35-37] In patients with hyperglycemia, feeding a diet containing limited digestible carbohydrates is warranted. In contrast, hypoglycemia can occur in patients with hepatic insufficiency and severe disease, dogs with portosystemic shunts, and some dogs with hepatocellular carcinoma (see chapter 39). In these cases, feeding a diet with a higher concentration of easily digestible carbohydrates is beneficial.

Indigestible carbohydrates are more commonly known as dietary fiber, which can be further classified as fermentable and nonfermentable fiber. Poorly fermentable fiber such as cellulose and hemicellulose increases the bulk of ingesta and promotes intestinal transit and turnover. This can be beneficial by limiting the amount of time fermentation occurs if nondigested proteins are present in the large intestines. The intestinal microbiota utilizes fermentable fibers such as pectin, gums, beta-glucans, and resistant starches. The resulting increase in volatile fatty acids acidifies the ingesta, trapping ammonia in the interstitial tract and promoting its excretion. Lactulose is a fermentable disaccharide commonly used to treat hepatic encephalopathy in dogs and cats. There are several mechanisms of action lactulose may have, including the reduction of the transit time of ingesta, promoting the uptake of ammonia by colonic bacteria, and acidifying the lumen, which traps ammonia and also reduces the presence of urease-producing bacteria.[38] Giving lactulose, in addition to feeding a hepatic support-type diet, was shown to have a better clinical effect than the diet alone.[39] However, in a retrospective study, there was no difference in the median survival time of dogs with CPSS managed with diet compared to those who also received lactulose in addition to the diet.[40] While there is no definitive study examining the efficacy of lactulose or fermentable fibers as a whole, it nonetheless remains a common treatment in patients with hepatic dysfunction.

Vitamins

Vitamin deficiencies can occur in patients with liver disease due to hepatic dysfunction, diminished reserves, poor intake, and/or malabsorption. In humans, vitamin A and D deficiencies are commonly reported, so monitoring serum 25-hydroxyvitamin D (25(OH)D) in patients with chronic liver disease is recommended.[3] In dogs with extrahepatic shunts, a reduction in serum vitamin A and D concentrations, which were improved following surgery, have also been reported.[41] Vitamin A is not a commonly available assay. Therefore, ensuring sufficient intake of these nutrients and monitoring concentrations of vitamin D is recommended.

Other vitamins of interest include vitamin E (α-tocopherol) and vitamin C. These vitamins function as antioxidants and protect cell membranes from oxidative damage. Vitamin C is not an essential nutrient for dogs and cats as it is for humans and other species, as they can endogenously synthesize vitamin C using the glucuronic acid pathway in the liver. This process may be impaired in cases of liver dysfunction. However, in dogs with CPSS, only a small portion were reported to have a lower plasma concentration of vitamin C.[42] In another study, no difference in circulating vitamin C was found in dogs with chronic liver disease compared to healthy dogs.[43] In a small study of dogs with chronic hepatitis, feeding a diet supplemented with vitamin E for three months increased concentrations in serum and the liver and improved glutathione redox cycling, but there were no changes in histological findings.[44] However, in human medicine, a meta-analysis found that higher circulating vitamin E concentrations were associated with lower concentrations of liver enzymes.[45] Although there is still limited evidence of the clinical efficacy of supplementation of these vitamins in veterinary medicine, the supplementation of these nutrients is commonly performed, particularly in cases of necroinflammatory liver disease.[46]

B vitamins participate as cofactors in several metabolic reactions. Prolonged hyporexia or anorexia can quick diminish reserves, especially if there is increased urinary output, as they are stored in limited quantities in the body. A reduction in serum folic acid and an increase in cobalamin has been reported in dogs with extrahepatic shunts.[41] The serum cobalamin concentration was not improved following surgery, whereas folic acid concentrations were. Deficiencies of B vitamins can be hard to measure, and because they are relatively cheap and there is a high safety margin, general recommendations are to supplement these nutrients in the diets of patients with liver disease.

Unlike some of the other more subtle signs of vitamin deficiencies, vitamin K deficiency is relatively easily detectable in liver disease by assessing bleeding times. A possibility of deficiency should be considered in cases of cholestatic liver disease and in those treated with oral antibiotic therapy. In cases of deficiencies, parenteral treatment is recommended over oral supplementation. Demonstrable vitamin K-responsive coagulopathy is much less common in dogs than in cats with liver disease.

Minerals

A few essential minerals warrant special consideration in patients with hepatic disease, namely copper, zinc, sodium, potassium, and manganese.

Copper and zinc

Normally, copper absorption, distribution, metabolism, and excretion are tightly regulated in the body. However, copper can accumulate in the liver as the result of excessive dietary copper intake or decreased biliary excretion, for example, with severe cirrhosis.[47] Copper storage disease in dogs is caused by an interaction between the environment (i.e., dietary copper intake) and genetic predisposition. A tendency to build up excess copper in the liver has been described in several breeds, including Bedlington Terriers, Labrador Retrievers, Dobermans, West Highland White Terriers, and Dalmatians.[48] The pathophysiology of these conditions is examined in a previous chapter (chapter 33).

Commercially available copper-restricted diets contain approximately 1.2 mg copper/1,000 kcal. The addition of zinc to the diet can also reduce copper absorption by stimulating the synthesis of metallothionein in enterocytes, which binds copper and promotes its loss in the intestinal tract.[49] A diet with 1.2 mg copper and 25.5 mg zinc/1,000 kcal reduced hepatic copper concentrations below 400 mg/kg dry weight.[50] In dogs with high hepatic copper concentrations, however, the addition of copper chelators such as D-penicillamine in addition to feeding a copper-restricted diet is likely needed.[51] Supplementing a diet with zinc can also have additional benefits. Zinc deficiencies can occur as a result of reduced intake and impaired intestinal absorption. In addition, a positive zinc status has been found to be associated with overall survival in human patients with liver cirrhosis.[52] However, zinc should not be supplemented while using copper chelators.

Recently, a discussion has been ongoing about whether there should be a limit set for dietary copper in pet food for healthy dogs.[53] There is currently no recommended safe upper limit for copper in dog food in the US. In Europe, the organizing body representing the pet food industry (FEDIAF) has set a legal maximum copper concentration in pet food, which is approximately 139% of minimum requirements on a dry matter basis. However, this legal limit is related to reducing environmental contamination rather than to animal health. A recent study analyzed the mineral content of dog foods and found that some diets were below the minimum copper requirement, whereas one diet was above the legal maximum.[54] The current status of not setting a maximum for copper in the US was upheld by an expert panel convened by the Association of American Feed Control Officials (AAFCO).[55] The panel recommended that further studies are required to determine a clearer cause and effect of dietary copper content and a rise in copper-associated hepatopathy in dogs and to determine what safe upper limit to set if needed ultimately.

Sodium and potassium

Other minerals of interest are sodium and potassium. Restriction of sodium is only recommended in patients with portal hypertension and ascites. Generally, feeding <0.5 g sodium/1,000 kcal is recommended as a low-sodium diet. However, concurrent use of aldosterone inhibitors in these dogs may increase the risk of hyponatremia, so sodium concentrations should be carefully monitored. Occurrence of hypokalemia can be common due to vomiting, diarrhea, and reduced food intake. In these cases, supplementing potassium through the diet or with intravenous fluid therapy is warranted.

Manganese

Manganese concentrations in whole blood have been described to be increased in dogs with CPSS.[56] An excess of manganese is thought to contribute to the clinical signs of hepatic encephalopathy, which is corrected by feeding manganese-restricted diets in rats.[57] Further research is needed to understand the role manganese plays in hepatic encephalopathy in dogs and whether a reduction in intake can improve signs.

Conclusion

Nutritional support is a mainstay treatment in the management of hepatobiliary disease in veterinary patients. There are overall nutritional goals, such as providing adequate caloric intake and carefully monitoring nutritional status, which are applicable to all disease types. However, certain conditions (such as hepatic encephalopathy or copper-associated hepatopathy) have their own nutritional nuances, so a tailored approach to each patient is necessary.

KEY POINTS

- Nutrition plays a vital role in the management and progression of hepatobiliary disease.
- Commercial hepatic support-type diets are mainly designed to address hepatic encephalopathy and copper-associated hepatopathy and will not be appropriate for all patients.
- Providing adequate (but not excessive) calories and proteins is important to maintain muscle mass, which is relevant, particularly in patients with hepatic encephalopathy.
- Dietary fat increases the caloric density of a diet, which reduces the amount of food needed to be eaten to achieve a caloric target.
- Carbohydrates have different functions when provided in their digestible vs. nondigestible forms.
- The specific requirements and goals for vitamins and minerals should be tailored to the individual and their disease state.

References

1. Freeman L, Becvarova I, Cave N, et al. WSAVA nutritional assessment guidelines. *J Small Anim Pract* 52(7):385-396, 2011.
2. Cederholm T, Barazzoni R, Austin P, et al. ESPEN guidelines on definitions and terminology of clinical nutrition. *Clin Nutrition* 36(1):49-64, 2017.
3. Merli M, Berzigotti A, Zelber-Sagi S, et al. EASL Clinical Practice Guidelines on nutrition in chronic liver disease. *J Hepatol* 70(1):172-193, 2019.
4. Laviano A, Inui A, Marks DL, et al. Neural control of the anorexia-cachexia syndrome. *Am J Physiol Endocrinol Metab* 295(5):1000-1008, 2008.
5. Reichenberg A, Kraus T, Haack M, Schuld A, Pollmächer T, Yirmiya R. Endotoxin-induced changes in food consumption in healthy volunteers are associated with TNF-α and IL-6 secretion. *Psychoneuroendocrinology* 27(8):945-956, 2002.
6. Freeman L, Becvarova I, Cave N, et al. WSAVA nutritional assessment guidelines. *J Small Anim Pract* 52(7):385-396, 2011.
7. Leung YB, Cave N, Wester TJ. Loss of body weight and lean mass in long-stay, hospitalized canine patients. *J Anim Physiol Anim Nutr (Berl)* 107(6):1444-1455, 2023.
8. Brunetto MA, Gomes MOSS, Andre MR, et al. Effects of nutritional support on hospital outcome in dogs and cats. *J Vet Emerg Crit Care* 20(2):224-231, 2010.
9. Liu DT, Brown DC, Silverstein DC. Early nutritional support is associated with decreased length of hospitalization in dogs with septic peritonitis: A retrospective study of 45 cases (2000-2009). *J Vet Emerg Crit Care* 22(4):453-459, 2012.
10. Mohr AJ, Leisewitz AL, Jacobson LS, Steiner JM, Ruaux CG, Williams DA. Effect of early enteral nutrition on intestinal permeability, intestinal protein loss, and outcome in dogs with severe parvoviral enteritis. *J Vet Intern Med* 17(6):791-798, 2003.
11. Montano-Loza AJ, Meza-Junco J, Prado CMM, et al. Muscle wasting is associated with mortality in patients with cirrhosis. *Clin Gastroenterol Hepatol* 10(2):166-173, 2012.
12. Tivers MS, Handel I, Gow AG, Lipscomb VJ, Jalan R, Mellanby RJ. Hyperammonemia and systemic inflammatory response syndrome predicts

presence of hepatic encephalopathy in dogs with congenital portosystemic shunts. *PLoS One* 9(1):1-7, 2014.

13. Weber FL, Veach GL. The importance of the small intestine in gut ammonium production in the fasting dog. *Gastroenterology* 77(2):235-240, 1979.
14. Wright G, Noiret L, Olde Damink SWM, Jalan R. Interorgan ammonia metabolism in liver failure: The basis of current and future therapies. *Liver International* 31(2):163-175, 2011.
15. Chatauret N, Desjardins P, Zwingmann C, Rose C, Rao KVR, Butterworth RF. Direct molecular and spectroscopic evidence for increased ammonia removal capacity of skeletal muscle in acute liver failure. *J Hepatol* 44(6):1083-1088, 2006.
16. Laflamme DP, Allen SW, Huber TL. Apparent dietary protein requirement of dogs with portosystemic shunt. *Am J Vet Res* 54(5):719-723, 1993.
17. Proot S, Biourge V, Teske E, Rothuizen J. Soy protein isolate versus meat-based low-protein diet for dogs with congenital portosystemic shunts. *J Vet Intern Med* 23(4):794-800, 2009.
18. Amodio P, Bemeur C, Butterworth R, et al. The nutritional management of hepatic encephalopathy in patients with cirrhosis: International society for hepatic encephalopathy and nitrogen metabolism consensus. *Hepatology* 58(1):325-336, 2013.
19. Greenberger NJ, Carley J, Schenker S, Bettinger I, Stamnes C, Beyer P. Effect of vegetable and animal protein diets in chronic hepatic encephalopathy. *Am J Dig Dis* 22(10):845-855, 1977.
20. James JH. Branched chain amino acids in hepatic encephalopathy. *Am J Surg* 183(4):424-429, 2002.
21. Marrone G, Serra A, Miele L, et al. Branched chain amino acids in hepatic encephalopathy and sarcopenia in liver cirrhosis: Evidence and uncertainties. *World J Gastroenterol* 29(19):2905-2915, 2023.
22. Swansson WD, Anderson BM, Yeoh SW, Lewis DJ. Management of minimal and overt hepatic encephalopathy with branched-chain amino acids: a review of the evidence. *Eur J Gastroenterol Hepatol* 35(8):812-821, 2023.
23. Schaeffer MC, Rogers QR, Leung PMB, Wolfe BM, Strombeck DR. Changes in cerebrospinal fluid and plasma amino acid concentrations with elevated dietary protein concentration in dogs with portacaval shunts. *Life Sci* 48(23):2215-2223, 1991.
24. Devriendt N, Paepe D, Serrano G, et al. Plasma amino acid profiles in dogs with closed extrahepatic portosystemic shunts are only partially improved 3 months after successful gradual attenuation. *J Vet Intern Med* 35(3):1347-1354, 2021.
25. Gow AG. Hepatic encephalopathy. *Vet Clin North Am Small Anim Pract* 47(3):585-599, 2017.
26. Roberts MT, Bermingham EN, Cave NJ, Young W, McKenzie CM, Thomas DG. Macronutrient intake of dogs, self-selecting diets varying in composition offered ad libitum. *J Anim Physiol Anim Nutr (Berl)* 102(2):568-575, 2018.
27. Watkins BA. Importance of essential fatty acids and their derivatives in poultry. *J Nutrition* 121(9):1475-1485, 1991.
28. Lauritzen L, Brambilla P, Mazzocchi A, Harsløf LBS, Ciappolino V, Agostoni C. DHA effects in brain development and function. *Nutrients* 8(1):1-17, 2016.
29. Pawlosky R, Barnes A, Salem N. Essential fatty acid metabolism in the feline: relationship between liver and brain production of long-chain polyunsaturated fatty acids. *J Lipid Res* 35(11):2032-2040, 1994.
30. Céspedes N, Tamayo A, Rodriguez MJ, Zúñiga-Hernández J. EPA plus DHA improves survival related to a decrease of injury after extended liver ischemia in Sprague-Dawley rats. *Ann Hepatol* 19(2):172-178, 2020.
31. Kilpatrick S, Dreistadt M, Frowde P, et al. Presence of systemic inflammatory response syndrome predicts a poor clinical outcome in dogs with a primary hepatitis. *PLoS One* 11(1):1-10, 2016.
32. Puchalska P, Crawford PA. Multi-dimensional roles of ketone bodies in fuel metabolism, signaling, and therapeutics. *Cell Metab* 25(2):262-284, 2017.
33. McGarry JD, Foster DW. Ketogenesis and cholesterol synthesis in normal and neoplastic tissues of the rat. *J Biological Chemistry* 244(15):4251-4256, 1969.
34. Li K, Wang WH, Wu JB, Xiao WH. β-hydroxybutyrate: A crucial therapeutic target for diverse liver diseases. *Biomed Pharmacother* 165:115191, 2023.
35. Center SA, Crawford MA, Guida L, Erb HN, King J. A retrospective study of 77 cats with severe hepatic lipidosis: 1975-1990. *J Vet Intern Med* 7(6):349-359, 1993.
36. DeMarle KB, Webster CRL, Penninck D, Ferrer L. Approach to the diagnosis of hepatocutaneous syndrome in dogs: A retrospective study and literature review. *J Am Anim Hosp Assoc* 57(1):15-25, 2021.
37. Queau Y, Larsen JA, Kass PH, Glucksman GS, Fascetti AJ. Factors associated with adverse outcomes during parenteral nutrition administration in dogs and cats. *J Vet Intern Med* 25(3):446-452, 2011.
38. Alimirah M, Sadiq O, Gordon SC. Novel therapies in hepatic encephalopathy. *Clin Liver Dis* 24(2):303-315, 2020.
39. Serrano G, Devriendt N, de Rooster H, Paepe D. Comparison of diet, lactulose, and metronidazole combinations in the control of pre-surgical clinical signs in dogs with congenital extrahepatic portosystemic shunts. *J Vet Intern Med* 36(4):1258-1266, 2022.
40. Favier RP, de Graaf E, Corbee RJ, Kummeling A. Outcome of non-surgical dietary treatment with or without lactulose in dogs with congenital portosystemic shunts. *Vet Quart* 40(1):108-114, 2020.
41. Devriendt N, Serrano G, Paepe D, Vandenabeele S, Stock E, de Rooster H. Persistent hypercobalaminemia three months after successful gradual attenuation of extrahepatic shunts in dogs: a prospective cohort study. *BMC Vet Res* 18(1):1-8, 2022.
42. Hishiyama N, Kayanuma H, Matsui T, et al. Plasma concentration of vitamin C in dogs with a portosystemic shunt. *Can J Vet Res* 70(4):305-307, 2006.
43. Galler A, Tran JL, Krammer-Lukas S, et al. Blood vitamin levels in dogs with chronic liver disease. *Vet Med Austria* 100(5-6):133-139, 2013.
44. Twedt DC, Webb C, Tetrick M. The effect of dietary vitamin E on the clinical laboratory and oxidant status of dogs with chronic hepatitis. *J Vet Intern Med* 17:418A, 2003.
45. Vogli S, Naska A, Marinos G, Kasdagli MI, Orfanos P. The effect of vitamin E supplementation on serum aminotransferases in non-alcoholic fatty liver disease (NAFLD): A systematic review and meta-analysis. *Nutrients* 15(17):3733, 2023.
46. Webster CRL, Center SA, Cullen JM, et al. ACVIM consensus statement on the diagnosis and treatment of chronic hepatitis in dogs. *J Vet Intern Med* 33(3):1173-1200, 2019.
47. Aburto EM, Cribb AE, Fuentealba IC. Effect of chronic exposure to excess dietary copper and dietary selenium supplementation on liver specimens from rats. *Am J Vet Res* 62(9):1423-1427, 2001.
48. Dirksen K, Fieten H. Canine copper-associated hepatitis. *Vet Clin North Am Small Anim Pract* 47(3):631-644, 2017.
49. Hall AC, Young BW, Bremner I. Intestinal metallothionein and the mutual antagonism between copper and zinc in the rat. *J Inorg Biochem* 11(1):57-66, 1979.
50. Hoffmann G, Jones PGG, Biourge V, et al. Dietary management of hepatic copper accumulation in labrador retrievers. *J Vet Intern Med* 23(5):957-963, 2009.
51. Fieten H, Biourge VC, Watson AL, Leegwater PAJ, Van den Ingh TSGAM, Rothuizen J. Nutritional management of inherited copper-associated hepatitis in the Labrador retriever. *Vet J* 199(3):429-433, 2014.
52. Nishikawa H, Enomoto H, Yoh K, et al. Serum zinc level classification system: usefulness in patients with liver cirrhosis. *J Clin Med* 8(12), 2019.
53. Center SA, Richter KP, Twedt DC, Wakshlag JJ, Watson PJ, Webster CRL. Is it time to reconsider current guidelines for copper content in commercial dog foods? *J Am Vet Med Assoc* 258(4):357-364, 2021.
54. Pacelik JK, Biel W, Witkowicz R, Podsiadło C. Mineral and heavy metal content in dry dog foods with different main animal components. *Sci Rep* (0123456789):1-15, 2023.
55. Burkholder W, Fascetti A, Thompson A, et al. Copper in dog foods expert panel final report with recommendations to the pet food committee. AAFCO Guidelines for Copper Concentrations in Foods for Normal Dogs, 2022.
56. Gow AG, Marques AIC, Yool DA, Duncan A, Mellanby RJ. Whole blood manganese concentrations in dogs with congenital portosystemic shunts. *J Vet Intern Med* 24(1):90-96, 2010.
57. Li Y, Mei LH, Qiang JW, Ji CX, Ju S. Reduction of manganese intake improves neuropsychological manifestations in rats with minimal hepatic encephalopathy. *Neuroscience* 347:148-155, 2017.

Index